Infectious Disease

Antimalarial Chemotherapy

*Mechanisms of Action, Resistance,
and New Directions in Drug Discovery*

Edited by

Philip J. Rosenthal, MD

School of Medicine, University of California, San Francisco, CA

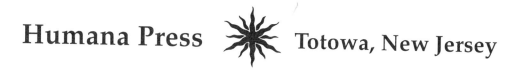

Humana Press ✳ Totowa, New Jersey

This publication is printed on acid-free paper. ∞
ANSI Z39.48-1984 (American Standards Institute) Permanence of Paper for Printed Library Materials.

Cover design by Patricia F. Cleary.
Production Editor: Kim Hoather-Potter.

For additional copies, pricing for bulk purchases, and/or information about other Humana titles, contact Humana at the above address or at any of the following numbers: Tel: 973-256-1699; Fax: 973-256-8341; E-mail: humana@humanapr.com, or visit our Website: http://humanapress.com

Printed in the United States of America. 10 9 8 7 6 5 4 3 2 1

Library of Congress Cataloging in Publication Data

Antimalarial chemotherapy : mechanisms of action, resistance, and new directions in drug discovery / edited by
    Philip J. Rosenthal.
        p. ; cm. -- (Infectious disease)
    Includes bibliographical references and index.
    ISBN 0-89603-670-7 (alk. paper)
        1. Antimalarials. I. Rosenthal, Philip J. II. Infectious
disease (Totowa, N.J.)
        [DNLM: 1. Antimalarials—pharmacology. 2. Drug Resistance. 3.
Malaria—drug therapy. QV 256 A6307 2001]
    RC159.A5 A58 2001
    616.9'362061--dc21
                                                                    00-059762

Preface

We who are engrossed in the study of antimalarial chemotherapy are fond of repeating certain maxims. Malaria is one of the most important disease problems in the world. The control of malaria is increasingly limited by resistance to available drugs. New strategies for treating malaria are urgently needed. We should strive to identify new targets for antimalarial agents. Each of these maxims has reached the status of a cliché, but is nonetheless compelling. The complex biology of malaria parasites and extreme poverty in most malarious regions have locked us into an unrelenting continuation of endemic malaria in most of the tropical world. Meanwhile, drug resistance worsens, and it appears that the speed of efforts to develop new treatment strategies may not keep pace with the resourceful parasites. This rather bleak scenario presents us with major challenges. For the short term, as drug resistance worsens and standard therapies fail, how will we utilize existing agents to prevent worsening of worldwide malaria? Which strategies are likely to provide effective new antimalarial drugs? And for the future, how can we develop strategies incorporating old and new therapies and other control modalities to begin to lessen the worldwide burden of malaria?

Although challenges for the effective treatment and control of malaria are great, so are current opportunities. Our understanding of the biology of malaria parasites is growing rapidly. The entire genome of *Plasmodium falciparum* will soon be sequenced. New molecular technologies are allowing us to definitively assess the biological roles of key parasite molecules. There is good reason to believe that these advances will speed up the pace of antimalarial drug discovery and development. As is discussed throughout this book, recent progress has been impressive. New insights into the appropriate use of existing drugs and optimal means of attacking known targets are being gained, and new potential drug targets are being identified.

At this point, it seems appropriate to collect our current understanding of antimalarial chemotherapy in a single volume. Much has changed since earlier classic references on this subject. We have moved to a more rational approach to antimalarial chemotherapy, where we are attempting to logically use existing agents and to develop new drugs designed to target specific parasite pathways. For this approach, a much better understanding of parasite biology is needed.

Antimalarial Chemotherapy: Mechanisms of Action, Resistance, and New Directions in Drug Discovery offers detailed discussions from experts in many areas. As background, chapters on the biology of parasites highlight two key areas, the plasmodial food vacuole and plasmodial transport mechanisms. The public health consequences of current problems in antimalarial chemotherapy are also reviewed. Established antimalarial drugs and new agents under development are then discussed in detail. Our emphasis is not on summarizing established drug usages, but rather to present current understanding of the mechanisms of action and resistance of existing agents in order to help us design new strategies to use these or related compounds. The last section of the book presents information on new compounds. These include agents that are related to existing effective antimalarials and some new targets. The chosen targets represent a small sample of potential new avenues for chemotherapy. It is hoped that the discussions of parasite biology and chemotherapy provided in this book will help to stimulate additional ventures in this direction. As is often mentioned (in yet another cliché), additional funding for research on malaria will be essential for the breadth of study required to develop multiple new drugs.

My editing of *Antimalarial Chemotherapy: Mechanisms of Action, Resistance, and New Directions in Drug Discovery* has been rather time-consuming, but very rewarding in allowing me the opportunity to work with world leaders in all areas of malaria chemotherapy, and in providing me with a privileged look at the status of cutting edge research in this field. I wish to thank all of the authors for their hard work in preparing excellent discussions on their respective topics. Thanks are also in order to those who have helped me to choose specific topics and authors and offered advice through the course of the book preparation process. I'm afraid that I will certainly neglect some contributors, but special thanks go to Steve Meshnick, Irwin Sherman, Hagai Ginsburg, Ioav Cabantchick, Terrie Taylor, Peter Bloland, Chris Plowe, David Fidock, Tom Wellems, Mike Gottlieb, Lou Miller, Steve Ward, Leann Tilley, and Piero Olliaro. I thank members of my laboratory at UCSF and my collaborators in Kampala, Uganda, for their inspiration and useful ideas. I remain indebted to the late Jim Leech, who was the perfect mentor to start me on a path of antimalarial drug discovery. Lastly, I thank my wife, Kandice Strako, for her indulgence and support during the hectic and seemingly never-ending editing process. My hope is that this book will offer a useful review for those who study malaria, and, more importantly, an entry point into antimalarial chemotherapy for those new to this field. If this is the case, and we can help to expand efforts toward antimalarial drug discovery and development, our labors will certainly have been worthwhile.

Philip J. Rosenthal, MD

Contents

Contributors

THOMAS AKOMPONG, PhD • *Departments of Pathology and Microbiology-Immunology, Northwestern University Medical School, Chicago, IL*

J. KEVIN BAIRD, PhD • *US Navy Medical Research Unit, Parasitic Diseases Program, American Embassy, Jakarta, Indonesia*

RITU BANERJEE, BA • *Departments of Molecular Microbiology and Medicine, Howard Hughes Medical Institute, Washington University, St. Louis, MO*

PETER B. BLOLAND, DVM, MPVM • *Malaria Epidemiology Branch, Division of Parasitic Diseases, Center for Infectious Diseases, Centers for Disease Control and Prevention, Chamblee, GA*

RALF P. BRUECKNER, MD• *Division of Experimental Therapeutics, Walter Reed Army Institute of Research, Silver Spring, MD*

MICHÈLE CALAS, PhD • *Laboratoire des Aminoacides, Peptides et Proteines, Université de Montpellier II, Montpellier Cedex, France*

BARBARA CLOUGH, PhD • *Division of Parasitology, The National Institute for Medical Research, London, UK*

MARY J. DOBSON, DPHIL • *Wellcome Unit for the History of Medicine, Oxford University, Oxford, UK*

GRANT DORSEY, MD • *Department of Medicine, San Francisco General Hospital and University of California, San Francisco, CA*

JEFFREY S. ELIAS, BA • *Department of Chemistry, School of Arts and Sciences, Johns Hopkins University, Baltimore, MD*

DAVID A. FIDOCK, PhD • *Department of Microbiology and Immunology, Albert Einstein College of Medicine, Bronx, NY*

MICK FOLEY, PhD • *Department of Biochemistry, La Trobe University, Bundoora, Australia*

ANNETTE M. GERO, PhD • *School of Biochemistry and Molecular Genetics, University of New South Wales, Sydney, Australia*

DANIEL E. GOLDBERG, MD, PhD • *Departments of Molecular Microbiology and Medicine, Howard Hughes Medical Institute, Washington University, St. Louis, MO*

VICTOR R. GORDEUK, MD • *Center for Sickle Cell Disease, Howard University, Washington, DC*

KASTURI HALDAR, PhD • *Departments of Pathology and Microbiology-Immunology, Northwestern University Medical School, Chicago, IL*

MIKHAIL KRASAVIN, BA • *Department of Chemistry, School of Arts and Sciences, Johns Hopkins University, Baltimore, MD*

PAUL LORIA, BSc (HONS) • *Department of Biochemistry, La Trobe University, Bundoora, Australia*

MARK LOYEVSKY, PhD • *Center for Sickle Cell Disease, Howard University, Washington, DC*

MICHAEL MCCUTCHEN, BA • *Department of Chemistry, School of Arts and Sciences, Johns Hopkins University, Baltimore, MD*

JOHN P. MAXWELL, BA • *Department of Chemistry, School of Arts and Sciences, Johns Hopkins University, Baltimore, MD*

STEVEN R. MESHNICK, MD, PhD • *Department of Epidemiology, University of Michigan School of Public Health, Ann Arbor, MI*

WILBUR K. MILHOUS, PhD • *Division of Experimental Therapeutics, Walter Reed Army Institute of Research, Silver Spring, MD*

LOUIS H. MILLER, MD • *Laboratory of Parasitic Diseases, National Institute of Allergy and Infectious Diseases, National Institutes of Health, Bethesda, MD*

COLIN OHRT, MD • *Division of Experimental Therapeutics, Walter Reed Army Institute of Research, Silver Spring, MD*

PIERO L. OLLIARO, MD, PhD • *UNDP/WB/WHO Special Programme for Research and Training in Tropical Diseases (TDR), World Health Organization, Geneva, Switzerland*

MICHAEL H. PARKER, PhD • *Department of Chemistry, School of Arts and Sciences, Johns Hopkins University, Baltimore, MD*

CHRISTOPHER V. PLOWE, MD, MPH • *Malaria Section, Center for Vaccine Development, University of Maryland School of Medicine, Baltimore, MD*

POONSAKDI PLOYPRADITH, PhD • *Department of Chemistry, School of Arts and Sciences, Johns Hopkins University, Baltimore, MD*

GARY H. POSNER, PhD • *Department of Chemistry, School of Arts and Sciences, Johns Hopkins University, Baltimore, MD*

PRADIPSINH K. RATHOD, PhD • *Department of Biology, The Catholic University of America, Washington, DC*

KAYLENE J. RAYNES, MD • *Department of Pharmacology and Therapeutics, University of Liverpool, Liverpool, UK*

PHILIP J. ROSENTHAL, MD • *Department of Medicine, San Francisco General Hospital and University of California, San Francisco, CA*

PAUL A. STOCKS, MD • *Department of Pharmacology and Therapeutics, University of Liverpool, Liverpool, UK*

LEANN TILLEY, PhD • *Department of Biochemistry, La Trobe University, Bundoora, Australia*

AKHIL B. VAIDYA, PhD • *Department of Microbiology and Immunology, MCP Hahnemann School of Medicine, Philadelphia, PA*

HENRI JOSEPH VIAL, PhD • *Dynamique Moléculaire des Interactions Membranaires, CNRS, Université Montpellier II, Montpellier Cedex, France*

STEPHEN A. WARD, MD • *Department of Pharmacology and Therapeutics, University of Liverpool, Liverpool, UK*

ALEXANDER L. WEIS, MD • *Lipitek International Inc., San Antonio, TX*

THOMAS E. WELLEMS, MD, PhD • *Malaria Genetics Section, Laboratory of Parasitic Diseases, National Institute of Allergy and Infectious Diseases, National Institutes of Health, Bethesda, MD*

R. J. M. (IAIN) WILSON, PhD • *The National Institute for Medical Research, London, UK*

I
INTRODUCTION

The Need for New Approaches to Antimalarial Chemotherapy

Philip J. Rosenthal and Louis H. Miller

INTRODUCTION

Malaria has been a major cause of human suffering for thousands of years, and despite important advances in our understanding of the disease, it continues to be one of the greatest causes of serious illness and death in the world. Ironically, at a time when exciting scientific advances are offering the opportunity to successfully manage many previously untreatable diseases, our ability to reliably treat malaria has actually diminished over the last half-century. At present, a number of antimalarial drugs are available, but their use is limited by high cost, toxicity, and increasing parasite resistance. Thus, there is a great need for the optimal use of available drugs and the development of new approaches to antimalarial chemotherapy.

THE CURRENT MALARIA SITUATION

In 1955, the World Health Organization launched a program to eradicate malaria. This effort included some important successes, but, for the most part, it was a major disappointment (1). Indeed, over recent decades, morbidity and mortality caused by malaria have increased in many parts of the world and most of the world's population remains at risk of contracting this disease (Figs. 1 and 2). Hundreds of millions of clinical episodes of malaria occur each year, and it was estimated that 1.5–2.7 million deaths resulted from these infections in 1996 (3). Thus, malaria is one of the great infectious disease killers, and it exerts an enormous toll on developing countries throughout the tropics (4). In particular, falciparum malaria is an overwhelming problem in sub-Saharan Africa, where most malarial morbidity and mortality occurs. Numerous factors contribute to the persistence of a severe worldwide malaria problem. First, efforts to control mosquito vectors, which were quite successful in some areas many years ago, have been limited by financial constraints and insecticide resistance. Second, programs to treat and control malaria, especially in highly vulnerable young children and pregnant women, are severely limited by poverty in most endemic regions. Third, despite significant efforts, an effective malaria vaccine is not yet available and is unlikely to be available to those most at need in the near future. Fourth, malaria parasites have consistently demonstrated the ability to develop resistance to available

From: *Antimalarial Chemotherapy: Mechanisms of Action, Resistance, and New Directions in Drug Discovery*
Edited by: P. J. Rosenthal © Humana Press Inc., Totowa, NJ

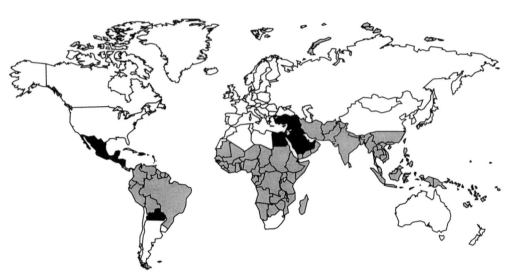

Fig. 1. Distribution of malaria, 1997. Regions endemic for malaria are shaded. Endemic areas with known chloroquine-resistant falciparum malaria are gray, and those without known chloroquine resistance are black. (Map from Centers for Disease Control and Prevention.)

drugs. Fifth, although great strides have been made in our understanding of malaria in recent years, our ability to develop new strategies to control the disease remains significantly limited by an incomplete understanding of the biology of the parasite and of the host response to parasite infection.

CURRENT MALARIA CONTROL EFFORTS

Most likely, the successful control of malaria will require advances in many areas, including the control of mosquito vectors, the development of effective vaccines, and the identification of new chemotherapeutic agents. Although the toll of malaria morbidity and mortality remains unacceptably high, important advances are being made. Inexpensive vector control measures, notably the use of insecticide-impregnated bednets, have proven effective and are currently being implemented in many endemic areas *(5)*. Great progress is being made in the characterization of the host immune response against malaria parasites, and a number of classes of vaccines are in different stages of testing *(6)*. An appreciation of the value of antimalarial drug combinations to improve efficacy and limit the development of resistance has recently arisen *(7)*. Extensive studies of drug combinations, in particular those including derivatives of the new drug artemisinin, are currently underway.

A promising recent change is the development of a consensus that bold new efforts are urgently needed to control malaria. International agencies have recently initiated new programs that will provide increased funds for malaria control and research. The Roll Back Malaria initiative was formed in 1998 to expedite and coordinate worldwide malaria control efforts. The principal focus of this initiative is to address the pressing needs of those most at risk of severe malaria: children and pregnant women in Africa and other highly endemic regions. Two important focused programs were established in 1999: the Malaria Vaccine Initiative and the Medicines for Malaria Venture. Impor-

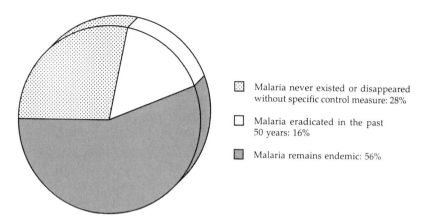

Fig. 2. Worldwide malaria endemicity. Percentages of populations living in areas with present or past malaria endemicity are shown. (Adapted from ref. *2*.)

tantly, these programs will be much better funded than older national and international efforts at malaria control. As a disease of the poorest of nations, malaria remains a poor cousin of the major health problems of the developed world, and funding for malaria control and research is dwarfed by that for heart disease, cancer, AIDS, and asthma (Table 1). However, the new consensus offers some promise that the pace of advances toward malaria control will increase. This issue is of great relevance to the subject of this volume, as drug discovery and development are very expensive.

Antimalarial drug development has been severely limited by a lack of interest of pharmaceutical companies in investing large sums for the development of drugs for a disease of disadvantaged populations. Indeed, nearly all available antimalarials have been developed through government (including military) research programs (chloroquine, primaquine, mefloquine, Fansidar, halofantrine), the fortuitous identification of efficacy in a natural product (quinine, artemisinins), or the identification of antimalarial potency in drugs marketed for other indications (folate antagonists, sulfas, antibiotics, atovaquone). No drug has been fully developed as an antimalarial by industry, although industry–government collaborations are currently playing key roles in the introduction of some new agents. In addition, a key strategy of the new Medicines for Malaria Venture is to finance collaborations that combine the drug discovery expertise of industry and the malaria expertise of academic groups to pursue antimalarial drug discovery without major investment by pharmaceutical companies.

THE BIOLOGY OF MALARIA PARASITES

Humans become infected with malaria parasites after the bite of an anopheline mosquito harboring plasmodial sporozoites (Fig. 3). The sporozoites circulate to the liver, where hepatocytes are invaded, and an asymptomatic pre-erythrocytic phase of infection begins. After one to several weeks, merozoites are released into the circulation. These parasites invade erythrocytes to begin the erythrocytic cycle of infection, which includes rapid, asexual multiplication of parasites, and is responsible for all of the clinical manifestations of malaria. Some parasites also develop into gametocytes, which

Table 1
Estimated Annual Global Research
Expenditure and Mortality for Three Diseases, 1990–1992

Disease	Expenditure (millions of US dollars)	Mortality (thousands)	Expenditure per fatality (U.S. dollars)
HIV/AIDS	952	290.8	3274
Asthma	143	181.3	789
Malaria	60	926.4	65

Source: Adapted from ref. *8*.

subsequently infect mosquitoes, allowing completion of the life cycle. Four species of *Plasmodium* cause human disease. *Plasmodium falciparum* is, by far, the most important species, as it is responsible for nearly all severe malaria. This parasite is an enormous problem in Africa and is endemic in most malarious regions of the world. *P. falciparum* uniquely infects erythrocytes of all ages, and mature parasite-infected erythrocytes adhere to endothelial cells to avoid splenic clearance. Of additional great importance, *P. falciparum* has demonstrated the ability to develop resistance to most available antimalarial drugs *(9)*. Infection with *P. vivax* is also very common, and although this infection causes relatively little severe disease, it is one of the most important causes of morbidity among parasitic infections, particularly in Southeast Asia, the Indian subcontinent, South and Central America, and parts of Oceania. Drug resistance in *P. vivax* has been recognized only recently, but it is increasing, with vivax malaria resistant to chloroquine and other antimalarials noted in Southeast Asia, Oceania, India, and South America. *P. malariae* and *P. ovale* are relatively uncommon causes of human malaria. In *P. vivax* and *P. ovale* malaria, parasites have a chronic liver phase (hypnozoite), in addition to the transient hepatic phase that precedes erythrocyte infection (Fig. 3). Hypnozoites require specific therapy for eradication.

THE HOST RESPONSE TO INFECTION WITH MALARIA PARASITES

Initial infections with *P. falciparum* are commonly fatal, but patients who survive develop some antiparasitic immunity. This immunity, which includes humoral and cellular responses against multiple parasite life-cycle stages, allows improved outcomes after subsequent infections. After multiple infections, *P. falciparum* causes relatively mild disease or is asymptomatic in many older children and adults. However, antimalarial immunity is incomplete, strain-specific, and short-lived, and is only maintained by frequent reinfection. In regions of very high transmission (greater than one infectious mosquito bite per day in parts of Africa), severe malaria occurs mostly in young children; older individuals are protected against life-threatening disease. In contrast, individuals living in regions of low transmission and travelers from nonendemic areas are at great risk of developing a severe illness after infection with *P. falciparum*, regardless of age. Another group at high risk is pregnant women, even if antimalarial immunity was previously high. Responses to plasmodial infection are also affected by genetic factors. Individuals that are heterozygous for sickle hemoglobin and those with certain major histocompatibility complex (MHC) polymorphisms are partially protected against

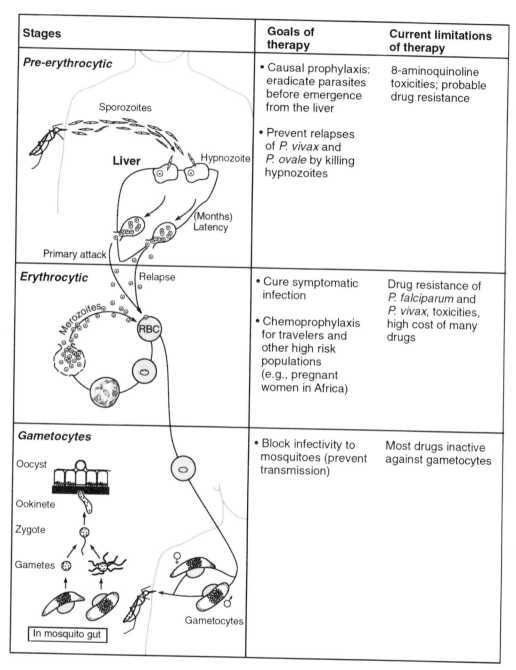

Stages	Goals of therapy	Current limitations of therapy
Pre-erythrocytic	• Causal prophylaxis: eradicate parasites before emergence from the liver	8-aminoquinoline toxicities; probable drug resistance
	• Prevent relapses of *P. vivax* and *P. ovale* by killing hypnozoites	
Erythrocytic	• Cure symptomatic infection	Drug resistance of *P. falciparum* and *P. vivax*, toxicities, high cost of many drugs
	• Chemoprophylaxis for travelers and other high risk populations (e.g., pregnant women in Africa)	
Gametocytes	• Block infectivity to mosquitoes (prevent transmission)	Most drugs inactive against gametocytes

Fig. 3. Life cycle of malaria parasites.

severe falciparum malaria. Indeed, it is likely that numerous polymorphisms in erythrocyte proteins, immune mediators, and other proteins have been selected for by the severe pressure of lethal falciparum malaria over thousands of years of human evolution.

The complexity of host responses to infection with malaria parasites makes the study of antimalarial drug efficacy difficult. Drug effects must be judged with consideration of the host antiparasitic immune response. Indeed, the current situation in sub-Saharan Africa is that chloroquine remains the drug of choice in most countries despite widespread resistance of parasites to this agent, in part due to financial constraints, but also due to the fact that this drug is often at least partially effective in treating populations with significant antimalarial immunity. Thus, as new antimalarial agents are evaluated, the major role of host immunity in responses to plasmodial infection must always be considered.

AVAILABLE ANTIMALARIAL DRUGS

The first chemically characterized antimicrobial agent was quinine, which was purified by Peletier and Caventou from the bark of the Cinchona tree in 1820. In the 20th century, numerous other effective antimalarials were identified, as is reviewed in Chapter 2. At present, important antimalarial drugs include a number of quinolines, inhibitors of enzymes required for folate metabolism, some antibiotics, a series of endoperoxides related to the natural product artemisinin, and the hydroxynaphthoquinone atovaquone (Table 2).

No existing antimalarial drug was developed in a fully rational manner, with a focused attempt to inhibit a known drug target. Rather, in all cases, antimalarial potency has been identified clinically in animal models or in vitro, and subsequent studies have attempted to identify drug targets. Of note, as will be discussed in other chapters, for most available agents the target of action within the malaria parasite remains uncertain.

Our limited understanding of the biochemistry of malaria parasites hinders rational approaches to new drug development. Of available agents, the antimalarial mechanism of action is fully established only for inhibitors of enzymes required for folate biosynthesis. An improved appreciation of the mechanisms of action of drugs, even of agents such as chloroquine that are often no longer effective, should be helpful in the identification of new drugs. Indeed, one appealing strategy for new drug development is to improve on existing drugs by engineering chemical modifications that improve activity or limit resistance to existing agents.

Resistance to most available antimalarial agents has developed. Resistance developed slowly to chloroquine, but that to other drugs, including other quinolines and folate antagonists, developed more rapidly after the drugs were introduced. Resistance to new derivatives of artemisinin has not yet been identified, and these drugs are expected to play a major role in the treatment of falciparum malaria in the near future. However, with increased use of these drugs, it is likely that resistant parasites will be selected.

As is the case with mechanisms of antimalarial action, mechanisms of resistance are poorly understood for most drugs (*see* Chapter 8). Exceptions to this rule are inhibitors of folate pathway enzymes, where recent work has identified specific mutations in genes encoding target enzymes as mediators of resistance to these drugs (*10*) (*see* Chapter 9). Very recent work has also identified mutations that appear, in part, to mediate chloroquine resistance. A better understanding of the mechanisms by which malaria parasites develop drug resistance should aid in the design of new agents that circumvent or reverse known parasite resistance mechanisms.

Table 2
Available Antimalarial Drugs

Drug	Class	Use
Chloroquine	4-Aminoquinoline	Treatment and chemoprophylaxis of sensitive parasites
Amodiaquine	4-Aminoquinoline	Treatment of some chloroquine-resistant *P. falciparum*
Quinine/quinidine	Quinoline methanol	Treatment of chloroquine-resistant *P. falciparum*
Mefloquine	Quinoline methanol	Chemoprophylaxis and treatment of *P. falciparum*
Primaquine	8-Aminoquinoline	Radical cure and terminal prophylaxis of *P. vivax* and *P. ovale*
Pyrimethamine/sulfadoxine	Folate antagonist, sulfa combination	Treatment of some chloroquine-resistant *P. falciparum*
Proquanil	Folate antagonist	Chemoprophylaxis (with chloroquine)
Doxycycline	Tetracycline antibiotic	Treatment of *P. falciparum* (with quinine); chemoprophylaxis
Halofantrine	Phenanthrene methanol	Treatment of some chloroquine-resistant *P. falciparum*
Artemisinins	Sesquiterpene lactone endoperoxides	Treatment of multidrug-resistant *P. falciparum*
Atovaquone/proguanil (Malarone)	Quinone/folate antagonist combination	Treatment and chemoprophylaxis of *P. falciparum*

NEW APPROACHES TO ANTIMALARIAL CHEMOTHERAPY

We are presently at a critical juncture in the history of the chemotherapy of malaria, as increasing drug resistance is leading to the need to rethink therapeutic approaches. Replacement of chloroquine as the standard antimalarial agent has increasingly become necessary because of the gradual spread of resistance in *P. falciparum* populations. The replacement of chloroquine as presumptive therapy for falciparum malaria has already occurred in many areas, in particular Southeast Asia and parts of South America. However, chloroquine remains the first-line therapy for uncomplicated falciparum malaria in most of Africa. Despite a very high prevalence of resistant parasites in some areas, chloroquine is often at least partially effective in highly immune populations, but clinical failures are common, and increased mortality resulting from drug resistance has been documented *(11)*. No clear consensus exists as to the appropriate approach to address increasing chloroquine resistance in Africa. Although chloroquine continues to be heavily used, new agents must be considered for routine presumptive therapy *(12)* (*see* Chapter 5). In a few countries chloroquine has been replaced by pyrimethamine/sulfadoxine as the first-line drug, but resistance to this combination appears to be increasing rapidly.

Multiple general approaches to the identification of new antimalarials are being pursued at this time (Table 3). A first approach is to optimize therapy with existing agents. New dosing regimens or formulations of some agents may optimize activity. Combination therapies, including new agents (e.g., artemisinin derivatives, atovaquone) and new combinations of older agents (e.g., chlorproguanil/dapsone) are under study as first-line therapies for Africa and other areas with widespread drug resistance (*see* Chapter 12). Combinations of two effective agents should improve antimalarial efficacy. In the case of both the artemisinin derivatives and atovaquone, the new agents have had unacceptable failure rates when used as single agents to treat falciparum malaria, but they have been highly effective in combination with other established antimalarials. Importantly, the use of combination antimalarial therapy should also slow the progression of parasite resistance to the new agents.

A second approach to antimalarial chemotherapy is to evaluate compounds that are chemically related to existing agents. This approach does not require knowledge of the mechanism of action or the biological target of the parent compound. Indeed, this approach was responsible for the development of many existing antimalarials. For example, chloroquine, primaquine, and mefloquine were discovered as a result of chemical strategies to improve upon quinine. More recently, 4-aminoquinolines that are closely related to chloroquine appear to offer the antimalarial potency of the parent drug, even against chloroquine-resistant parasites (*see* Chapter 13), and the 8-aminoquinoline tafenoquine offers improved activity against hepatic-stage parasites over that of the parent compound primaquine (*see* Chapter 7). New folate antagonists (*see* Chapter 16) and new endoperoxides related to artemisinin (*see* Chapter 14) are also under study. Some new agents that are already under clinical evaluation, including lumefantrine and pyronaridine, were developed based on strategies to improve on existing agents (*see* Chapter 12).

Natural-product-derived compounds offer a third approach to chemotherapy. This approach has identified the most important drugs currently available to treat severe

Table 3
General Approaches to the Discovery
of New Antimalarial Agents Discussed in This Volume

Approach	Examples	Chapter
Optimize therapy with existing agents	Artemisinin-derivative combinations	12
	Atovaquone/proguanil (Malarone)	11
	Chlorproguanil/dapsone	12
Develop analogs of existing agents	Chloroquine, amodiaquine, mefloquine	6
	New quinolines	13
	Primaquine, tafenoquine	7
	Lumefantrine, pyronaridine	12
	New endoperoxides	14
	New folate antagonists	16
Natural products and their derivatives	Quinine, quinidine	6
	Artemisinin and derivatives	10
Compounds active against other diseases	Folate antagonists	9
	Antibiotics	15
	Atovaquone	11
	Iron chelators	17
Drug-resistance reversers	Chlorpheniramine and others	8
Compounds active against new targets	Protease inhibitors	18
	Phospholipid-metabolism inhibitors	19
	Inhibitors of transport mechanisms	20

falciparum malaria, quinine, and derivatives of artemisinsin. In the case of artemisinin, relatively simple chemical modifications of the natural-product parent compound have led to a series of highly potent antimalarials that will probably play a critical role in the treatment of severe malaria over the next decade (*see* Chapter 10). Extensive evaluations of natural products as potential new therapies for human diseases are underway. It is important that such trials include the evaluation of the antimalarial potency of plant extracts and potential drugs purified from these extracts.

A fourth approach to antimalarial chemotherapy is to identify agents that are developed or marketed as treatments for other diseases. Folate inhibitors and other antibiotics were developed for their antibacterial properties and were later found to be active against malaria parasites. Atovaquone was initially identified as an antimalarial, but its development was expedited by the discovery of its activity against *Pneumocystis carinii*. More recently, its potential as an antimalarial (as a component of the combination drug Malarone) has been re-explored (*see* Chapter 11). Iron chelators, which are used to treat iron-overload syndromes, have documented antimalarial efficacy (*see* Chapter 17). These examples suggest that it is appropriate to screen new antimicrobial agents and other available compounds as antimalarial drugs. This approach is facilitated by the presence of high-throughput assays for potential antimalarials. As suggested by the recent development of Malarone, the consideration of compounds with activity against other, more economically attractive microbial targets may provide a relatively inexpensive means of identifying new antimalarials.

A fifth approach to chemotherapy is to combine previously effective agents with compounds that reverse parasite resistance to these agents. Many drugs have been shown to reverse the resistance of *P. falciparum* to chloroquine in vitro. Although, in many cases, unacceptably high concentrations of the resistance reversers are needed for their effects, the commonly used antihistamine chlorpheniramine and other agents have been shown to reverse resistance at clinically acceptable dosing levels (*see* Chapter 8). Evaluation of these compounds and other potential reversers of resistance to chloroquine is ongoing.

The most scientifically appealing new approach to chemotherapy is the identification of new targets and subsequent discovery of compounds that act on these targets. Our rapid progress in the characterization of the biology of malaria parasites suggests that this last approach is most likely to identify important new antimalarial compounds in the future. Some potential targets for new drugs are likely the targets of existing agents that were developed without knowledge of their specific biological effects. Chloroquine probably causes parasite toxicity by blocking the polymerization of free heme in the parasite food vacuole (*see* Chapter 6). New inhibitors of this process are of interest as potential antimalarials (*see* Chapter 13). Some antibiotics probably exert their antimalarial effects via inhibition of protein synthesis or other processes in the prokaryote-like plastid organelle. New inhibitors of plastid metabolism may also exert specific antimalarial effects (*see* Chapter 15). As the mechanisms of action of established antimalarials are better characterized, the identified sites of action of these drugs will be logical additional targets for new antimalarial compounds. Additional potential targets, for which inhibitors with antimalarial activity have been identified, include parasite proteases (*see* Chapter 18), parasite phospholipid metabolism (*see* Chapter 19), and novel transport mechanisms (*see* Chapter 20). Many others are under study (*13*). The identification of new targets should be dramatically expedited by the malaria genome project, which, within a few years, will identify the sequences of all proteins of *P. falciparum*.

In summary, multiple approaches have proven track records for the development of antimalarial drugs. It is essential that these older approaches continue and that they are supplemented by the rational development of new agents directed against newly identified parasite targets. The continued control of malaria will likely require multiple new effective agents. A recently stated goal of the Medicines for Malaria Venture is to develop one new effective antimalarial drug every 5 yr. Our ultimate goal, of course, is not merely to continue malaria control at its current rate of success, but to move toward the elimination of this health problem. This goal will likely require major advances in vector control, vaccinology, and the development of new drugs, each a daunting task. However, recent advances in many areas of vector, host, and parasite biology are encouraging, and there is good reason to believe that, with increasing broad support of research efforts, important gains against malaria can be achieved in the near future.

REFERENCES

1. Oaks SC, Mitchell VS, Pearson GW, Carpenter CCJ (eds). Malaria: Obstacles and Opportunities. Washington, DC: National Academy Press, 1991.
2. Knell AJ. Malaria. Oxford: Oxford University Press, 1991.
3. World Health Organization. The World Health Report 1997. Geneva: World Health Organization, 1997.
4. Olliaro P, Cattani J, Wirth D. Malaria, the submerged disease. JAMA 1996;275:230–233.
5. D'Alessandro U, Olaleye BO, McGuire W, Langerock P, Bennett S, Aikins MK, Thomson MC, et al. Mortality and morbidity from malaria in Gambian children after introduction of an impregnated bednet programme. Lancet 1995;345:479–483.
6. Miller LH, Hoffman SL. Research toward vaccines against malaria. Nat Med 1998;4: 520–524.
7. White N. Antimalarial drug resistance and combination chemotherapy. Philos. Trans R Soc Lond B: Biol Sci 1999;354:739–749.
8. Anderson J, MacLean M, Davies C. Malaria Research: An Audit of International Activity. London:The Wellcome Trust, 1996.
9. White NJ. Drug resistance in malaria. Br Med Bull 1998;54:703–315.
10. Plowe CV, Cortese JF, Djimde A, Nwanyanwu OC, Watkins WM, Winstanley PA, et al. Mutations in *Plasmodium falciparum* dihydrofolate reductase and dihydropteroate synthase and epidemiologic patterns of pyrimethamine-sulfadoxine use and resistance. J Infect Dis 1997;176:1590–1596.
11. Trape JF, Pison G, Preziosi MP, Enel C, Desgrees du Lou A, Delaunay V, et al. Impact of chloroquine resistance on malaria mortality. C R Acad Sci III 1998;321:689–697.
12. Bloland PB, Lackritz EM, Kazembe PN, Were JBO, Steketee R, Campbell CC. Beyond chloroquine: implications of drug resistance for evaluating malaria therapy efficacy and treatment policy in Africa. J Infect Dis 1993;167:932–937.
13. Olliaro PL, Yuthavong Y. An overview of chemotherapeutic targets for antimalarial drug discovery. Pharmacol Ther 1999;81:91–110.

2

The History of Antimalarial Drugs

Steven R. Meshnick and Mary J. Dobson

INTRODUCTION

Physicians have diagnosed and treated fevers for thousands of years. Until Robert Koch, Louis Pasteur, and their contemporaries uncovered the "germs" that cause most febrile illnesses, fevers were considered diseases, not results of diseases. Fevers were treated with a variety of remedies, such as bloodletting or herbs, most of which were ineffective. Malaria-like febrile illnesses (with names like "the ague" or "paludism") have been described since Hippocrates as fevers that were periodic and associated with marshes and swamps. The word "malaria" comes from the Italian "mal'aria" for "bad airs." It was not until the 1880s and 1890s that Alphonse Laveran, Ronald Ross, Battista Grassi, and others were able to identify the malaria parasite and link the transmission of malaria to mosquitoes. Although the understanding of the mosquito cycle led to a number of new approaches in vector control in the early 20th century, malaria prophylaxis and therapy continued to draw on earlier remedies. Indeed, what is remarkable about malarial fevers is that two herbal treatments, cinchona bark and qinghao, were used to treat malaria effectively for hundreds of years prior to the understanding of the mosquito cycle. Today both quinine (derived from the cinchona bark) and artemisinin (from qinghao) remain of prime importance in the control of malaria.

The practice of Western medicine changed dramatically during the 19th and 20th centuries, as herbal remedies were gradually replaced by pure chemical compounds and, later, synthetic drugs. So, too, did the treatment of malaria undergo important scientific developments. Malaria was among the first diseases to be treated by a pure chemical compound—quinine—isolated from the cinchona bark in 1820. It was, subsequently, the first disease to be treated by a synthetic compound—methylene blue. In addition, malaria parasites were among the first pathogenic microbes to out-smart medical intervention and become drug resistant.

Malaria was one of the best-studied diseases in Western medicine until the middle of the 20th century. Until that time, malaria was still endemic in North America and Europe. It also had great importance because it represented an obstacle to the expansion of European nations into the tropical world. It also played an important role in the major wars of both the 19th and 20th centuries. The situation has changed, and, until recently, interest in malaria in Western nations has waned even though the disease at a global scale has not.

From: *Antimalarial Chemotherapy: Mechanisms of Action, Resistance, and New Directions in Drug Discovery*
Edited by: P. J. Rosenthal © Humana Press Inc., Totowa, NJ

QUININE

The compound quinine occurs naturally in the bark of Cinchona trees, originally found in high altitudes of South America (Fig. 1). Cinchona bark was introduced into Europe as a treatment for the ague in the early 17th century by Jesuit priests returning from Peru. Peruvian Indians chewed on cinchona bark—but, as far as we know, not to treat malaria. Indeed, malaria may not have existed in the New World prior to Columbus *(1,2)*. There have been many speculations about the South American Indians' knowledge and use of the cinchona bark. According to one account, Indians used it while working in cold streams in Spanish-owned mines in order to stop shivering. This effect was probably the result of quinine's direct effects on skeletal muscle and neuromuscular junctions *(3)*. Some physicians and Jesuit priests in Peru reasoned that the bark might be able to stop the shivering associated with attacks of the ague. They tried the bark of the "fever tree" on malarial patients and found that the feverish symptoms of ague sufferers were relieved.

The Countess of Chinchon and her husband are credited with bringing the bark back to Spain (Fig. 2) although like several of the myths and mysteries associated with the early history of cinchona, this story is probably fallacious. Linnaeus in 1742 named the tree, cinchona, after her, although the bark was more commonly known as Jesuits' powder or Peruvian bark *(4)*.

A number of European physicians and quack doctors had remarkable successes with the bark *(5)*, but its use initially met with a great deal of skepticism. First, many people were skeptical of anything associated with the Jesuits. In fact, Oliver Cromwell suffered severely from malaria, apparently because he refused to ingest "the powder of the devil" *(6)*. Second, because merchants were frequently unable to distinguish cinchona from other trees, many types of bark were used as long as they were bitter. Finally, different cinchona species vary greatly in quinine content *(7)* and there was considerable confusion concerning the "best" bark to administer. These last two factors made therapeutic results inconsistent.

Richard Morton, who published his *Pyretologia* in 1692, became a firm advocate of Peruvian bark. He claimed it was a "Herculean antidote" to the poison of intermittent fevers and, when given in proper dosage, usually returned the patient to health immediately *(8)*. He also used the therapeutic results of the bark as a guide to diagnosis. His ideas were further developed by Francesco Torti who, in his classic work of 1712, *Therapeutice Specialis,* designed a "tree of fevers." Different fevers, shown as branches of the tree, were divided into categories: On the left were those that responded to cinchona (shown as branches covered with bark) and on the right were those that did not (depicted as denuded leafless branches) *(8)*. Torti's classification and differentiation of fevers and his recognition that only certain fevers could be treated by cinchona was of major importance. By the late 18th century, formulations became more standardized and cinchona was more widely accepted as a treatment for specific intermittent fevers *(3,9)*.

Cinchona had become so popular by the eighteenth century that several species of cinchona trees were becoming extinct *(6,10)*. In 1820, two young French chemists, Pierre Pelletier and Joseph Caventou, isolated the alkaloids quinine and cinchonine from cinchona bark. Within a year, several French physicians were successfully using pure quinine to treat patients with intermittent fever *(11)*. Explorers and scientists then

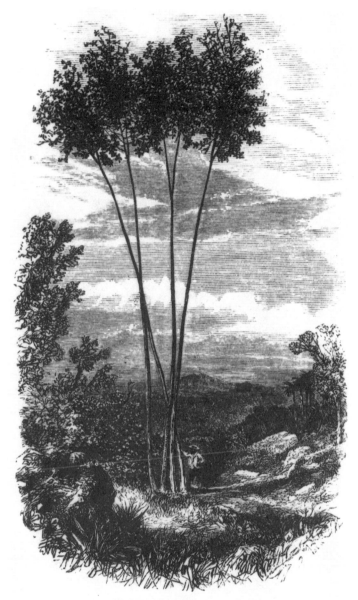

CHINCHONA NITIDA TREES.

(From a sketch by Mr. Pritchett.)

Fig. 1. Cinchona tree. (From Markham, CR. Peruvian Bark: The Introduction of Chinchona Cultivation into British India. London: John Murray, 1860. Reproduced with the permission of the Wellcome Institute Library, London, UK.)

began to search for the cinchona species with the highest quinine content. Charles Ledger and his faithful Bolivian servant, Manuel Incra Mamani, found a variety of cinchona with a high quinine content (*Cinchona ledgeriana*); after the British rejected Ledger's offer, he sold some seeds to the Dutch government for a few guilders in 1865

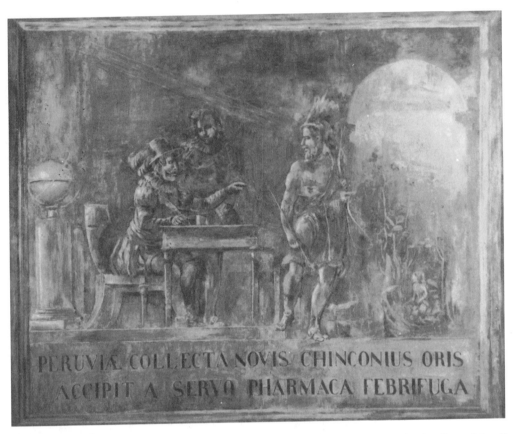

Fig. 2. The Count of Chinchon receives cinchona. (From a fresco in the Ospedale di Santo Spirito in Rome. Reproduced with the permission of the Wellcome Institute Library, London, UK.)

(9,12). These seeds were one of the best investments in history. Within a short time, the Dutch plantations of Java were producing 97% of the world's supply of quinine and had a virtual monopoly, producing in the 1930s about 10 million kilograms of bark a year (Fig. 3). From the mid-19th century to the 1940s, quinine became the standard therapy for intermittent fever throughout the world.

Prior to the isolation of quinine, the bark was usually administered as a suspension in wine or spirits to counteract its bitterness. This recipe may have evolved into the gin and tonic, a daily staple of British colonialists throughout the world *(13)* (Fig. 4). Tonic water today only contains 15 mg of quinine per liter *(14),* so the drink has little antimalarial benefit.

SYNTHETIC ANTIMALARIALS

The science of synthetic organic chemistry underwent a revolution in the late 19th century, partly in response to the need for new antimalarials. In 1856, William Henry Perkins, an 18-yr-old English chemist, set out to synthesize quinine, but failed. (Indeed, the synthesis of quinine was not accomplished until 1944 and, even to this day, has not been achieved on a commercially economic scale.) However, Perkins succeeded in

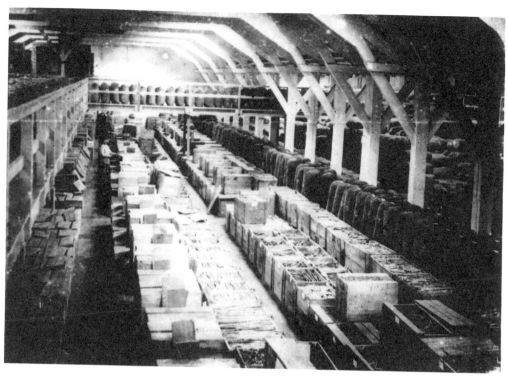

Fig. 3. Photograph of a warehouse in Amsterdam, cases filled with cinchona bark. (Reproduced with the permission of the Wellcome Institute Library, London, UK.)

synthesizing "mauve," the first synthetic textile dye that did not wash off in water. This advance sparked the development of a huge German synthetic dye industry *(6)*.

The new dye industry helped promote the advancement of medicine. When microbial pathogens were first identified, they were difficult to see under the microscope. Newly synthesized dyes were then used by microbiologists as stains to enhance visualization and classification. Paul Ehrlich, a German scientist, noticed that methylene blue was particularly effective in staining malaria parasites. He reasoned that because the parasite avidly took up the dye, it might be poisoned by it in vivo. In 1891, Ehrlich cured two patients of malaria using methylene blue, the first time a synthetic drug was ever used in humans *(15)*.

Bayer, one of the leading German dye companies, soon became a leading pharmaceutical company. A team of chemists and biologists was assembled by Bayer to develop new synthetic antimalarials using methylene blue as a prototype. In 1925, they developed plasmoquine (also called pamaquine). Plasmoquine, the first 8-aminoquinoline, proved to be the first compound capable of preventing relapses in vivax malaria. In 1932, they developed mepacrine (atebrine) which was effective against falciparum malaria.

In 1934, H. Andersag, working at the Elberfield labs of Bayer IG Farbenindustrie AG developed a compound known as resochin *(16,17)*. Although the compound looked promising, it was felt to be too toxic. In 1936, Andersag synthesized a derivative of resochin known as sontochin, which seemed to be less toxic.

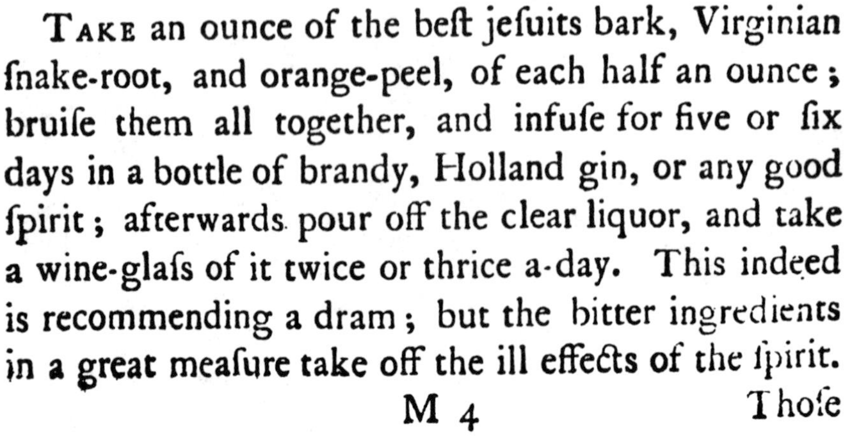

TAKE an ounce of the beſt jeſuits bark, Virginian
ſnake-root, and orange-peel, of each half an ounce;
bruiſe them all together, and infuſe for five or ſix
days in a bottle of brandy, Holland gin, or any good
ſpirit; afterwards pour off the clear liquor, and take
a wine-glaſs of it twice or thrice a-day. This indeed
is recommending a dram; but the bitter ingredients
in a great meaſure take off the ill effects of the ſpirit.

M 4   Thoſe

Fig. 4. An early recipe for the gin and tonic. (From Buchan W. Domestic Medicine: or, a Treatise on the Prevention and Cure of Diseases by Regimen and Simple Medicines. London: W. Strachan & T. Cadell, 1781. Reproduced with the permission of the Wellcome Institute Library, London, UK.)

During World War II, the world supply of quinine was cut off as the Japanese took over Java. Plasmoquine and mepacrine (atebrine) were manufactured and widely used by both sides. As part of the war effort, American, British, and Australian scientists cooperated in a large-scale attempt to develop new synthetic antimalarials. Sixteen thousand compounds were synthesized and tested. Surprisingly, Allied scientists had been informed about resochin and it was one of the first tested compounds. It had the acquisition number SN-183. For the second time, it was considered too toxic and dropped. Meanwhile, French Vichy physicians were carrying out clinical trials on sontochin in Tunis. After the allies captured North Africa, they obtained samples of sontochin and data from the study. Interest was rekindled in resochin, which was renamed chloroquine (and renumbered SN-7618). By 1946, US clinical trials showed that this compound was far superior to atebrine *(16,17)*. The eventual recognition of chloroquine as a powerful antimalarial is one of the most fascinating stories in the history and development of synthetic drugs. As Coatney has commented, "the main story of chloroquine, 1934 to 1946, involves investigators of six countries on five continents and embraces its initial discovery, rejection, re-discovery, evaluation and acceptance" *(17)*.

Chloroquine proved to be the most effective and important antimalarial ever and was used widely throughout the world. In the 1950s, Mario Pinotti in Brazil introduced the strategy of putting chloroquine into common cooking salt as a way of distributing the drug as a prophylactic on a wide scale. This medicated salt program (using either chloroquine or pyrimethamine) became known as "Pinotti's method" and was employed in South America as well as parts of Africa and Asia. Chloroquine was the main drug of choice in the WHO Global Eradication Programme of the 1950s and 1960s, and although somewhat overshadowed by the widespread use of the residual insecticide DDT, chemoprophylaxis with chloroquine tablets or chloroquine-medicated salt was an important supplementary component of eradication and control programs in many areas of the world. Its use was only curtailed beginning in the 1960s with the advent of chloroquine resistance in *Plasmodium falciparum* (which may have been caused, in part, by the medicated salt program). Chloroquine resistance has now spread to many of the areas of the world where the infection is endemic *(18)*.

Chloroquine was one of many antimalarials resulting from scientific advances made during World War II. The American effort also included attempts to make more effective versions of the 8-aminoquinoline plasmaquine. Soon after the war, primaquine was introduced, and proved to be the standard drug for the prevention of relapses in vivax malaria *(16)*. Interestingly, 50 yr later, American military scientists have found yet another promising 8-aminoquinoline, WR 238605 or tafenoquine *(19)*.

The British war effort led to the development of proguanil (Paludrine). After the war, proguanil served as a prototype for the development of pyrimethamine (Daraprim) in 1950 by Burroughs–Wellcome *(16)*. Pyrimethamine, in combination with sulfadoxine, was introduced in the 1970s and named Fansidar *(20)*. Fansidar is still in wide use, particularly in Africa.

Several compounds discovered during the American war effort later served as prototypes for the development of other antimalarials. One such compound, SN 10275, was a prototype for mefloquine, which was introduced in the mid-1970s *(21)*. Mefloquine (Lariam) is widely used throughout the world. Another class of compound developed during World War II were the 2-hydroxynaphthoquinones. These served as prototypes for a drug that was introduced only recently—atovaquone. Atovaquone is now being manufactured by Glaxo-Wellcome Pharmaceuticals in combination with proguanil and sold as Malarone *(22)*.

ARTEMISININ

Artemisia annua—sweet wormwood or qinghao (pronounced "ching-how")—was used by Chinese herbal medicine practitioners for at least 2000 yr, initially to treat hemorrhoids. In 1596, Li Shizhen, a famous herbalist, recommended this herb for fever, and specified that the extract be prepared in cold water *(23)*.

In 1967, the government of the People's Republic of China established a program to screen traditional remedies for drug activities *(24)* in an effort to professionalize traditional medicine. Qinghao was tested in this program and found to have potent antimalarial activity. In 1972, the active ingredient was purified and named qinghaosu (essence of qinghao). Qinghaosu and derivatives were then tested on thousands of patients. Summaries of these studies were published in the late 1970s and early 1980s *(25,26)*. Artemisinin derivatives are now widely used in Southeast Asia and are starting to be used elsewhere (reviewed in ref. *27*).

ANTIMALARIALS AND THEIR IMPACT ON HISTORY

Quinine had a profound influence on modern colonial history and a number of historians have highlighted the importance of this single drug as one of the "tools of empire" *(28)*. Falciparum malaria was a major problem for missionaries, explorers, colonists, and the military in many parts of the tropical and subtropical world. As Europeans began to settle the coasts, penetrate the interiors, and colonize the lands of Africa and Asia, they were frequently struck down with tropical diseases, including malaria.

Malaria in West Africa, a region often typified as "White Man's Grave," was especially severe. For example, almost half of the British soldiers stationed in Sierra Leone between 1817 and 1836 died of infectious disease, mostly malaria (28). The introduction of quinine, however, contributed to a marked reduction of colonial military mortality in certain areas from the mid-19th century (29). Its use was encouraged by some, although not all, doctors as imperative for survival in the tropics. In Alexander Bryson's text of 1847, *Report on the Climate and Principal Diseases of the African Station*, he recommended and noted the importance of quinine as a prophylaxis amongst Europeans:

> So general has the use of quinine now become, that there is hardly any part of Western Africa, where there are resident Europeans, in whose houses it is not to be found; it is in fact considered to be one of the necessaries of life, where life is of all things the most uncertain.

Later, when malaria and other tropical diseases were shown to be the result of infectious agents rather than an inherently bad climate, the use of quinine as a prophylactic and effective treatment for malaria was advocated in the scientific literature, advice manuals, and travel guides for Europeans venturing into the tropics. Although death rates in the early 20th century remained high among Europeans in malarial areas, the use of quinine, as well as mosquito control, bed-nets, screening, and other forms of prevention and protection, helped alleviate the misery caused by malaria. Indigenous populations were often viewed as "reservoirs" of infection and it was suggested by a number of leading malariologists in the early twentieth century that the "immune" adult did not suffer from the debilitating effects of malaria. However, as Europeans increasingly relied on local and imported labor forces to work on European plantations, estates, and mines, it was soon recognized that malaria was a problem for indigenous as well as colonial populations. Gradually, the use of quinine was recommended more widely for humanitarian as well as economic reasons and demands for the drug increased in the first half of the twentieth century.

Concerns about the correct dosage, the cost, and the side effects of long-term prophylaxis with quinine, and especially its possible connection with blackwater fever, however, gave rise to scientific debates concerning its use. Moreover, for many of the poorest rural populations of the world, the drug was not readily available. In 1925, the Malaria Commission of the Health Committee of the League of Nations estimated that no less than 26,441,000 kg of quinine would be required annually in order to provide a therapeutic dose of 2.6 g to every malaria case in the world. The actual consumption remained considerably less, reaching a figure of only 610,000 kg in the 1930s (30).

It has been particularly during the military campaigns and the major wars of the past 150 yr that quinine and, later, synthetic antimalarials have been employed most rigorously and on a wide scale (Fig. 5). Quinine played an important role in American military history. The American Civil War might have ended in its first year if malaria had not ravaged General McClellan's troops invading Virginia (31). Although Union troops vastly outnumbered Confederate troops, "Chickahominy fever," a combination of malaria and typhoid, made Union troops unable to fight. During the war, the Union army used over 25,000 kg of quinine or other cinchona products (9).

Antimalarials also played a crucial role in World War II, especially in the Southwest Pacific. In many cases, malaria posed a far greater health risk than battlefield injuries

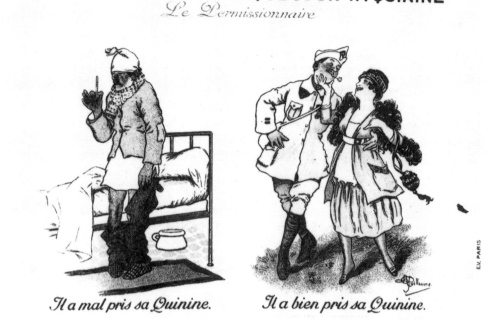

SOLDAT : PRENDS CHAQUE JOUR TA QUININE

Le Permissionnaire

Il a mal pris sa Quinine.   *Il a bien pris sa Quinine.*

Fig. 5. The results of taking quinine contrasted with the results of not taking it. (Postcard, Paris circa 1914. Reproduced with the permission of the Wellcome Institute Library, London, UK.)

(32). Daily prophylaxis with atebrine was required for all Allied troops, even though it turned the skin yellow and was reputed to cause impotence. This drug helped protect the health of the Allied troops fighting in some of the most malarious areas of the world and, as Bruce-Chwatt has said, "there is no exaggeration in saying that this probably changed the course of modern history" *(33)*. Interestingly, Japanese troops fighting in this area also used atebrine, but at an inadequate dose. This may have contributed to the development of atebrine resistance in New Guinea *(32)*.

During the Vietnam War, malaria was the single greatest cause of casualties even though all troops received prophylaxis with chloroquine and primaquine *(21)*. An estimated 390,000 sick days were lost to malaria among the American forces and the emergence of strains of falciparum that were resistant to available antimalarial drugs caused considerable concern and a renewed interest in the search for new antimalarial agents at the Walter Reed Army Institute of Research in Washington *(16)*.

The American military maintained a strong program in antimalarial drug development through the early 1990s. They synthesized and tested over 250,000 compounds *(21)*. Several drug companies such as Wellcome and Roche also maintain active programs. However, the economics of drug development have changed dramatically in recent years as have methods of warfare. As a result, the American military's antimalarial development program has been cut, and many drug companies have stopped attempting to develop new antimalarials. As fears of drug resistance are becoming more pervasive, it is essential that new drugs or combinations of older drugs be developed for the future.

CONCLUSION

As the development costs of pharmaceuticals have escalated, the Western pharmaceutical industry has lost interest in antimalarial development. Once resistance to artemisinin and Malarone develop, there may be no new antimalarials ready to take their places.

In the last few years there has been a renewed concern for malaria as a global problem with programs such as WHO's Roll Back Malaria and the Multilateral Initiative on Malaria. History tells us that many of our past breakthroughs in malaria control were driven by the needs of the military and of the colonial powers. Can malaria control in the tropical and subtropical parts of the world advance in the absence of war or colonialism?

REFERENCES

1. Dunn FL. On the antiquity of malaria in the western hemisphere. Hum Biol 1965;37:385–393.
2. McNeill WH. Plagues and Peoples. Penguin, London: 1976.
3. Guerra F. The introduction of cinchona in the treatment of malaria. J Trop Med Hyg 1977;80:112–118, 135–140.
4. Bruce-Chwatt LJ. Cinchona and its alkaloids: 350 years later. NY State J Med 1988; 88:318–322.
5. Dobson MJ. Bitter-sweet solutions for malaria: exploring natural remedies from the past. Parassitologia 1998;40:69–81.
6. Hobhouse H Seeds of Change. Five Plants that Transformed Mankind. New York: Harper and Row, 1986.
7. Smit EHD Quinine is not what it used to be. . . . Acta Leidensia 1987;55:21–27.
8. Jarcho S. Quinine's Predecessor. Francesco Torti and the Early History of Cinchona. Baltimore: Johns Hopkins University Press, 1993.
9. Russell PF Man's Mastery of Malaria. London: Oxford University Press, 1955.
10. Taylor N Cinchona in Java; the Story of Quinine. New York: Greenberg, 1945.
11. Smith DC. Quinine and fever: the development of the effective dosage. J Hist Med 1976;31:343–367.
12. Gramiccia G. The Life of Charles Ledger (1818–1905). London: Macmillan, 1988.
13. McHale D. The Cinchona tree. Biologist 1986;33:45–53.
14. Meshnick SR. Why does quinine still work after 350 years of use? Parasitol Today 1997;13:89–90.
15. Weatherall M. In Search of a Cure. A History of Pharmaceutical Discovery. Oxford: Oxford University Press, 1990.
16. Greenwood D. Conflicts of interest: the genesis of synthetic antimalarial agents in peace and war. J Antimicrob Chemother 1995;36:857–872.
17. Coatney GR. Pitfalls in a discovery: the chronicle of chloroquine. Am J Trop Med Hyg 1963;12:121–28.
18. Peters, W. Chemotherapy and Drug Resistance in Malaria. London: Academic Press, 1987.
19. Brueckner RP, Coster T, Wesche DL, Shmuklarsky M, Schuster BG. Prophylaxis of *Plasmodium falciparum* infection in a human challenge model with WR 238605, a new 8-aminoquinoline antimalarial. Antimicrob Agents Chemother 1998;42:1293–1294.
20. Shanks GD, Karwacki JJ, Singharaj P. Malaria prophylaxis during military operations in Thailand. Mil Med. 1989;154:500–502.
21. Shanks GD. The rise and fall of mefloquine as an antimalarial drug in South East Asia Mil Med 1994;4:275–281.
22. Looareesuwan S, Chulay JD, Canfield CJ, Hutchinson DB. Malarone (atovaquone and proguanil hydrochloride): a review of its clinical development for treatment of malaria. Malarone Clinical Trials Study Group. Am J Trop Med Hyg 1999;60:533–541.

23. Klayman D. Qinghaosu (artemisinin): an antimalarial drug from China. Science 1985;228: 1049–1055.
24. Lusha X. A new drug for malaria. China Reconstructs 1979;28:48–49.
25. China Cooperative Research Group on Qinghaosu and Its Derivatives as Antimalarials. Chemical studies on qinghaosu (artemisinine). J Trad Chin Med 1982;2:3–8.
26. China Cooperative Research Group on Qinghaosu and Its Derivatives as Antimalarials. The chemistry and synthesis of qinghaosu derivatives. J Trad Chin Med. 1982;2:9–16.
27. Meshnick SR, Taylor TE, Kamchonwongpaisan, S. Artemisinin and the antimalarial endo-peroxides: from herbal remedy to targeted chemotherapy. Microbiol Rev 1996;60:301–315.
28. Headrick DR. The Tools of Empire. Oxford: Oxford University Press, 1981.
29. Curtin PD. The end of the "white man's grave"? Nineteenth-century mortality in West Africa. J Interdisciplin His 1990;21:663–688.
30. Russell AJH. Quinine supplies in India. Rec Malaria Survey India 1937;7:233–244.
31. Simpson HN. Invisible Armies. The Impact of Disease on American History. Indianapolis, IN: Bobbs-Merrill Co., 1980.
32. Sweeney AW. The possibility of an "X" factor. The first documented drug resistance of human malaria. Int J Parasitol 1996;26:1035–1061.
33. Bruce-Chwatt LJ (ed). Chemotherapy of Malaria. Geneva: World Health Organization, 1986.

3

Transport and Trafficking
in *Plasmodium*-Infected Red Cells

Kasturi Haldar and Thomas Akompong

INTRODUCTION

The organism at the focus of antimalarial chemotherapy is *Plasmodium falciparum*. It causes the most virulent of human malarias and shows rapidly emerging drug resistance. The main targets of antimalarials are blood-stage parasites that are responsible for all of the symptoms and pathologies associated with the disease. These stages reside in the mature erythrocyte, a terminally differentiated, simple, host cell that is devoid of all intracellular organelles and are surrounded by a parasitophorous vacuolar membrane (PVM: *see* Fig. 1). The host erythrocyte is incapable of *de novo* protein or lipid synthesis and does not engage in the internalization of its surface membrane (*1*). There is a complete lack of endocytic machinery, which is lost as the reticulocyte matures into the erythrocyte. Hence, antimalarials need to enter an unusual intracellular niche.

Entry and survival of the parasite in this specialized niche is intimately linked to secretory trafficking of its proteins and lipids. Ongoing studies have shown that *P. falciparum* induces unique structural changes, protein and waste export, and nutrient import in infected red cells. There is evidence both for a nonspecific ion pore and an anion-selective channel that mediate solute transport in the PVM and the infected red cell membrane, respectively (*2,3*). An interconnected network of tubovesicular membranes (TVM) permeant to exogenous nutrients and drugs appears to connect the lumen of the vacuole to the extracellular plasma (*4*). Some of the solute transport pathways may be exploited to efficiently deliver antimalarials (*5*). Their resident components (*6,7*) as well as additional parasite secretory determinants (such as those within organelles like the food vacuole [Chapter 4] or the apicoplast [Chapter 17]) may provide targets for antimalarials. In this chapter, we will provide an overview on secretory transport mechanisms of *P. falciparum* and their implications for both the delivery of antimalarials and the development of new targets for chemotherapy.

ASEXUAL BLOOD-STAGE DEVELOPMENT, SECRETORY ORGANIZATION, AND TRANSPORT FUNCTIONS

Plasmodium species, like other members of the phylum apicomplexa, contain apical organelles, secretion from which underlies the entry of extracellular merozoites into

From: *Antimalarial Chemotherapy: Mechanisms of Action, Resistance, and New Directions in Drug Discovery*
Edited by: P. J. Rosenthal © Humana Press Inc., Totowa, NJ

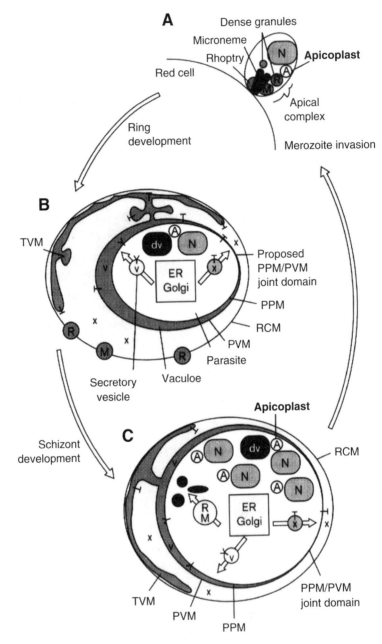

Fig. 1. Secretory development in the asexual cycle in *P. falciparum*. **(A)** Merozoite invasion. Daughter merozoites lyse out of a schizont infected red cell with each daughter inheriting a complete set of secretory organelles. The contents of the apical complex (such as protein M and R of the microneme and rhoptry) in the merozoite are discharged to the red cell membrane during invasion and/or early ring development. After invasion, the apical organelles are disorganized and no longer detected in the ring-infected red cell. **(B)** Secretory membrane development in ring and trophozoite-infected red cells. Within the red cell, the parasite is bounded by its own plasma membrane (PPM). The parasitophorous vacuolar membrane (PVM) surrounds the PPM and is continuous with the TVM, which extends up to the red cell membrane (RCM). Secretory vesicles shown export protein V to the vacuole, protein Y to the PPM, protein T to

the red cell. Unlike other apicomplexans (such as *Toxoplasma* and *Cryptosporidium*), in *Plasmodium*, apical secretory structures disappear immediately after invasion (*see* Fig. 1) and can no longer be detected in ring-stage parasites (0–24 h after invasion). Invasion is rapid, but exogenous antibodies [especially those bound to the parasite *(8)*] can enter at this time, suggesting an opportunity to deliver macromolecules to the infected red cell. Within 12 h of ring development, new solute-transport activities emerge. These have been ascribed to a parasite-induced anion-selective channel (reviewed in ref. *9*). Secretory development of a single, large, digestive food vacuole (FV) within the parasite (*see* Chapter 4) and a network of TVMs in the red cell are initiated in the ring stage, but mature forms of both organelles are not detected prior to the trophozoite stage (24–36 h after invasion) *(10)*. By the trophozoite stage, the parasite also exports proteins to multiple destinations in the red cell and inserts nonspecific nutrient pores in the vacuolar membrane *(11,12)*.

From 36 to 48 hr after invasion, the parasite enters schizogony to undergo mitosis and develop secretory structures of the apical secretory complex. This is also the time of plastid biogenesis and multiplication. The plastid is an unusual chloroplast relic (*see* Chapter 17) that is a secondary endosymbiont. It lies within the parasite plasma membrane, but proteins targeted to this organelle must be recruited into the secretory pathway *(13)*. Thus, it appears that the development of parasite-induced transport functions in the red cell precedes the development of organellar secretory functions. It is possible that this is required to satisfy high levels of metabolic demand needed during karyokinesis and cytokinesis and that temporal regulation of plasmodial secretory development is key to parasite proliferation in the red cell.

At about 48 h after invasion, the PVM and red cell membranes lyse, and the released merozoites invade fresh erythrocytes to reinitiate the asexual cycle. Little is known of mechanisms that underlie the rupture of the PVM and the red cell at these terminal stages of development. However, it is possible that changes in the flux or specificities of solute or macromolecule transport in the PVM and/or the red cell membrane play a role in erythrocyte rupture.

Channels, Pores, and a TVM Network Function in Solute and Nutrient Transport Between the Red Cell and the Parasite

As indicated earlier, during ring and trophozoite development, there are numerous changes in solute and nutrient transport properties of *P. falciparum*-infected red cells (Table 1). Accruing evidence suggests that these changes may be accounted for by solute channels induced in the PVM and infected red cell membrane as well as the TVM. However, although many of the characteristics of solute transport of each of these pathways are known, their organization relative to each other is still not fully

---

(*continued*) the TVM, and protein X to the red cell cytosol. Late ring- and trophozoite-stage parasites contain a prominent digestive (food) vacuole (dv). **(C)** Secretory maturation in schizont-stage parasites. Schizonts are actively growing multinucleated cells with a fully developed TVM. Protein export to the PPM is dominant (shown as protein Y). The formation of the apical secretory organelles and the accumulation of proteins (such as R and M) in these organelles by a pathway of regulated secretion are also detected at this stage. N = nucleus; A = apicoplast.

Table 1
Summary of Putative Transport Pathways in *Plasmodium*

Transport pathway	Transported molecules
Anion-selective channel	Prefers anions but can transport cations, glucose, amino acids, purines, pyrimidines, and vitamins
Nonspecific ion pore	Anions and cation <1400 Dalton
TVM	Amino acids, nucleosides, and drugs

Note: See text for references.

understood. The molecular identities of components of these pathways are beginning to emerge (greatly facilitated by the sequencing of the malaria genome) and this should provide a better understanding of their mechanisms of action and coordinate function in the infected red cell.

The anion-selective channel may underlie the first steps of parasite-induced solute transport into infected red cells *(9)*. An unusual feature of this channel is that although it has the characteristics of a chloride transporter and prefers anions, it can also support a substantial flux of cations such as K^+ and Rb^+ as well as choline *(3)*. The transport of cations is strongly dependent on the nature of anions in the suspending media. Strikingly, the substitution of NO_3^- for Cl^- results in a severalfold increase in the influx and efflux of Rb^+ and choline. This channel has been shown to transport glucose, purines, pyrimidines, amino acids, vitamins (e.g., pantothenic acid), and an antiplasmodial protease inhibitor *(14–16)*. In addition to its broad specificity, other features of the anion-selective channel include nonsaturable transport and inhibition by organic ions such as 5-nitro-2-(3-phenylpropylamino)benzoic acid (NPPB) *(3,6)*. There is no direct evidence that the channel can take up nutrients present at low extracellular concentrations, although recent data suggest that in the rodent parasite *P. vinckei,* a similar channel contributes to a third of choline influx *(14)*. In these studies, choline was also transported by the choline carrier of erythrocytes, indicating that host pathways are employed, but parasite nutrient demand may outstrip the capacity of host transporters even early in intraerythrocytic development. The anion-selective channel is likely to reside at the infected red cell surface, although there is no direct evidence for its localization in cells.

The non specific ion pore transports both cations and anions with a cutoff size of 1400 Daltons and an effective pore size diameter of 23 Å *(12)*. It was originally identified by patch-clamping permeabilized infected red cells *(2)*. It is similar to a pore in the vacuole of *Toxoplasma gondii (17)*, suggesting that a novel class of channels may be used by intracellular parasites to acquire nutrients from the host cytosol. Characterization of this PVM pore activity by reconstitution of parasite membranes into black lipid membranes suggests that under "open"-channel conditions, ion transport is not saturable or sensitive to the lipid environment of the bilayer *(12)*. Thus, the pore may influence bulk flux of ions across the PVM.

The TVM is a complex, parasite-induced organelle that contains multiple protein and lipid domains *(18)*. It was originally identified by three-dimensional reconstruction of consecutive high-resolution optical sections through live, infected erythrocytes labeled with fluorescent lipids *(19,20)*. Both confocal and scanning electron micro-

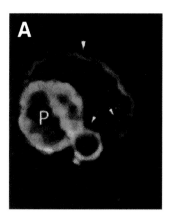 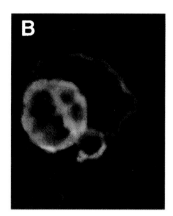 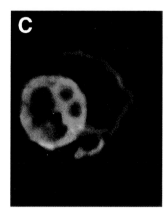

Fig. 2. Localization of PFGCN20 (an ATP-binding cassette protein) to the TVM. Infected erythrocytes were labeled with 4,4-difloro-4-bora-3a,4a-diaza-*s*-indacene (BODIPY)–ceramide and antibodies to PFGCN20 and examined by deconvolution microscopy. Green delineates lipid staining, red indicates distribution of PFGCN20, and yellow-orange shows the relative overlap between the two. Three consecutive optical sections **(A–C)**, 400 nm apart are shown for a late trophozoite. P denotes parasite; arrowhead indicates red cell membrane, and arrows indicate TVM. (From ref. *24*.)

graphs *(21)* confirmed that the TVM emerges from the parasitophorous vacuole and extends to the periphery of the red cell. Lipid and protein colabeling assays showed that Maurer's clefts and intraerythrocytic loops [seen as isolated structures in transmission electron micrographs *(22)*] form subdomains of the TVM. How individual structural units and domains are maintained as separate membrane entities in a continuous network is poorly understood.

A parasite sphingomyelin synthase is known to be an important constituent activity of the TVM *(19)*. Inhibition of this enzyme by the sphingolipid analog *dl*-threo-1-phenyl-2-palmitoylamino-3-morpholino-1-propanol (PPMP) and/or its dodecyl homolog PDMP blocked tubular development in the network *(7)*. A parasite fatty acyl coenzyme A synthetase is also likely to be a resident molecule of the TVM *(23)*, although this localization needs to be confirmed by high-resolution microscopy. Additional studies show that a parasite homolog of an ATP-binding cassette (ABC) transporter is located in the periphery of the TVM and its junctions with the red cell membrane (*see* Fig. 2) *(24)*. There is increasing evidence for the role of ABC transporters in lipid transport *(25)*. Taken together, these observations, suggest that *de novo* lipid synthesis and transport are important to the assembly and regulation of the TVM. PPMP-induced inhibition of tubular development in the TVM does not result in a block in biosynthetic protein export from the parasite to destinations in the red cell *(4)*. It does, however, retard the movement of low-molecular-weight chromogenic substrates (such as lucifer yellow) and nutrient solutes (such as nucleosides and amino acids) from the extracellular medium to the parasite *(4)*, suggesting that the TVM can function under physiological conditions to deliver low-molecular-weight nutrients to the parasite.

Like the anion-selective channel, the TVM transports a broad range of amino acids and nucleosides and the pathway may increase the efficiency of delivery of at least a subset of essential nutrients to the parasite. This may explain why the TVM is only essential at the later stages of intraerythrocytic development *(4)*. Although there is no direct evidence that the nonsaturable, anion-selective solute channels are integral to the TVM, they may function at TVM–red cell junctions. The TVM is not a duct *(26)* [a structure whose existence is debated *(27,28)*] that enables extracellular macromolecules to diffuse into infected red cells. If the nonspecific ion-channel is present on the TVM, it may enable solute flux from the red cell cytosol to the TVM. A dilution in concentration that is expected when solutes move from the lumen of the TVM into the red cell cytosol may not be a significant disadvantage given the presence of high-affinity transporters in the parasite plasma membrane (Chapter 22). If restricted to the vacuolar membrane alone, the nonspecific channel may transport solutes from the red cell cytosol, whereas the TVM (in conjunction with the nonsaturable anion-selective channel) delivers exogenous solutes to the parasite.

Our understanding of nutrient transport into the plasmodial vacuole is still evolving. A general consensus has emerged over the last 5 yr to suggest that parasite-induced transport pathways in the red cell traffic a wide range of low-molecular substances and this broad specificity precludes high-affinity interactions characteristic of substrate-specific transporters. This situation contrasts with solute uptake at the parasite plasma membrane (Chapter 22), where transport is stereospecific and dissociation constants are in the nanomolar range.

DELIVERY OF ANTIMALARIALS

The induction by the parasite of a broad-specificity, low-affinity transport pathway in the red cell would, at first glance, bode well for the delivery of antimalarials to infected erythrocytes. However, not all low-molecular-weight solutes enter infected cells; surprisingly, sucrose is excluded. This observation underlies the notion that the PVM–TVM functions as a sieving endosome and that defining its substrate specificity is likely to have profound implications for drug delivery. Chloroquine is a weak base and, at neutral pH, can efficiently diffuse across membranes. However, other antimalarials such as the folate derivatives and artemisinin are relatively impermeant, but, nonetheless, gain access to the parasite.

The transport of nucleosides by the TVM suggested that the network may also deliver toxic nucleotide compounds. 5-Fluoroorotate (5-FO) was the first inhibitor shown to be transported by the TVM *(4)*. It is of interest as an antimalarial because orotic acid is the only pyrimidine that is incorporated into the parasite *(29)*. PPMP treatment inhibited accumulation of radiolabeled 5-FO by approx 90%, these TVM-arrested cells displayed more than a 15-fold resistance to killing by 5-FO. Thus, it is possible that the resistance to 5-FO seen in some mutants *(30)* is the result of alterations in transport by the TVM. The transport of 5-FO is not saturable, suggesting that it may use the anion-selective channel to cross the infected red cell membrane and enter the TVM.

Artemisinin is a second drug transported by the TVM. It is a sesquiterpene endoperoxide that is active against multidrug-resistant parasites *(31)* (Chapter 11). Although artemisinin accumulates at high levels in infected red cells *(32)*, very little is known of the mechanisms by which it is taken up by the infected red cell or potential cellular targets. In studies with the inhibitor of TVM development, PPMP, there was a close correlation between the degree of TVM inhibition and the reduction in artemisinin accumulation, strongly suggesting that the TVM accounts for 70% of dihydroartemisinin transport in infected red cells *(5)*. This uptake is saturable and temperature dependent, suggesting that it is a carrier-mediated process with a K_m of 276 ± 34. PPMP treatment had no effect on the K_m, but reduced the V_{max} of transport by approx 40% (from 3.12 to 1.81 ± 0.13 nmol/min/10^6 parasites). Thus, PPMP does not alter the initial interaction of dihydroartemisinin with its carrier and, hence, the carrier must reside at the infected red cell surface rather than within the TVM. In delivering artemisinin and its derivatives to the TVM, the carrier may interact with another parasite transporter and/or channel in the TVM or possibly span both red cell and TVM membranes at specialized junctions of interaction. Thus, artemisinin transport contrasts with the uptake of purines, pyrimidines and amino acids into the TVM, which is nonsaturable, arguing for the absence of a carrier *(4)*. The data suggest that the TVM may interact with multiple transporters at the infected red cell surface.

The protease inhibitor pepstatin appears to be transported by the anion-selective channel *(16)*. Although pepstatin is not likely to be an effective drug, these data suggest that peptidic inhibitors of food vacuole proteases may utilize this pathway to enter infected red cells and subsequently cross into the vacuole via the TVM or nonspecific channels in the PVM. In all cases, it is not known how antimalarials are delivered from the lumen of the PVM into the cytoplasm of the parasite.

Protein Export and Secretory Destinations of Interest in Infected Erythrocytes

How solute channels, TVM components, and other parasite proteins are exported to various destinations in the infected red cell remains largely unknown. Because the mature red cell does not have any transport machinery, there is general agreement that export mechanisms must be regulated by the parasite. There is reasonable evidence for multiple pathways of protein and membrane delivery from the parasite to the red cell and a number of models for parasite protein export have been proposed *(20,33,34)*. The molecular characterization of these pathways is still sketchy. Because the destinations are unique, the molecular pathways may not be present in other cells and, hence, could present antiparasite targets. Further, even when general principles of eukaryotic secretion are preserved, differences between plasmodial and human homologs may be exploited to selectively target the parasite. The food vacuole and apicoplast are parasite secretory organelles whose constituent molecules provide recognized targets (Chapters 4 and 17). However, unique parasite-specific characteristics of secretory pathways that target to these organelles should also be examined as potential chemotherepeutic targets.

Parasite-adhesion molecules exported to the red cell include the var and rif antigens *(35,36)*. VARs are better studied, and they appear to be a family of molecules that underlie adhesion of mature infected red cells to endothelial cells *(37–39)* placenta *(40,41)*, and other red cells *(42)*. VARs have domains that are homologous to the Duffy binding domains (DBL) of other parasite molecules that mediate invasion of red cells by *P. vivax (43–45)*. This observation suggests that the molecular basis of parasite-induced cell interactions may be conserved, with variations in the DBL domains giving rise to a unique substrate-binding specificity of a VAR.

VARs are synthesized early in ring-stage development, although they are required to mediate cell interaction at the late trophozoite and schizont stages. Protein complexes called "knobs" that assemble underneath the red cell cytoskeleton serve to cluster VAR antigens into focal adhesion zones and, thereby, increase the net avidity of infected red cells for endothelial substrates *(46)*. VARs lack an amino-terminal endoplasmic recticulum (ER) signal sequence. A single transmembrane domain may function as an internal signal sequence, but definitive evidence for signals that recruit VARs into the secretory pathway and then export them from the parasite to the red cell membrane have yet to be obtained. Merozoite proteins with DBLs are located in apical organelles. They have canonical signal sequences for their cotranslational recruitment into the ER, but the signals that target them (and other secretory polypeptides) to the apical organelles at schizogony have yet to be elucidated.

Studies using a marker of PVM, EXP-1, suggest that targeting to the PVM requires signal-mediated recruitment into the secretory pathway, followed by vesicular transport to the parasite plasma membrane and then the PVM *(47,48)*. However, it is not known why parasite plasma membrane proteins are simultaneously not exported to the vacuolar membrane and why there are no vesicles detected between the parasite plasma membrane and the vacuolar membrane. In vitro studies suggest that a newly synthesized glycophorin-binding protein (GBP) can be detected in the lumen of the vacuole *(49)*. Because GBP is a secretory protein *(50)* that is exported to the red cell cytosol, this observation suggests that GBP undergoes posttranslational translocation across the vacuolar membrane.

As is the case for many secretory organelles, assembly of the FV requires expression of its resident enzymes. These enzymes may be taken up from the PVM by the cytostome during ingestion of erythrocyte cytosol. In the case of the apicoplast, many of its proteins are encoded by nuclear DNA and secretory transport of these proteins to the plastid is expected to require a bipartite signal sequence coupled to an apicoplast targeting sequence. This mechanism has been described in *Toxoplasma (13)*, *Euglena (51)* and recently also in *P. falciparum* (Cheresh and Haldar, unpublished data). Studies with *Euglena* suggest that targeting of apicoplast proteins occurs by recruitment into the ER, through the Golgi complex prior to transport to the apicoplast *(51)*. Signals that mediate localization to the FV, as well as the PVM–TVM and red cell membrane are not known.

In addition to unique targeting signals that might be present on cargo proteins (proteins in a secretory vesicle), it is possible that there is temporal regulation of the secretory apparatus. Specific components may be turned on or off to differentially regulate protein targeting at different developmental stages. The best example of this is the prominent role of the apical organelles in invasion and their subsequent dissolution in ring-stage parasite. The fate of the apicoplast during this process is not known. Secretory reorganization in ring-stage parasites may be linked to the selective export of the resident Golgi enzyme sphingomyelin synthase *(19)* that is critical to TVM development *(7)*.

A Novel Golgi in Asexual Parasites

The Golgi is the major organelle for sorting proteins and lipids. In mammalian cells, it is functionally and structurally separated into cis, medial, and trans cisternae arranged in stacks. The Golgi ribbon arises from corresponding cisternae of adjacent stacks that are connected by tubular elements *(52)*. Camillo Golgi identified the organelle during his study of neuronal cells, after he studied the malaria parasite (he discovered the relationship between chills and the release of merozoites [Golgi's rule] and providing the first detailed description of *P. vivax* and *P. malariae*). Ironically, infected red cells lack classical Golgi cisternae, especially in the ring and trophozoite stages, and thus the first clues about secretory properties of the plasmodial Golgi came from the identification of plasmodial homologs of proteins that reside and regulate traffic in mammalian Golgi. *P. falciparum* homolog of receptors for protein retention in ER (PfERD2) *(53)*, sphingomyelin synthase *(54)*, and, recently, rabs 1, 6, and 11 *(55,56)* have been found in *P. falciparum*. Plasmodial homologs for resident ER markers have also been identified *(57–59)*. The gene-encoding plasmodial ADP-ribosylation factor (ARF) has been cloned *(60,61)*, but its sites of concentration are unknown.

Because of the difficulty of identifying cisternae, Lingelbach and colleagues suggested that plasmodial ring and trophozoite stages lack a Golgi complex *(62)*. Subsequently, a combination of deconvolution microscopy and immunoelectron microscopy has provided sufficient resolution to separate early and late Golgi membranes within the parasite and to show that they are, indeed, segregated into distinct structures in rings. They have unusual morphological features, however, in that they are unstacked and lack cisternae *(56)*. Because ring-stage parasites engage in classical secretory export *(63,64)*, these observations suggest that a stacked, cisternal Golgi apparatus is not fundamental to organizing secretion. At schizogony, when the parasite targets proteins to multiple organelles of the apical complex, and each newly assembled daughter merozoite must inherit its own secretory apparatus (Fig. 1), the Golgi may be "restacked." It would be interesting to investigate whether unstacking to a clustered, tubovesicular Golgi in the merozoite-to-ring transition underlies secretion of the apical organelles, Golgi compartment that contains sphingomyelin synthase, and/or other compartments.

SECRETORY TARGETS FOR ANTIMALARIAL CHEMOTHERAPY

Multiple potential drug targets involve secretory pathways, including food vacuole proteases (Chapters 4 and 20), components of the apicoplast (Chapter 17), the anion-selective channel, and the TVM. We will restrict the discussion in this chapter to targets in the TVM and red cell membrane.

The action of the anion-selective channel can be inhibited by organic cations such as NPPB. These cations also block parasite proliferation in vitro *(6)*. Thus, a channel could be a therapeutic target, but there is a need to develop reagents that do not affect host ion channels. Differential sensitivity to sphingolipid analogs led to the discovery that inhibition of the exported sphingomyelin synthase caused a block in TVM assembly during ring-to-trophozoite development. Although toxicity from short-term treatments with PPMP are reversible, exposure of cultured malaria parasites over 48 h blocked TVM development, nutrient transport, and parasite development. In long-term cultures, PPMP can block parasite growth at very low concentrations ($0.05\ \mu M$) *(7)*, suggesting that sphingolipid synthesis provides a potential target for chemotherapy. Other TVM components that underlie the organization and function of the network as well as additional molecular processes that regulate aspects of solute import *(6,12)* or protein export *(11)* in the infected red cell may also be targets for new antimalarials.

Table 2
Parasite-Induced Accumulation of [^{3}H]dihydroartemisinin,
Its Inhibition by PPMP, and Competition with Cold Artemisinin

| | Cell-associated [^{3}H]dihydroartemisinin (picomoles/10^6 parasites) | |
Incubation	37°C	4°C
PPMP		
Uninfected cells	6	3
Young (ring: 6–12 h)	133	15
Mature (trophozoites: 30–36 h)	625	38
Infected + PPMP		
0.0 μM	581	28
1.0 μM	384	25
3.3 μM	208	23
5.0 μM	162	163
Infected + cold artemisinin		
0.0 μM	420	41
1.0 μM	242	36
10 μM	103	19

Note: Uninfected, ring or trophozoite-infected red cells were incubated with [^{3}H] dihydroartemisinin in RPMI 1640 at 4°C or 37°C for 1 h. To determine the effects of PPMP on artemisinin accumulation, the cells were treated with 0, 1, 3.3, and 5 μM PPMP prior to their incubation with [^{3}H]dihydroartemisinin. In the competition assay, 1.5X and 15X cold artemisinin was added together with radiolabeled dihydroartemisinin. The results are the mean of triplicate determinations expressed as picomoles artemisinin/10^6 parasites.
Source: Ref. 5.

Artemisinin enters the TVM (competes with dihydroartemisinin; *see* Table 2) and affects membrane properties there. The endoperoxide bridge is believed to be essential for artemisinin's antimalarial activity as it allows interaction with heme and hemozoin (Chapter 11), but it has been suggested that these interactions themselves may not lead to parasite killing (65,66). Instead, membrane damage caused by free radicals may be critical. Low, pharmacologically effective concentrations of artemisinin induce aberrant membrane budding in the PVM–TVM (Fig. 3) when there is no ultrastructural effect on the food vacuole or its contents (5). Higher concentrations show damage to the food vacuole. Thus, although artemisinin may act elsewhere in the cell, at low concentrations it can act on PVM and/or TVM membranes and affect membrane protein export from the vacuolar network. Because the export of Maurer's clefts was not affected at these concentrations, these observations suggest that the observed export was not the result of nonspecific degeneration of the entire tubovesicular network.

Combining PPMP with artemisinin has an additive effect in cell killing, suggesting that the two drugs may act on a common process (5). Because PPMP is known to specifically block the TVM, artemisinin may also (at least in part) target the TVM. Hence, anti-TVM reagents used in combination with artemisinin and/or its derivatives may provide a new, combinatorial chemotherapeutic approach to treating malaria.

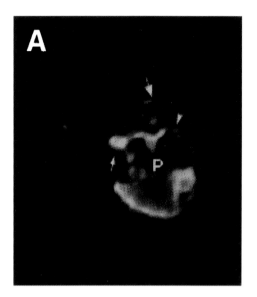 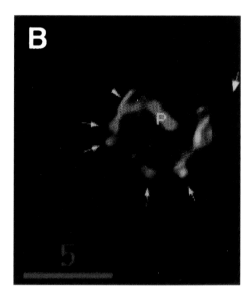

Fig. 3. Effect of artemisinin on membrane transport in the PVM and TVM of infected red cells. **(A–B)** Single optical sections taken through infected red cells mock treated **(A)** or incubated with artemisinin **(B)** and labeled with BODIPY C_5–ceramide (green) and anti-EXP-1 antibodies (red). A large EXP-1-labeled loop is marked by a small thin arrow in **(A)** and seen at the top right-hand-side corner of the parasite in **(B)**. In **(B)**, small thin arrows indicate additional sites of EXP-1 budding. For both panels, the arrowhead indicates EXP-1 in the periphery of the parasite; the large arrow indicates the position of the red cell membrane, P denotes parasite, and parasite nuclei appear purple/blue. Scale bar = 5 µm. (From ref. *5*.)

Recent studies suggest that inhibitors of acyl CoA synthetases block parasite growth *(67)*; thus, these enzymes may also provide new targets for chemotherapy. Interestingly, although multiple synthetases exist, only one is exported to the red cell *(23)* and may be resident in the TVM. This enzyme is structurally distinct from its mammalian homologs, but it is still unclear whether the inhibitors target the enzyme in TVM rather than an intracellular location.

CONCLUSIONS

The novel organization of plasmodial secretory organelles has led to the suggestion that they are difficult to study relative to related apicomplexans like *Toxoplasma (68)*. However, the unique membrane properties of *Plasmodium* are likely to reveal novel functions underlying their organization. What has emerged from recent studies is the identification of important, exported secretory determinants that regulate metabolism, transport, and adherence properties of infected red cells and may be exploited to deliver drugs and provide new targets. However, this is likely to be the tip of the iceberg underlying the complex phenotypes of solute transport and cytoadherence that are linked to virulence and disease pathology. In addition, there are major unanswered questions related to the signals that target parasite determinants to various destinations in the host cell and apical complex (and thereby regulate organelle biogenesis) that could be targets of new antimalarials.

ACKNOWLEDGMENTS

This work was supported by NIH grants (AI26670, 39071) and a Burroughs Wellcome New Initiatives in Malaria Award to Kasturi Haldar.

REFERENCES

1. Chasis JA, Prenant M, Leung A, Mohandas N. Membrane assembly and remodelling during reticulocyte maturation. Blood 1989;74:1112–1120.
2. Desai SA, Krogstad DJ, McCleskey EW. A nutrient-permeable channel on the intraerythrocytic malaria parasite. Nature 1993;362:643–646.
3. Kirk K, Horner HA, Elford BC, Ellory JC, Newbold C. Transport of diverse substrates into malaria infected erythrocytes via pathway showing functional characteristics of a chloride channel. Biol J Chem 1994;269:3339–3347.
4. Lauer SA, Rathod PK, Ghori N, Haldar K. A membrane network for nutrient import in red cells infected with the malaria parasite. Science 1997;276:1122–1125.
5. Akompong T, VanWye J, Ghori N, Haldar K. Artemisinin and its derivatives are transported by a vacuolar network of *P. falciparum* and their anti-malarial activities are additive with toxic sphingolipid analogues that block the network. Mol Biochem Parasitol 1999;100:71–79.
6. Kirk K, Horner HA. In search of a selective inhibitor of the induced transport of small solutes in *Plasmodium falciparum*-infected erythrocytes: effects of arylaminobenzoates. Biochem J 1995;311:761–768.
7. Lauer S, Ghori N, Haldar K. Sphingolipid synthesis as a novel target for chemotherapy against malaria parasites. Proc Natl Acad Sci USA 1995;92:9181–9185.
8. Blackman MJ, Scott-Finnigan TJ, Shai S, Holder AA. Antibodies inhibit the protease-mediated processing of a malaria merozoite surface protein. J Exp Med 1994;180:389–393.
9. Elford BC, Cowman GM, Ferguson DJP. Parasite regulated membrane transport processes and metabolic control in malaria-infected erythrocytes. Biochem J 1995;308:361–374.
10. Haldar K, Holder AA. Export of parasite proteins to the erythrocyte in *Plasmodium falciparum*-infected cells. Semin Cell Biol 1993;4:345–353.
11. Deitsch KW, Wellems TE. Membrane modifications in erythrocytes parasitized by *Plasmodium falciparum*. Mol Biochem Parasitol 1996;76:1–10.
12. Desai SA, Rosenberg RL. Pore size of the malaria parasite's nutrient channel. Proc Natl Acad Sci USA 1997;94:2045–2049.
13. Waller RF, Keeling PJ, Donald RG, Striepen B, Handman E, Lang-Unnasch N, Cowman AF, Besra GS, Roos DS, McFadden GI. Nuclear-encoded proteins target to the plastid in *Toxoplasma gondii* and *Plasmodium falciparum*. Proc Natl Acad Sci USA 1998;95:12,352–12,357.
14. Staines HM, Kirk K. Increased choline transport in erythrocytes from mice infected with the malaria parasite *Plasmodium vinckei vinckei*. Biochem J 1998;334:525–530.
15. Saliba KJ, Horner HA, Kirk K. Transport and metabolism of the essential vitamin pantothetic acid in human erythrocytes infected with the malaria parasite *Plasmodium falciparum*. J Biol Chem 1998;273:10,190–10,195.
16. Saliba KJ, Kirk K. Uptake of an antiplasmodial protease inhibitor into *Plasmodium falciparum*-infected human erythrocytes via a parasite-induced pathway. Mol Biochem Parasitol 1998;94:297–301.
17. Schwab JC, Beckers CJ, Joiner KA. The parasitophorous vacuole membrane surrounding intracellular *Toxoplasma gondii* functions as a molecular sieve. Proc Natl Acad Sci USA 1994;91:509–513.

18. Haldar K. Intracellular trafficking in *Plasmodium*-infected erythrocytes. Curr Opin Microbiol 1998;1:466–471.

19. Elmendorf HG, Haldar K. *Plasmodium falciparum* exports the Golgi marker sphingomyelin synthase into a tubovesicular network in the cytoplasm of mature erythrocytes. J Cell Biol 1994;124:449–462.

20. Elmendorf HG, Haldar K. Secretory activities in *Plasmodium*. Parasitol Today 1993;9:98–102.

21. Elford BC, Ferguson DJP. Secretory Processes in *Plasmodium*. Parasitol Today 1993;9:80–81.

22. Langreth SG, Jensen JB, Reese RT, Trager W. Fine structure of human malaria in vitro. J Protozool 1978;443–452.

23. Matesanz F, Duran-Chica I, Alcina A. The cloning and expression of Pfacs1, a *Plasmodium falciparum* fatty acyl coenzyme A synthetase-1 targeted to the host erythrocyte cytoplasm. J Mol Biol 1999;291:59–70.

24. Bozdech Z, VanWye J, Haldar K, Schurr E. The human malaria parasite *Plasmodium falciparum* exports the ATP-binding cassette protein PFGCN20 to membrane structures in the host red blood cell. Mol Biochem Parasitol 1998;100:217–222.

25. Freeman MW. Effluxed lipids: Tangier Island's latest report. Proc Natl Acad Sci USA 1999;96:10,950–10,952.

26. Pouvelle B, et al. Direct access to serum macromolecules by intraerythrocytic malaria parasites. Nature 1991;353:73–75.

27. Hibbs AR, Stenzel DJ, Saul A. Macromolecular transport in malaria—does the duct exist? Eur J Cell Biol 1997;72:182–188.

28. Haldar K. Ducts channels and transporters in *Plasmodium*-infected erythrocytes. Parasitol Today 1994;10:393–395.

29. Rathod PK, Khatri A. Synthesis and antiproliferative activity of threo-5-fluoro-L-dihydroorotate. J Biol Chem 1990;265:14,242–14,249.

30. Rathod PK, Khosla M, Gassis S, Young RD, Lutz C. Selection and characterization of 5-fluoroorotate-resistant *Plasmodium falciparum*. Antimicrob Agents Chemother 1994;38:2871–2876.

31. Jiang JB, Li GQ, Guo XB, Kong YC, Arnold K. Antimalarial activity of mefloquine and qinghaosu. Lancet 1982;2:285–288.

32. Gu HM, Warhurst DC, Peters W. Uptake of [3H]dihydroartemisinine by erythrocytes infected with *Plasmodium falciparum in vitro*. Trans Soc R Trop Med Hyg 1984;78:265–270.

33. Gormley JA, Howard RJ, Taraschi TF. Trafficking of malarial proteins to the host cell cytoplasm and erythrocyte surface membrane involves multiple pathways. J Cell Biol 1992;119:1481–1495.

34. Lingelbach K. Protein trafficking in the *Plasmodium falciparum*-infected erythrocyte—from models to mechanisms. Annal Trop Med Parasitol 1997;91:543–549.

35. Fernandez V, Hommel M, Chen Q, Hagblom P, Wahlgren M. Small, clonally variant antigens expressed on the surface of the *Plasmodium falciparum*-infected erythrocyte are encoded by the rif gene family and are the target of human immune responses. J Exp Med 1999;190:1393–1404.

36. Kyes SA, Rowe JA, Kriek N, Newbold CI. Rifins: a second family of clonally variant proteins expressed on the surface of red cells infected with *Plasmodium falciparum*. Proc Natl Acad Sci USA 1999;96:9333–9338.

37. Smith JD, Chitnis CE, Craig AG, Roberts DJ, Hudson-Taylor DE, Peterson DS, Piches R, Newbold CI, Miller LH. Switches in expression of *Plasmodium falciparum* var genes correlate with changes in antigenic and cytoadherent phenotypes of infected erythrocytes. Cell 1995;82:101–110.

38. Su X-Z, Heatwole VM, Wertheimer SP, Buinet F, Herrfeldt JA, Peterson DS, Ravetch JA, Wellems TE. The large diverse gene family var encodes proteins involved in cytoadherence and antigenic variation of *Plasmodium falciparum*-infected erythrocytes. Cell 1995;82:89–100.

39. Baruch DI, Pasloske BL, Singh HB, Bi X, Ma XC, Feldman M, Taraschi TF, Howard RJ. Cloning of the *P. falciparum* gene encoding PfEMP1, a malarial variant antigen and adherence receptor on the surface of parasitized human erythrocytes. Cell 1995;82:77–87.

40. Reeder JC, Cowman AF, Davern KM, Beeson JG, Thompson JK, Rogerson SJ, Brown GV. The adhesion of *Plasmodium falciparum*-infected erythrocytes to chondroitin sulfate A is mediated by *P. falciparum* erythrocyte membrane protein 1. Proc Natl Acad Sci USA 1999;96:5198–5202.

41. Buffet PA, Gamain B, Scheidig C, Batuch D, Smith JD, Hernandez-Rivas R, Pouvelle B, Oishi S, Fuji N, Fusai T, Parzy D, Miller LH, Gysin J, Scherf A. *Plasmodium falciparum* domain mediating adhesion to chondroitin sulfate A: A receptor for human placental infection. Proc Natl Acad Sci USA 1999;96:12,743–12,748.

42. Rowe JA, Moulds JM, Newbold CI, Miller LH. *P. falciparum* rosetting mediated by a parasite-variant erythrocyte membrane protein and complement-receptor. Nature 1997;388: 292–295.

43. B. Sim KL, Chitnis CE, Wasniowska K, Hadley TJ, Miller LH. Receptor and ligand domains for invasion of erythrocytes by *Plasmodium falciparum*. Science 1994;264:1941–1944.

44. Chitnis CE, Miller LH. Identification of the erythrocyte binding domains of *Plasmodium vivax* and *Plasmodium knowlesi* proteins involved in erythrocyte invasion. J Exp Med 1994;180:497–506.

45. Kappe SHI, Curley GP, Noe AR, Dalton JP, Adams JH. Erythrocyte binding protein homologues of rodent malaria parasites. Mol Biochem Parasitol 1997;89:137–148.

46. Crabb BS, et al. Targeted gene disruption shows that knobs enable malaria-infected red cells to cytoadhere under physiological shear stress. Cell 1997;89:287–296.

47. Günther K, et al. An exported protein of *Plasmodium falciparum* is synthesized as an integral membrane protein. Mol Biochem Parasitol 1991;46:149–158.

48. Ansorge I, Paprotka K, Bhakdi S, Lingelbach K. Permeabilization of the erythrocyte with streptolysin O allows access to the vacuolar membrane of *Plasmodium falciparum* and molecular analysis of membrane topology. Mol Biochem Parasitol 1997;84:259–261.

49. Ansorge I, Benting J, Bhakdi S, Lingelbach K. Protein sorting in *Plasmodium falciparum*-infected red blood cells permeablised with the pore forming protein streptolysin O. Biochem J 1996;315:307–314.

50. Benting J, Mattei D, Lingelbach K. Brefeldin A inhibits transport of glycophorin binding protein from *Plasmodium falciparum* into the host erythrocyte. Biochem J 1994; 300:821–826.

51. Sulli C, Schwartzbach SD. The polyprotein precursor to the Euglena Light-harvesting chlorophyll a/b-binding protein is transported to the Golgi apparatus prior to chloroplast import and polyprotein processing. J Biol Chem 1995;270:13,084–13,090.

52. Warren G. Intracellular membrane morphology. Trans R Soc Lond Series B Biological Studies 1995;349:291–295.

53. Elmendorf HG, Haldar K. Identification and localization of ERD2 in the malaria parasite *Plasmodium falciparum*: separation of sites of sphingomyelin synthesis and implications for the organization of the Golgi. EMBO J. 1993;12:4763–4773.

54. Haldar K, Uyetake L, Ghori N, Elmendorf HG, Li W-L. The accumulation and metabolism of a fluorescent ceramide derivative in *Plasmodium falciparum*-infected erythrocytes. Mol Biochem Parasitol 1991;49:143–156.

55. Alves de Castro F, Ward GE, Jambou R, Attal G, Mayau V, Jaureguiberry G, Braun-Breton C, Chakrabarti D, Langsley G. Identification of a family of Rab G-proteins in *Plasmodium falciparum* and a detailed characterization of pfrab6. Mol Biochem Parasitol 1996;80:77–88.

56. VanWye J, Ghori N, Webster P, Mitschler RR, Elmendorf HG, Haldar K. Identification and localization of rab6, separation of rab6 from ERD2 and implications for an "unstacked" Golgi in *falciparum* P. Mol Biochem Parasitol 1996;83:107–120.

57. Kumar N, Syin C, Carter R, Quakyi I, Miller LH. *Plasmodium falciparum* gene encoding a protein similar to the 78-kDa rat glucose-regulated stress protein. Proc Natl Acad Sci USA 1988;85:6277–6281.
58. Greca NL, Hibbs AR, Riffkin C, Foley M, Tilley L. Identification of an endoplasmic reticulum-resident calcium-binding protein with multiple EF-hand motifs in asexual stages of *Plasmodium falciparum*1. Mol Biochem Parasitol 1997;89:283–293.
59. Albano FR, Berman A, La Greca N, Hibbs AR, Wickham M, Foley M, Tilley L. A homologue of Sar1p localizes to a novel trafficking pathway in malaria-infected erythrocytes. Eur J Cell Biol 1999;78:453–462.
60. Stafford WH, Stockley RW, B LS, AA H. Isolation A, expression and characterization of the gene for an ADP-ribosylation factor from the human malaria parasite, *Plasmodium falciparum*. Eur J Biochem 1996;242:104–113.
61. Truong RM, Francis SE, Chakrabarti D, Goldberg DE. Cloning and characterization of *Plasmodium falciparum* ADP-ribosylation factor and factor-like genes. Mol Biochem Parasitol 1997;84:247–253.
62. Banting G, Benting J, Lingelbach K. A minimalist view of the secretory pathway in *Plasmodium falciparum*. Trends Cell Biol. 1995;5:340–343.
63. Crary JL, Haldar K. Brefeldin A inhibits protein secretion and parasite maturation in the ring stage of *Plasmodium falciparum*. Mol Biochem Parasitol 1992;53:185–192.
64. Hinterberg K, Scherf A, Gysin G, Toyoshima T, Aikawa M, Mazie JC, da Silva LP, Mattei D. *Plasmodium falciparum*: the Pf. 332 antigen is secreted by a brefeldin A dependent pathway and is translocated to the erythrocyte membrane via Maurer's clefts. Exp Parasitol 1994;79:279–291.
65. Meshnick SR, Thomas A, Ranz A, Xu CM, Pan HZ. Artemisinin (qinghaosu): the role of intrcellualr hemin in its mechanism of antimalarial action. Mol Biochem Parasitol 1991;49:181–189.
66. Hong YL, Yang YZ, Meshnick SR. The interaction of artemisinin with malarial hemozoin. Mol Biochem Parasitol 1994;63:121–128.
67. Beaumelle BD, Vial HJ. Correlation of the efficiency of fatty acid derivatives in suppressing *Plasmodium falciparum* growth in culture with their inhibitory effect on acyl-CoA synthetase activity. Mol Biochem Parasitol 1998;28:39–42.
68. Roos DS, Crawford MJ, Donald RGK, Fohl LM, Hager KM, Kissinger JC, Reynolds MG, Striepen B, Sullivan WJ. Transport and trafficking: *Toxoplasma* as a model for *Plasmodium*. Novartis Foundation Symposium, 1998.

4

The *Plasmodium* Food Vacuole

Ritu Banerjee and Daniel E. Goldberg

INTRODUCTION

The *Plasmodium* food vacuole is a sophisticated organelle optimized for hemoglobin metabolism. It is the site of acidification, hemoglobin proteolysis, peptide transport, heme polymerization, detoxification of oxygen radicals, and quinoline action. A number of proteins that function in the food vacuole are known. Among them are aspartic, cysteine, and metalloproteases, an ATP-binding cassette (ABC) transporter, an ATPase, a heme polymerase, and several oxidant defense enzymes. In this chapter, we review the molecular details of food vacuole function and highlight potential targets for antimalarial drug development.

AMINO ACID UTILIZATION

Intraerythrocytic stages of *Plasmodium* are capable of very limited *de novo* amino acid synthesis *(1,2)*. To obtain amino acids for protein synthesis, the malaria parasite must degrade host cell hemoglobin as well as import extracellular nutrients. Much evidence suggests that a major amino acid source for the parasite is hemoglobin, which is present at 340 mg/mL in the red cell cytosol *(3)*. In approx 12 h, the trophozoite-stage parasite degrades 75% of host cell hemoglobin *(4–6)*. Radiolabeled amino acids derived from hemoglobin degradation are incorporated into parasite proteins *(7,8)*. For normal growth in culture, intraerythrocytic *Plasmodium* requires exogenously supplied amino acids that are either limiting (methionine, cysteine, glutamic acid, and glutamine) or absent (isoleucine) in hemoglobin *(9)*. The most significant growth retardation of parasites in culture occurs when isoleucine is omitted from the medium *(9,10)*. Cultures grown in medium containing only these five amino acids (forced to rely on hemoglobin degradation) are more sensitive to hemoglobin-degradation inhibitors than cultures grown in complete medium *(11)*. Nevertheless, cultures in complete medium are still susceptible to a wide range of protease inhibitors *(12–16)* (*see* Chapter 20).

Retarding hemoglobin degradation by genetic or chemical modification of substrate interferes with parasite growth. Erythrocytes containing fetal hemoglobin, which is poorly cleaved by parasite proteases, do not support normal parasite development *(17,18)*. Further, transgenic mice overexpressing fetal hemoglobin are protected against malaria infections. Hemoglobin degradation is slowed and parasite growth delayed in this model *(19)*. Treatment of cultured parasites with the hemoglobin crosslinker

From: *Antimalarial Chemotherapy: Mechanisms of Action, Resistance, and New Directions in Drug Discovery*
Edited by: P. J. Rosenthal © Humana Press Inc., Totowa, NJ

dibromoaspirin, inhibits parasite growth, perhaps because it makes host cell hemoglobin less susceptible to degradation *(20)*.

Several studies suggest that hemoglobin catabolism may serve a purpose other than amino acid generation. All amino acids, even those present in hemoglobin, are readily taken up by the parasite from the culture medium and incorporated into parasite proteins *(2,7)*. The amount of hemoglobin degradation is similar whether parasites are cultured in rich or minimal medium. Although vast amounts of hemoglobin are degraded by the parasite, it has been found that resealed erythrocyte ghosts containing only 7% of the total red cell hemoglobin support normal parasite development *(21)*. Also, hemoglobin degradation results in the production of excess amino acids, which are not utilized by the parasite, but rather diffuse into the erythrocyte *(22)*. This has raised the possibility that hemoglobin degradation occurs in order to reduce host cell volume and create a physical space for the parasite *(23)*, which increases its volume 25-fold in one intraerythrocytic cycle *(24)*.

Thus, hemoglobin catabolism is clearly essential for parasite survival. The degree of reliance on hemoglobin as an amino acid source is not well defined and may vary with culture conditions. Whether degradation of hemoglobin is to provide nutrients, to make room in the host cell, or for some other purpose, impeding this process has dire consequences for the parasite. For this reason, hemoglobin metabolism is an attractive target for pharmacologic intervention.

CELL BIOLOGY OF HEMOGLOBIN INGESTION

Hemoglobin ingestion and digestion vary with intraerythrocytic stage. In very early ring stages, the parasite abuts the erythrocyte membrane and may obtain nutrients directly through a passageway or "metabolic window" in the apposed membranes *(25,26)*. There is evidence that host cell cytosol is taken up by micropinocytosis, although hemoglobin digestion and hemozoin production are minimal at this stage *(27)*.

In the more metabolically active trophozoite stage, hemoglobin catabolism is a complex and efficient process. Host cell cytosol is taken up through the cytostome, a pear-shaped structure that is formed by invagination of the parasitophorous vacuolar membrane and parasite plasma membrane (Fig. 1) *(25,27,29,30)*. In *P. falciparum*, double-membrane transport vesicles bud off from the cytostome and migrate toward and fuse with the large, central food vacuole *(27,30,31)*. Within the food vacuole, a single-membrane transport vesicle can sometimes be seen, especially if parasites are treated with chloroquine *(30,32–34)*. A phospholipase is hypothesized to lyse the remaining membrane of the transport vesicle, releasing its contents *(35)*. It is unclear if hemoglobin digestion begins within the food vacuole or in acidified transport vesicles en route to the food vacuole. Electron microscopy studies have shown that in other *Plasmodium* species, multiple smaller food vacuoles exist, and the cytostome is a tortuous, tubular structure *(36,37)*.

The food vacuole is an acidic (pH 5.0–5.4), degradative organelle *(38,39)* that appears more specialized than its homologs, the lysosome, and yeast vacuole. Unlike these organelles, the *P. falciparum* food vacuole does not contain nonproteolytic hydrolases such as β-galactosidase, β-glucuronidase, and acid phosphatase *(28)*. The food vacuole appears devoted to the catabolism of hemoglobin and is probably not involved in gen-

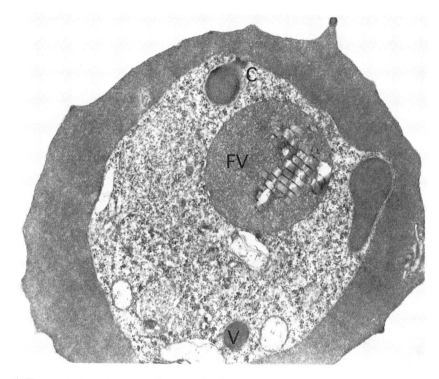

Fig. 1. Transmission electron micrograph of a P. falciparum trophozoite within an erythrocyte. C = cytostome; V = transport vesicle; FV = food vacuole. (From ref. *28.*)

eral protein degradation. Erythrocyte proteins like superoxide dismutase and catalase accumulate in the food vacuole but are not broken down, highlighting the specificity of food vacuole proteases (*see* next section).

HEMOGLOBIN-DEGRADING PROTEASES

Overview

Many early studies reported acid hemoglobinase activities in parasitized erythrocyte extracts or purified parasite extracts *(40–50)*. However, some of these activities may have been derived from the host cell or the parasite cytoplasm. The identification and characterization of proteases whose physiological function is hemoglobin catabolism was achieved after it became possible to isolate pure food vacuoles *(28)*. Differential centrifugation and Percoll density gradient separation yielded pure food vacuoles as assessed by electron microscopy and marker enzyme analysis *(28,30)*. Extracts of purified food vacuoles contained globin-degrading activity *(28,51)*. A combination of pepstatin, an aspartic protease inhibitor, and E64, a cysteine protease inhibitor, completely blocked globin degradation, suggesting important roles for aspartic and cysteine proteases *(28,52,53)*.

To date, four distinct proteases have been purified from the food vacuole and shown to act in a semiordered fashion in vitro to degrade the hemoglobin tetramer. Two aspartic proteases, termed plasmepsins, appear to initiate the degradative process. A cysteine protease, falcipain, plays a vital downstream role. A metalloprotease, falcilysin, acts even further downstream.

Plasmepsins

Substrate Specificity

Two homologous aspartic proteases called plasmepsins I (PM I) and II (PM II) were purified from isolated food vacuoles *(11,52)*. At the amino acid level, plasmepsins I and II are 73% identical to each other and approximately 35% identical to mammalian aspartic proteases like renin and cathepsin D *(11,54)*. They have pH optima near 5, consistent with their location within the acidic vacuole *(11,54)*. Mass spectroscopic analysis revealed that both proteases initially cleave the same site within the native hemoglobin tetramer, between residues 33Phe-34Leu in the α-chain *(51,52)*. This is also the site where food vacuole extracts initially cleave hemoglobin *(51)*. Cleavage in this highly conserved hinge region of hemoglobin is hypothesized to unravel the globin fold. The 33Phe–34Leu site is probably accessible to the proteases only after hemoglobin dissociates from the tetramer to the dimer. Interestingly, hemoglobin F has less propensity to dissociate to dimer form *(55)* and is cleaved poorly by the plasmepsins *(19)*. Transgenic mice expressing human hemoglobin F are protected from malaria *(19)*. This could be the basis of poor growth of *P. falciparum* in hemoglobin F-containing red blood cells and could even contribute to the protection from malaria seen in the first few months of newborn life, as levels of hemoglobin F slowly decrease *(17,18)*.

The plasmepsins appear to make different secondary cleavages once the hemoglobin has denatured. PM I prefers Phe at the P1 position, whereas PM II prefers hydrophobic residues on either side of the scissile bond, especially Leu at P1' *(52)*. This specificity is borne out using a combinatorial library of peptidic inhibitors *(56)*. When PM II is assessed with a series of chromogenic peptides, the cleavage specificities overall fit well with those determined for hemoglobin *(57,58)*. Interestingly, in this assay basic residues are not tolerated in the P3 position even though this residue is arginine in the primary globin cleavage site and even though fluorogenic peptides with P3 arginine are well recognized *(59)*.

Expression

Surprisingly, PM I and II have different patterns of expression during the intraerythrocytic cycle. Messenger RNA for PM I is expressed in early ring stages, whereas that of PM II is undetectable in rings and abundant in trophozoites *(60,61)*. It is possible that only PM I is required to perform the limited hemoglobin degradation that occurs in the ring stage. In contrast, both plasmepsins may be needed for the dramatic hemoglobin catabolism of the trophozoite. It is also possible that PM I performs a function other than hemoglobin degradation during the ring stage.

Biosynthesis and Processing

Like other aspartic proteases, both plasmepsins are expressed as zymogens. However, unlike most other aspartic proteases, they lack a signal sequence and have a very long propiece that contains a single membrane-spanning domain. Proplasmepsins are 51-kDa type II integral membrane proteins that are proteolytically processed to generate 37-kDa soluble, mature enzymes (Fig. 2) *(60)*. The plasmepsins appear to be secre-

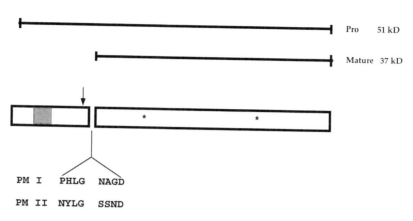

Fig. 2. Schematic of plasmepsins I and II. The 51-kDa proforms are proteolytically processed to generate 37-kDa mature forms. A 21-amino-acid transmembrane domain exists within each propiece (shaded). Catalytic aspartic acids are marked with asterisks (*). An arrow depicts the autocatalytic site used by recombinant PM II, 12 amino acids upstream from the cleavage site determined for native PM II. The sequence of the site where each propiece is cleaved is indicated. (From ref. *60.*)

tory proteins, as the fungal metabolite Brefeldin A blocks their maturation, presumably by preventing their targeting to a compartment downstream of the Golgi. In vivo pulse-chase studies followed by immunoprecipitation with specific PM I and PM II antibodies reveal that both proenzymes are processed rapidly, with a $t_{1/2}$ of 20 min (Fig. 3). The site at which the propiece is cleaved from the mature enzyme is conserved between the plasmepsins : LG * XXXD. As this site does not match the substrate specificity of either plasmepsin, it is appealing to think that activation of both proplasmepsins is mediated by a novel, unidentified protease. In culture, pulse-chase experiments show that processing is blocked only by lysosomotropic agents, a proton-pump inhibitor, and tripeptide aldehyde inhibitors *(60).* In a cell-free assay using parasite extract to cleave radiolabeled proplasmepsins, processing requires acidic conditions and is blocked only by tripeptide aldehydes (Banerjee R and Goldberg DE, unpublished). These results suggest that an unusual protease activates both proenzymes upon their arrival in the food vacuole. Although most aspartic proteases undergo autocatalytic activation, a few, like renin, must be processed in trans by other proteases *(62,63).*

Structure

Both proplasmepsins I and II have been expressed in recombinant form in *Escherichia coli,* where they are generated as N-terminally truncated, insoluble products *(54,59,64,65).* They can be solubilized in urea and refolded. Recombinant PM I does not autoactivate detectably. At acidic pH, a slight activity toward peptide substrate is found, although the recombinant and native forms display very different kinetic properties *(59,65).* Recently, a PM I mutant with a single valine for lysine 110 substitution in the propiece was expressed and yielded an autoactivatable, functional protein that may be useful in inhibitor screens *(61).*

Recombinant PM II makes a fortuitous but erroneous autocatalytic cleavage, processing itself 12 amino acids NH$_2$ terminal to the start of the mature protein *(54,59,64).*

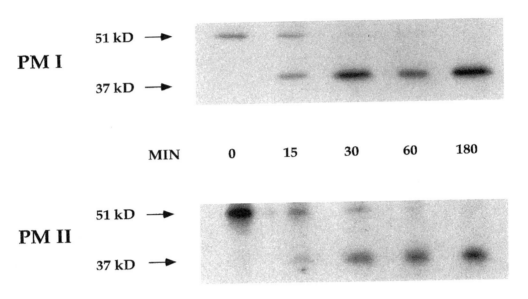

Fig. 3. Maturation of Plasmepsins I and II. In a pulse-chase experiment, *P. falciparum* tro-phozoites were labeled with ^{35}S-methionine/cysteine for 10 min and chased for various times in nonradioactive medium. Lysates were immunoprecipitated with specific PM I or PM II anti-bodies. Both plasmepsins are processed with a $t_{1/2}$ of approx 20 min. (From ref. *60*.)

Even so, recombinant PM2 is active and displays kinetic properties similar to the native enzyme *(59)*. It is abundantly expressed and was crystallized, complexed with the inhibitor pepstatin *(66)*. The structure of PM II revealed that it had the typical bilobal structure of eukaryotic aspartic proteases. PM II crystals contains two molecules in different conformations, related by a rotation of 5° between the N- and C-terminal domains. This indicates that PM II has a high degree of interdomain flexibility and may suggest how it is able to recognize and cleave a large, proteinaceous substrate. The second active site motif in PM II is DSG instead of DTG, and the flap over the active site contains a valine substitution for Gly 79. These substitutions cause pepstatin to bind to PM II in a slightly different conformation than it binds to other eukaryotic aspartic proteases, providing hope for the design of nontoxic inhibitors of PM II. The identifi-cation of low-molecular-weight inhibitors that are more specific for PM II than cathe-psin D has been reported *(67)* (*see* Chapter 20).

Recently, the crystal structure of an N-terminally truncated proplasmepsin II was solved and revealed that proplasmepsin II has a novel mechanism of maintaining inac-tivity before maturation *(68)*. Instead of the propiece occluding the active site as is seen in other aspartic protease zymogens, the long propiece of the proPM II acts as a "har-ness" that interacts with the C-terminal domain, opening and severely distorting the active site such that the two lobes of the protein are kept apart *(68)*.

Also, unlike some other aspartic proteases, the polyproline loops of plasmepsins I and II appear not to be involved in substrate recognition. Replacing the loop of PM II with that of PM I resulted in a hybrid with substrate specificity similar to PM II *(59)*.

Plasmepsins May Have Nonredundant Functions in Addition to Hemoglobin Degradation

In the schizont stages, hemoglobin degradation is complete, yet plasmepsin I and II protein levels remain high. This may be because they are simply not degraded or because they are playing additional roles in the schizont stage. It was recently found that PM II may be a spectrinase that degrades the erythrocyte membrane and facilitates merozoite rupture *(69,70)*. A spectrinase activity in parasite extracts was found to copurify with PM II and cleave spectrin exactly where it is cleaved by PM II. In vitro, PM II can digest spectrin at pH 6.8, although its optimal activity is at pH 5. In schizont stages, PM II is located at the periphery of the parasite, a location consistent with a spectrinase function *(70)*. It is unclear if or how PM I is functioning during the schizont stage, although it may have other functions during the metabolically less active ring stage.

Inhibitor studies also suggest that PM I and II do not have redundant functions. When cultures are treated with PM I-specific inhibitors, SC-50083 *(11)* or RO-40-4388 *(61)*, parasites die, demonstrating that PM II cannot compensate for PM I function. PM II-specific inhibitors have not yet been identified.

Other Plasmodium *Species*

A single plasmepsin homolog has been identified from each of the other human malaria species. These homologs have been expressed in recombinant form. When the kinetic properties and substrate specificities of the various plasmepsins are compared, it is apparent that the proteases from *P. vivax* and *P. malariae* more closely resemble *P. falciparum* PM I than PM II *(57)*.

Falcipain

When cultured intraerythrocytic parasites are treated with cysteine protease inhibitors, their food vacuoles swell and fill with undegraded globin, implicating a cysteine protease in hemoglobin catabolism *(12,15,71,72)*. Using gelatin-substrate polyacrylamide gel electrophoresis (PAGE), a 28-kDa cysteine protease activity called falcipain was identified in trophozoite extracts *(71)*. A cysteine protease activity believed to be falcipain was purified from food vacuole extracts, although its N-terminal sequence could not be obtained *(53)*. The substrate specificity of falcipain is similar to that of cathepsin L *(16)*.

The gene for falcipain has been cloned *(73)*. It predicts a 67-kDa proform and a 26.8-kDa mature enzyme that is 37% identical to cathepsin L. Northern blot analysis revealed that falcipain mRNA was expressed in ring-stage parasites. The predicted amino acid sequence of falcipain was used to make peptide antibodies that recognize a 28-kDa protein in trophozoite extracts. This suggests that the 28-kDa cysteine protease activity originally identified in trophozoite extract was likely to be the product of this gene *(73)*.

Like the plasmepsins, falcipain is synthesized as a proenzyme with an extremely long propiece containing a hydrophobic stretch of 20 amino acids that may be a membrane-spanning domain *(73,74)*. Recombinant falcipain expressed in baculovirus was not processed correctly, appeared in a precursor form, and had different kinetic properties from native falcipain *(53,74)*. Homologous cysteine protease genes have been

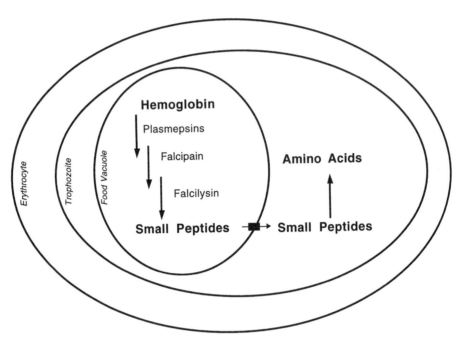

Fig. 4. Order and compartmentalization of hemoglobin degradation. Within the food vacuole, hemoglobin is degraded first by the plasmepsins, followed by falcipain and then falcilysin, generating peptides. These peptides are transported out of the food vacuole, to the parasite cytoplasm where they are terminally degraded to amino acids by exopeptidases.

identified in *P. vivax*, *P. malariae*, and a variety of avian and rodent malarias *(75,76)*. Inhibitors that block falcipain in vitro kill cultured *P. falciparum (13,14,16)* and cure *P. vinckei* infections in mice *(77,78)* (*see* Chapter 20), suggesting a crucial role for this protease.

Falcilysin

A zinc metalloprotease called falcilysin was recently purified from food vacuoles and determined to function downstream of the plasmepsins and falcipain in the hemoglobin-degradation pathway *(79)*. Purified falcilysin does not cleave hemoglobin or globin but will degrade fragments of hemoglobin that have been generated by PM II action. Using mass spectroscopy, it was determined that falcilysin preferred to cleave sites in which the P1, P1', and/or P4' residues are polar.

The gene for falcilysin has been cloned and predicts a 138.8-kDa protein, although falcilysin purified from the food vacuole is 125-kDa in size. Reasons for this size discrepancy are unclear. The predicted amino acid sequence of falcilysin revealed a HXXEX active-site motif, a defining feature of the M16 family of the clan ME metallopeptidases. Unlike the other hemoglobin-degrading proteases characterized, there do not appear to be any membrane-spanning domains in the falcilysin protein *(79)*.

Order of Action

Hemoglobin degradation in the *Plasmodium* food vacuole appears to proceed in a semiordered pathway (Fig. 4). In vitro, plasmepsins I and II are capable of cleaving native hemoglobin, whereas under nonreducing conditions, falcipain will only cleave globin that has been denatured *(52,53,74)*. Falcilysin will cleave neither hemoglobin nor denatured globin. Rather, it will only recognize peptide fragments (10–15 amino acids in length) generated by upstream proteases. Falcilysin cleaves at polar residues, in contrast to the upstream enzymes, which prefer hydrophobic sites *(79)*. The complementarity of these specificities ensures efficiency of proteolysis.

Only aspartic protease inhibitors will effectively block the initial steps of hemoglobin degradation by purified food vacuole extracts *(28,52)*. It is possible that there could be an accumulation of erythrocyte glutathione in the food vacuole and a highly reducing environment that would rapidly denature hemoglobin and allow falcipain to work early in the process. However, the catalase that accumulates in the vacuole limits the reducing ability of glutathione *(53)*; in addition, the available data suggest a strong oxidizing environment in the food vacuole *(50)* (*see* Oxidant Defense Enzymes and Chapter 11). Perhaps the best evidence for order in the degradative pathway comes from the work of Bray and colleagues, who have shown that plasmepsin inhibitors prevent heme release during short- or long-term incubations, in culture or in extracts *(80)*.

Cysteine protease inhibitors (*see* Chapter 20) still have a dramatic effect on cultured *Plasmodium* parasites. They cause swelling of the food vacuole to an enormous size, resulting in parasite death *(12,15)*. A logical interpretation of this finding is that plasmepsin-generated hemoglobin fragments cannot be further degraded without falcipain action and therefore build up to levels that cause osmotic swelling *(53)*. Therefore, during falcipain inhibition, the parasite, which is trying to create more room for itself outside by degrading red blood cell hemoglobin, winds up with less room inside and cannot develop normally. A paradoxical finding is that parasites treated with cysteine protease inhibitors for long periods of time accumulate undigested hemoglobin in the swollen vacuoles *(15)*. This may be the result of gross vacuolar dysfunction such as ionic and pH dysregulation that prevent general proteolysis from occurring.

When food vacuole extracts are incubated with hemoglobin, peptides are generated with cleavage sites throughout the α and β-chains, an average of eight amino acids apart *(81)*. No free amino acids are generated and there is no end-point heterogeneity. This suggests a lack of exopeptidase action. Further, no exopeptidases can be detected in the vacuole using colorimetric substrates *(81)*. This suggests further order and compartmentalization of the degradative pathway. It is likely that peptide transporters exist to export digestion products out of the food vacuole for terminal degradation by cytoplasmic exopeptidases. *Plasmodium* neutral exopeptidases have been characterized *(82–85)*.

Other Proteases

Several lines of evidence suggest the existence of uncharacterized proteases within the food vacuole. Hemoglobin incubated in vitro with food vacuole lysates is cleaved at novel sites that are not attributable to plasmepsins I and II, falcipain, or falcilysin *(81)*. An additional food vacuole aspartic protease activity has been reported *(50)*. A gene for a third aspartic protease has been identified using low-stringency Southern analysis *(11)*.

The cloning of an unusual *P. falciparum* plasmepsin homolog was recently reported *(86)*. Although 60% identical to PM I, it has several active-site substitutions, including replacement of a catalytic aspartate with a histidine, as well as changes in the flap

region that lies over the binding cleft. This protease, called HAP or histo-aspartic protease could be inactive and similar to the pregnancy-associated glycoproteins (PAGs)
of ungulates. These PAGs are aspartic protease homologs, some of which have histidine residues replacing one of the catalytic aspartic acids. They appear to be catalytically inactive but still capable of binding pepstatin (87–90). Alternatively, HAP might
be an active protease acting through a novel catalytic mechanism. Work in our laboratory supports this latter hypothesis. HAP-specific monoclonal antibodies were generated and used to purify native HAP from isolated food vacuoles. Native HAP was
capable of cleaving a fluorogenic peptide, with a pH optimum higher than those of PM
I and II (Banerjee R and Goldberg DE, unpublished). A fourth aspartic protease is also
present in the *Plasmodium* database. All four of these genes are present in a cluster on
chromosome 14 (TIGR) (61). A motif (LG * XXXD) appears where the propieces of
PM I and II are cleaved from the mature enzymes and this sequence is conserved in the
predicted coding regions of the two other homologs. This suggests that a single
maturase is responsible for activating all of these proteins.

TARGETING TO THE FOOD VACUOLE

Very little is known about protein secretion and targeting in *Plasmodium*. Unlike
mammalian secretory systems, the malaria parasite lacks a morphologically distinct
Golgi (36,91–93). It is also puzzling that secretion of some plasmodial proteins appears
to be Brefeldin A-sensitive (93,94), whereas secretion of others appears resistant
(95,96). Also, N- or O-glycosylation in *Plasmodium* are minor or nonexistent modifications of proteins (97–100).

The extremely long propieces of the plasmepsins and falcipain may contain targeting
information, as is the case in other organisms. The propeptides of the yeast vacuolar
proteins proteinase A, carboxypeptidase Y, and aminopeptidase 1 all contain vacuolar
targeting signals (101–103). When the propieces of proteinase A and carboxypeptidase Y
are fused to invertase, the fusion proteins are redirected to the yeast vacuole (101,104).
On the other hand, it is possible that vacuolar targeting signals do not exist in *Plasmodium* and proteins are brought to the food vacuole by bulk flow through the hemoglobin-
ingestion pathway. ImmunoEM studies have shown that PM I is concentrated within the
food vacuole (FV), but it is also present at the parasite plasma membrane, cytostome, and
hemoglobin-laden transport vesicles coming in from the surface (11). This suggests that
newly synthesized PM I is secreted to the parasite plasma membrane and then internal-
ized along with hemoglobin and trafficked to the food vacuole (Fig. 5). Integral membrane proteins PGH1 and VAP-B also might take this indirect route to the food vacuole,
as both are found on the parasite plasma membrane, as well as in the food vacuole
(105,106). It appears that HRP II, a soluble protein, is also delivered to the food vacuole
through the hemoglobin-ingestion pathway (107). With the recent ability to transfect
Plasmodium, targeting requirements and pathways should become clearer.

OTHER PROTEINS IN THE FOOD VACUOLE

ATPase

The acidic conditions of the food vacuole are most likely maintained by an ATP-
driven proton pump, as is the case in lysosomes (108). An ATPase activity has been

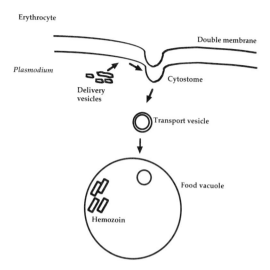

Fig. 5. Proposed vacuolar targeting pathway for the plasmepsins. After synthesis in the ER as type II integral membrane proteins, proplasmepsins enter the secretory pathway and are trafficked to the parasite surface. Then, along with hemoglobin, they are ingested through the cytostome and travel via transport vesicles to the food vacuole. Within the vacuole, acidic conditions and a processing enzyme affect their maturation and cleavage from the membrane. (From ref. *11*.)

found to be enriched in food vacuole membranes *(109,110)*. It appears capable of hydrolyzing ATP, GTP, UTP, and CTP, has a neutral pH optimum, and is inhibited by NEM and NBD-Cl. Both the *Plasmodium* A and B subunits of the vacuolar ATPase have been cloned *(105,111)*. Whereas the A subunit (VAP A) has not been localized, the B subunit (VAP B) shows a heterogeneous localization throughout the parasite, including in the food vacuole *(105)*.

PGH-1

Several genes with homology to the ABC transporter family have been found in *P. falciparum* *(112,113)*. One of these, mdr1, encodes a 160-kDa protein called P-glycoprotein homolog 1 (PGH1) which localizes to the food vacuole membrane *(106)*. PGH1 looks like a typical ABC transporter, with 12 transmembrane domains and 2 hydrophilic domains capable of nucleotide binding. Photoaffinity labeling studies have shown that PGH1 is capable of binding ATP, ADP, GTP, and GDP *(114)*. It is expressed and phosphorylated on serine and threonine residues throughout the intraerythrocytic cycle *(115)*.

PGH1 was presumed to mediate transport across the food vacuole, because homologous mammalian ABC transporters can act as energy-dependent transporters that efflux drugs in multidrug-resistant tumor cells. Heterologous expression studies have proven that PGH1 can function as a transporter. Overexpressed PGH1 in CHO cells localizes to lysosomal membranes and causes accumulation of chloroquine in lysosomes *(116)*. Pfmdr1 can complement Ste6-null mutants in yeast and restore mating, presumably by transporting mating peptide *(117,118)*. A physiological role in transporting hemoglobin peptides is possible but has not been established. A role in mediating drug resistance has been proposed but not yet clarified *(113,119,120) (see* Chapters 5 and 9).

Oxidant Defense Enzymes

Intraerythrocytic stages of *Plasmodium* are microaerophilic and grow best under reduced oxygen pressure. Oxidant drugs like hydrogen peroxide and hydroxyl radicals kill parasites in culture *(121)*. Ironically, the process of hemoglobin degradation produces great oxidative stress on the parasite as well as the host cell *(122)*. Upon release from hemoglobin, the heme iron is oxidized, reacting with molecular oxygen to generate superoxide anions, hydroxyl radicals, and hydrogen peroxide. Under the acidic conditions of the food vacuole, oxyhemoglobin can also auto-oxidize in a reaction yielding methemoglobin and a superoxide anion *(123)*. Methemoglobin is found in unusually high proportions in the food vacuole, perhaps reflecting a strong oxidizing environment *(50)*.

Remarkably, *Plasmodium* is capable of usurping host oxidant defense enzymes for protection from activated oxygen species. Erythrocyte superoxide dismutase (SOD) and catalase are ingested along with hemoglobin and function within the food vacuole in *P. falciparum* and *P. berghei (53,124–126)*. The SOD was determined to be host derived based on inhibitor sensitivity, molecular weight, and electrophoretic mobility. It was possible to determine that *P. berghei* isolated from mouse erythrocytes contain mouse SOD, whereas parasites isolated from rat erythocytes contain rat SOD *(125)*. Presumably, the food vacuole also contains reducing equivalents like NADPH and glutathione, which are abundant in the host cell cytosol *(127)*.

Plasmodium also appears to have genes encoding endogenous oxidant defense enzymes. The genes for glutathione peroxidase and superoxide dismutase have been identified in *P. falciparum,* although their gene products have not yet been localized *(128,129)*. A glutathione peroxidase activity that increases in more mature asexual stages has been detected in *P. falciparum (128)*.

Erythrocytes infected with malaria parasites have weakened oxidant defenses. The parasite depletes the host cell's enzymes and reducing equivalents and produces activated oxygen species that can diffuse into the erythrocyte cytosol *(122)*. Erythrocytes from patients with glucose-6-phosphate dehydrogenase deficiency and thalassemia are especially sensitive to oxidative stress and are overwhelmed by additional parasite-generated oxidants, making them prone to lysis before parasite maturation *(121,130,131)*. This may, in part explain why patients with these disorders are less vulnerable to malaria, although other mechanisms are also likely to be important *(132,133)*.

CG2

From the products of a genetic cross, it was determined that a chloroquine-resistance determinant maps to a 36-kb region of chromosome 7 *(134)*. One of the expressed open reading frames has been called candidate gene 2 (cg2). Candidate gene 2 encodes a 330-kDa protein that bears no significant homology to other proteins. It is expressed in late ring-stage and early trophozoite-stage parasites and localizes to the parasite periphery and the food vacuole where it appears associated with hemozoin *(134)*. It is unclear if cg2 is a membrane protein *(135,136)*. The physiological function of cg2 and a possible role in chloroquine resistance have not been established.

Histidine-Rich Proteins

Two of the three known histidine-rich proteins (HRPs) in *P. falciparum* are found within the food vacuole. HRP II and III are homologous, soluble proteins that contain greater than 30% histidine *(137)*. They are secreted out and beyond the erythrocyte but also appear to be trafficked to the food vacuole through the hemoglobin ingestion pathway *(107,138,139)*.

In the food vacuole, HRP II and III may function in heme polymerization *(107)* (*see* Chapter 7). Both proteins can bind heme and promote formation of hemozoin in vitro, in a reaction that is inhibitable by chloroquine. It is postulated that HRP II and III initiate heme polymerization, as an extension of the polymer can occur in the absence of protein *(140)*. A laboratory clone that lacks HRP II and III grows poorly but still polymerizes heme *(107)*. It may have other redundant HRPs or it is possible that other polymerization systems are of physiological importance. HRP II has a very high affinity for zinc and could have other metal/heme-binding roles *(141)*.

HEME METABOLISM

Free heme is a toxic by-product of hemoglobin degradation. Free heme can cause enzyme inhibition, peroxidation of membranes, production of free oxygen radicals, and impaired leukocyte function *(142,143)*. *Plasmodium falciparum* has little or no heme oxygenase (the enzyme used by vertebrates to catabolize heme), although it has been reported in other species *(144)*. All *Plasmodium* species have a unique capability to detoxify heme in the food vacuole by polymerizing it into a crystalline structure called hemozoin, or malarial pigment *(145–147)* (discussed in Chapter 7). The blood-sucking insect, *Rhodnius prolixus*, a vector for *Trypanosoma cruzi (148)*, and Schistosomes *(149)* are the only other organisms known to polymerize heme. Additionally, in *Plasmodium,* some of the heme may be degraded instead of polymerized, and a portion of the heme iron may be released *(6,150)*. The fate of this iron and its contribution to the parasite's iron requirements are unknown.

CONCLUSIONS

The *Plasmodium* food vacuole houses the specialized components of malarial hemoglobin catabolism (Fig. 6). We are only beginning to unravel the molecular details of food vacuole function, but it is clear that it has capabilities unlike any other degradative organelle known. Much like a nuclear reactor, the food vacuole generates energy, yet sequesters toxic by-products. Inhibiting hemoglobin degradation within the food vacuole is a valid approach to antimalarial chemotherapy. Completion of the *P. falciparum* genome sequencing project in the near future will undoubtedly reveal more proteins that function in the food vacuole and are promising targets for antimalarial drug development.

ACKNOWLEDGMENTS

This work was supported by NIH grants A1-31615 and A1-37977. DEG is a recipient of the Burroughs Wellcome Fund Scholar Award in Molecular Parasitology. We thank Kathleen Kolakovich Eggleson for providing Fig. 4.

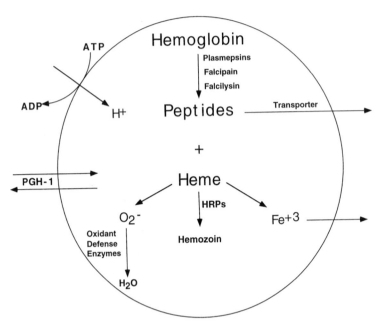

Fig. 6. Proteins and metabolic processes within the *Plasmodium* food vacuole. Hemoglobin is degraded by proteases, generating peptides and free heme. Peptides are transported out of the food vacuole to the cytoplasm for terminal degradation. The heme has three fates: (1) It is polymerized to hemozoin, possibly by the action of histidine-rich proteins; (2) it reacts with molecular oxygen, generating reactive oxygen species that are scavenged by host-derived as well as endogenous oxidant defense enzymes like SOD and catalase; (3) it is degraded, liberating iron, some of which is probably utilized by the parasite. A vacuolar ATPase acidifies the food vacuole, and P-glycoprotein homolog-1 or PGH-1 may act as a transporter in the vacuole membrane, although its physiological role is unknown.

REFERENCES

1. Ting IP, Sherman IW. Carbon dioxide fixation in malaria—I. Kinetic studies in *Plasmodium lophurae*. Comp Biochem Physiol 1966;19:855–869.
2. Sherman IW. Amino acid metabolism and protein synthesis in malarial parasites. Bull WHO 1977;55:265–276.
3. Stryer L Biochemistry. New York: WH Freeman;1988:143–176.
4. Morrison DB, Jeskey HA. Alterations in some constituents of the monkey erythrocyte infected with *Plasmodium knowlesi* as related to pigment formation. J Natl Malar Soc 1948;7:259–264.
5. Ball EG, McKee RW, Anfinsen CB, Cruz WO, Geiman Q M. Studies on malarial parasites: IX. Chemical and metabolic changes during growth and multiplication *in vivo* and *in vitro*. J Biol Chem 1948;175:547–571.
6. Loria P, Miller S, Foley M, Tilley L. Inhibition of the peroxidative degradation of haem as the basis of action of chloroquine and other quinoline antimalarials. Biochem J 1999;339:363–370.
7. McCormick GJ. Amino acid transport and incorporation in red blood cells of normal and *Plasmodium knowlesi*-infected Rhesus monkeys. Exp Parasitol 1970;27:143–149.
8. Sherman IW, Tanigoshi L. Incorporation of 14C-amino acids by malaria (*Plasmodium lophurae*). Int J Biochem 1970;1:635–637.

9. Divo AD, Geary TG, Davis NL, Jensen JB. Nutritional requirements of *Plasmodium falciparum* in culture. I. Exogenously supplied dialyzable components necessary for continuous growth. J Protozool 1985;32:59–64.
10. Pollet H, Conrad ME. Malaria: extracellular amino acid requirements for *in vitro* growth of erythrocytic forms of *Plasmodium knowlesi*. Proc Soc Exp Biol Med 1968;127:251–253.
11. Francis SE, Gluzman IY. Oksman A, Knickerbocker A, Mueller R, Bryant ML, et al. Molecular characterization and inhibition of a *Plasmodium falciparum* aspartic hemoglobinase. EMBO J 1994;13:306–317.
12. Bailly E, Jambou R, Savel J, Jaureguiberry G. *Plasmodium falciparum*: differential sensitivity in vitro to E-64 (cysteine protease inhibitor) and pepstatin A (aspartyl protease inhibitor). J Protozool 1992;39:593–599.
13. Rosenthal PJ, Olson JE, Lee GK, Palmer JT, Klaus JL, Rasnick D. Antimalarial effects of vinyl sulfone cysteine proteinase inhibitors. Antimicrob Agents Chemother 1996;40: 1600–1603.
14. Rosenthal PJ, Wollish WS, Palmer JT, Rasnick D. Antimalarial effects of peptide inhibitors of a *Plasmodium falciparum* cysteine proteinase. J Clin Invest 1991;88:1467–1472.
15. Rosenthal PJ. *Plasmodium falciparum*: effects of proteinase inhibitors on globin hydrolysis by cultured malaria parasites. Exp Parasitol 1995;80:272–281.
16. Rosenthal PJ, McKerrow JH, Rasnick D, Leech JH. *Plasmodium falciparum*: inhibitors of lysosomal cysteine proteinases inhibit a trophozoite proteinase and block parasite development. Mol Biochem Parasitol 1989;35:177–184.
17. Pasvol G, Weatherall DJ, Wilson RJM. Effects of foetal haemoglobin on susceptibility of red cells to *Plasmodium falciparum*. Nature 1977;270:171–173.
18. Wilson, R.J.M., Pasvol G, Weatherall DJ. Invasion and growth of *Plasmodium falciparum* in different types of human erythrocyte. Bull WHO 1977;55:179–186.
19. Shear HL, Grinberg L, Gilman J, Fabry ME, Stamatoyannopoulos G, Goldberg DE, et al. Transgenic mice expressing human fetal globin are protected from malaria by a novel mechanism. Blood 1998;92:2520–2526.
20. Geary TG, Delaney EJ, Klotz IM, Jensen JB. Inhibition of the growth of *Plasmodium falciparum in vitro* by covalent modification of hemoglobin. Mol Biochem Parasitol 1983;9:59–72.
21. Rangachari K, Dluzewski AR, Wilson RJ. M., Gratzer WB. Cytoplasmic factor required for entry of malaria parasites into RBC's. Blood 1987;70:77–82.
22. Zarchin S, Krugliak M, Ginsburg H. Digestion of the host erythrocyte by malaria parasites is the primary target for quinoline-containing antimalarials. Biochem Pharmacol 1986;35:2435–2442.
23. Ginsburg H. Some reflections concerning host erythrocyte–malarial parasite interrelationships. Blood Cells 1990;16:225–235.
24. Desai SA, Krogstad DJ, McCleskey EW. A nutrient-permeable channel on the intraerythrocytic malaria parasite. Nature 1993;362:643–646.
25. Langreth SG, Jensen JB, Reese RT, Trager W. Fine structure in human malaria *in vitro*. J Protozool 1978;25:443–452.
26. Olliaro PL, Goldberg DE. The *Plasmodium* digestive vacuole: Metabolic headquarters and choice drug target. Parasitol Today 1995;11:294–297.
27. Slomianny C. Three-dimensional reconstruction of the feeding process of the malaria parasite. Blood Cells 1990;16:369–378.
28. Goldberg DE, Slater AFG, Cerami A, Henderson GB. Hemoglobin degradation in the malaria parasite *Plasmodium falciparum*: an ordered process in a unique organelle. Proc Natl Acad Sci USA 1990;87:2931–2935.
29. Aikawa M, Hepler PK, Huff CG, Sprinz H. The feeding mechanism of avian malarial parasites. J Cell Biol 1966;28:355–373.

30. Goldberg DE. Hemoglobin degradation in *Plasmodium*-infected red blood cells. Semin Cell Biol 1993;4:355–361.

31. Aikawa M, Thompson PE. Localization of acid phosphatase activity in *Plasmodium* berghei and *P. gallinaceum*: an electron microscopic observation. J Parasitol 1971;57:603–610.

32. Macomber P, Sprinz H. Morphological effects of chloroquine on *Plasmodium berghei* in mice. Nature 1967;214:937–939.

33. Aikawa M. High-resolution autoradiography of malarial parasites treated with ^{3}H-chloroquine. Am J Pathol 1972;67:277–284.

34. Yayon A, Timberg R, Friedman S, Ginsburg H. Effects of chloroquine on the feeding mechanism of the intraerythrocytic human malarial parasite *Plasmodium falciparum*. J Protozool 1984;31:367–372.

35. Krugliak M, Waldman Z, Ginsburg H. Gentamicin and amikacin repress the growth of *Plasmodium falciparum* in culture, probably by inhibiting a parasite acid phospholipase. Life Sci 1987;40:1253–1257.

36. Slomianny C, Prensier G. A cytochemical ultrastructural study of the lysosomal system of different species of malaria parasites. J Protozool 1990;37:465–470.

37. Rudzinska M, Trager W, Bray RS. Pinocytotic uptake and digestion of hemoglobin in malaria parasites. J Protozool 1965;12:563–576.

38. Krogstad DJ, Schlesinger PH, Gluzman IY. Antimalarials increase vesicle pH in *Plasmodium falciparum*. J Cell Biol 1985;101:2302–2309.

39. Yayon A, Cabantchik ZI, Ginsburg H. Identification of the acidic compartment of *Plasmodium falciparum*-infected human erythrocytes as the target of the antimalarial drug chloroquine. EMBO J 1984;3:2695–2700.

40. Gyang FN, Poole B, Trager W. Peptidases from *Plasmodium falciparum* cultured *in vitro*. Mol Biochem Parasitol 1982;5:263–273.

41. Vander Jagt DL, Hunsaker LA, Campos NM. Comparison of proteases from chloroquine-sensitive and chloroquine-resistant strains of *Plasmodium falciparum*. Biochem Pharmacol 1987;36:3285–3291.

42. Bailly E, Savel J, Mahouy G, Jaureguiberry G. *Plasmodium falciparum*: isolation and characterization of a 55-kDa protease with a cathepsin D-like activity from *P. falciparum*. Exp Parasitol 1991;72:278–284.

43. Vander Jagt DL, Hunsaker LA, Campos NM. Characterization of a hemoglobin-degrading, low molecular weight protease from *Plasmodium falciparum*. Mol Biochem Parasitol, 1986;18:389–400.

44. Levy MR, Siddiqui WA, Chou SC. Acid protease activity in *Plasmodium falciparum* and *P. knowlesi* and ghosts of their respective host red cells. Nature 1974;247:546–549.

45. Sherman IW, Tanigoshi L. Purification of *Plasmodium lophurae* cathepsin D and its effects on erythrocyte membrane proteins. Mol Biochem Parasitol 1983;8:207–226.

46. Levy MR, Chou SC. Activity and some properties of an acid proteinase from normal and *Plasmodium berghei*-infected red cells. J Parasitol 1973;59:1064–1070.

47. Aissi E, Charet P, Bouquelet S, Biguet J. Endoprotease in *Plasmodium yoelii nigeriensis*. Comp Biochem Physiol 1983;74B:559–566.

48. Hempelmann E, Wilson RJM. Endopeptidases from *Plasmodium knowlesi*. Parasitology 1980;80:323–330.

49. Sato K, Fukabori Y, Suzuki M. *Plasmodium berghei*: a study of globinolytic enzyme in erythrocytic parasite. Zbl Bakt Hyg 1987;264:487–495.

50. Vander Jagt DL, Hunsaker LA, Campos NM, Scaletti JV. Localization and characterization of hemoglobin-degrading aspartic proteinases from the malarial parasite *Plasmodium falciparum*. Biochim Biophys Acta 1992;1122:256–264.

51. Goldberg DE, Slater AFG, Beavis R, Chait B, Cerami A, Henderson GB. Hemoglobin degradation in the human malaria pathogen *Plasmodium falciparum*: a catabolic pathway initiated by a specific aspartic protease. J Exp Med 1991;173:961–969.

52. Gluzman IY, Francis SE, Oksman A, Smith CE, Duffin KL, Goldberg DE. Order and specificity of the *Plasmodium falciparum* hemoglobin degradation pathway. J Clin Invest 1994;93:1602–1608.

53. Francis SE, Gluzman IY, Oksman A, Banerjee D, Goldberg DE. Characterization of native falcipain, an enzyme involved in *Plasmodium falciparum* hemoglobin degradation. Mol Biochem Parasitol 1996;83:189–200.

54. Dame JB, Reddy GR, Yowell CA, Dunn BM, Kay J, Berry C. Sequence, expression, and modeled structure of an aspartic proteinase from the human malaria parasite *Plasmodium falciparum*. Mol Biochem Parasitol 1994;64:177–190.

55. Manning JM. Remote contributions to subunit interactions: lessons from adult and fetal hemoglobins. TIBS 1999;24:211–212.

56. Dianni Carroll C, Patel H, Johnson TO, Guo T, Orlowski M, He Z, et al. Identification of potent inhibitors of *Plasmodium falciparum* plasmepsin II from an encoded statine combinatorial library. Bioorg Med Chem. Lett 1998;8:2315–2320.

57. Westling J, Yowell CA, Majer P, Erickson JW, Dame JB, Dunn BM. *Plasmodium falciparum, P. vivax, P. malariae*: a comparison of the active site properties of plasmepsins cloned and expressed from three different species of the malaria parasite. Exp Parasitol 1997;87:185–193.

58. Berry C, Dame JB, Dunn BM, Kay J. Aspartic proteinases from the human malaria parasite *Plasmodium falciparum*. In: Takahashi K (ed). Aspartic Proteinases: Structure, Function, Biology, and Biomedical Implications, New York: Plenum 1995, pp. 511–518.

59. Luker KE, Francis SE, Gluzman IY, Goldberg DE. Kinetic analysis of plasmepsins I and II, aspartic proteases of the *Plasmodium falciparum* digestive vacuole. Mol Biochem Parasitol 1996;79:71–78.

60. Francis SE, Banerjee R, Goldberg DE. Biosynthesis and maturation of the malarial aspartic hemoglobinases plasmepsins I and II. J Biol Chem 1997;272:14,961–14,968.

61. Moon RP, Tyas L, Certa U, Rupp K, Bur D, Jacquet C, et al. Expression and characterization of plasmepsin I from *Plasmodium falciparum*. Eur J Biochem 1997;244:552–560.

62. Shinagawa T, Do YS, Baxter JD, Carilli C, Schilling J, Hsueh WA. Identification of an enzyme in human kidney that correctly processes prorenin. Proc Natl Acad Sci USA 1990;87:1927–1931.

63. Kim W, Hatsuzawa K, Ishizuka Y, Hashiba K, Murakami K, Nakayama K. A processing enzyme for prorenin in mouse submandibular gland. J Biol Chem 1990;265:5930–5933.

64. Hill J, Tyas L, Phylip LH, Kay J, Dunn BM, Berry C. High level expression and characterisation of plasmepsin II, an aspartic proteinase from *Plasmodium falciparum*. FEBS Lett 1994;352:155–158.

65. Tyas L, Gluzman IY, Moon RP, Rupp K, Westling J, Ridley RG, et al. Naturally-occurring and recombinant forms of the aspartic proteinases plasmepsins I and II from the malaria parasite *Plasmodium falciparum*. FEBS Lett 1999;454:210–214.

66. Silva AM, Lee AY, Gulnik SV, Majer, P. et al. Structure and inhibition of plasmepsin II, a hemoglobin-degrading enzyme from *Plasmodium falciparum*. Proc Natl Acad Sci USA 1996;93:10,034–10,039.

67. Haque TS, Skillman G, Lee CE, Habashita H, Gluzman IY, Ewing TJ. et al. Potent low-molecular weight non-peptide inhibitors of malarial aspartyl protease plasmepsin II. J Med Chem 1999;42:1428–1440.

68. Bernstein NK, Cherney MM, Loetscher H, Ridley RG, James MNG. Crystal structure of the novel aspartic proteinase zymogen proplasmepsin II from *Plasmodium falciparum*. Nature Struct Biol 1999;6:32–37.

69. Deguercy A, Hommel M, Schrevel J. Purification and characterization of 37-kilodalton proteases from *Plasmodium falciparum* and *Plasmodium berghei* which cleave erythrocyte cytoskeletal components. Mol Biochem Parasitol 1990;38:233–244.

70. Le Bonniec S, Deregnaucourt C, Redeker V, Banerjee R, Grellier P, Goldberg DE, et al. Plasmepsin II, an acidic hemoglobinase from the *Plasmodium falciparum* food vacuole is active at neutral pH on the host erythrocyte membrane skeleton. J Biol Chem 1999;274: 14,218–14,223.

71. Rosenthal PJ, McKerrow JH, Aikawa M, Nagasawa H, Leech JH. A malarial cysteine proteinase is necessary for hemoglobin degradation by *Plasmodium falciparum*. J Clin Invest 1988;82:1560–1566.

72. Gamboa de Dominguez ND, Rosenthal PJ. Cysteine proteinase inhibitors block early steps in hemoglobin degradation by cultured malaria parasites. Blood 1996;87: 4448–4454.

73. Rosenthal PJ, Nelson RG. Isolation and characterization of a cysteine proteinase gene of *Plasmodium falciparum*. Mol Biochem Parasitol 1992;51:143–152.

74. Salas F, Fichmann J, Lee GK, Scott MD, Rosenthal PJ. Functional expression of falcipain, a *Plasmodium falciparum* cysteine proteinase, supports its role as a malarial hemoglobinase. Infect Immun 1995;63:2120–2125.

75. Rosenthal PJ. A *Plasmodium vinckei* cysteine proteinase shares unique features with its *Plasmodium falciparum* analogue. Biochim Biophys Acta 1993;1173:91–93.

76. Rosenthal PJ. Conservation of key amino acids among the cysteine proteinases of multiple malarial species. Mol Biochem Parasitol 1996;75:255–260.

77. Olson JE, Lee GK, Semenov A, Rosenthal PJ. Antimalarial effects in mice of orally administered peptidyl cysteine protease inhibitors. Bioorg Med Chem 1999;7:633–638.

78. Rosenthal PJ, Lee GK, Smith RE. Inhibition of a *Plasmodium vinckei* cysteine proteinase cures murine malaria. J Clin Invest 1993;91:1052–1056.

79. Eggleson KK, Duffin KL, Goldberg DE. Identification and characterization of falcilysin, a metallopeptidase involved in hemoglobin catabolism within the malaria parasite *Plasmodium falciparum*. J Biol Chem 1999;274:32,411–32,417.

80. Bray PG, Janneh O, Raynes KJ, Mungthin M, Ginsburg H, Ward SA. Cellular uptake of chloroquine is dependent on binding to ferriprotoporphyrin IX and is independent of NHE activity in *Plasmodium falciparum*. J Cell Biol 1999;145:363–376.

81. Kolakovich KA, Gluzman IY, Duffin KL, Goldberg DE. Generation of hemoglobin peptides in the acidic digestive vacuole of *Plasmodium falciparum* implicates peptide transport in amino acid production. Mol Biochem Parasitol 1997;87:123–135.

82. Florent I, Derhy Z, Allary M, Monsigny M, Mayer R, Schrevel J. A *Plasmodium falciparum* aminopeptidase gene belonging to the M1 family of zinc-metallopeptidases is expressed in erythrocytic stages. Mol Biochem Parasitol 1998;97:149–160.

83. Vander Jagt DL, Baack BR, Hunsaker LA. Purification and characterization of an aminopeptidase from *Plasmodium falciparum*. Mol Biochem Parasitol 1984;10:45–54.

84. Curley GP, O'Donovan S, McNally J, Mullally M, O'Hara H, Troy A, et al. Aminopeptidases from *Plasmodium falciparum*, *Plasmodium chabaudi chabaudi*, and *Plasmodium berghei*. J Euk Microbiol 1994;41:119–123.

85. Nankya-Kitaka MF, Curley GP, Gavigan CS, Bell A, Dalton JP. *Plasmodium chabaudi chabaudi* and *P. falciparum*: inhibition of aminopeptidase and parasite growth by bestatin and nitrobestatin. Parasitol Res 1998;84:552–558.

86. Berry C, Humphreys MJ, Matharu P, Granger R, Horrocks P, Moon RP, et al. A distinct member of the aspartic proteinase gene family from the human malaria parasite *Plasmodium falciparum*. FEBS Lett 1999;447:149–154.

87. Xie S, Low BG, Nagel RJ, Kramer KK, Anthony RV, Zoli AP, et al. Identification of the major pregnancy-specific antigens of cattle and sheep as inactive members of the aspartic proteinase family. Proc Natl Acad Sci USA 1991;88:10,247–10,251.

88. Xie S, Green J, Beckers J, Roberts RM. The gene encoding bovine pregnancy-associated glycoprotein-1, an inactive member of the aspartic proteinase family. Gene 1995;159: 193–197.

89. Guruprasad K, Blundell TL, Xie S, Green J, Szafranska B, Nagel RJ, et al. Comparative modelling and analysis of amino acid substitutions suggests that the family of pregnancy-associated glycoproteins includes both active and inactive aspartic proteinases. Protein Engin 1996;9:849–856.

90. Xie S., G., J., Bixby JB, Szafranska B, DeMartini JC, Hecht S, Roberts RM. The diversity and evolutionary relationships of the pregnancy-associated glycoproteins, an aspartic proteinase subfamily consisting of many trophoblast-expressed genes. Proc Natl Acad Sci USA 1997;94:12,809–12,816.

91. Elmendorf HG, Haldar K. Identification and localization of ERD2 in the malaria parasite *Plasmodium falciparum*: separation from sites of sphingomyelin synthesis and implication for organization of the Golgi. EMBO J 1993;12:4763–4773.

92. Van Wye J, Ghori N, Webster P, Mitschler RR, Elmendorf HG, Haldar K. Identification and localization of rab6, separation of rab6 from ERD2 and implications for an unstacked Golgi, in *Plasmodium falciparum*. Mol Biochem Parasitol 1996;83:107–120.

93. Mattei D, Ward GE, Langsley G, Lingelbach K. Novel secretory pathways in *Plasmodium*? Parasitol Today 1999;15:235–237.

94. Crary JL, Haldar K. Brefeldin A inhibits protein secretion and parasite maturation in the ring stage of *Plasmodium falciparum*. Mol Biochem Parasitol 1992;53:185–192.

95. Moura IC, Pudles J. A *Plasmodium chabaudi chabaudi* high molecular mass glycoprotein translocated to the host cell membrane by a non-classical secretory pathway. Eur J Cell Biol 1999;78:186–193.

96. Elmendorf HG, Bangs JD, Haldar K. Synthesis and secretion of proteins by released malarial parasites. Mol Biochem Parasitol 1992;52:215–230.

97. Kimura EA, Couto AS, Peres VJ, Casal OL, Katzin AM. N-Linked glycoproteins are related to schizogony of the intraerythrocytic stage in *Plasmodium falciparum*. J Biol Chem 1996;271:14,452–14,461.

98. Dieckmann-Schuppert A, Bause E, Schwarz RT. Studies on O-glycans of *Plasmodium falciparum*-infected human erythrocytes: evidence for O-GlcNAc and transferase in malaria parasites. Eur J Biochem 1993;216:779–788.

99. Dieckmann-Schuppert A, Bender S, Odenthal-Schnittler M, Bause E, Schwarz RT. Apparent lack of N-glycosylation in the asexual intraerythrocytic stage of *Plasmodium falciparum*. Eur J Biochem 1992;205:815–825.

100. Gowda DC, Gupta P, Davidson EA. Glycosylphosphatidylinositol anchors represent the major carbohydrate modification in proteins of intraerythrocytic stage *Plasmodium falciparum*. J Biol Chem 1997;272:6428–6439.

101. Klionsky DJ, Banta LM, Emr SD. Intracellular sorting and processing of a yeast vacuolar hydrolase: proteinase A propeptide contains vacuolar targeting information. Mol Cell Biol 1988;8:2105–2116.

102. Valls LA, Hunter CP, Rothman JH, Stevens TH. Protein sorting in yeast: the localization determinant of yeast vacuolar carboxypeptidase Y resides in the propeptide. Cell, 1987;48:887–897.

103. Oda MN, Scott SV, Hefner-Gravink A, Caffarelli AD, Klionsky DJ. Identification of a cytoplasm to vacuole targeting determinant in aminopeptidase I. J Cell Biol 1996;132:999–1010.

104. Johnson LM, Bankaitis VA, Emr SD, Distinct sorting determinants direct intracellular sorting and modification of a yeast vacuolar protease. Cell 1987;48:875–885.

105. Karcz SR, Herrmann VR, Trottein F, Cowman AF. Cloning and characterization of the vacuolar ATPase B subunit from *Plasmodium falciparum*. Mol Biochem Parasitol 1994;65:123–133.

106. Cowman AF, Karcz S, Galatis D, Culvenor JG. A P-glycoprotein homologue of *Plasmodium falciparum* is localized on the digestive vacuole. J Cell Biol 1991;114:1033–1042.

107. Sullivan DJ, Gluzman IY, Goldberg DE. *Plasmodium* hemozoin formation mediated by histidine-rich proteins. Science 1996;271:219–222.
108. Choi I, Mego JL. Intravacuolar proteolysis in *Plasmodium falciparum* digestive vacuoles is similar to intralysosomal proteolysis in mammalian cells. Biochim Biophys Acta 1987;926:170–176.
109. Choi I, Mego JL. Purification of *Plasmodium falciparum* digestive vacuoles and partial characterization of the vacuolar membrane ATPase. Mol Biochem Parasitol 1988;31:71–78.
110. Saliba KJ, Folb PI, Smith PJ. Role for the *Plasmodium falciparum* digestive vacuole in chloroquine resistance. Biochem Pharm 1998;56:313–320.
111. Karcz SR, Herrmann VR, Cowman AF. Cloning and characterization of a vacuolar ATPase A subunit homologue from *Plasmodium falciparum*. Mol Biochem Parasitol 1993;58:333–344.
112. Rubio JP, Cowman AF. The ATP-binding cassette (ABC) gene family of *Plasmodium falciparum*. Parasitol Today 1996;12:135–140.
113. Wilson CM, Serrano AE, Wasley A, Bogenschutz MP, Shankar AH, Wirth DF. Amplification of a gene related to mammalian mdr genes in drug-resistant *Plasmodium falciparum*. Science 1989;244:1184–1186.
114. Karcz SR, Galatis D, Cowman AF. Nucleotide binding properties of a P-glycoprotein homologue from *Plasmodium falciparum*. Mol Biochem Parasitol 1993;58:269–276.
115. Lim A, Cowman AF. Phosphorylation of a P-glycoprotein homologue in *Plasmodium falciparum*. Mol Biochem Parasitol 1993;62:293–302.
116. Van Es H, Karcz S, Chu F, Cowman AF, Vidal S, Gros P, et al. Expression of the plasmodial pfmdr1 gene in mammalian cells is associated with increased susceptibility to chloroquine. Mol Cell Biol 1994;14:2419–2428.
117. Volkman SK, Cowman AF, Wirth DF. Functional complementation of the ste6 gene of *Saccharomyces cerevisiae* with the pfmdr1 gene of *Plasmodium falciparum*. Proc Natl Acad Sci USA 1995;92:8921–8925.
118. Volkman S, Wirth D. Functional analysis of pfmdr1 gene of *Plasmodium falciparum*. Methods Enzymol 1998;292:174–181.
119. Cowman AF, Karcz S. Drug resistance and the P-glycoprotein homologues of *Plasmodium falciparum*. Semin Cell Biol 1993;4:29–35.
120. Cowman AF, Galatis D, Thompson JK. Selection for mefloquine resistance in *Plasmodium falciparum* is linked to amplification of the pfmdr1 gene and cross-resistance to halofantrine and quinine. Proc Natl Acad Sci USA 1994;91:1143–1147.
121. Vennerstrom JL, Eaton JW. Oxidants, oxidant drugs, and malaria. J Med Chem 1988;31:1269–1277.
122. Atamna H, Ginsburg H. Origin of reactive oxygen species in erythrocytes infected with *Plasmodium falciparum*. Mol Biochem Parasitol 1993;61:231–242.
123. Wallace WJ, Hourchens RA, Maxwell JC, Caughey WS. Mechanism of autooxidation for hemoglobins and myoglobins. J Biol Chem 1982;257:4966–4977.
124. Arias AE, Walter RD. *Plasmodium falciparum*: association with erythrocyte superoxide dismutase. J Protozool 1988;35:348–351.
125. Fairfield AS, Meshnick SR. Malaria parasites adopt host cell superoxide dismutase. Science, 1983;221:764–766.
126. Fairfield AS, Eaton JW, Meshnick SR. Superoxide dismutase and catalase in the murine malaria, *Plasmodium berghei*: content and subcellular distribution. Arch Biochem Biophys 1986;250:526–529.
127. Williams WJ, Beutler E, Erslev AJ, Lichtman MA. Hematology. New York: McGraw-Hill, 1990, p. 319.
128. Fairfield AS, Abosch A, Ranz A, Eaton JW, Meshnick SR. Oxidant defense enzymes of *Plasmodium falciparum*. Mol Biochem Parasitol 1988;30:77–82.

129. Gamain B, Langsley G, Fourmaux MN, Touzel JP, Camus D, Dive D, et al. Molecular characterization of the glutathione peroxidase gene of the human malaria parasite *Plasmodium falciparum*. Mol Biochem Parasitol 1996;78:237–248.

130. Friedman MJ. Oxidant damage mediates variant red cell resistance to malaria. Nature 1979;280:245–247.

131. Eckman JR, Eaton JW. Dependence of plasmodial glutathione metabolism on the host cell. Nature 1979;278:754–756.

132. Weatherall DJ. Host genetics and infectious disease. Parasitology, 1996;112:S23–S29.

133. Destro-Bisol G, Giardina B, Sansonetti B, Spedini G. Interaction between oxidized hemoglobin and the cell membrane: a common basis for several *falciparum* malaria-linked genetic traits. Yearbook Phys Anthropol 1996;39:137–159.

134. Su X, Kirkman LA, Fujioka H, Wellems TE. Complex polymorphisms in a 330-kDa protein are linked to chloroquine-resistant *P. falciparum* in southeast Asia and Africa. Cell 1997;91:593–603.

135. Sanchez CP, Horrocks P, Lanzer M. Is the putative chloroquine resistance mediator CG2 the Na+/H+ exchanger of *Plasmodium falciparum*? Cell 1998;92:601–602.

136. Wellems TE, Wootton JC, Fujioka H, Su X, Cooper, R., Baruch D, et al. *P. falciparum* CG2, linked to chloroquine resistance, does not resemble Na+/H+ exchangers. Cell 1998;94:285–286.

137. Wellems TE, Howard RJ. Homologous genes encode two distinct histidine-rich proteins in a cloned isolate of *Plasmodium falciparum*. Proc Natl Acad Sci USA 1986;83:6065–6069.

138. Howard RJ, Uni S, Aikawa M, Aley SB, Leech JH, Lew AM, et al. Secretion of a malarial histidine-rich protein (PfHRP II) from *Plasmodium falciparum*-infected erythrocytes. J Cell Biol 1986;103:1269–1277.

139. Parra ME, Evans CB, Taylor DW. Identification of *Plasmodium falciparum* histidine-rich protein II in the plasma of humans with malaria. J Clin Microbiol 1991;29:1629–1634.

140. Dorn A, Stoffel R, Matile H, Bubendorf A, Ridley RG. Malarial haemozoin/β-haematin supports haem polymerization in the absence of protein. Nature 1995;374:269–271.

141. Panton LJ, McPhie P, Maloy WL, Wellems TE, Taylor DW, Howard RJ. Purification and partial characterization of an unusual protein of *Plasmodium falciparum*: histidine-rich protein II. Mol Biochem Parasitol 1989;35:149–160.

142. Schwarzer E, Turrini F, Ulliers D, Giribaldi G, Ginsburg H, Arese P. Impairment of macrophage functions after ingestion of *Plasmodium falciparum*-infected erythrocytes or isolated malarial pigment. J Exp Med 1992;176:1033–1041.

143. Banyal HS, Chevli R, Fitch CD. Hemin lyses malaria parasites. Science 1981;214:667–669.

144. Srivastava P, Pandey VC. Heme oxygenase and related indices in chloroquine-resistant and sensitive strains of *Plasmodium berghei*. Int J Parasitol 1995;25:1061–1064.

145. Slater A, Swiggard WJ, Orton BR, Flitter WD, Goldberg DE, Cerami A, et al. An iron-carboxylate bond links the heme units of malaria pigment. Proc Natl Acad Sci USA 1991;88:325–329.

146. Slater AFG, Cerami A. Inhibition by chloroquine of a novel haem polymerase enzyme activity in malaria trophozoites. Nature 1992;355:167–169.

147. Francis SE, Sullivan DJ, Goldberg DE. Hemoglobin metabolism in the malaria parasite *Plasmodium falciparum*. Annu. Rev. Microbiol 1997;51:97–123.

148. Oliveira MF, Silva JR, Dansa-Petretski M, de Souza W, Lins U, Braga CM. S., et al. Haem detoxification by an insect. Nature 1999;400:517–518.

149. Homewood CA, Jewsbury JM. Comparison of malarial and schistosome pigment. Trans R Soc Trop Med Hyg 1972;66:1–2.

150. Ginsburg H, Famin O, Zhang J, Krugliak M. Inhibition of glutathione-dependent degradation of heme by chloroquine and amodiaquine as a possible basis for their antimalarial mode of action. Biochem Pharmacol 1998;56:1305–1313.

5

Clinical and Public Health Implications of Antimalarial Drug Resistance

Piero L. Olliaro and Peter B. Bloland

INTRODUCTION

With 41% of the world's population at risk of malaria, with as many as 400 million new clinical cases and 1.5–2.7 million deaths occurring each year, malaria is a major public health threat *(1)*. In the fight against malaria, antimalarial chemotherapy is, and will remain for the foreseeable future, the most fundamental component of malaria control *(2)*. Although other control strategies have shown promise in reducing malaria-associated morbidity and mortality, the need for people living in areas with malaria transmission to have ready access to effective antimalarial drugs remains essential.

Drug resistance poses an enormous challenge to continued efforts to bring malaria under control *(3)*. In some areas of the world, malaria is resistant to nearly every anti-malarial drug currently available. However, in most of the malarious world, the risk of malaria becoming essentially untreatable is the result of more fundamental causes; for people living in the poorest areas of the world, it is not a lack of effective antimalarial drugs that poses the greatest threat, as much as the lack of antimalarial drugs that are both effective and affordable, or lack of access to drugs at all.

Any discussion of developing or deploying new drugs for malaria should be con-ducted with a solid understanding of the human side of malarial illness: not only an understanding of the clinical consequences of drug resistance and therapy failure but also an understanding of the impact of drug resistance on public health and a careful consideration of how drugs are actually used. Issues such as adherence, availability, cost, perceived value, and acceptability will influence how drugs are used and, there-fore, will also determine their ultimate usefulness. These factors also have an impact on how rapidly resistance will develop. People's perceptions of illness and their treat-ment-seeking behavior will also determine not only how drugs are used but when and for what set of symptoms they are used.

The problem is tremendously complex. Not only is the public sector of most malaria endemic countries unable to deliver the correct drugs efficiently and reliably, but the majority of cases are treated outside of the formal health services. In various surveys conducted in Africa, the proportion of patients seeking malaria treatment outside of the official health sector ranges from a low of 12% to a high of 82% *(4)*. In one verbal

From: *Antimalarial Chemotherapy: Mechanisms of Action, Resistance, and New Directions in Drug Discovery*
Edited by: P. J. Rosenthal © Humana Press Inc., Totowa, NJ

autopsy study in Tanzania, only 45% of children who died had been brought to public-sector health facility during their illness *(5)*. Most people (> 90% in most studies) with fever in malaria-endemic countries do, however, receive treatment for malaria at some time during the course of their illness *(4)*. Drugs used are either provided through the health service or bought from shops, chemical sellers, and private practitioners. The private sector accounts for between 40% and 60% of all antimalarials distributed, and "unofficial" sources (e.g., street sellers, market stalls) account for as much as 25% of all antimalarial distribution *(6)*. The outcome of treatment, whether obtained in the formal health system or not, depends not only on the efficacy of the drug used but also on the correctness of the diagnosis, the quality and appropriateness of the advice given, and the willingness of the patient/guardian to purchase and use an appropriate dose. Innovative strategies must be identified to maximize the success of treatments provided through the national health services, the private sector, informal sources, and the household.

Misuse of drugs, for whatever reason, greatly increases the probability of parasite drug resistance. The speed at which resistance develops is the main determinant of the length of the useful life-span of antimalarial drugs. Therefore, measures to protect drugs against parasite resistance through the twin goals of maximizing appropriate use and discouraging misuse should be central to any strategy developed to control malaria. This chapter discusses antimalarial drug therapy and drug development in the context of the challenges facing malaria control activities.

DEFINITIONS

Antimalarial drug resistance has been defined as the "ability of a parasite strain to survive and/or multiply despite the administration and absorption of a drug given in doses equal to or higher than those usually recommended but within tolerance of the subject." This definition was later modified to specify that the drug in question must "gain access to the parasite or the infected red blood cell for the duration of the time necessary for its normal action" *(7)*. Most researchers interpret this as referring only to persistence of parasites after treatment doses of an antimalarial rather than prophylaxis failure, although the latter can be a useful tool for early warning of the presence of drug resistance *(8)*.

A distinction must be made among failure to clear malarial parasitemia, failure to resolve clinical disease following a treatment with an antimalarial drug, and true anti-malarial drug resistance. Although drug resistance can cause treatment failure, not all treatment failure is caused by drug resistance. Many factors can contribute to apparent treatment failure, including incorrect dosing, nonadherence to the dosing regimen, poor drug quality, drug interactions, poor or erratic absorption, and misdiagnosis. Probably all of these factors, while causing treatment failure (or apparent treatment failure) in the patient, may also contribute to the development and intensification of true drug resistance through increasing the likelihood of exposure of parasites to suboptimal drug levels. Conversely, drug-resistant parasites can be cleared from the body by the immune system. This partially explains discrepancies between clinical outcomes and in vitro sensitivity or presence of resistance-conferring mutations.

DETERMINANTS OF DRUG RESISTANCE AND TREATMENT FAILURE

Clinically relevant resistance to antimalarial drugs emerges primarily through increases in the prevalence of resistance-conferring gene mutations in an environment of selective drug pressure. Parasites survive the presence of drugs through mutation. Mutations occur at random because of replication errors. Many of those mutations are lethal and the parasite will die. Occasionally, a mutation will confer on a parasite a survival advantage when a given drug is present. This parasite, provided it is not cleared by the host's immune system, will proliferate and its progeny carry that mutation. Additional survival advantage could be gained by further mutations. This process generates populations of parasites with different abilities to survive a drug. Over time, the parasite populations with the greatest survival advantage will predominate.

The length of time that a drug will remain therapeutically useful is primarily determined by how frequently such mutations develop, the baseline prevalence of mutations that exist before significant selective drug pressure is exerted, how quickly they spread within a parasite population, and the degree of resistance to a given drug conferred by these mutations.

Although it is not obvious whether *Plasmodia* are effectively clonal or whether they undergo outcrossing at a high rate *(9)*, it is clear that natural parasite populations exhibit considerable variability in their susceptibility to antimalarial drugs *(10)*. The range of naturally occurring drug susceptibilities within a parasite population is a function of the size of the circulating population of parasites (the "biomass" or "parasite burden"); a larger parasite biomass increases the chances for parasite mutation, broadening the distribution of parasite susceptibilities within that population *(11)*. If a mutation does not compromise other biologic functions or confers a net survival advantage in the presence of a given drug, the possibility exists, provided the parasite carrying that mutation escapes the host's immune defenses, that the parasites with the mutation will be selected for and transmitted.

Factors Involved in the Generation of Drug Resistance

The frequency at which these mutation events occur and the speed at which resistance develops and spreads is influenced by a variety of factors related to pharmacological characteristics of the drugs used, the local epidemiological context in which they are used, and the manner in which the drugs are deployed and used operationally *(12)*.

The buildup of resistance is not indefinite and stops at an equilibrium that gives the parasite the best trade-off between surviving a given drug and the loss of biologic performance ("parasite fitness"). A critical issue to understand is if and when the process can be reversed. This understanding would allow, at least in theory, the formulation of policies designed to alternate (or "rotate") drug use before full, nonreversible resistance is acquired. So far, there is no definitive evidence of a significant shift to restored sensitivity of parasites at the human population level, although increased in vitro susceptibility to chloroquine (CQ) is normally found in areas where this drug has not been in use for several years (e.g., Thailand and areas of China) *(13,14)*.

Pharmaco-Biological Factors

Pharmacological factors that influence the rate of development of resistance include the drug's pharmacokinetic and pharmacodynamic characteristics, as well as the drug's intrinsic propensity to generate resistance. Drugs with a long residence time in the organism and a slow rate of reduction of the parasite "biomass" are more vulnerable to resistance. Equally vulnerable are drugs against which resistance develops through single-point mutations in the target molecule (also referred to as single nucleotide polymorphysm, or SNP), such as the antifolates *(15)* and atovaquone *(16)*. By contrast, the quinolines (chloroquine [CQ], quinine) have enjoyed a longer therapeutic life-span because resistance to these drugs is apparently multigenic—the greater the number of genes involved, the slower resistance will evolve.

Epidemiological Factors

One determinant of resistance development is the self-fertilization that occurs between male and female gametocytes when they are picked up by a mosquito during a blood meal. Such reassortment determines the mutations that are carried by the ensuing generation of parasites that are transmitted to the next individual(s). In this process, the intensity of transmission plays a critical, yet undetermined, role, which is principally related to the number of parasite clones carried by each individual *(17)*.

Mathematical models have been generated, although with conflicting results as to the likelihood for resistance to occur at different transmission rates *(18,19)*. The size of the parasite genetic pool depends on intensity of transmission and the probability of genetic rearrangement during the sexual phase of parasite development in the vector. It is possible that resistance emerges and spreads more rapidly in areas of low transmission, where limited numbers of parasites are exposed to intense drug pressure. Mathematical models, however, also suggest that there is an increased development of resistance in situations with high transmission rates as well *(20,21)*.

The intensity of transmission may influence resistance indirectly, via mechanisms such as immunity and drug use. Intense, continuous transmission favors the early acquisition of immunity, at the cost of increased mortality. This should, in theory, confine use of antimalarial drugs—thus limiting the ensuing selection pressure on parasites—to the younger age groups (primarily, children under 5 yr). In practice, this is not always true, and antimalarials are often used by all age groups to treat fever. Additionally, high rates of transmission increase the probability that parasites will be exposed to subtherapeutic drug levels, especially drugs with long half-lives. People living in areas where transmission occurs at lower rates have fewer malaria attacks but, because the level of acquired immunity is far less, remain at greater risk of severe malarial illness for their entire lives.

Operational and Behavioral Factors

The way that drugs are used by both health care providers and patients plays an important role in determining drugs' useful life-spans. Of particular concern are the manner in which drug policies are formulated and implemented and the extent to which official policy can influence practice: specifically, whether drugs are available only with a physician's prescription or whether they are readily available on the open market; whether antimalarials are prescribed only to patients with a proven malaria infection or whether they are prescribed on the basis of a clinical suspicion alone; the extent to which providers (whether formal or informal) and users of antimalarial drugs adhere to official recommendations; and whether the cost or complexity of the recommended regimen might encourage incomplete dosing.

The way that people use antimalarial drugs greatly affects the degree of selective drug pressure; many behaviors result in exposure of parasites to inadequate or subtherapeutic drug levels, which, in turn, facilitates development of resistance. One example is the interplay between people's perceptions of illness and the likelihood of completing a full treatment course. Because people from many cultures perceive illness in terms of symptoms rather than causes, community perceptions of illness and their beliefs and practices related to treating those symptoms can differ greatly from Western biomedical definitions of malaria-related illness. Once the symptoms are gone, the illness is perceived to be gone as well. Patients treating themselves with drugs that produce rapid relief of symptoms, such as artemisinin compounds apparently do, may be more likely to stop before the complete regimen is completed, thereby exposing parasites to a subtherapeutic dose. Conversely, drugs such as sulfadoxine/pyrimethamine (SP), that have no apparent direct antipyretic effect, may be perceived by patients as failing even when they are effective at killing malaria parasites. Other causes of poor compliance include long-duration regimens, complex regimens, high cost, and frequent side effects.

MEASUREMENT AND DIAGNOSIS OF DRUG RESISTANCE

There are a number of methods to characterize or predict parasite response to drug therapy. There is a tendency to consider that only the simplest procedures have a place in malaria control and that all others are too sophisticated for use outside research. Although there are reasons for this, such as the technical and practical difficulties in performing some of these tests under field conditions, a more comprehensive approach is needed if we want to affect the course of resistance. Current research and field testing of various "indicators" aim at evaluating their relative role and use for drug policy-making and monitoring of control programs. Their relevance might vary depending on the intended use. In practice, however, none of the following tests offer a practical method for bedside evaluation of drug resistance; all available tests either do not give results quickly enough to influence treatment decisions or do not give results that are interpretable in terms of individual patient treatment. Traditionally, clinical response to treatment among infected individuals has been selected as the reference.

In nonmalarious areas, treatment is typically based on a worst-case assumption about the resistance patterns of the area in which the patient acquired the malaria infection. In the United States, for instance, if resistance to a given antimalarial drug is known to occur with any degree of frequency, then all infections are assumed to be resistant and a different drug is recommended.

In many endemic areas, however, therapy recommendations lag behind the current status of drug resistance. For example, many countries in Africa are still officially recommending the use of CQ even though resistance to this drug occurs frequently. Optimally, treatment recommendations are based on studies or surveillance that give a reasonable estimate of the frequency of drug resistance or treatment failure that occurs in a given population. Drug recommendations are then based on providing effective treatment to the greatest proportion of patients possible, given the financial resources of the country.

In Vivo Tests

These tests are intended to assess patients' responses to a given treatment. Response includes both clinical and parasitological parameters. Tests following patients for 7, 14, or 28 d have been used to monitor drug efficacy in vivo since 1964 (22). More recently, in an attempt to simplify and standardize procedures, WHO prepared and disseminated a 14-d test primarily based on clinical response to be used at sentinel sites in country programs (23).

A degree of disagreement continues about some aspects of these tests, particularly regarding the most appropriate outcome measures (clinical and/or parasitological clearance) and the best duration of follow-up. The focus in sub-Saharan Africa has been on clinical response to treatment rather than parasitologic clearance. As a result, clinical outcome measures derived from in vivo tests drive policy decisions and create situations in which a drug will be retained because of good clinical response to treatment even though a high degree of parasitologic failure might be occurring. There is reasonable evidence that such practice is contributing to resistance.

Duration of follow-up can also affect interpretation of the results of an in vivo test. Follow-up should be sufficiently long to detect recrudescence of parasites or symptoms over time. The duration of in vivo tests should be extended when testing a drug with a long residence time. On the other hand, intensity of transmission in a given area at a given time determines the probability that a reinfection will occur. Recrudescence and reinfection cannot be distinguished clinically or parasitologically. To some extent, polymorphic genes of *Plasmodium falciparum* (glurp, msp-1, msp-2) can be used to discriminate between the two by genotyping pretreatment and posttreatment isolates. Obviously, such techniques cannot be used routinely in most places. However, with expanding access to polymerase chain reaction (PCR) technology, such data are increasingly available.

In Vitro Tests

In vitro tests have been used to conduct surveillance, support clinical trials, and assist in patient management. The use that is most relevant to this chapter, however, is surveillance. For this purpose, samples are obtained from a series of patients and are tested in order to estimate the resistance patterns found among parasites circulating in a given area. In general terms, in vitro tests reflect intrinsic drug susceptibility of a given isolate, strain, or clone, whereas in vivo tests reflect the interaction between drug efficacy and host immune response that determines overall therapeutic efficacy. As such, in vivo and in vitro tests are complementary.

At present, in vitro tests are adapted to *P. falciparum* only, although some progress is being made with *P. vivax*. Current in vitro tests are as follows:

1. The WHO Mark II test in which patients' blood is inoculated into plates that are predosed with decreasing concentrations of drug. Giemsa-stained slides are prepared after 24-h of culture, and the degree to which maturation of the parasite is inhibited is calculated. Although this test is widely used and requires minimal equipment, it is cumbersome and somewhat lacking precision.
2. Radiolabeled hypoxanthine. Various adaptations of the original method developed by Dejardins et al. *(24–26)* exist. This test allows semiquantitative assessments but is limited because of the use of radiolabeled material (raising disposal problems) and the need for expensive equipment (a β-counter).
3. pLDH microtest. An enzymatic test, originally developed by Makler and colleagues *(27,28)* requires minimal equipment (spectrophotometer) and appears to correlate well with radiolabel methods.

Currently, there is no general agreement as to the place, if any, the in vitro test would have in control programs. There are, in the first place, technical limitations, including the artificial time-course of drug exposure, and the definition of cutoff values between sensitive and resistant parasites. Also, the different methods and analyses lead to different results, thus making interpretation and comparison of data across studies difficult. Several factors may affect results, including (1) technical elements that can modulate the in vitro concentration response (e.g., hematocrit, age of red cells, CO_2/O_2 tension, humidity), (2) parasite factors (mostly dependent on mixed population dynamics [resistant strains tend to outgrow sensitive ones], synchronicity of parasite cycle, parasite density, etc.), (3) drug factors (protein binding, lipid solubility, partition coefficients, solubility, stereochemistry, and molecular weight).

Second, there is the question of the relative role of in vitro versus in vivo testing. One concern that is often raised is the variability of the correlation between the two tests in different studies. One of the reasons for such unpredictable results is the different methodology used between researchers. Correlation varies also with the drug used: it is generally more problematic with antifolate drugs than with CQ *(29)*. The discrepancies can be explained, in part, by the role of the host's immune system.

In reality, the role of the in vitro test in control programs has never been assessed adequately. In part, this is the result of the above-mentioned technical problems that can be corrected if a more adequate test is introduced; currently, an improved version of the pLDH test (Druilhe P, et al., unpublished data) is being tested under the auspices of the European Commission and WHO/TDR. Moreover, attention is being given to the predictive value of in vitro parasite resistance with respect to the clinical failures, as well as to malaria morbidity and mortality.

Molecular Markers

We have a limited understanding of the molecular basis of resistance, paralleled by an almost equally limited knowledge of how drugs work. The availability of validated "early" markers of resistance would be of great value in predicting which drug option to select in a particular context, and thus in guiding drug policies.

Some of the mutations associated with resistance to specific drugs are known *(30)*. For instance, there is broad correlation between increased frequency of mutations in areas of the dihydrofolate reductase (DHFR) (at codons 108, 51, 59, and 164) and dihydropteroate synthase (DHPS) (codons 436, 437, 540, 581 and 613) genes and SP resistance across the world *(31)* (Chapter 9). We also know that DHFR and DHPS mutations occur in a progressive, stepwise fashion; resistance builds up by the accumulation of mutations under drug pressure. However, the relative contribution of individual mutations or series of mutations to in vitro and clinical resistance is controversial, in particular for DHPS. Thus, for the time being, we cannot correlate exactly clinical failure and predict evolution of resistance with molecular markers. The situation is far more complex with CQ and other quinolines (Chapter 8).

Research is attempting to validate the markers that are known and to identify new ones. With the rapid evolution of and increased access to technology, PCR testing for molecular markers may have a place in an "alert system" that monitors mutations and predicts incumbent resistance, as is already happening to an extent with SP.

CLINICAL CONSEQUENCES OF DRUG RESISTANCE AND TREATMENT FAILURE

Because of obvious ethical problems with closely studying the clinical results of failed treatment, existing knowledge of what happens when malaria drugs fail to clear malaria parasitemia is incomplete. Some data exist from the use of malaria infection as a treatment for neurosyphilis, in which subcurative doses of antimalarial drugs were given to maintain parasitemia but prevent death *(32)*. However, because this treatment was studied under controlled conditions among adults with a pre-existing, severe illness, these data are limited in their ability to assist in understanding the impact and consequences of failed treatment under natural conditions. Most of what is known about the impact of drug resistance and treatment failure comes from indirect sources, such as observational studies, short-term treatment trials, and public health surveillance.

Reduced Treatment Efficacy

The most obvious consequence of antimalarial drug resistance is a failure of the drug to produce a rapid and complete cure. This consequence can be manifested in a variety of ways.

Delayed Initial Therapeutic Response

This is considered by many to be the first sign of resistance. The rate of parasite and fever reduction is influenced not only by parasite susceptibility but also by host factors and the drug's pharamacokinetic and pharmacodynamic characteristics *(33,34)*. On the Thai–Burmese borders, clinical and parasitological response on d 3 after mefloquine monotherapy predicted subsequent treatment failure *(35)*. A similar correlation was found in Africa with CQ on d 2 *(36)*.

Parasitologic Recrudescence and Return of Clinical Symptoms

In some settings, recrudescent infections tend to be clinically silent *(37)*. Nonetheless, the return of clinical symptoms associated with recrudescent parasitemia is probably the most common clinical consequence of failed treatment. In Malawi, Kenya, and Zambia, febrile, anemic children with *P. falciparum* infections were enrolled and treated with either CQ or SP. In spite of parasitologic failure rates after CQ treatment that ranged from 75% to 80%, more than 90% of children became afebrile within 48 h of initiation of treatment *(31,38,39)*. However, the duration of this clinical improvement was short; the median time until a return of clinical symptoms was as few as 10–14 d. The greater the in vivo resistance exhibited by the parasite, the shorter the duration of clinical improvement after initial treatment *(33)*.

The time at which recrudescence occurs depends on a drug's half-life. With long-half-life drugs, such as mefloquine, recrudescent infections can occur up to 63 d after treatment, or even longer in pregnant women *(40)*. In the early stages of resistance, short-term follow-up (14 d) would underestimate the real incidence of treatment failures that would occur only later.

Complications

Anemia

Anemia is a common and important complication of malaria in children, potentially leading to reduced exercise tolerance, impaired growth rate, impaired neurologic and cognitive development, delayed healing of wounds, and death *(41)*. Anemia in young children can be exacerbated by treatment failure. In the studies described earlier, hematologic response was studied over 14–28 d after treatment. Children who received a treatment that was highly effective at removing parasites (SP in these studies) had increases in hemoglobin concentration greater than those seen among CQ-treated children at each of 4 wk of follow-up. This difference in hemoglobin levels after treatment was as much as 1–4 g/dL between treatment groups *(33)*.

In Zaire (now the Democratic Republic of Congo), in 1986, malaria was the leading cause of anemia requiring blood transfusion, with 87% of transfusions being given to malaria patients. CQ resistance was first identified in Kinshasa in 1984, and by 1986, 82% of falciparum infections among children demonstrated in vitro resistance to CQ *(42)*. Between 1982 and 1986, this increase in CQ resistance was accompanied by a two-fold increase in pediatric blood transfusions *(43)*. Compared with children who did not get transfused, the likelihood of children being seropositive for human immunodeficiency virus (HIV) increased from 2.8 times higher after one transfusion to 21.9 times higher after three transfusions *(38)*. Although blood screening practices have greatly improved since this study, the association among malaria, anemia, and HIV continues to be of great concern for both children and pregnant women *(44,45)*.

Complications During Pregnancy

Plasmodium falciparum infections occurring during pregnancy among semi-immune women have been associated with an increased risk of delivering low-birth-weight babies. Malaria parasites will sequester in the placenta in large numbers. The exact mechanism by which this placental malaria causes low birth weight is not fully understood; however, it is likely to be related to interference with nutrient transport across the placenta to the fetus. Malaria during pregnancy is a well-known risk factor for maternal anemia and some studies have also shown an association between placental malaria and the development of anemia during the infant's first 6 months of life *(46,47)*. In endemic areas, malaria may be responsible for as much as 30% of preventable low birth weight. Low birth weight, in turn, is the greatest single risk factor for infant mortality *(48)*. Women in their first and second pregnancies and all HIV-infected women regardless of parity are at greatest risk for malaria *(49)*.

Traditionally, prevention strategies for malaria during pregnancy involved providing women with weekly CQ prophylaxis. The potential usefulness of this intervention has been nearly eliminated by the advent of CQ resistance in much of the world. In one study in Malawi, separate groups of women were provided with either CQ or mefloquine prophylaxis; compliance was assured by directly observed treatment *(50)*. Women who received CQ prophylaxis had placental malaria rates that were not significantly different from women from the general population who had not received any intervention (32% and 38%, respectively) *(51)*. Those women receiving an effective intervention, either mefloquine or SP (given in two treatment doses in the second and third trimester), had a significantly lower rate of placental malaria (6.2% for mefloquine and 9% for SP) *(52)*.

Alternative strategies have been promoted as an affordable, effective, and implementable intervention to prevent placental malaria based on preventive intermittent treatment with SP during the second and third trimester *(53)*. Although this strategy has been shown to be effective in several settings, spreading SP resistance will increasingly undermine this strategy, further eroding currently available and affordable drugs usable for intervention during pregnancy.

The list of antimalarial drugs that are available, safe, and currently effective for use as regular prophylaxis during pregnancy is relatively short. Although there are some areas that could continue to use CQ, SP, or combinations of proguanil + CQ until newer approaches to chemotherapy during pregnancy are proven, mefloquine is the most obvious successor. Although mefloquine might be able to replace CQ in this type of intervention, it is currently far more expensive than CQ and is beyond the financial reach of most of the highest-risk countries, especially in Africa. Admittedly, prevention of malaria during pregnancy through prophylaxis was never particularly effective because of generally poor adherence; however, the advent of CQ resistance has essentially eliminated this as an option.

Plasmodium falciparum infections among pregnant nonimmune women can be more severe than those among women who are not pregnant. Failure of malaria treatment among these women could result in the progression of illness to cerebral malaria, pulmonary edema, renal failure, and maternal or fetal death *(54)*. Having highly effective drugs to treat these women will continue to be a priority.

PUBLIC HEALTH CONSEQUENCES

Increases in Malaria Transmission

At the simplest level, poor therapeutic efficacy fails to remove parasites from infected individuals, thereby maintaining a larger population of parasitemic individuals in a given area and maintaining a larger biomass of parasites contributing to malaria transmission. Drug resistance has been implicated, at least partially, for malaria epidemics observed in Somalia *(55)* and highland areas of Kenya *(56)*.

Drug resistance is also more directly associated with a potential for increased transmission by enhancing gametocyte carriage *(57)*. This can be a result of longer parasite clearance times, which are associated with increase gametocyte carriage, or increased frequency of recrudescent infections, which are twice as likely to carry gametocytes compared with primary infections *(58,59)*. There are, however, major differences among antimalarial drugs. Some drugs (e.g., SP) generate larger amounts of gametocytes than others (e.g., CQ). For CQ, gametocytes from drug-resistant isolates appear to transmit infection to mosquitoes more efficiently than gametocytes from drug-susceptible parasites *(32,60)*.

Chloroquine resistance has been shown to confer a survival advantage to parasites that appears to be independent of drug pressure (e.g., schizont maturation may be more efficient among resistant parasites) *(61,62)*. Similarly, there exist some data to suggest that a genetic plasticity develops that allows resistant parasites to adapt more quickly to new drugs than would normally be expected and even when the new drug is not pharmacologically related *(63)*.

There is some evidence that certain combinations of drug-resistant parasites and vector species enhance the transmission of drug resistance, whereas other combinations inhibit transmission of resistant parasites. In Southeast Asia, two important vectors, *Anopheles stephensi* and *A. dirus,* appear to be more susceptible to drug-resistant malaria than to drug-sensitive malaria *(64,65)*. In Sri Lanka, researchers found that patients with CQ-resistant malaria infections were more likely to have gametocytemia than those with sensitive infections and that the gametocytes from resistant infections were more infective to mosquitoes *(32)*. The reverse may also be true: Some malaria vectors may be somewhat refractory to drug-resistant malaria, which may partially explain the pockets of CQ sensitivity that remain in the world in spite of very similar human populations and drug pressure (e.g., Haiti) *(66)*.

The implications of these findings on the burden of disease in human populations are not clear. However, increases in overall parasite prevalence rates from treatment failure or from increased levels of transmission would likely result in increases in human morbidity and mortality.

Frequency of Severe Illness

On an individual basis, the primary concern with failed malaria treatment is progression to severe, potentially life-threatening or fatal illness. Crude estimates of the number of clinical attacks of malaria among African children range from 1 to 5 per year; of these, an estimated 2% of these attacks are severe *(67)*. The risk of a given febrile illness caused by *P. falciparum* actually progressing to a fatal illness, however, is unknown. White *(68)* has argued that although case-fatality rates for severe malaria have remained stable because of the continued efficacy of quinine and artemisinin compounds, malaria morbidity and mortality has nonetheless increased because of the number of severe malaria cases that develop because of ineffective first-line treatment. Progression from mild, acute febrile illness to severe disease is also related to the level of acquired immunity of the patient, human and possibly parasite genetic characteristics, treatment-seeking behavior on the part of the patient or caretaker, and the infecting dose *(69)*.

Malawi changed its national malaria treatment policy from CQ to SP in March 1993. Surveillance data from 1991 until the implementation of the new policy in 1993 showed that hospital admissions because of uncomplicated malaria, anemia, and cerebral malaria increased by 14%, 22% and 10%, respectively. After the policy change, from 1993 to 1995, the rate of admission for uncomplicated malaria continued to increase; however, the rates for admission because of anemia and cerebral malaria decreased by 39% and 5%, respectively (O. Nwanyanwu, unpublished data; P. Kazembe, personal communication).

Mortality Rates

Estimates of the impact of effective treatment on the mortality rate of malaria range from a 50-fold decrease in probability of mortality among uncomplicated malaria cases (from about 5% to 0.1%) to a 5-fold decrease in probability of mortality among patients with severe illness (from nearly 100% to 15–20%) *(58)*. As treatment fails, the overall case-fatality rate undoubtedly rises.

Actual data illustrating either a decrease in mortality rates because of effective treatment or a rise in mortality rates because of ineffective treatment are limited. One study of hospital-based data with postdischarge monitoring in western Kenya spanned a period of time when in-hospital treatment was slowly changing from CQ (the officially recommended treatment throughout this period) to other forms of more efficacious antimalarial treatment (mostly quinine, SP, and cotrimoxazole) *(70)*. Children who had been admitted to the hospital were evaluated at discharge and at 4 and 8 wk postdischarge. Whereas malaria had an overall case-fatality rate of 20%, children treated with CQ had a 33% case-fatality rate, and children treated with an effective antimalarial treatment had an 11% case-fatality rate. Overall, 60% of deaths among these children was attributed to ineffective treatment. Surveillance data from this same hospital collected between 1991 and 1994 showed a progressive drop in in-hospital case-fatality rates from 9.9% to 2.8% as use of efficacious antimalarial therapy increased from 37% to 97% (Zucker, unpublished data).

In Malawi, deaths caused by malaria and anemia increased 31% and 36%, respectively, between 1991 and March 1993 (while CQ was still being used for treatment of uncomplicated malaria). After a policy change to SP for treatment of uncomplicated malaria, deaths attributed to malaria and anemia decreased 8% and 26%, respectively (Nwanyanwu O, unpublished data; Kazembe P, personal communication).

A study conducted in three epidemiologically different areas of Senegal from 1984 to 1995 tracked malaria mortality rates among children 0–9 yr of age *(71)*. CQ resistance was first demonstrated in Senegal in 1988 and the first treatment failures in the study areas occurred between 1990 and 1993. During the period following the advent of CQ resistance, malaria mortality rates in these study areas increased by 2.1-, 2.5-, and 5.5-fold. However, such a correlation has not been found in Asia *(72)*.

Sociobehavioral and Economic Implications of Increasing Treatment Failure

In the context of the studies mentioned earlier, there was no indication that the recrudescent illness was more severe than the initial illness. However, with the relatively small numbers and the speed at which recrudescent illnesses were identified and retreated, this is not surprising. At best, recrudescent illnesses will result in increased costs associated with higher patient loads and the cost of retreatment. Additionally, high rates of treatment failure may erode the confidence of patients in the health care system, causing further delays in seeking treatment and potentially increases in the rates of severe malaria and death.

To properly assess the true economic impact of resistance, a wide range of costs, including both direct and indirect costs, and health effects need to be considered. Direct costs, borne individually or by the health system, or both, include the cost of the drug itself, the cost of repeat treatments with antimalarial and ancillary drugs (such as antipyretics) when symptoms are not relieved, second-line therapy with either oral or injectable medications, and management of any complications. Examples of indirect costs include transportation costs, work/school days lost, lost income for individuals, and personnel and supply costs at the health facility.

Economic evaluation is becoming a key element in evaluating interventions *(73)*. Models to assess the cost-effectiveness of interventions are being developed *(74)*. However, only recently have we started to realize the economic ramifications of resistance and appreciate the importance of these elements for policy-level decision making. Such evaluation is particularly important when countries are confronted with the problem of switching from a failing first-line drug to an alternative treatment. Policy-level decision-makers need data to compare the cost-effectiveness of different heath care interventions in terms of costs and health outcome, such as the cost per death or disability-adjusted life year (DALY) *(75)* averted, potential treatment cost savings, and reduction in indirect costs to households, such as those resulting from faster return to productive activities. Models have been proposed to analyze these trade-offs with both antimalarial drugs *(76–78)* and antibiotics *(79,80)*.

APPROACHES TO COUNTER ANTIMALARIAL DRUG RESISTANCE

Rational antimalarial drug policies are critical for creating an environment that does limits the development of resistance. Even though they are crucial, the factors that influence the process of formulating national antimalarial drug policies and the types of evidence (biomedical, behavioral, or economic) that are needed to inform policy development are poorly understood, and research to improve this situation is inadequate and poor. It is essential that appropriate means are allocated to investigate such factors as drug use, cost-effectiveness, and patient and provider behavior to be able to facilitate the policy development process. After antimalarial-drug-use policies are formulated, it is equally important to provide resources to improve adherence to recommendations and to monitor drug efficacy and tolerability over time.

Policy alone is unlikely to meet the challenge of antimalarial drug resistance. Policy makers and malaria control programs need new tools and new approaches to counter the parasite's ability to resist drug action. For new tools and approaches to be developed, it is important to recognize several interacting factors that inhibit this process:

- Limitations of the current chemotherapeutic armamentarium imposed by the expense and time required to research, develop, and market new antimalarial compounds *(81)*, resulting in an overreliance on the 4-aminoquinoline and folate-inhibitor families of compounds
- The ramifications of malaria treatment policies and practices (such as the widespread, uncontrolled availability of antimalarial drugs in the private sector and reliance on presumptive treatment of malaria)
- Inadequate investments in basic parasite biochemistry, molecular biology, and new drug development

Various approaches can be envisaged to prevent or reduce the pace at which resistance develops. In practice, the feasibility of any given approach depends on its affordability, implementability, and sustainability. Short- and long-term measures should be envisaged.

One clear need is to develop new drugs. Although drug development output for malaria and other "tropical diseases" has been rather low *(82)*, in the long run, this rate can be improved with new technology. Recent advances in science and in the synthesis and screening of compounds (combinatorial chemistry, high-throughput screening) will facilitate the discovery of new targets and newer drugs with novel mechanisms of actions and chemical characteristics unrelated to existing drugs that may avoid cross-resistance. Some of these are known *(83)*. The malaria genome project is delivering information that can be exploited to identify putative new targets *(84)*. The "postgenomic agenda" is already reality *(85)*.

Whereas the principles above would apply to virtually any drug development, what the malaria resistance story is teaching us is that specific additional characteristics should be sought, namely those related to the drug's propensity to generate resistance. In particular, the trade-offs between long and short residence times in humans become critical. Although drugs with long half-lives are useful for directly observed therapy (which can prevent the effects of poor patient compliance), chemoprophylaxis (because the dosage interval can be lengthened), and for their posttreatment "chemoprophylactic" effect (e.g.,

SP), they are particularly vulnerable to developing resistance, as they are likely to produce subtherapeutic plasma concentrations of drug for significant periods of time, providing "selection pressure" for the emergence of drug resistance. Conversely, drugs with short half-lives require multiple-day dosing, which is known to significantly decrease dosing completion rates and facilitate development of resistance.

Discovering and developing new chemicals takes time and is expensive; various initiatives are being tried to speed up drug research and development for antimalarial drugs, such as the Medicines for Malaria Venture. Yet, solutions are needed urgently *(86)*. In general, countries need improved malaria-treatment policies and case management (improving the diagnosis of malaria, enhancing compliance, and detecting and treating treatment failures). More specifically, there are ways of gaining "extra mileage" from currently available drugs to prolong their life-spans. Recently, emphasis is being put on new combinations of currently available drugs *(3)*. This strategy could provide effective regimens less likely to promote the development of resistance. Combining different drugs with independent modes of action can prevent the emergence of resistance to both drugs because the probability that an infected patient will have parasites resistant to both drugs is enormously reduced (the product of the probability of resistance to either drug). Artesunate and its main metabolite, dihydroartemisinin, are highly effective and rapidly acting against multidrug-resistant *P. falciparum* and have very short half-lives; the latter property is inherently protective against the development of resistance. Although declines in susceptibility to artemisinin drugs have been seen in areas where they are used extensively *(87)*, no clinically significant artemisinin resistance has been identified to date. On the Thai–Burmese border, the combination of artesunate and mefloquine has reportedly stopped the progression of mefloquine resistance *(88)*. There are several reasons for this: artesunate eliminates most of the infection and the remaining parasites are then exposed to high concentrations of the slow-acting mefloquine; because of the rapid reduction of parasites, the selective pressure for the emergence of mutant parasites is greatly reduced; and artesunate also decreases gametocyte carriage (the sexual form required to complete the parasite life cycle) *(89)*, thus reducing malaria transmission and the spread of resistance *(90)*. Although it is unclear to what extent combination-therapy approaches can be exported to very different epidemiologic, cultural, and economic settings, these strategies do offer tremendous hope to places such as sub-Saharan Africa.

REFERENCES

1. World Health Organization. World malaria situation in 1993, part I. Weekly Epidemiol Rec 1996;71:17–22.
2. Olliaro P, Cattani J, Wirth D. Malaria: the submerged disease. JAMA, 1996;275(3):230–234.
3. White NJ. Drug resistance in malaria. Br Med Bull 1998;54(3):703–715.
4. McCombie SC Treatment seeking for malaria: a review of recent research. Soc Sci Med 1996;43:933–945.
5. Mtango FDE, Neuvians D, Broome CV, Hightower AW, Pio A. Risk factors for deaths in children under 5 years old in Bagamoyo District, Tanzania. Trop Med Parasitol 43:1992; 229–233.
6. Foster SD. Pricing, distribution, and use of antimalarial drugs. Bull WHO 1991;69:349–363.
7. Bruce-Chwatt LJ, Black RH, Canfield CJ, Clyde DF, Peters W, Wernsdorfer WH. Chemotherapy of Malaria. Geneva: World Health Organization, 1986.

8. Lobel HO, Campbell CC. Malaria prophylaxis and distribution of drug resistance. Clin Trop Med Commun Dis 1986;1:225–242.

9. Hey J. Parasite populations: the puzzle of *Plasmodium*. Curr Biol 1999;9:565–567.

10. Druilhe P, Daubersies P, Patarapotikul J, Gentil C, Chene L, Chongsuphajaisiddhi T, et al. A primary malarial infection is composed of a very wide range of genetically diverse but related parasites. J Clin Invest 1998;101(9):2008–2016.

11. White NJ. Assessment of the pharmacological properties of antimalarial drugs in vivo. Antimicrob Agents Chemother. 1997;41(7):1413–1422.

12. White NJ, Olliaro PL. Strategies for the prevention of antimalarial drug resistance: rationale for combination chemotherapy for malaria. Parasitol Today,12 1996;(19):399–401.

13. Thaithong S, Suebsaeng L, Rooney W, Beale GH. Evidence of increased chloroquine sensitivity in Thai isolates of *Plasmodium* falciparum. Trans R Soc Trop Med 1988;Hyg; 82:37–38.

14. Liu D, Liu R, Ren D, Gao D, Zhang C, Qui C, et al. Changes in the resistance of *Plasmodium falciparum* to chloroquine in Hainan, China. Bull WHO 1995;73:483–486.

15. Watkins WM, Mberu EK, Winstanley PA, Plowe CV. The efficacy of antifolate antimalarial combinations in Africa: a predictive model based on pharmacodynamic and pharmacokientic analyses. Parasitol Today 1997;13(12):459–464.

16. Looareesuwan S, Viravan C, Webster HK, Kyle DE, Hutchinson DB, Canfield CJ. Clinical studies of atovaquone, alone or in combination with other antimalarial drugs, for treatment of acute uncomplicated malaria in Thailand. Am J Trop Med 1996;Hyg;54(1):62–66.

17. Hill WG, Babiker HA, Ranford-Cartwright LC, Walliker D. Estimation of inbreeding coefficients from genotypic data on multiple alleles, and application to estimation of clonality in malaria parasites. Genet Res 1995;65(1):53–61.

18. Dye C, Willimas BG. Multigenic resistance among inbred malaria parasites. Proc R Soc London Ser B 1997;264:61–67.

19. Hastings IM. A model for the origins and spread of drug resistant malaria. Parasitology 1997;115:133–141.

20. Hastings IM, Mackinnon MJ. The emergence of drug-resistant malaria. Parasitology 1998;117:411–417.

21. Mackinnon MJ, Hastings IM. The evolution of multiple drug resistance in malaria parasites. Trans R Soc Trop Med Hyg 92:1998;188–195.

22. WHO Resistance of malaria Parasites to Drugs. Report of a WHO Scientific Group. Geneva: WHO, 1965.

23. WHO Assessment of therapeutic efficacy of antimalarial drugs—for uncomplicated falciparum malaria in areas with intense transmission. WHO Report WHO/MAL/96.1077 (1996).

24. Dejardins RE, Canfield CJ, Haynes JD, Chulay JD. Quantitative assessment of antimalarial activiy in vitro by a semiautomated microdilution technique. Antimicrob Agents Chemother. 1979;16:710–718.

25. Druilhe P, Mazier D, Brandicourt O, Gentilini M. One-step *Plasmodium falciparum* cultivation—application to in vitro drugs testing. Tropenmed Parasitol 34:1983;233–234.

26. Le Bras J, Deloron P. In vitor study of drug sensitivity of *Plasmodium falciparum*: evaluation of a new semi-micro test. Am J Trop Med Hyg 1983;32:447–451.

27. Makler MT, Ries JM, Williams JA, Bacroft JE, Piper RC, Gibbins BL, et al. Parasite lactate dehydrogenase as an assay for *Plasmodium falciparum* drug susceptibility assay. Am J Trop Med Hyg 1993;48:739–741.

28. Basco LK, Marquet F, Makler MT, Le Bras J. *Plasmodium falciparum* and *Plasmodium vivax*: lactate dehydrogenase activity and its application for in vitro drug susceptibility assay. Exp Parasitol 1995;80:260–271.

29. Ringwald P, Basco LK. Comparison of in vivo and in vitro tests of resistance in patients treated with chloroquine in Yaounde, Cameroon. Bull WHO 1999;77(1):34–43.

30. Plowe C, Kublin JG, Doumbo OK. P. falciparum dihydrofolate reductase and dihydropteroate synthase mutations: epidemiology and role of clinical resistance to antifolates. Drug Resist Updates 1998;1:389–396.
31. Wang P, Lee CS, Bayoumi R, Djimde A, Doumbo O, Swedberg G, et al. Resistance to antifolates in *Plasmodium falciparum*, monitored by sequence analysis of dihydropteroate synthetase and dihydrofolate reductase alleles in large number of field samples of diverse origins. Mol. Biochem. Parasitol. 1997;8:161–177.
32. Collins WE, Jeffrey GM. A retrospective examination of sporozoite- and trophozoite-induced infections with *Plasmodium falciparum*. Am J Trop Med Hyg 1999;61(Suppl 1):1–48.
33. White NJ, Krishna S. Treatment of malaria; some considerations and limitations of the current methods of assessment. Trans R Soc Trop Med Hyg 1989;83:767–777.
34. White NJ. Assessment of the pharmacodynamic properties of antimalarial drugs in vivo. Antimicrob Agents Chemother 1997;41(7):1413–1422.
35. Ter Kuile FO, Nosten F, Luxemburger C, Phaipun L, Chongsuphajaisiddhi T, White NJ. Predictors of mefloquine treatment failure: a prospective study in 1590 patients with uncomplicated falciparum malaria. Trans R Soc Trop Med Hyg 1995;660–664.
36. Bloland PB, Kazembe PN, Oloo AJ, Himonga B, Barat LM, Ruebush TK. Chloroquine in Africa: critical assessment and recommendations for monitoring and evaluating chloroquine therapy efficacy in sub-Saharan Africa. Trop Med Int Health 1998;3:543–552.
37. Handunnetti SM, Gunewardena DM, Pathirana PP, Ekanayake K, Weerasinghe SM. Features of recrudescent chloroquine-resistant *Plasmodium falciparum* infections confer a survival advantage on parasites and have implications for disease control. Trans R Soc Trop Med 1996;Hyg;90:563–567.
38. Bloland PB, Lackritz EM, Kazembe PN, Were JBO, Steketee R, Campbell CC. Beyond chloroquine: implications of drug resistance for evaluating malaria therapy efficacy and treatment policy in Africa. J Infect Dis 1993;167:932–937.
39. Barat LM, Hinonga B, Nkunika S, Ettling M, Ruebush TK, Kapelwa W, et al. A systematic approach to the development of a rational malaria treatment policy in Zambia. Trop Med Int Health 1998;3:535–542.
40. Smithuis FM, van Woensel JBM, Nordlander E, Sok Vantha W, ter Kuile FO. Comparison of two mefloquine regimens for treatment of falciparum malaria on the north-eastern Thai–Cambodian border. Antimicrob Agents Chemother 1993;37:1977–1981.
41. Luby SP, Kazembe PN, Redd SC, Ziba C, Nwanyanwu OC, Hightower AW, et al. Using clinical signs to diagnose anaemia in African children. Bull WHO 1995;73:477–482.
42. Greenberg AE, Ntumbanzondo M, Ntula N, Mawa L, Howell J, Davachi F. Hospital-based surveillance of malaria-related paediatric morbidity and mortality in Kinshasa, Zaire. Bull WHO 1989;67(2):189–196.
43. Greenberg AE, Nguyen-Dinh P, Mann JM, Kabote N, Colebunders RL, Francis H, et al. The association between malaria, blood transfusions, and HIV seropositivity in a pediatric population in Kinshasa, Zaire. JAMA 1988;259:545–549.
44. Zucker JR, Lackritz EM, Ruebsuh TK, Hightower AW, Adungosi JE, Were JBO, et al. Anaemia, blood transfusion practices, HIV and mortality among women of reproductive age in western Kenya. Trans R Soc Trop Med Hyg 1994;88:173–176.
45. Lackritz EM. Prevention of HIV transmission by blood transfusion in the developing world: achievements and continuing challenges. AIDS 12(Suppl A);1998:S81–S86.
46. Redd SC, Wirima JJ, Steketee RW. Risk factors for anemia in young children in rural Malawi. Am J Trop Med Hyg. 1994;51:170–174.
47. Cornet M, Le Hasran J-Y, Fievet N, Cot M, Personne P, Gounoue R, et al. Prevalence of and risk factors for anemia in young children in South-Cameroon. Am J Trop Med Hyg 1998;58:606–611.
48. McCormick MC. The contribution of low birth weight to infant mortality and childhood mortality. N Engl J Med 1985;312:82–90.

49. Steketee RW, Wirima JJ, Bloland PB, Chilima B, Mermin JH, Chitsulo L, et al. Impairment of a pregnant woman's acquired ability to limit *Plasmodium falciparum* by infection with human immunodeficiency virus type 1. Am J Trop Med Hyg 1996;55(Suppl 1):33–41.

50. Steketee RW, Wirima JJ, Slutsker L, Roberts JM, Khoromana CO, Heymann DL, et al. Malaria parasite infection during pregnancy and at delivery in mother, placenta, and newborn: efficacy of chloroquine and mefloquine in rural Malawi. Am J Trop Med Hyg 1996;55,(Suppl 1):24–32.

51. Steketee RW, Wirima JJ, Slutsker L, McDermott JM, Hightower AW, et al. Malaria Prevention in Pregnancy. The Effects of Treatment and Chemoprophylaxis on Placental Malaria Infection, Low Birth Weight, and Fetal, Infant, and Child Survival (African Child Survival Initiative—Combating Childhood Communicable Diseases Project Document 099-4048). Atlanta, GA: Centers for Disease Control and Prevention, 1993.

52. Schultz LJ, Steketee RW, Macheso A, Kazembe P, Chitsulo L, Wirima JJ. The efficacy of antimalarial regimens containing sulfadoxine-pyrimethamine and/or chloroquine in preventing peripheral and placental *Plasmodium falciparum* infection among pregnant women in Malawi. Am J Trop Med Hyg 1994;51:515–522.

53. Parise ME, Ayisi JG, Nahlen BL, Schultz LJ, Roberts JM, Misore A, et al. Efficacy of sulfadoxine–pyrimethamine for prevention of placental malaria in an area of Kenya with a high prevalence of malaria and human immunodeficiency virus infection. Am J Trop Med Hyg 1998;59:813–822.

54. Menedez C. Malaria during pregnancy: a priority area for malaria research and control. Parasitol Today 1995;11:178–183.

55. Warsame M, Wernsdorfer WH, Ericsson Ö, Björkman A. Isolated malaria outbreak in Somalia: role of chloroquine-resistant *Plasmodium falciparum* demonstrated in Balcad epidemic. J Trop Med Hyg 1990;93:284–289.

56. Malakooti MA, Biomndo K, Shanks GD. Reemergence of epidemic malaria in the highlands of western Kenya. Emerg Infect Dis 1998;4(4):671–676.

57. Price R, Nosten F, Simpson JA, Luxemburger C, Phaipun L, ter Kuile F, et al. Risk factors for gametocyte carriage in uncomplicated falciparum malaria. Am J Trop Med Hyg 1999;60(6):1019–1023.

58. Price RN, Nosten F, Luxemberger C, ter Kuile FO, Paiphun L, Chongsuphajaisiddhi T, et al. Effects of artemisinin derivatives on malaria transmissibility. Lancet 1996;347:1654–1658.

59. Handunnetti SM, Gunewardena, Pathirana PPSL, Ekanayake K, Weerasinghe S, Mendis KN. Features of recrudescent chloroquine-resistant *Plasmodium falciparum* infections confer a survival advantage on parasites and have implications for disease control. Trans R Soc Trop Med 1996;Hyg;90:563–567.

60. Hogh B, Gamage-Mendis A, Butcher GA, Thompson R, Begtrup K, Mendis C, et al. The differing impact of chloroquine and pyrimethamine/sulfadoxine upon the infectivity of malaria species to the mosquito vector. Am J Trop Med Hyg. 1998;58(2):176–182.

61. Wernsdorfer WH, Landgraf B, Wiedermann G, Kollaritsch H. Chloroquine resistance of *Plasmodium falciparum*: a biological advantage? Trans R Soc Trop Med 1995;Hyg;89:90–91.

62. Warsame M, Wernsdorfer WH, Payne D, Björkman A. Susceptibility of *Plasmodium falciparum* in vitro to chloroquine, mefloquine, quinine and sulfadoxine/pyrimethamine in Somalia: relationships between the responses to the different drugs. Trans R Soc Trop Med 1991;Hyg;85:565–569.

63. Rathod PK, McErlean T, Lee PC. Variations in frequencies of drug resistance in *Plasmodium* falciparum. Proc Natl Acad Sci USA 1997;94:9389–9393.

64. Wilkinson RN, Noeypatimanondh S, Gould DJ. Infectivity of falciparum malaria patients for anopheline mosquitoes before and after chloroquine treatment. Trans R Soc Trop Med Hyg 1976;70:306–307.

65. Sucharit S, Surathin K, Tumrasvin W, Sucharit P. Chloroquine resistant *Plasmodium falciparum* in Thailand: susceptibility of *Anopheles*. J Med Assoc Thai 1977;60:648–654.

66. Kachur SP, Nicholas E, Jean-Francois V, Benitez A, Bloland PB, Saint Jean Y, et al. Prevalence of malaria parasitemia and accuracy of microscopic diagnosis in Haiti, October 1995. Pan Am J Public Health 1998;3:35–39.
67. Greenwood B, Marsh K, Snow R. Why do some African children develop severe malaria? Parasitology Today 1991;7:277–281.
68. White N. Antimalarial drug resistance and mortality in falciparum malaria. Trop Med Int Health 1999;4:469–470.
69. Marsh K. Malaria—a neglected disease? Parasitology 1992;104:S53–S69.
70. Zucker JR, Lackrtiz EM, Ruebush TK, Hightower AW, Adungosi JE, Were JBO, et al. Childhood mortality during and after hospitalization in western Kenya: effect of malaria treatment regimens. Am J Trop Med Hyg 1996;55:655–660.
71. Trape J-F, Pison G, Preziosi M-P, Enel C, Desgrées du Loû A, Delaunay V, et al. Impact of chloroquine resistance on malaria mortality. CR Acad Sci Paris, Sci Vie 1998;321: 689–697.
72. Hoffman SL, Masbar S, Hussein PR, Soewart A, Harun S, Marwoto HA, et al. Absence of malaria mortality in villagers with chloroquine-resistance *Plasmodium falciparum* treated with chloroquine. Trans R Soc Trop Med Hyg 1984;78:175–178;.
73. Evans DB, Hurley SF. The application of economic evaluation techniques in the health sector: the state of the art. J Int Dev 7(3):1995;503–524.
74. Goodman CA, Coleman PG, Mills AJ. Cost-effectiveness of malaria control in sub-Saharan Africa. Lancet 1999;354(9176):378–385.
75. Murray CJL, Lopez AD. The Global burden of disease: A Comprehensive Assessment of Mortality and Disability from Diseases, Injuries and Risk Factors in 1990 and Projected to 2020. Cambridge, MA: Harvard School of Public Health (on behalf of WHO and the World Bank), 1996.
76. Phillips M, Phillips-Howard PA. Economic implications of resistance to antimalarial drugs. Pharmacoeconomics 1996;10(3):225–238.
77. Sudre P, Breman JG, McFarland D, Koplan JP. Treatment of chloroquine-resistant malaria in African children: a cost-effectiveness analysis. Int J Epidemiol 1992;21(1):146–154.
78. Schapira A, Beales PF, Halloran ME. Malaria—living with drug-resistance. Parasitol Today 1993;9(5):168–174.
79. Coast J, Smith RD, Millar MR. Superbugs—should antimicrobial resistance be included as a cost in economic-evaluation. Health Econ 1996;5(3):217–226.
80. Coast J, Smith RD, Millar MR. An economic perspective on policy to reduce antimicrobial resistance. Soc Sci Med 1998;46(1):29–39.
81. Ridley RG. *Plasmodium*: drug discovery and development—an industrial perspective. Exp Parasitol, 1997;87:293–304.
82. Trouiller P, Olliaro PL. Drug development output: what proportion for tropical diseases? Lancet 1999;354(9173):164.
83. Olliaro PL, Yuthavong Y. An overview of chemotherapeutic targets for antimalarial drug discovery. Pharmacol Ther. 1999;81(2):91–110.
84. Gardner MJ The genome of the malaria parasite. Curr Opin Genet Dev 1999;9(6):704–708.
85. Melton L. From DNA to drugs. Novartis Foundation Symposium. From genome to therapy: integrating new technologies with drug development. Mol Med Today 1999;5(11):468–469.
86. White NJ, Nosten F, Looareesuwan S, Watkins WM, Marsh K, Snow RW, et al. Averting a malaria disaster. Lancet 1999;353(9168):1965–7.
87. Wongsrichanalai C, Wimonwattrawatee T, Sookto P, Laboonchai A, Heppner DG, Kyle DE, et al. In vitro sensitivity of *Plasmodium falciparum* to artesunate in Thailand. Bull WHO 1999;77:392–98.
88. Price RN, Nosten F, Luxemburger C, van Vugt M, Phaipun L, Chongsuphajaisiddhi T, White NJ. Artesunate/mefloquine treatment of multi-drug resistant falciparum malaria. Trans R Soc Trop Med Hyg 1997;91(5):574–577.

89. Price RN, Nosten F, Luxemburger C, ter Kuile FO, Paiphun L, Chongsuphajaisiddhi T, et al. Effects of artemisinin derivatives on malaria transmissibility. Lancet 1996;347(9016): 1654–1658.
90. White N. Antimalarial drug resistance and combination chemotherapy. Phil Trans R Soc London B 1999;354:739–749.

II
Established Antimalarial Drugs and Compounds Under Clinical Development

6

Chloroquine and Other Quinoline Antimalarials

Leann Tilley, Paul Loria, and Mick Foley

INTRODUCTION

In the blood stages of infections with *Plasmodium* species, the malaria parasite finds a sanctuary from the immune system within its host's erythrocytes. The mature human erythrocyte, which is essentially a "sack" of hemoglobin, provides the parasite with a ready supply of amino acids and other nutrients, but presents the parasite with certain logistical problems with respect to disposal of waste products. For example, the parasite's diet of hemoglobin leads to the production of toxic heme. The problem of heme disposal represents an "Achilles' heel" that leaves the parasite susceptible to attack by drugs, such as the quinoline antimalarials, that interfere with heme detoxification.

Quinoline-containing antimalarial drugs, such as chloroquine, quinine, and mefloquine, are vital compounds in our chemotherapeutic armory against malaria. Quinine (Fig. 1) has been used for 300 yr—ever since extracts of the bark of the *Cinchona* tree were first shown to have antimalarial activity (*see* Chapter 2 for a more detailed history). Early synthetic work in Germany produced the 8-aminoquinolines, primaquine (Fig. 1) and pamaquine. Primaquine is still used to eradicate the liver-stage hypnozoites of *P. vivax* and *P. ovale* (*see* Chapter 8). In further work, the basic side chain of pamaquine was attached to a number of heterocyclic ring systems, which led to the synthesis of the acridine derivative, quinacrine (also known as atebrine or mepacrine, Fig. 1) (*1*). During World War II, the synthetic 4-aminoquinoline, chloroquine (CQ) was introduced (Fig. 1) (*2*). Because of its low toxicity and, for many years, its effectiveness, CQ has been a mainstay in the fight against malaria ever since. As CQ resistance began to appear, massive screening programs were initiated in the United States, producing three new antimalarial drugs, a 4-aminoquinoline (amodiaquine), a quinolinemethanol (mefloquine), and a phenanthrene methanol (halofantrine) (Fig. 1). Unfortunately, resistance to each of these drugs has now been reported in many areas of the world (*see* Chapter 8) and in some areas, multidrug resistance has become such a serious problem that, for the first time in 300 yr, we are in danger of having no effective quinolines for use in the fight against malaria.

The alarming spread of malaria, particularly drug-resistant malaria, has led to an urgent need for the development of novel antimalarial drugs. This process would be greatly enhanced by a detailed molecular knowledge of the modes of action of current antimalarial drugs. Somewhat surprisingly, the precise modes of action of the quinoline antimalarials are still not completely understood. This chapter reviews the current

From: *Antimalarial Chemotherapy: Mechanisms of Action, Resistance, and New Directions in Drug Discovery*
Edited by: P. J. Rosenthal © Humana Press Inc., Totowa, NJ

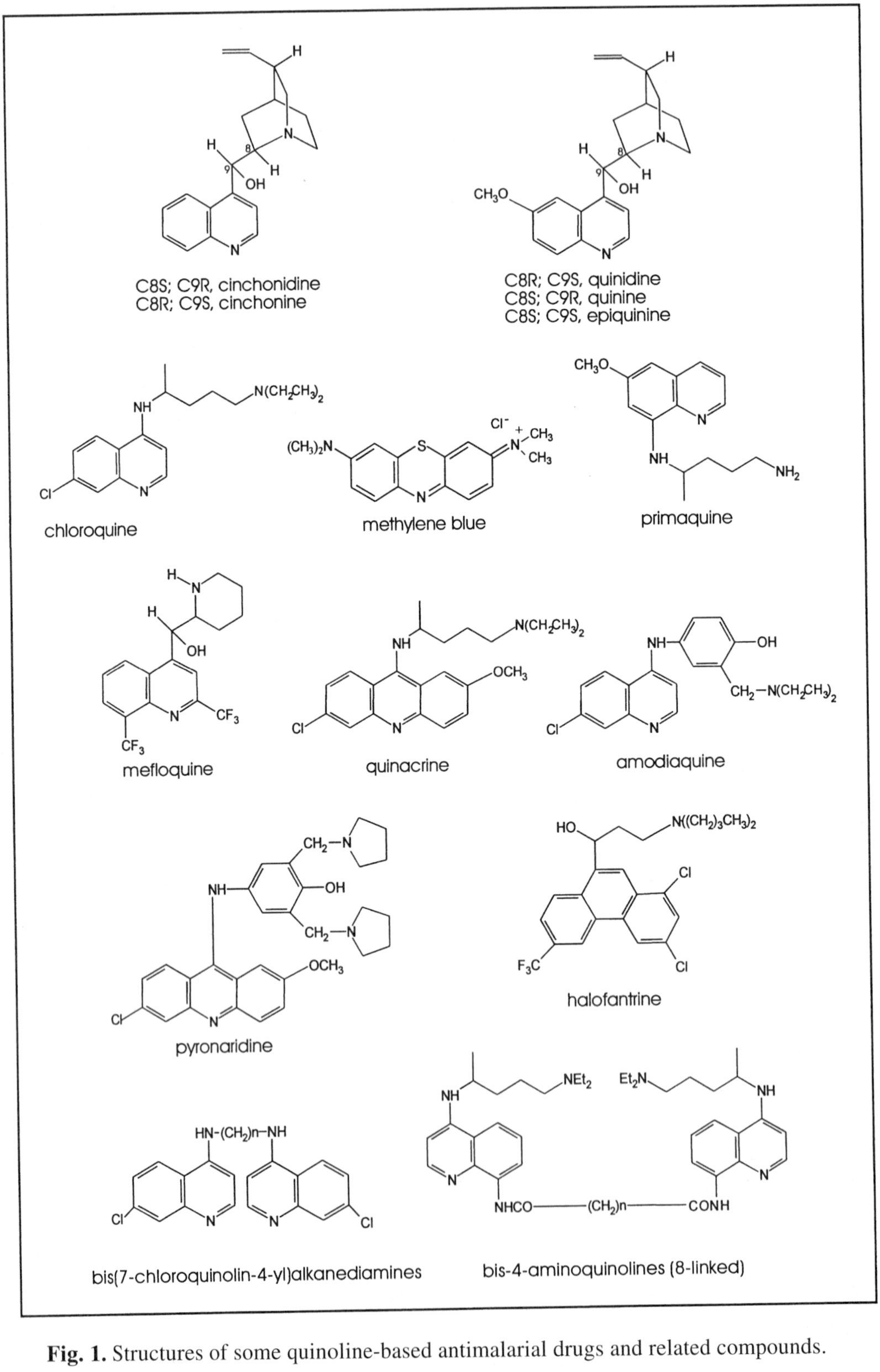

C8S; C9R, cinchonidine
C8R; C9S, cinchonine

C8R; C9S, quinidine
C8S; C9R, quinine
C8S; C9S, epiquinine

chloroquine

methylene blue

primaquine

mefloquine

quinacrine

amodiaquine

pyronaridine

halofantrine

bis(7-chloroquinolin-4-yl)alkanediamines

bis-4-aminoquinolines (8-linked)

Fig. 1. Structures of some quinoline-based antimalarial drugs and related compounds.

state of knowledge about the targets and modes of action of the quinoline drugs and examines some recent proposals that may lead to the development of improved derivatives.

MECHANISMS OF ACTION OF CQ

Site of Action of CQ Within the Parasite

Chloroquine has pharmacological effects against a wide range of cells as evidenced by the fact that, in addition to its effects on malaria, it can be used to treat a range of auto-immune diseases, including rheumatoid arthritis and systemic lupus erythematosus (see refs. *3–6* for reviews). Its wide range of activities is also indicated by the various side effects experienced when the drug is taken even at moderate doses *(7–12)* and by the fatal effects of the drug when taken as an overdose *(9,13,14)*. The multiple effects of CQ have hindered efforts to establish the molecular basis for its inhibitory activity against the malaria parasite. Early studies suggested that interactions of CQ with DNA *(15,16)*, proteases *(17,18)*, phospholipases *(19,20)*, or metabolic enzymes *(21–23)* might underlie its antimalarial potency. However, these models failed to explain the ability of CQ to kill plasmodia at a concentration three orders of magnitude lower than the concentration at which it is toxic to mammalian cells *(24,25)*.

A clue to the mechanism of action of CQ came from the observation that it is active only against the erythrocytic stages of malaria parasites. It is not active against pre-erythrocytic or hypnozoite-stage parasites in the liver *(26)*, nor against mature gametocytes *(27–29)*. Indeed, CQ acts exclusively against those stages of the intraerythrocytic cycle during which the parasite is actively degrading hemoglobin *(26)*. It has been inferred, therefore, that CQ must interfere with the feeding process. The proposal that the food vacuole is the site of CQ action is supported by ultrastructural studies. The first changes that are seen after treatment of malaria parasites with pharmacologically relevant concentrations of CQ are swelling of the parasite food vacuole and accumulation of undigested hemoglobin in endocytic vesicles *(30–33)*. Thus, the selectivity of action of quinoline drugs appears to derive from the fact that they target a parasite-specific process, namely some aspect of hemoglobin digestion.

Accumulation of CQ in the Parasite Food Vacuole: Ion Gradients or a Receptor?

Chloroquine is taken up only to a very limited extent (to concentrations about two-fold those in the plasma) by uninfected erythrocytes *(34)*. By contrast, CQ is thought to be concentrated several thousandfold inside the malaria parasite *(32,35,36)*. CQ accumulation follows a biphasic pattern, with a high-affinity, low-capacity component, which is saturated at an external CQ concentration of 20–100 nM, plus a lower-affinity, higher-capacity component operating at higher external concentrations of CQ *(37,38)*. Similar profiles of CQ uptake have been observed for isolated food vacuoles *(39)*. Three major hypotheses have been put forward to account for CQ accumulation, and debate still rages over the precise mechanism.

A number of early studies suggested that CQ accumulation is driven by an "ion-trapping" or "weak-base" mechanism *(38,40–42)*. CQ is a diprotic weak base (pK_{a_1} = 8.1, pK_{a_2} = 10.2) and according to the weak base model, an unprotonated form of CQ readily traverses the membranes of the parasitized erythrocyte and moves down the pH gradient to accumulate in the acidic food vacuole (pH 5–5.2) *(35,37,38,41,43,44)*. Once protonated, the drug becomes membrane impermeable and is trapped in the acidic compartment of the parasite. According to this weak-base model, the level of CQ accumulation depends only on the difference in pH between the external medium and the food vacuole *(24,35,37,38)*. Equation (1) *(45)* describes the relationship between the external and intravacuolar concentrations of CQ:

$$\frac{(CQ)_v}{(CQ)_0} = \frac{1 + 10^{(pK_{a_1} - pHv)} + 10^{(pK_{a_1} + pK_{a_2} - 2pHv)}}{1 + 10^{(pK_{a_1} - pHo)} + 10^{(pK_{a_1} + pK_{a_2} - 2pHO)}} \qquad (1)$$

where pH_v and $(CQ)_v$ are the pH and concentration of CQ in the food vacuole, and pH_0 and $(CQ)_0$ are the pH and concentration of CQ in the medium.

In agreement with the predictions of this model, the concentration of CQ required for 50% inhibition of parasite growth has been shown to be pH-dependent *(46)* and proton-pump inhibitors have been shown to be antagonistic to CQ action *(47,48)*. CQ uptake is an active process requiring metabolic energy *(24,37,46,47,49)*; the weak-base model assumes that this energy is required for the maintenance of the electrochemical gradient across the food vacuole membrane. Early estimates by Krogstad et al. *(24)* suggested that the weak-base effect was insufficient to account for CQ uptake. However, more recent measurements by Hawley et al. *(38)* indicated that experimentally measured levels of CQ accumulation can be adequately explained by the weak-base effect. Making certain assumptions about the vacuolar pH and volume, these authors estimated that the overall cellular accumulation ratio for CQ would be 1700-fold, if accumulation was driven solely by the weak-base effect. At an external concentration of 10 n*M*, the cellular accumulation ratio for CQ was shown to be 1800-fold *(38)*. Nonetheless, the level of accumulation has been reported to be higher in the food vacuoles of malaria-infected erythrocytes than in the acidic compartments of mammalian cells, which has been taken as evidence for additional mechanisms for uptake of quinolines in parasite-infected erythrocytes *(24)*.

Various studies have suggested that the kinetics and saturability of the high-affinity component of CQ uptake are best explained by the involvement of a specific transporter *(43,50–52)*. The existence of a CQ "permease" was first proposed by Warhurst *(53)* and recent studies have provided further support for a carrier-mediated mechanism for CQ uptake. CQ accumulation has been shown to be inhibited in a dose-dependent and competitive manner by 5-(*N*-ethyl-*N*-isopropyl)amiloride (EIPA), an inhibitor of Na^+/H^+ exchange *(54)*. The parasite has a Na^+/H^+ exchanger located on the parasite plasma membrane where it is thought to be involved in the export of protons generated during glycolysis *(55)*. It has been proposed that CQ binds to the Na^+ site on the antiporter and stimulates the Na^+/H^+ antiporter to undergo a burst of activity that transports CQ through the exchanger *(54,56)*. More recent work, however, has argued against this proposal. In a sodium-free medium that would completely disable the parasite Na^+/H^+ exchanger, CQ uptake was not altered and amiloride was still able to inhibit uptake *(57,58)*. These data argue that the plasmodial Na^+/H^+ exchanger does not play a major role in CQ uptake. Indeed, it has been suggested that the parasite relies on a V-type H^+-ATPase for pH regulation rather than a Na^+/H^+ exchanger *(59)*. Moreover, the effect of EIPA on CQ uptake may result from its weak base and heme-binding properties rather than from its effect on the Na^+/H^+ exchanger (*see* refs. *60* and *61*, for reviews). Nonetheless, it is still formally possible that alterations in ion gradients could indirectly affect CQ uptake. For example, Martiney et al. *(62)* suggested that an alteration of the activity of a membrane anion channel could indirectly affect CQ transit. Alternatively, ion channels may play a role in restoring normal cellular pH following CQ uptake *(63)*.

The other major hypothesis that has been put forward to account for the saturability of CQ accumulation is the presence of a cellular "receptor." The suggestion that free heme (ferriprotoporphyrin IX, FP) molecules in the food vacuole might act as an intravacuolar receptor for CQ was originally put forward by Chou et al. *(64)*. This suggestion initially met with little support because of the lack of evidence for a pool of FP in the parasite in a form that would be capable of binding CQ *(65)*. More recently, however, estimates of the level of detergent-soluble (i.e., unpolymerized) FP in parasitized erythrocytes have been reported. The pool of "free" FP was measured to be 100–400 nmol/mL of packed *P. falciparum*-infected erythrocytes *(66,67)*. This is sufficient to account for the high-affinity component of CQ uptake. The "FP receptor" hypothesis is strongly supported by the work of Bray et al. *(57,58)*, who have shown that treatment of infected erythrocytes with a protease inhibitor, which inhibits hemoglobin breakdown and therefore FP production, decreases the uptake of CQ.

Overall, the currently available data suggest that both ion trapping and receptor binding may contribute to CQ uptake at pharmacologically important concentrations of CQ. Whereas the difference in pH between the external and food vacuole compartments is likely to contribute to the total level of CQ uptake, the rate of uptake may be influenced by the activities of different ion channels and the saturable component of CQ uptake is probably determined by FP binding.

Degradation of Hemoglobin: An Achilles Heel?

The mature human erythrocyte contains 310–350 mg/mL hemoglobin *(68)*, which equates to a FP concentration of about 20 mM. *P. falciparum* degrades at least 75% of the erythrocyte hemoglobin during intraerythrocytic growth *(67)* to provide nutrients and to create the physical space required for its development. The intraerythrocytic parasite feeds by the endocytic uptake of hemoglobin from the host cytoplasm (Fig. 2). Hemoglobin-containing vesicles are transported to a modified secondary lysosome known as the food vacuole. The outer membrane of the endocytic vesicle fuses with that of the food vacuole and the inner membrane of the vesicle is degraded by phospholipases to release its contents *(69)*. The hemoglobin is digested by the action of a series of proteases (*see* Chapter 4 for a review). This diet of hemoglobin creates a waste-disposal problem for the parasite as each hemoglobin monomer contains a molecule of FP (Fig. 2). FP is relatively innocuous in the ferrous [Fe(II)] form within hemoglobin, but becomes toxic upon release from globin. The malaria parasite may have some heme oxygenase activity *(70–72)*. However, this appears to be a minor pathway, as measurable levels of carbon monoxide, a characteristic product of FP degradation by heme oxygenase, are not formed during growth of *P. falciparum* in vitro *(73)*. Thus, the parasite lacks the machinery for enzymic degradation of the potentially lytic FP molecules and is faced with a significant toxic-waste problem. If 75% of the 20-mM hemoglobin protomers were quantitatively converted to free FP, the cellular concentration of free FP could reach 15 mM. If this pool of free FP was concentrated within the food

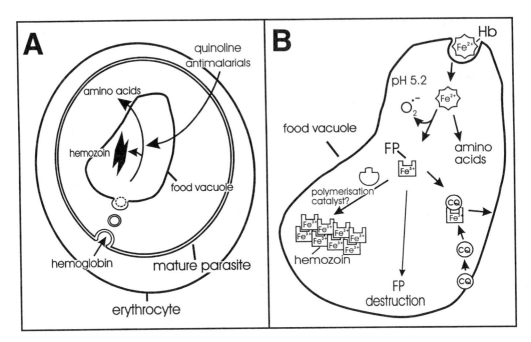

Fig. 2. The digestive process in the malaria-infected erythrocyte and the putative mode of action of CQ. **(A)** Hemoglobin degradation. Hemoglobin is taken up by a process of endocytosis and degraded by a series of proteases within the acidic food vacuole. Heme is produced as a toxic by-product. **(B)** Heme (FP) detoxification. Toxic FP moieties are polymerized into insoluble granules of hemozoin. The polymerization process may be facilitated by "heme polymerization catalysts." Alternatively, FP may be destroyed by reaction with H_2O_2 in the food vacuole or it may diffuse into the parasite cytosol where it is destroyed by reaction with GSH. CQ is proposed to bind to FP and inhibit FP polymerization and FP destruction, thereby leading to a buildup of FP molecules that is toxic to parasite proteins and membranes.

vacuole, which represents only 3–5% of the total parasite volume *(69)*, the intravacuolar FP level could reach 300–500 mM. As the cellular "free" FP in *P. falciparum*-infected erythrocytes only reaches 0.1–0.4 mM *(66,67)*, the parasite must possess a mechanism for the disposal of the released FP molecules. Nonetheless, the data suggest that the parasite is living on a "knife edge," whereby its mechanisms for detoxifying FP may only be just sufficient to prevent the toxic effects of its own metabolic waste.

A second toxic insult derives from the fact that when oxyhemoglobin is released into the food vacuole of the parasite at about pH 5, it is rapidly converted to methemoglobin *(74)*, with the concomitant production of a superoxide anion (Figs. 2B and 3A) *(75)*. At pH 5, the superoxide will spontaneously dismutate to H_2O_2 (Fig. 3A) *(76,77)*. The parasite possesses a series of oxidant defense enzymes that will protect the parasite cytoplasm. Plasmodial superoxide dismutase and glutathione peroxidase *(78–80)* have been identified and characterized and a catalase activity has also been observed *(81)*. The food vacuole will be under particular oxidative stress, although it might be partially protected by antioxidant enzymes adopted from the host along with the blood meal. Several studies have shown decreased levels of catalase and superoxide dismutase activities in malaria-infected erythrocytes compared with controls *(82–86)*, indicating

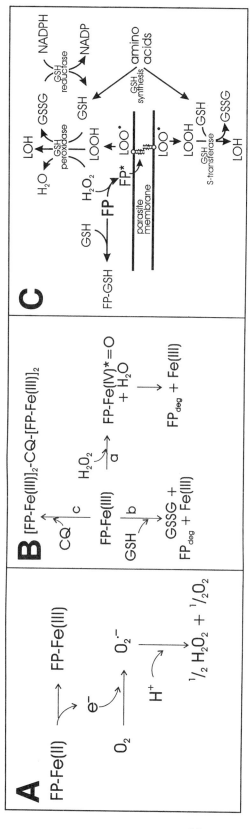

Fig. 3. **(A)** Generation of H_2O_2 in the food vacuole. In the acid conditions of the food vacuole, FP-Fe(II) in oxyhemoglobin is rapidly oxidized to the Fe(III) state with the transfer of an electron to oxygen to generate a superoxide radical. The superoxide is spontaneously converted to H_2O_2. **(B)** Putative mechanisms for FP destruction. FP can interact with H_2O_2 to form an activated intermediate that undergoes intramolecular cleavage with degradation of the porphyrin ring (FP_{deg}) [pathway a, (67,122)]. Alternatively, FP can form a complex with GSH and be destroyed by a poorly defined oxidative reaction [pathway b, (66)]. CQ can form a tight complex with FP (pathway c) which prevents FP destruction (Note: the μ-oxo dimer of FP is represented as $(FP-Fe(III))_2$). **(C)** Possible role of GSH in protection against FP-induced lipid peroxidation. The activated intermediate (FP*), formed by reaction of FP with H_2O_2, can catalyze the formation of lipid peroxides (LOOH). These lipid peroxides (and secondary lipid peroxidation products, such as aldehydes) can be destroyed by the action of GSH peroxidase or GSH transferase. Alternatively, GSH can bind FP and prevent its activation. GSH is regenerated in the parasite by the action of GSH reductase and by *de novo* GSH synthesis.

that the parasite is under substantial oxidative stress. Thus, the degradation of hemoglobin produces a heavy burden of reactive oxygen species, which leaves the parasite very susceptible to further oxidative insult *(87,88)*.

Polymerization of FP: Spontaneous or Facilitated?

The process whereby FP is detoxified in the malaria parasite has been the subject of intense study over the last few years. A prominent route for the detoxification of FP is polymerization into crystals of hemozoin, the characteristic malaria pigment (Fig. 2B). FP is present in hemozoin as a polymer of β-hematin (i.e., a noncovalent coordination complex with the ferric iron of each FP moiety chelated onto a carboxyl side chain of the adjacent moiety) *(89–92)*. The hemozoin polymer can be distinguished from other FP aggregates by its insolubility in solvents such as sodium bicarbonate, chloroform, and 2.5% sodium dodecyl sulfate (SDS) at low pH *(93)* and by its characteristic infrared spectrum *(94)*. The hemozoin accumulates in the food vacuole within the maturing parasite and is released during rupture of schizonts and finally degraded by the host *(95)*.

The molecular mechanism for the formation of hemozoin has been the subject of much controversy. A "heme-polymerizing" activity was demonstrated in preparations of insoluble material from malaria-infected erythrocytes *(94)*. It was initially proposed that this indicated the presence of a parasite-encoded enzyme that catalyzed the polymerization of FP (i.e., a "heme polymerase") (Fig. 2B) *(94,96)*. More recently, however, it has been shown that this "polymerase" activity can survive extensive boiling and protease treatments *(97,98)*. The robust nature of the activating agent is more consistent with a nonproteinaceous catalyst and, indeed, it has been proposed that the FP polymerizing activity of parasite preparations is the result of the presence of preformed FP polymers *(97,99)*. These polymers of FP are thought to act as nucleation centers, allowing the efficient addition of further FP monomers.

The presence of preformed hemozoin templates is likely to make a significant contribution to the catalysis of FP polymerization in mature-stage parasites. However, in the initial stages of FP polymerization (i.e., when a ring-stage parasite commences hemoglobin breakdown), FP sequestration must occur in the absence of preformed nucleation sites. Spontaneous formation of β-hematin polymers can be induced during incubation at elevated temperatures (e.g., 70°C) *(89,100)*; however, the rate of uncatalyzed polymerization of FP in vitro is slow under "physiological" conditions *(98,100,101)*. For example, Raynes et al. *(98)* reported that spontaneous FP polymerization (in 1-mL of a 1-mM FP preparation) occurs at a rate of less than 1 nmol/h. This is, at best, sufficient to allow polymerization of about 3% of the free FP molecules over a 24-h period and cannot account for the known efficiency of FP polymerization in vivo. These data suggest that additional polymerization-enhancing factors must facilitate the initial phase of hemozoin formation in the food vacuole.

Fitch and Chou *(102)* demonstrated heat-stable and heat-labile polymerizing activities in *P. berghei* extracts, but these activities have not been characterized at the molecular level. Bendrat et al. *(103)* proposed that specific lipid components in parasite preparations may contribute to the catalysis of FP polymerization; however, Dorn et al. *(104)* and Fitch et al. *(105)* have shown that catalytic activity of acetonitrile extracts of malarial trophozoites can be mimicked by extracts of uninfected erythrocytes or purified lipids. Other work has indicated that histidine-rich proteins may also contribute to the catalysis of FP polymerization *(106)*. HRPII and HRPIII are histidine- and alanine-rich proteins that have been shown to bind FP *(106–108)*. The repetitive hexapeptide sequence (Ala-His-His-Ala-Ala-Asp) of the HRPII protein appears to be responsible for binding FP *(109,110)*. FP is bound as a six-coordinate, low-spin *bis*-histidyl ligand *(111)*, although the extent of binding has been shown to decrease at pH values below the pKa for histidine (i.e., at less than pH 6.5) *(112)*. The role of HRPII in FP polymerization in vivo is still somewhat speculative. HRPII is located in several cellular compartments *(106,108)*, indicating that it may have functions additional to its putative role in enhancing FP polymerization. The existence of a parasite clone, 3B-D5, that lacks both HRPII and HRPIII *(113)* also argues against an essential role for these proteins in FP detoxification. The 3B-D5 clone has been shown to be CQ resistant *(113)*, which suggests that if histidine-rich proteins are involved in protection against the toxic effects of FP, there must be multiple proteins that perform the same role in *P. falciparum*. HRPIV has been suggested as a possible candidate for an additional protective histidine-rich protein *(106,114)*.

Even in the presence of lipid or histidine-rich protein catalysts, FP polymerization in vitro is rather sluggish relative to the rate at which it must occur in vivo. Our inability to reproduce efficient FP polymerization in the absence of parasite material may indicate the involvement of additional, as-yet uncharacterized, enzymic or chemical catalysts or may simply reflect our inability to reproduce experimentally the metabolic conditions that prevail in the food vacuole. Further work is still needed to completely characterize the FP polymerization process.

FP Degradation: An Alternative Means of FP Detoxification?

Recently, evidence has emerged to suggest that FP polymerization is not the only or even the major means of FP detoxification in malaria-infected erythrocytes. FP balance sheets, accounting for the fate of FP moieties liberated during hemoglobin catabolism, have been prepared. In *P. falciparum*-infected erythrocytes, about 75% of the hemoglobin molecules are digested during growth, but only about one-third of the released FP molecules are polymerized to form hemozoin *(66,67,115)*. The remaining population of FP molecules appears to be disposed of by an alternative mechanism. Similarly, for *P. berghei* in rat reticulocytes, only 20–30% of the FP appears to be sequestered into hemozoin *(116)*. The "missing" FP molecules do not appear to simply diffuse out of the cell, as the total content of iron in mature parasite-infected erythrocytes is similar to that in uninfected erythrocytes *(67)*. This suggests that the FP must be destroyed within the parasite with the release of the iron moiety. In the absence of extensive heme oxygenase activity, a nonenzymic route of FP destruction must be envisaged (Fig. 2B).

Two mechanisms have been put forward to account for the destruction of FP (Fig. 3B). Ginsburg et al. *(66)* have proposed that nonpolymerized FP exits the food vacuole and is subsequently degraded by reaction with glutathione (GSH) in the parasite cytosol. The thiol group of GSH has been shown to bind to the FP iron with an association constant of $3 \times 10^4 \ M^{-1}$ *(117)*. The reaction of FP with GSH has been studied in vitro *(66,118)* and appears to lead to the release of iron and oxidation of GSH. The molecular mechanism and the products of the reaction have not been completely characterized; however, the reaction produces oxidative radicals and is enhanced in

HEPES buffer and somewhat inhibited by the presence of protein *(66,118)*. Auto-oxidation of iron has previously been shown to produce radicals from Good's buffers, such as HEPES *(119)*, suggesting that an oxidative mechanism may be involved. A role for peroxy radicals in the mechanism of FP destruction is further indicated by the inhibitory effect of superoxide dismutase *(118)*.

A role for GSH in FP destruction is supported by studies using murine parasites. CQ-resistant *P. berghei* show reduced hemozoin production, but normal levels of hemoglobin degradation *(116)*, indicating that the resistant parasites have developed an efficient mechanism for the disposal of FP. Using NK65-derived lines that display a range of levels of CQ resistance, an inverse relationship between hemozoin content and GSH and glutathione *S*-transferase levels was observed *(120,121)*. These authors conclude that GSH of erythrocytic origin detoxifies FP within the food vacuole, although it is not clear if this could occur via GSH-mediated FP destruction, as this process occurs only very slowly at low pH *(118)*.

An alternative mechanism for FP destruction has been put forward by Loria et al. *(67)*. These authors have suggested that free FP in the food vacuole reacts with H_2O_2 that is formed during the conversion of oxyhemoglobin to methemoglobin. When the contents of an endocytic vesicle (containing 20 mM hemoglobin) are released into the food vacuole at pH 5, oxyhemoglobin undergoes spontaneous auto-oxidation with the production of a superoxide anion (Fig. 3A) *(75,76)*. At pH 5, superoxide spontaneously dismutates to H_2O_2 and the concentration of H_2O_2 may reach a transient local level of several millimolars. FP has previously been shown to react with H_2O_2 to form a ferryl intermediate with the ultimate destruction of the porphyrin ring (Fig. 3B) *(122–124)*. Loria et al. *(67)* have shown that free FP undergoes rapid peroxidative decomposition under conditions designed to resemble those found in the food vacuole (i.e., at pH 5.2), in the presence of protein.

Both the peroxidative and GSH-mediated pathways may contribute to the destruction of FP in malaria-infected erythrocytes. The relative contributions of these pathways could be determined by estimating the amount of Fe(III) in the different subcellular compartments of parasitized erythrocytes. It should be noted that the released Fe(III) is itself potentially toxic. In the presence of reducing agents such as GSH, ferric iron can be converted to the ferrous form, which can participate in pathways such as the Fenton reaction. Presumably, the parasite has developed systems for protection against the Fe(III) that is released. For example, HRPII is known to bind tightly to metal ions *(125)* and may play a role in sequestering the Fe(III) and preventing it from participating in destructive reactions.

FP Polymerization: The Target of CQ Action?

In spite of the various mechanisms that the parasite uses to detoxify FP, it is clear that the process of hemoglobin degradation, with its associated production of FP and reactive oxygen species, represents an "Achilles' heel" that leaves the parasite susceptible to attack by drugs that interfere with detoxification or enhance the toxicity of the waste products. In very early studies, Mackerras and Ercole *(126)* noted that treatment of *P. falciparum*-infected patients with quinacrine led to the production of gametocytes with reduced pigment. Later, CQ-resistant *P. berghei* were shown to produce less pigment than CQ-sensitive strains *(34,127)*. These observations suggested that the mechanism of action of CQ is connected with the process of hemozoin formation. This idea was supported by the early ultrastructural studies of Warhurst and Hockley *(31)* and Macomber and Sprinz *(30)* which showed that CQ causes morphological alterations (clumping) of pigment granules in murine parasites.

Chloroquine has been shown to form a complex with FP *(64,128–132)*. Early studies suggested a 1 : 2 stoichiometry for CQ binding to FP *(64)*. However, recent studies by Dorn et al. *(133)* confirmed the previous suggestion of Moreau et al. *(134)* that CQ forms a complex with the μ-oxo dimeric form of FP with a stoichiometry of 1 CQ : 2 μ-oxo dimers. Studies using nuclear magnetic resonance (NMR) have been taken to suggest that the interaction of CQ with FP involves π–π stacking *(134)*, although crystals of the complex have never been obtained to confirm this model. The binding constant for the FP–CQ complex is difficult to measure experimentally, because of the tendency of FP to form higher-order aggregates. This problem is exacerbated under the low-pH conditions that exist in the food vacuole, as, in the absence of protein, FP is largely insoluble at pH 5. Early studies suggested a high-affinity interaction of CQ and FP *(64)*, but recent studies by Dorn et al. *(133)*, using isothermal titration microcalorimetry to measure binding at pH 6.5, found a relatively low-association constant ($K_A = 4.0 \times 10^5 \; M^{-1}$). The strength of binding of CQ to FP may be somewhat lower again at pH 5 *(133)*. Nonetheless, given the submillimolar concentration of CQ that probably is achieved in the food vacuole *(38)*, all of the available "free" FP is likely to be in a complex with CQ.

The ability of CQ to bind to FP led Fitch *(135)* to propose that CQ acts by forming a toxic complex with free FP (Fig. 2B). The ability of CQ to interfere with FP detoxification in vitro was first demonstrated by Slater and Cerami *(94)*. They showed that the polymerization of FP was inhibited by CQ at concentrations in the high micromolar range. These data suggested a scenario whereby CQ-induced inhibition of FP polymerization leads to a buildup of toxic FP molecules and/or FP–CQ complexes within the parasite. Inhibition of FP polymerization is thus envisaged to poison the parasite with its own metabolic debris. The ability of CQ and a number of other quinoline antimalarial drugs to inhibit both spontaneous FP polymerization and parasite extract-catalyzed polymerization of FP has since been confirmed by a number of workers *(97,98,100,136)*. The mechanism of inhibition appears to involve competition for the FP substrate. Dorn et al. *(133)* found that inhibitory quinolines bind primarily to the μ-oxo dimer form of FP and proposed that this binding inhibits hemozoin formation by moving the equilibrium away from the monomeric form of FP that participates in the polymerization process. There is also evidence that CQ can cap FP polymers, thereby preventing elongation of the polymer *(137,138)*.

The idea that quinoline compounds act by inhibiting FP polymerization is supported by a number of structure–function studies. The antimalarial activities of a range of compounds have been shown to be well correlated with their abilities to inhibit FP polymerization *(98,133,139–141)*, especially if the efficiency of drug accumulation by parasites is taken into account *(142,143)*. Despite these favorable structure–activity correlations, there is still some debate as to whether FP polymerization is the primary target of quinoline action in vivo *(144)*. Some workers have shown a decrease in the amount of hemozoin formed when plasmodium-infected erythrocytes are treated with CQ *(96,115)*, but other workers *(145)* found that the inhibition of hemozoin formation was secondary to parasite killing.

FP Degradation: Another Target of CQ Action?

More recently, CQ has been shown to efficiently inhibit destruction of FP (Fig. 3B). The GSH-mediated pathway for FP destruction is inhibited by CQ, even when the FP is membrane associated *(66,115,146)*. Ginsburg et al. *(66)* have proposed that the reaction of FP with GSH occurs outside the food vacuole (FV) and that this is where CQ effects its action. By contrast, Loria et al. *(67)* have proposed that the reaction of FP with H_2O_2 occurs inside the food vacuole. This reaction is also inhibited by CQ at concentrations similar to those required to inhibit FP polymerization and well within the concentration that it is likely to be reached in the food vacuole *(67)*. Inhibition of this reaction would lead to a buildup of FP and H_2O_2. The abilities of a range of quinolines and related drugs to inhibit both GSH-mediated and H_2O_2-mediated FP destruction have been shown to correlate well with their antimalarial activities *(66,67,115,146)*. For example, the 9-aminoacridine, quinacrine, has been shown to be as efficient an inhibitor of the peroxidative destruction of FP as CQ, whereas epiquinine (Fig. 1), a quinoline compound with very low antimalarial activity, has little inhibitory effect *(67)*. Furthermore, treatment of *P. falciparum*-infected erythrocytes with CQ has been shown to lead to a buildup of membrane-associated FP within the parasite *(66,67)*. The involvement of H_2O_2 in the mechanism of action of CQ is supported by the finding that the activity of CQ against *P. falciparum* is enhanced in the presence of hydrogen peroxide *(147)*. The involvement of GSH in the mechanism of action of CQ is supported by the finding that treatment of *P. falciparum-* or *P. berghei*-infected erythrocytes with a GSH antagonist enhances CQ action *(66,120)*. Assuming that the peroxidative and GSH-mediated destruction pathways are major routes for FP destruction in the parasite, inhibition of these pathways by CQ, in combination with the inhibition of FP polymerization, could lead to an accumulation of FP moieties that would eventually overwhelm the parasite's defense mechanisms.

Oxidative Defense Mechanism: Yet Another Target of CQ Action?

A number of processes operate in the food vacuole to decompose the H_2O_2 that is produced in parasitized erythrocytes as a consequence of the conversion of oxyhemoglobin to methemoglobin. Host-derived glutathione peroxidase would have very little activity at the pH of the food vacuole *(148)*; however, catalase remains active at pH 5 *(149)* and may contribute to H_2O_2 decomposition until it is digested by vacuolar proteases. Another possible route for H_2O_2 breakdown comes from the observation that FP itself can decompose H_2O_2 via catalase-like and peroxidase-like activities *(123,124,150,151)*. This reaction occurs efficiently under the conditions of the food vacuole *(67)*. Thus, the enzyme-like activities of free FP may contribute to the detoxification of reactive oxygen species. It has been shown that CQ is an efficient inhibitor of the catalase-like and peroxidase-like activities of FP *(67,124,151)*. The formation of CQ–FP complexes in the food vacuole could prolong the half-life of any hydrogen peroxide that is produced. This buildup of H_2O_2 would exacerbate the oxidative stress caused by hemoglobin breakdown.

FP Toxicity: The Final Mediator of CQ Action?

As detailed earlier, the available evidence indicates that one of the major consequences of CQ treatment is likely to be a buildup of free FP molecules. The question remains: What is the final target of this CQ-induced accumulation of FP? Moderate FP concentrations have been shown to inhibit parasite enzymes *(18,152)*, to disrupt membrane ion gradients *(153)*, and to lyse cells *(130,154,155)*, presumably the result of the detergent-like properties of this amphipathic molecule. The direct chemical toxicity of FP, however, is greatly diminished in the presence of excess protein *(156)*. Given that the food vacuole environment is likely to be rich in intact and partially digested protein components, including the FP-binding histidine-rich proteins, free FP may not be toxic unless it reaches very high concentrations. The available estimates suggest that, even in the absence of CQ, *P. falciparum*-infected erythrocytes contain 0.1–0.4 mM unpolymerized (i.e., detergent-soluble) FP *(66,67)*. This level is approximately doubled upon treatment with CQ *(66,67)*. If this FP is localized to the food vacuole, it could reach concentrations of several millimolars even in the absence of CQ. Such a high concentration of "free" FP seems unlikely, as this would be sufficient to destroy most cellular membranes. This suggests that most of the nonpolymerized FP is probably sequestered into a nontoxic state either by aggregation at the low pH of the food vacuole or by binding to proteins. Nonetheless, toxic effects of the FP moieties may eventuate when FP builds up to a level that overwhelms the parasite's defense systems. Alternatively, the FP–CQ complex may be significantly more toxic than FP alone.

Apart from its direct detergent-like effects, FP has cytotoxic activity via a free-radical-dependent mechanism *(157)*. Free FP can catalyze the peroxidation of a wide range of substrates *(67,123,151)*. The ability of FP to intercalate into lipid bilayers allows it to catalyze the peroxidation of unsaturated lipids, which can destroy membrane integrity (Fig. 3C) *(158)*. The increased oxidative stress in parasite-infected erythrocytes is indicated by decreased levels of antioxidant defense molecules *(82–86,159)* and by the fact that they are significantly more susceptible to free-radical-mediated damage to lipids *(87,160,161)*. CQ has been shown to inhibit FP-catalyzed peroxidation of soluble substrates *(67,151)*. However, CQ enhances the ability of FP to intercalate into membranes *(67,162)* and, under some conditions, can enhance the ability of FP to catalyze lipid peroxidation *(163)* (Loria P, Tilley L, 1999, unpublished data). Thus, the buildup of CQ–FP complexes may enhance the toxicity of the reactive oxygen species produced during hemoglobin degradation. If peroxidative damage to membrane lipids or membrane-embedded proteins is the final target of CQ action, this would explain the irreversible nature of CQ activity against the parasite *(20)*.

It will be clear from the above discussion that despite significant advances in our understanding of CQ action over the last few years, the precise mechanism of parasite killing by CQ is still not completely understood. Part of the difficulty in attempts to unravel the mechanism(s) of action of CQ is the complex interplay between the malarial parasite and its erythrocytic host. It is likely that CQ inhibits parasite growth by a number of additive or synergistic effects that are difficult to reproduce in studies on parasite components. Nonetheless, it seems very likely that FP–CQ interactions provide an essential key to understanding the molecular mechanism of CQ action. This allows us to define the following characteristics as being important in the design of an active quinoline antimalarial drug. The drug should (1) show tight binding to FP, (2) be able to inhibit FP polymerization, (3) be able to inhibit FP destruction, and (4) be able to promote FP-induced membrane or protein damage. In addition, the drug needs to be able to gain ready access to FP within the parasite.

Mechanisms of CQ Resistance

The molecular basis for the development of resistance to CQ has been the subject of much scientific dispute. One interesting early observation was that quinoline drug resistance in *P. falciparum* has some parallels with multidrug resistance (MDR) in tumor cells, the most striking of which is the ability of verapamil and a number of other molecules to modulate both CQ resistance and tumor MDR *(164,165)*. MDR in tumor cells can be the result of the overexpression of an ATP-dependent drug transporter, known as P-glycoprotein *(166)* and excitement was generated when a homolog, designated *pfmdr1*, was amplified from *P. falciparum* genomic DNA *(167,168)*. Early studies suggested a correlation between the presence of specific *pfmdr1* alleles and CQ resistance *(167,168)*. A number of further studies did not support a tight correlation *(113,169)*; however, recent transfection studies demonstrate that particular *pfmdr1* alleles are responsible, at least in part, for the CQ-resistance phenotype *(170)*. Chapter 8 provides an in-depth analysis of the different mechanisms that have been put forward to account for CQ resistance. It also includes a discussion of the genetic studies indicating that proteins encoded by a region on chromosome 7 are involved in CQ resistance *(171,172)*. In this chapter, we will concentrate on those studies that may further our understanding of the mechanism of action of CQ.

Chloroquine-resistant parasites accumulate CQ in their acidic food vacuoles less efficiently than CQ-sensitive strains, suggesting that drug-resistance results, at least in part, from exclusion of the drug from the site of action rather than an alteration in the CQ target *(35,37,39)*, although a decrease in target susceptibility may also be involved *(40,42,173,174)*. A number of studies have indicated that the decreased steady-state levels of CQ are the result of a diminished level of accumulation rather than a drug export mechanism *(20,42,47,175,176)*. As detailed earlier, it appears that effective CQ action relies on efficient CQ uptake, tight binding to the μ-oxo form of FP and, eventually, FP-mediated lytic or peroxidative damage. Thus, CQ resistance could arise as a result of interference with one or more of these events. For example, changes in vacuolar conditions or the physical state and accessibility of the FP molecules could affect the uptake of CQ and the efficiency of formation of CQ–FP complexes. Alternatively, increased expression of FP-binding proteins or alterations in parasite oxidant defense mechanisms could protect the parasite against the downstream effects of CQ. In reality, it is likely that CQ resistance is a multigenic phenotype whereby several separate mutational events contribute to a decreased sensitivity to CQ.

Recent data by Bray et al. *(57)* suggests that the decreased uptake of CQ by CQ-resistant parasites is the result of an alteration in the access of CQ to free FP in the food vacuole. According to their analysis, the decreased uptake of CQ does not result from a decrease in the number of binding sites, but from a decrease in the apparent affinity of CQ for these sites. There are several possible molecular explanations for this decreased affinity. First, FP-binding proteins in the parasite food vacuole could compete with CQ for binding sites; FP-binding proteins, including the histidine-rich proteins, have been identified in plasmodia *(106,177)*. However, no candidate proteins associated with CQ resistance have yet been identified. Second, a change in the apparent affinity of CQ for FP could arise from a modified vacuolar pH *(42,47)*. For example, an increase in vacuolar pH of 0.5 units would be sufficient to decrease CQ accumulation by 10-fold

(45,175). Studies on digitonin-permeabilized infected erythrocytes did not reveal large differences in the pH of the vacuoles of CQ-sensitive and CQ-resistant parasites *(43)*, however, further studies using intact parasitized erythrocytes may be needed to detect the small pH changes that may be involved. Ursos et al. have recently reported that the pH of the food vacuole of a CQ-resistant strain of *P. falciparum* (Dd2) is lower than that of a CQ-sensitive strain (HB3). They propose that aggregation of FP in the more acid pH conditions prevents CQ binding to FP and thus decreases CQ uptake. Further studies are required to confirm this finding in other parasite strains. Third, the apparent binding affinity might decrease if the "free" FP in the food vacuole was converted to an aggregated form that bound CQ less tightly. Finally, the FP could be transferred to the parasite cytosol, where the concentration of CQ would be lower and the amount of competing FP-binding moieties higher.

Some insights into CQ action may be gained from studies of CQ-resistant strains of murine parasites. CQ-resistant *P. berghei* produces less visible pigment than CQ-sensitive strains; however, the extent of hemoglobin digestion is not decreased *(116,179)*. Thus, FP is still released at the same rate, but the parasite presumably has developed alternative CQ-insensitive mechanisms for its disposal. CQ-resistant murine parasites have been shown to have increased levels of GSH and glutathione *S*-transferase activity *(120,180)*. Moreover, buthionine sulfoximine, a specific inhibitor of glutathione synthesis, partially reverses CQ resistance and leads to a significant increase in hemozoin production *(120,121)*. This suggests that GSH plays a very important role in the development of CQ resistance in *P. berghei*.

In *P. falciparum*-infected erythrocytes, the level of hemozoin production does not appear to correlate with CQ resistance *(115)*. However, loading of parasitized erythrocytes with GSH has been shown to decrease susceptibility to CQ, whereas treatment with buthionine sulfoximine increases susceptibility to CQ *(66)*. Thus, the GSH level appears to be at least one factor that can regulate CQ resistance in *P. falciparum*. It is interesting to speculate on the multiple roles that GSH might play in producing a CQ-resistant phenotype. There is no evidence to suggest that GSH reacts with CQ and CQ resistance does not appear to be associated with drug metabolism *(181)*. However, GSH can bind FP *(117,182)* and may compete with CQ for access to FP. This could lead to a decrease in the level of CQ accumulation. Moreover, the binding of GSH to FP has been shown to protect cells against FP-mediated lysis *(182)* and against FP-catalyzed lipid peroxidation *(117)*. GSH also can bring about the direct destruction of FP molecules (*see* the subsection FP Degradation—An Alternative Means of FP Detoxification).

In addition to these enzyme-independent interactions, GSH is involved in a range of enzyme-mediated detoxification mechanisms. For example, glutathione *S*-transferase (GST) can catalyze the reaction of FP with GSH *(183,184)*. GST can also destroy lipid peroxides *(185)* and catalyze the conjugation of GSH with a variety of secondary substrates of lipid peroxidation *(186,187)*. A further beneficial effect may derive from the removal of H_2O_2 via the glutathione peroxidase reaction *(188)*. Some possible points of interaction of the GSH-mediated detoxification pathways with the pathways for FP-induced lipid damage are indicated in Fig. 3C. It is important to note that treatment with CQ does not increase flux through the hexose–monophosphate shunt *(81,189)*, as might be predicted from this scheme and that GSH reductase activity is reduced by CQ treatment *(180)*. This may result from inhibition of GSH reductase by FP or FP–CQ complexes *(190)*, which would exacerbate the toxic effects of FP. Clearly, further work is required to fully understand the interplay between FP and GSH. This may lead to the development of synergistic treatments that target both GSH metabolism and the FP detoxification pathways.

The above considerations allow us to speculate on the possible roles for Pgh-1, which has been shown to play a role in CQ resistance (*[170]*; and also the subsection Mechanisms of Resistence to the Quinolinemethanols and Chapter 8 for further details). Pgh-1 is probably not involved in direct transport of CQ (for a review, *see* ref. *178*); however, it is possible that it might control ion gradients and thus indirectly regulate the localization of CQ. Alternatively, Pgh-1 may be involved in the transport of hydrophobic toxins into the food vacuole for detoxification. Conceivably, Pgh-1 might be responsible for the retrieval of FP that has leaked out of the food vacuole, perhaps in the form of FP-GSH complexes. A mutated form of Pgh-1 may allow the FP to escape to the larger volume of the cytosol, thus decreasing the concentration of the FP below the K_D for binding to CQ. A third possibility is that Pgh-1 might be involved in protecting membranes against FP-induced damage. Enhanced transport of oxidized lipid products or complexes of these products with GSH into the food vacuole might help protect the parasite against oxidative damage. Members of the P-glycoprotein family have previously been shown to act as transporters of lipids and GSH conjugates *(191,192)*. Clearly, further work is required to test these various possibilities.

MECHANISMS OF ACTION OF OTHER QUINOLINE ANTIMALARIALS

In the face of increasing CQ resistance, a number of quinoline antimalarial drugs that are active against CQ-resistant parasites have been developed. Massive screening programs in the United States, at the end of the Second World War, produced the 4-aminoquinoline amodiaquine (*see* ref. *193*, for a review). Amodiaquine has been used as an alternative to CQ for the prophylaxis of malaria for over 40 yr. In 1963, because of problems in Vietnam with CQ-resistant malaria, the Walter Reed Army Institute for Research initiated a further large-scale screening program to identify additional antimalarial drugs. From the 300,000 compounds that were screened (*see* ref. *194* for a review), only a handful of useful drugs emerged. The most promising group of compounds were the 4-quinolinemethanols, which are structural analogs of quinine (see ref. *195* for a review). Mefloquine has proven to be effective in antimalarial chemotherapy in the field over the last 30 yr, especially against CQ-resistant strains of malaria parasites, although resistance and worries about toxicity are now limiting its use *(196,197)*. A related class of compounds to emerge from the Walter Reed screening program were compounds in which the quinoline portion of the 4-quinolinemethanols was replaced by a different aromatic ring system to form the aryl(amino)carbinols. The subclass of 9-phenanthrenemethanols showed the most promise and halofantrine (Fig. 1) has been used to treat CQ-resistant malaria *(198,199)*, although its usefulness has been restricted by reports of serious cardiotoxicity *(200)*. More recently, another aminoalcohol, benflumetol, and the azacrine-type Mannich base, pyronaridine (Fig. 1), have been introduced into the field (for a review, see ref. *201*). Although these drugs are not quinoline based, the available evidence suggest that they have similar mechanisms of action (*see* Chapter 13 for a more extensive description of these novel antimalarial drugs). In this chapter, we will concentrate on some of the quinoline-containing drugs that have been proven in the field in the hope that an analysis of the mechanisms of action of these drugs may reveal structure–function relationships that will lead to the development of novel and more active drugs.

Mechanism of Action of Other 4-Aminoquinolines

Chloroquine is a member of a general class of 4-aminoquinolines, in which the quinoline nucleus is substituted in the 4-position with a basic side chain. This class also includes amodiaquine and a number of amodiaquine derivatives *(143)*, as well as a series of novel bisquinolines (Fig. 1) *(98,202,203)* and a series of quinolines with shortened side chains *(204,205)*. These drugs probably all have a similar mechanism of action. Amodiaquine is closely related to CQ, differing only by having a *p*-hydroxyanilino aromatic ring in its side chain (Fig. 1). Amodiaquine is a more active inhibitor of the growth of *P. falciparum* in vitro than CQ *(206)*; however, amodiaquine is rapidly metabolized in vivo to its desethyl derivative *(207)*, which has a significantly reduced activity. Amodiaquine competitively inhibits CQ accumulation and vice versa, suggesting that these compounds share a similar mechanism of accumulation *(208)*. Like CQ, amodiaquine is a diprotic weak base, but the pK_a values are lower (pK_{a_1} = 7.1, pK_{a_2} = 8.1), so that amodiaquine might be expected to be accumulated less efficiently in the parasite food vacuole, on the basis of ion trapping. In fact, amodiaquine is accumulated more efficiently than CQ, indicating that uptake is enhanced by an additional mechanism *(38)*.

Amodiaquine has been shown to bind to FP *(133,143,209)* with a slightly lower affinity than CQ ($K_A = 10^5$ M^{-1} at pH 6.5). However, it inhibits FP polymerization in vitro with a similar efficiency to CQ *(133,210)*, suggesting that it also exerts its activity by interfering with FP detoxification. Amodiaquine has also been shown to inhibit hemozoin formation and cause FP accumulation in parasitized erythrocytes and to efficiently inhibit the GSH-mediated destruction of FP in vitro *(66,115)*. Mungthin et al. *(211)* showed that inhibition of hemoglobin degradation antagonizes the action of amodiaquine, further indicating a role for FP binding in the action of amodiaquine. Thus, amodiaquine and other 4-amioquinolines probably act in a manner similar to CQ.

Mechanism of Resistance to Other 4-Aminoquinolines

When amodiaquine was first introduced into the field as an alternative to CQ, it appeared to be active against CQ-resistant *P. falciparum*. Resistance to amodiaquine and its derivatives has, however, inevitably followed in the path of CQ resistance *(212)*. Furthermore, there is substantial evidence in both field and laboratory studies for cross-resistance between CQ and amodiaquine or its metabolites *(26,173,174,207)* as well as between CQ and the 9-aminoacridine quinacrine and the Mannich base pyronaridine *(213,214)*.

Some 4-aminoquinolines appear, however, to at least partially escape the CQ resistance mechanism. For examples, a series of CQ analogs with shortened side chains *(204,205)* and a series of *bis*-4-aminoquinolines *(98,202,203,215–218)* have been shown to have activity against CQ-resistant parasites. More extensive testing of these novel 4-aminoquinolines against a large number of strains of *P. falciparum* revealed a degree of cross-resistance with CQ *(203,219)*. However, these studies suggest that the CQ-resistance mechanism can be overcome, at least partially, by minimal changes in the CQ structure. In the absence of a clear understanding of the mechanism of resistance to CQ, it is difficult to predict structural features that might be associated with activity against CQ-resistant strains. However, clearly, it is essential to undertake further studies of the ability of these drugs to interact with FP. In particular, it may be useful to examine these interactions in the presence of GSH or FP-interacting proteins, such as HRPII *(106)*. This may lead to information that will be useful in the design of new 4-aminoquinolines that overcome the mechanism of CQ resistance.

Mechanism of Action of the Quinolinemethanols

The quinolinemethanol antimalarial drugs comprise a quinoline nucleus with an amino alcohol side chain. Quinine and cinchonine, and their respective stereoisomers, quinidine and cinchonidine *(see* Fig. 1*)*, were first identified as the major alkaloids of the *Cinchona* bark, and all possess antimalarial properties *(see* ref. *220* for a review). Quinine and quinidine continue to be important in the therapy of malaria *(194,221)*, either alone or in combination with antibiotic antimalarials *(222)*. Quinidine is a more potent antimalarial than quinine, but it has a higher cardiotoxicity *(194)*. The synthetic quinolinemethanol mefloquine is more active and better tolerated than quinine and is effective as a single-dose therapy *(195,196,223)*.

Mefloquine and quinine are lipophilic drugs that bind tightly to serum components, including high-density lipoproteins *(224,225)*. This may facilitate the delivery of mefloquine to the parasite, as plasmodia have been shown to accumulate lipids and other hydrophobic molecules from the serum *(226,227)*. Mefloquine also binds with high affinity to membranes *(228)* and uninfected erythrocytes *(229,230)*, equilibrating between saline solution and erythrocyte membranes with a partition coefficient of 60 *(224,229)*. High-affinity binding to erythrocytes and other cells may provide a reservoir of mefloquine and contribute to the very long half-life of mefloquine in the body *(225,231)*.

Mefloquine and quinine competitively inhibit CQ accumulation, suggesting that these compounds share a similar mechanism of accumulation *(231,232)*, although, unlike CQ, quinine action is not inhibited by proton-pump inhibitors *(48)*. Moreover, mefloquine and quinine are much weaker bases than CQ. Mefloquine has a pK_{a_1} value below 2 and a pK_{a_2} value of 8.6 *(224,233)*, whereas quinine has a pK_{a_1} value of approx 4.2 *(234)* and a pK_{a_2} value of 8.2–8.5 *(224,234)*. The quinolinemethanols will, therefore, be monoprotonated under physiological conditions. According to Eq. (1), the quinolinemethanols will be concentrated in the food vacuole only about 200-fold *(35,41)*. Despite this, mefloquine is a more potent inhibitor than CQ of the growth of drug-sensitive strains of *P. falciparum (235–237)*. One possible explanation for this apparent discrepancy is that the uptake of the quinolinemethanols is enhanced by the action of a specific transport system *(225,232)*. Quantitative studies on the uptake of quinine and mefloquine by parasitized erythrocytes are complicated by the hydrophobic nature of these drugs, but available estimates indicate that quinolinemethanols are accumulated much less efficiently than CQ *(49)*. A second alternative is that the quinolinemethanols may act on a different molecular target to CQ. This suggestion is supported by the finding that mefloquine and quinine are antagonistic in action with CQ *(48,238)*.

Like CQ, the quinolinemethanols act primarily on the intraerythrocytic asexual stages of the parasite *(239–241)*. Ultrastructural studies indicate that mefloquine causes morphological changes in the food vacuole of *P. falciparum*. The changes resemble the alterations observed after CQ treatment, except that mefloquine appears to cause degranulation of hemozoin rather than the clumping of pigment observed in murine parasites treated with CQ *(236,242,243)*. Blocking FP release with a protease inhibitor has been shown to be antagonistic to mefloquine action, as it is to CQ action *(138,211)*. These finding have led some authors to suggest that the mechanism of action of the quinolinemethanols may be similar to that of CQ *(see* refs. *138* and *210* for reviews). However, although evidence that FP interactions underpin the mode of action of the 4-aminoquinolines is quite compelling, it is not clear that FP is the only or even the major target for the antimalarial action of the quinolinemethanols.

Mefloquine interacts only weakly with free FP, with a recently reported K_A value of $1.2 \times 10^4 \ M^{-1}$ at pH 6.5 *(133)*. Mefloquine inhibits FP polymerization in vitro, with an efficiency that is similar to or somewhat less than that of CQ *(98,133,136)*, although mefloquine has been reported to cap FP polymers with a higher efficiency than CQ *(138)*. High concentrations of mefloquine are reported to inhibit hemozoin formation in *P. falciparum*-infected erythrocytes in vitro *(115)*; however, treatment of *P. berghei*-infected mice with mefloquine and quinine had no effect on hemozoin production *(136)*. Mefloquine has also been shown to be a less potent inhibitor than CQ of the peroxidative destruction of FP *(67)* and GSH-mediated FP destruction *(66)*, especially for membrane-associated FP *(115)*. Furthermore, mefloquine does not enhance FP-catalyzed lipid peroxidation to the same extent as CQ *(163)* and has been shown to interfere with the ability of CQ to enhance FP-induced cell lysis *(244)*.

The available data suggest, therefore, that mefloquine may interfere with a different step in the parasite feeding process than that inhibited by CQ *(241)*. Desneves et al. *(225)* used the technique of photoaffinity labeling to identify two high-affinity mefloquine-binding proteins with apparent molecular masses of 22–23 kDa and 36 kDa in *P. falciparum*-infected erythrocytes. The identities of these proteins have not yet been established, but they may be involved in mefloquine uptake or action. There is also increasing evidence to suggest a role for the plasmodial P-glycoprotein (Pgh-1) in mefloquine resistance (see the next subsection and Chapter 8). This raises the possibility that Pgh-1 may be the target of action of mefloquine.

Quinine also interacts rather weakly with FP ($K_A = 2.1 \times 10^4 \ M^{-1}$ at pH 6.5) *(133)* and inhibits FP polymerization with a similar efficiency to mefloquine *(102,136)*. Quinine is less effective than CQ as an inhibitor of FP catalase-like and peroxidase-like activities *(124,151)*, and it is only a weak inhibitor of GSH-mediated FP destruction *(115)*. In the absence of a specific transporter, quinine is likely to be accumulated less efficiently in the food vacuole than CQ. These data indicate that the mechanism of uptake and action of quinine may be similar to that of mefloquine, and rather different to that of CQ.

Mechanisms of Resistance to the Quinolinemethanols

The first reports of decreased sensitivity to quinine occurred in Brazil as early as 1910 (*see* refs. *212* and *245*). However, as quinine has been used much less extensively than CQ, it has retained its efficacy in the field much longer *(246)*. Nonetheless, reports of quinine resistance are increasing *(247)* and efficacy with quinine treatment has fallen below 50% in some parts of Southeast Asia, where quinine has been used to treat CQ-resistant parasites *(248)*. Resistance to mefloquine has been rising inexorably ever since this drug was introduced in the 1970s *(249–252)*. A detailed analysis of the clinical and molecular aspects of quinolinemethanol resistance are given in Chapters 5 and 8. Here, we will concentrate only on those aspects that may shed some light on the mechanism of action of the quinolinemethanols.

Like CQ resistance, mefloquine resistance appears to have parallels with the MDR of tumor cells. Resistance to mefloquine is not reversed by verapamil or chlorpromazine, but it can be reversed by penfluridol *(253,254)*. In field isolates of *P. falciparum*, mefloquine resistance is associated with an amplification of the *pfmdr1* gene *(169,237,255)* and overexpression of its protein product, the P-glycoprotein homolog, Pgh-1 *(237)*. Moreover, selection for mefloquine resistance in vitro leads to an amplification and overexpression of the *pfmdr1* gene *(237,256,257)*. Pgh-1 is partially localized in the membrane of the parasite food vacuole *(258)*, which is consistent with a direct role in drug transport, and recent transfection studies confirm that the presence of particular *pfmdr1* alleles is associated with increased mefloquine resistance *(170)*. Resistance to halofantrine and quinine also increases during selection for mefloquine resistance, suggesting a similar underlying mechanism *(237,255,257)*. It is likely, however, that mefloquine resistance can arise by more than one mechanism, as some strains of *P. falciparum* have been found to become mefloquine resistant without an amplification or alteration of the *pfmdr1* gene *(259,260)*.

Mefloquine has been shown to interact with high affinity with human P-glycoprotein *(261)*. This may explain the neurotoxic side effects of this drug *(261)* and indicates that the quinolinemethanols may be good substrates for P-glycoprotein transporters. However, the precise mechanism by which *pfmdr1* might mediate mefloquine (MQ) resistance is still not clear. Pgh-1 is located mainly on the food vacuole membrane *(262)* and is oriented with its nucleotide-binding domain exposed to the parasite cytoplasm *(262)*, which suggests pumping of substrates into the food vacuole rather than out. An increase in copy number would result in an increased transport of mefloquine into the food vacuole. If the target of mefloquine is in the food vacuole, this increased transport would be expected to increase rather than decrease the sensitivity of the parasite to mefloquine. This argument suggests that the site of quinolinemethanol action is outside the food vacuole or within the food vacuole membrane itself. One possibility is that Pgh-1 itself is the target of action of the quinolinemethanols. If, as suggested in the subsection Mechanisms of CQ Resistance, Pgh-1 is involved in the detoxification of FP by transporting FP–GSH complexes into the food vacuole, MQ might interfere with this process. Overexpression of Pgh-1 might, however, allow it to function even in the presence of mefloquine. By contrast, if the lumen of the food vacuole is the major site of CQ uptake and action, increased expression of Pgh-1, and thus transport of FP into the food vacuole lumen, would be expected to enhance CQ sensitivity, as indeed has been observed *(167)*.

FUTURE DIRECTIONS

From the above discussion, it will be clear that the studies of the past decade have given a glimpse of the molecular basis of quinoline drug action, although the details are still somewhat murky. If the components involved in the action of the quinoline antimalarials could be identified and fully characterized, a functional approach to the design of novel antimalarials would become a possibility. If, for example, tight binding to FP was confirmed as an essential component of quinoline drug action, it should be possible to set up rapid and inexpensive assays of FP binding in vitro, that could be used in the search for potential new chemotherapeutic reagents. The assays for peroxidative and GSH-mediated FP degradation are very simple to perform and could easily be adapted to high-throughput screening. If it can be shown that the level of FP–quinoline interaction in vivo depends on competition with FP-binding proteins or GSH, then binding or activity assays should be set up in the presence of these components. These assays might decrease the need for costly empirical searches for new antimalarial drugs (*see* ref. *263* for a review).

The belief that FP detoxification processes play an important role in CQ action has already led to the identification of a number of potential new antimalarial compounds. Two series of aminoquinolines with different substituents *(264,265)*, several series of novel bisquinolines *(98,203,266)*, a series of FP analogs *(139,267)*, a series of xanthones *(268)*, a novel class of multidentate metal coordination complexes *(141)*, a series of 8-aminoquinolines *(269)*, as well as the original synthetic antimalarial drug, methylene blue, and derivatives *(140)* have all been shown to have antimalarial activities that at least are partially correlated with their abilities to inhibit FP polymerization. Moreover, recent evidence suggests that artemisinin also exerts its antimalarial activity by a similar mechanism to CQ *(270)*. The suggestion that a large number of the antimalarial drugs in our armory target a single metabolic pathway is somewhat disconcerting. However, available evidence suggests that although the modes of action of these drugs may be related, the mechanisms of resistance may be quite distinct. Thus, further analysis of the FP detoxification processes may point to further useful compounds that are active against CQ-resistant parasites.

A knowledge of the mechanism of quinoline drug resistance would also facilitate the design of drugs or drug combinations that overcome the resistance mechanism. If it can be shown that GSH-dependent pathways are important in the mechanism of CQ resistance, then enzymes involved in GSH synthesis and metabolism should be targeted. In this regard, it is useful to note that the genes for GSH reductase *(271,272)* and a related thioredoxin reductase *(273–275)*, as well as γ-glutamylcysteine synthetase *(276)* and GSH peroxidase *(80)* have already been identified. Of these, glutathione reductase (PfGR) appears to be a likely candidate for a novel antimalarial drug target. The parasite enzyme is distinguished from other glutathione reductase enzymes by the presence of a 34-amino-acid insertion between the flavin-adenine dinucleotide (FAD)-binding motif and the the conserved H8 helix, which could modulate the enzyme activity *(271)*. A functional recombinant version of PfGR has been produced and shown to be preferentially sensitive to methylene blue *(277)*. Interestingly, methylene blue (Fig. 1) has a basic side arm and was the precursor for the development of the synthetic quinoline antimalarials (*see* ref. *178* for a review). It inhibits FP polymerization and has been proposed to exert its antimalarial activity, in part, by an effect on FP detoxification

(140). This leads to the intriguing suggestion that commonly used quinoline anti-malarials might be enhanced by combination with drugs that inhibit PfGR.

Inevitably, given time and sufficient exposure to sublethal doses, the malaria parasite almost certainly will evolve the means to defeat any new chemotherapeutic strategy that can be devised. It is hoped that, eventually, an effective malaria vaccine will be available to help in the fight against the disease, although this still seems some way off. Meanwhile, it is essential that we keep one step ahead of the parasite—a task that will be greatly facilitated by our increasing understanding of the molecular mechanisms involved in drug action and resistance.

NOTES ADDED IN PROOF

1. The recent work of Pagola et al. *(92)* indicates that the crystals are composed of dimers linked through reciprocal iron-carboxylate bonds rather than true polymers, however the commonly used term, FP polymer, is retained throughout this review.
2. Usros et al. *(278)* have recently reported that the pH of the food vacuole of a CQ resistant strain of *P. falciparum* (Ddz) is lower than that of a CQ sensitive strain (HB3). They propose that aggregation o f FP in the more acid pH conditions prevents CQ binding to FP and thus decreases CQ uptake. Further studies are required to confirm this finding in other parasite strains.

ACKNOWLEDGMENTS

We are very grateful to Professor Hagai Ginsburg, Hebrew University of Jerusalem, Israel, Dr. Patrick Bray, The University of Liverpool, Liverpool, UK, and Dr. Katja Becker and Dr. Heiner Schirmer, Heidelberg University, Germany, for discussions and insightful input.

REFERENCES

1. Coatney GR. Pitfalls in a discovery: the chronicle of chloroquine. Am J Trop Med Hyg 1963;12:121–128.
2. Loeb RF, Clarke WM, Coateney GR, Coggeshall LT, Dieuaide FR, Dochez AR, et al. Activity of a new antimalarial agent, chloroquine (SN 7618). J Am Med Assoc 1946;130:1069–1070.
3. Davis MJ, Woolf AD. Role of antimalarials in rheumatoid arthritis—the British experience. Lupus 1996;(5 Suppl 1):S37–S40.
4. Khraishi MM, Singh, G. The role of anti-malarials in rheumatoid arthritis—the American experience. Lupus 1996;(5 Suppl 1):S41–S44.
5. Meinâo IM, Sato EI, Andrade LE, Ferraz MB, Atra E. Controlled trial with chloroquine diphosphate in systemic lupus erythematosus Lupus 1996;5:237–241.
6. Wallace DJ. The use of chloroquine and hydroxychloroquine for non-infectious conditions other than rheumatoid arthritis or lupus: a critical review. Lupus 1996;5:S59–S64.
7. Bernstein HN. Ophthalmologic considerations and testing in patients receiving long-term antimalarial therapy. Am J Med 1983;75:25–34.
8. Olatunde A, Obih PO. Use and misuse of 4-aminoquinoline antimalarials in tropical Africa and re-examination of itch reaction to these drugs. Trop Doct 1981;11:97–101.
9. Good MI, Shader RI. Lethality and behavioral side effects of chloroquine. J Clin Psychopharmacol 1982;2:40–47.
10. Fries JF, Williams CA, Ramey DR, Bloch DA. The relative toxicity of alternative therapies for rheumatoid arthritis: implications for the therapeutic progression. Semin Arthritis Rheum 1993;23:68–73.

11. Luzzi GA, Peto TE. Adverse effects of antimalarials. An update. Drug Safety 1993;8:295–311.
12. Baguet JP, Tremel F, Fabre M. Chloroquine cardiomyopathy with conduction disorders. Heart 1999;81:221–223.
13. Kelly JC, Wasserman GS, Bernard WD, Schultz C, Knapp J. Chloroquine poisoning in a child. Ann Emerg Med 1990;19:47–50.
14. Keller T, Schneider A, Lamprecht R, Aderjan R, Tutsch-Bauer E, Kisser W. Fatal chloroquine intoxication. Forensic Sci Int 1998;96:21–28.
15. Cohen SN, Yielding, K. Spectrophotometric studies of the interaction of chloroquine with deoxyribonucleic acid. J Biol Chem 1965;240:3123–3131.
16. Ciak J, Hahn FE. Chloroquine: mode of action. Science 1966;151:347–349.
17. Levy MR, Siddiqui WA, Chou SC. Acid protease activity in *Plasmodium falciparum* and *P knowlesi* and ghosts of their respective host red cells. Nature 1974;247:546–549.
18. Vander Jagt DL, Hunsaker LA, Campos NM. Characterisation of haemoglobin degrading, low molecular weight protease from *Plasmodium falciparum*. Mol Biochem Parasitol 1986;18:389–400.
19. Naor Z, Catt KJ. Mechanism of action of gonadotropin-releasing hormone. Involvement of phospholipid turnover in luteinizing hormone release. J Biol Chem 1981;256:2226–2229.
20. Ginsburg H, Krugliak M. Quinoline-containing antimalarials mode of action: drug resistance and its reversal. Biochem Pharmacol 1992;43:63–70.
21. Foley M, Deady LW, Ng K, Cowman AF, Tilley L. Photoaffinity labeling of chloroquine-binding proteins in *Plasmodium falciparum*. J Biol Chem 1994;269:6955–6961.
22. Menting, J.G.T, Tilley L, Deady LW, Ng K, Cowman AF, Foley M. The antimalarial drug, chloroquine, interacts specifically with lactate dehydrogenase from *Plasmodium falciparum*. Mol Biochem Parasitol 1997;88:215–224.
23. Read JA, Wilkinson KW, Tranter R, Sessions RB, Brady RL Chloroquine binds in the cofactor binding site of *Plasmodium falciparum* lactate dehydrogenase. J Biol Chem 1999;274:10,213–10,218.
24. Krogstad DJ, Gluzman IY, Herwaldt BL, Schlesinger PH, Wellems TE. Energy dependence of chloroquine accumulation and chloroquine efflux in *Plasmodium falciparum*. Biochem Pharmacol 1992;43:57–62.
25. van Es, H.H.G, Karcz S, Chu F, Cowman AF, Vidal S, Gros P, et al. Expression of the plasmodial *pfmdr1* gene in mammalian cells is associated with increased susceptibility to chloroquine. Molec Cell Biol 1994;14:2419–2428.
26. Peters W. (ed.) Chemotherapy and Drug Resistance in Malaria. London: Academic, 1970.
27. Langreth SG, Nguyen-Dinh P, Trager W. *Plasmodium falciparum*: merozoite invasion *in vitro* in the presence of chloroquine. Exp Parasitol 1978;46:235–238.
28. Sinden RE. Gametocytogenesis of *Plasmodium falciparum in vitro:* ultrastructural observations on the lethal action of chloroquine. Ann Trop Med Parasitol 1982;76:15–23.
29. Zhang Y, Asante KS, Jung A. Stage-dependent inhibition of chloroquine on *Plasmodium falciparum in vitro*. J Parasitol 1986;72:830–836.
30. Macomber PB, Sprinz H. Morphological effects of chloroquine on *Plasmodium berghei* in mice. Nature 1967;214:937–939.
31. Warhurst DC, Hockley DJ. Mode of action of chloroquine on *Plasmodium berghei* and *P. cynomolgi*. Nature 1967;214:935–936.
32. Aikawa, M. High-resolution autoradiography of malarial parasites treated with ^{3}H-chloroquine. Am J Pathol 1972;67:277–284.
33. El-Shoura SM. Falciparum malaria in naturally infected human patients: VIII. Fine structure of intraerythrocytic asexual forms before and during chloroquine treatment. Appl Parasitol 1994;35:207–218.
34. Macomber PB, O'Brien RL, Hahn FE. Chloroquine: physiological basis of drug resistance in *Plasmodium berghei*. Science 1966;152:1374–1375.

35. Yayon A, Cabantchik ZI, Ginsburg H. Identification of the acidic compartment of *Plasmodium falciparum*-infected human erythrocytes as the target of the antimalarial drug chloroquine EMBO J 1984;3:2695–2700.
36. De Duve C, De Barsy T, Poole B, Trouet A, Tulkens P, Van Hoof F. Lysosomotrophic agents. Biochem Pharmacol 1974;23:2495–2531.
37. Fitch CD, Yunis NG, Chevli R, Gonzales Y. High-affinity accumulation of chloroquine by mouse erythrocytes infected with *Plasmodium berghei* J Clin Invest 1974; 54:24–33.
38. Hawley S, Bray P, Park K, Ward S. Amodiaquine accumulation in *Plasmodium falciparum* as a possible explanation for its superior antimalarial activity over chloroquine. Mol Biochem Parasitol 1996;80:15–25.
39. Saliba KJ, Folb PI, Smith PJ. Role for the *Plasmodium falciparum* digestive vacuole in chloroquine resistance. Biochem Pharmacol 1998;56:313–320.
40. Geary TG, Jensen JB, Ginsburg H. Uptake of [^{3}H]chloroquine by drug-sensitive and -resistant strains of the human malaria parasite *Plasmodium falciparum* Biochem Pharmacol 1986;35:3805–3812.
41. Ginsburg H, Nissani E, Krugliak, M. Alkalinisation of the food vacuole of malaria parasites by quinoline drugs and alkylamines is not correlated with their antimalarial activity. Biochem Pharmacol 1989;38:2645–2654.
42. Geary TG, Divo AD, Jensen JB, Zangwill M, Ginsburg H. Kinetic modelling of the response of *Plasmodium falciparum* to chloroquine and its experimental testing *in vitro*. Implications for mechanism of action of and resistance to the drug. Biochem Pharmacol 1990;40:685–691.
43. Krogstad DJ, Schlesinger PH, Gluzman IY. Antimalarials increase vesicle pH in *Plasmodium falciparum*. J Cell Biol 1985;101:2301–2309.
44. Veignie E, Moreau S. The mode of action of chloroquine. Non-weak base properties of 4-aminoquinolines and antimalarial effects on strains of *Plasmodium*. Ann Trop Med Parasitol 1991;85:229–237.
45. Krogstad DJ, Schlesinger PH. A perspective on antimalarial action: effects of weak bases on *Plasmodium falciparum*. Biochem Pharmacol 1986;35:547–552.
46. Yayon A, Cabantchik ZI, Ginsburg, H. Susceptibility of human malaria parasites to chloroquine is pH dependent Proc Natl Acad Sci USA 1985;82:2784–2788.
47. Bray PG, Howells RE, Ward SA. Vacuolar acidification and chloroquine sensitivity in *Plasmodium falciparum*. Biochem Pharmacol 1992;43:1219–1227.
48. Skinner-Adams T, Davis TM. Synergistic *in vitro* antimalarial activity of omeprazole and quinine. Antimicrob Agents Chemother 1999;43:1304–1306.
49. Polet H, Barr CF. Chloroquine and dihydroquinine. *In vitro* studies of their antimalarial effect upon *Plasmodium knowlesi*. J Pharmacol Exp Ther 1968;164:380–386.
50. Schlesinger PH, Krogstad DJ, Herwaldt BL. Antimalarial agents: mechanisms of action. Antimicrob Agents Chemother 1988;32:793–798.
51. Ferrari V, Cutler DJ. Simulation of kinetic data on the influx and efflux of chloroquine by erythrocytes infected with *Plasmodium falciparum*. Evidence for a drug-importer in chloroquine-sensitive strains. Biochem Pharmacol 1991;42:S167–S179.
52. Ferrari V, Cutler DJ. Kinetics and thermodynamics of chloroquine and hydroxychloroquine transport across the human erythrocyte membrane. Biochem Pharmacol 1991;41:23–30.
53. Warhurst DC. Antimalarial schizontocides: why a permease is necessary. Parasitol Today 1986;4:211–213.
54. Sanchez CP, Wunsch S, Lanzer, M. Identification of a chloroquine importer in *Plasmodium falciparum* Differences in import kinetics are genetically linked with the chloroquine-resistant phenotype. J Biol Chem 1997;272:2652–2658.

55. Bosia A, Ghigo D, Turrini F, Nissani E, Pescarmona GP, Ginsburg H. Kinetic characterization of Na+/H+ antiport of *Plasmodium falciparum* membrane. J Cell Physiol 1993;154:527–534.

56. Wunsch S, Sanchez CP, Gekle M, Grosse-Wortmann L, Wiesner J, Lanzer M. Differential stimulation of the Na+/H+ exchanger determines chloroquine uptake in *Plasmodium falciparum* J Cell Biol 1998;140:335–334.

57. Bray PG, Mungthin M, Ridley RG, Ward SA. Access to hematin: the basis of chloroquine resistance. Mol Pharmacol 1998;54:170–179.

58. Bray PG, Janneh O, Raynes KJ, Mungthin M, Ginsburg H, Ward SA. Cellular uptake of chloroquine is dependent on binding to ferriprotoporphyrin IX and is independent of NHE activity in *Plasmodium falciparum*. J Cell Biol 1999;145:363–376.

59. Saliba KJ, Kirk, K. pH regulation in the intracellular malaria parasite, *Plasmodium falciparum*. H(+) extrusion via a v-type H+-ATPase. J Biol Chem 1999;274:33,213–33,219.

60. Raynes KJ, Bray PG, Ward SA. Altered binding of chloroquine to ferriprotoporphyrin IX is the basis for chloroquine resistance. Drug Res Updates 1999;2:97–103.

61. Bray PG, Ward SA, Ginsburg H. Na+/H+ antiporter, chloroquine uptake and drug resistance. Parasitol Today 1999;15:360–363.

62. Martiney JA, Cerami A, Slater AF. Verapamil reversal of chloroquine resistance in the malaria parasite *Plasmodium falciparum* is specific for resistant parasites and independent of the weak base effect. J Biol Chem 1995;270:22,393–22,398.

63. Ridley RG. Malaria: dissecting chloroquine resistance. Curr Biol 8:1998;R346–R349.

64. Chou AC, Chevli R, Fitch CD. Ferriprotoporphyrin IX fulfills the criteria for identification as the chloroquine receptor of malaria parasites. Biochemistry 1980;19:1543–1549.

65. Ginsburg H, Geary TG. Current concepts and new ideas on the mechanism of action of quinoline-containing antimalarials. Biochem Pharmacol 1987;36:1567–1576.

66. Ginsburg H, Famin O, Zhang J, Krugliak M. Inhibition of glutathione-dependent degradation of heme by chloroquine and amodiaquine as a possible basis for their antimalarial mode of action. Biochem Pharmacol 1998;56:1305–1313.

67. Loria P, Miller S, Foley M, Tilley L. Inhibition of the peroxidative degradation of haem as the basis of action of chloroquine and other quinoline antimalarials. Biochem J 1999;339:363–370.

68. Hellerstein S, Spees W, Surapathana LO. Hemoglobin concentration and erythrocyte cation content. J Lab Clin Med 1970;76:10–24.

69. Yayon A, Timberg R, Friedman S, Ginsburg H. Effects of chloroquine on the feeding mechanism of the intraerythrocytic human malarial parasite *Plasmodium falciparum*. J Protozool 1984;31:367–372.

70. Srivastava P, Pandey VC. Heme oxygenase and related indices in chloroquine-resistant and -sensitive strains of *Plasmodium berghei*. Int J Parasitol 1995;25:1061–1064.

71. Srivastava P, Pandey VC, Misra AP, Gupta P, Raj K, Bhaduri AP. Potential inhibitors of plasmodial heme oxygenase; an innovative approach for combating chloroquine resistant malaria. Bioorg Med Chem 1998;6:181–187.

72. Srivastava P, Pandey VC, Bhaduri AP. Evaluation of resistant-reversal, CDRI compound 87/209 and its possible mode of action in rodent experimental malaria. Trop Med Parasitol 1995;46:83–87.

73. Eckman JR, Modler S, Eaton JW, Berger E, Engel RR. Host heme catabolism in drug-sensitive and drug-resistant malaria. J Lab Clin Med 1977;90:767–770.

74. Wallace WJ, Houtchens RA, Maxwell JC, Caughey WS. Mechanism of autooxidation for hemoglobins and myoglobins. Promotion of superoxide production by protons and anions J Biol Chem 1982;257:4966–4977.

75. Carrell RW, Winterbourn CC, Rachmilewitz EA. Activated oxygen and haemolysis. Br J Haematol 1975;30:259–264.

76. Atamna, H, Ginsburg H. Origin of reactive oxygen species in erythrocytes infected with *Plasmodium falciparum* Mol Biochem Parasitol 1993;61:231–241.

77. Har-El R, Marva E, Chevion, M, Golenser J. Is hemin responsible for the susceptibility of Plasmodia to oxidant stress? Free Radic Res Commun 1993;18:279–290.

78. Fridovich I. Biological effects of the superoxide radical. Arch Biochem Biophys 1986;247:1–11.

79. Fairfield AS, Abosch A, Ranz A, Eaton JW, Meshnick SR. Oxidant defense enzymes of *Plasmodium falciparum* Mol Biochem Parasitol 1988;30:77–82.

80. GamainGamain B, Langsley G, Fourmaux MN, Touzel JP, Camus D, Dive, D, et al. Molecular characterization of the glutathione peroxidase gene of the human malaria parasite *Plasmodium falciparum*. Mol Biochem Parasitol 1996;78:237–248.

81. Atamna H, Pescarmona G, Ginsburg H. Hexose-monophosphate shunt activity in intact *Plasmodium falciparum*-infected erythrocytes and in free parasites. Mol Biochem Parasitol 1994;67:79–89.

82. Mohan K, Ganguly NK, Dubey ML, Mahajan RC. Oxidative damage of erythrocytes infected with *Plasmodium falciparum*. An *in vitro* study. Ann Hematol 1992;65:131–134.

83. Mohan K, Dubey ML, Ganguly NK, Mahajan RC. *Plasmodium falciparum* induced perturbations of the erythrocyte antioxidant system. Clin Chim Acta 1992;209:19–26.

84. Areekul S, Boonme Y. Superoxide dismutase and catalase activities in red cells of patients with *Plasmodium falciparum*. J Med Assoc Thai 1987;70:127–131.

85. Mathews ST, Selvam R. Effect of radical treatment on erythrocyte lipid peroxidation in *Plasmodium vivax*-infected malaria patients. Biochem Int 1991;25:211–220.

86. Srivastava P, Puri SK, Dutta GP, Pandey VC. Status of oxidative stress and antioxidant defences during *Plasmodium knowlesi* infection and chloroquine treatment in *Macaca mulatta*. Int J Parasitol 1992;22:243–245.

87. Stocker R, Hunt NH, Buffinton GD, Weidemann MJ, Lewis-Hughes PH, Clark IA. Oxidative stress and protective mechanisms in erythrocytes in relation to *Plasmodium vinckei* load. Proc Natl Acad Sci USA 1985;82:548–551.

88. Hunt NH, Stocker R. Oxidative stress and the redox status of malaria-infected erythrocytes. Blood Cells 1990;16:499–526.

89. Slater, A.F.G, Swiggard WJ, Orton BR, Flitter WD, Goldberg DE, et al. An iron-carboxylate bond links the heme units of malarial parasite pigment. Proc Natl Acad Sci USA 1991;88:325–329.

90. Bohle DS, Dinnebier RE, Madsen SK, Stephens PW. Characterization of the products of the heme detoxification pathway in malarial late trophozoites by x-ray diffraction. J Biol Chem 1997;272:713–716.

91. Blauer G, Akkawi M. Investigations of B- and β-hematin. J Inorg Biochem 1997;66:145–152.

92. Pagola S, Stephens PW, Bohle DS, Kosar AD, Madsen SK. The structure of malaria pigment β-haematin. Nature 2000;404:307–310.

93. Fitch CD, Kanjananggulpan P. The state of ferriprotoporphyrin IX in malaria pigment. J Biol Chem 1987;262:15,552–15,555.

94. Slater AFG, Cerami A. Inhibition by chloroquine of a novel haem polymerase enzyme activity in malaria trophozoites. Nature 1992;355:167–169.

95. Pandey AV, Tekwani BL, Pandey VC. Characterisation of hemozoin from liver and spleen of mice infected with *Plasmodium yoelii*, a rodent malaria parasite. Biomed Res 1995;16:115–120.

96. Chou AC, Fitch CD. Heme polymerase: modulation by chloroquine treatment of a rodent malaria. Life Sci 1992;51:2073–2078.

97. Dorn A, Stoffel R, Matile H, Bubendorf A, Ridely RG. Malarial haemozoin/β-haematin supports haem polymerisation in the absence of protein. Nature 1995;374:269–271.

98. Raynes KJ, Foley M, Tilley L, Deady L. Novel bisquinoline antimalarials: synthesis, antimalarial activity and inhibition of haem polymerisation. Biochem Pharmacol 1996;52:551–559.

99. Ridley RG. Haemozoin formation in malaria parasites: is there a haem polymerase? Trends Microbiol 1996;4:253–254.

100. Egan TJ, Ross DC, Adams PA. Quinoline antimalarial drugs inhibit spontaneous formation of β-haematin (malaria pigment). FEBS Lett 1994;352:54–57.

101. Pandey AV, Tekwani BL. Formation of haemozoin/beta-haematin under physiological conditions is not spontaneous. FEBS Lett 1996;393:189–193.

102. Fitch CD, Chou AC. Heat-labile and heat-stimulable heme polymerase activities in *Plasmodium berghei*. Mol Biochem Parasitol 1996;82:261–264.

103. Bendrat K, Berger BJ, Cerami A. Haem polymerisation in malaria. Nature 1995;378:138–139.

104. Dorn A, Vippagunta SR, Matile H, Bubendorf A, Vennerstrom JL, Ridley RG. A comparison and analysis of several ways to promote haematin (haem) polymerisation and an assessment of its initiation *in vitro*. Biochem Pharmacol 1998;55:737–747.

105. Fitch CD, Cai GZ, Chen YF, Shoemaker JD. Involvement of lipids in ferriprotoporphyrin IX polymerization in malaria. Biochim Biophys Acta 1999;1454:31–37.

106. Sullivan DJ, Gluzman IY, Goldberg DE. *Plasmodium* hemozoin formation mediated by histidine-rich proteins. Science 1996;271:219–222.

107. Stahl HD, Kemp DJ, Crewther PE, Scanlon DB, Woodrow G, Brown GV, et al. Sequence of a cDNA encoding a small polymorphic histidine- and alanine-rich protein from *Plasmodium falciparum* Nucleic Acids Res 1985;13:7837–7846.

108. Howard RJ, Uni S, Aikawa M, Aley SB, Leech JH, Lew AM, et al. Secretion of a malarial histidine-rich protein (Pf HRP II) from *Plasmodium falciparum*-infected erythrocytes. J Cell Biol 1986;103:1269–1277.

109. Pandey AV, Joshi R, Tekwani BL, Singh RL, Chauhan VS. Synthetic peptides corresponding to a repetitive sequence of malarial histidine rich protein bind haem and inhibit haemozoin formation *in vitro*. Mol Biochem Parasitol 1997;90:281–287.

110. Ziegler J, Chang RT, Wright DW. Multiple-antigenic peptides of histidine-rich protein II of *Plasmodium falciparum*: dendritic biomineralization templates. J Am Chem Soc 1999;121:2395–2400.

111. Choi CY, Cerda JF, Chu HA, Babcock GT, Marletta MA. Spectroscopic characterization of the heme-binding sites in *Plasmodium falciparum* histidine-rich protein 2. Biochemistry 1999;38:16,916–16,124.

112. Lynn A, Chandra S, Malhotra P, Chauhan VS. Heme binding and polymerization by *Plasmodium falciparum* histidine rich protein II: influence of pH on activity and conformation. FEBS Lett 1999;459:267–271.

113. Wellems TE, Walker-Jonah A, Panton LJ. Genetic mapping of the chloroquine-resistance locus on *Plasmodium falciparum* chromosome 7. Proc Natl Acad Sci USA 1991;88:3382–3386.

114. Lenstra R, d'Auriol L, Andrieu B, Le Bras J, Galibert F. Cloning and sequencing of *Plasmodium falciparum* DNA fragments containing repetitive regions potentially coding for histidine-rich proteins: identification of two overlapping reading frames. Biochem Biophys Res Commun 1987;146:368–377.

115. Zhang J, Krugliak M, Ginsburg H. The fate of ferriprotorphyrin IX in malaria infected erythrocytes in conjunction with the mode of action of antimalarial drugs. Mol Biochem Parasitol 1999;99:129–141.

116. Wood PA, Eaton JW. Hemoglobin catabolism and host–parasite heme balance in chloroquine-sensitive and chloroquine-resistant *Plasmodium berghei* infections. Am J Trop Med Hyg 1993;48:465–472.

117. Shviro Y, Shaklai N. Glutathione as a scavenger of free hemin. A mechanism of preventing red cell membrane damage. Biochem Pharmacol 1987;36:3801–3807.

118. Atamna H, Ginsburg H. Heme degradation in the presence of glutathione. A proposed mechanism to account for the high levels of non-heme iron found in the membranes of hemoglobinopathic red blood cells. J Biol Chem 1995;270:24,876–24,883.

119. Grady JK, Chasteen ND, Harris DC. Radicals from "Good's" buffers. Anal Biochem 1988;173:111–115.
120. Dubois VL, Platel DF, Pauly G, Tribouley-Duret J. *Plasmodium berghei*: implication of intracellular glutathione and its related enzyme in chloroquine resistance *in vivo*. Exp Parasitol 1995;81:117–124.
121. Platel DF, Mangou F, and Tribouley-Duret J. Role of glutathione in the detoxification of ferriprotoporphyrin IX in chloroquine resistant *Plasmodium berghei*. Mol Biochem Parasitol 1999;98:215–223.
122. Brown SB, Hatzikonstantinou H, Herries DG. The role of peroxide in haem degradation. A study of the oxidation of ferrihaems by hydrogen peroxide. Biochem J 1978;174:901–907.
123. Traylor TG, Kim C, Richards JL, Xu F, Perrin CL. Reaction of iron(III) porphyrins with oxidants. Structure-reactivity studies. J Am Chem Soc 1995;117:3468–3474.
124. Ribeiro MCA, Augusto O, Ferreira AMC. Influence of quinoline-containing antimalarials in the catalase activity of ferriprotoporphyrin IX. J Inorg Biochem 1997;65:15–23.
125. Panton LJ, McPhie P, Maloy WL, Wellems TE, Taylor DW, Howard RJ. Purification and partial characterization of an unusual protein of *Plasmodium falciparum*: histidine-rich protein II. Mol Biochem Parasitol 1989;35:149–160.
126. Mackerras MJ, Ercole QN. Observations on the action of quinine, atebrine and plasmoquine on the gametocytes of *Plasmodium falciparum*. Trans Soc Trop Med Hyg 1949;42:443–454.
127. Peters W. Morphological and physiological variations in chloroquine-resistant *Plasmodium berghei*. Ann Soc Belge Med Trop 1965;45:365–378.
128. Cohen SN, Phifer KO, Yielding K. Spectrophotomeric studies of the interaction of chloroquine with deoxyribonucleic acid. J Biol Chem 1964;240:3123–3131.
129. Schueler FW, Cantrell WF. Antagonism of the antimalarial action of chloroquine by ferrihemate and an hypothesis for the mechanism of chloroquine resistance. J Pharmacol Exp Therap 1964;143:278–281.
130. McChesney EW, Fitch CD. 4-Aminoquinolines. In: Peters W, Richards WHG (eds.). Antimalarial Drugs II: Current Antimalarials and New Drug Developments Berlin: Springer-Verlag, 1984, pp. 30–60.
131. Adams PA, Berman PA, Egan TJ, Marsh PJ, Silver J. The iron environment in heme and heme-antimalarial complexes of pharmacological interest. J Inorg Biochem 1996;63:69–77.
132. Egan TJ, Mavuso WW, Ross DC, Marques HM. Thermodynamic factors controlling the interaction of quinoline antimalarial drugs with ferriprotoporphyrin IX. J Inorg Biochem 1997;68:137–145.
133. Dorn A, Vippagunta SR, Matile H, Jaquet C, Vennerstrom JL, Ridley RG. An assessment of drug-haematin binding as a mechanism for inhibition of haematin polymerisation by quinoline antimalarials. Biochem Pharmacol 1998;55:727–736.
134. Moreau S, Perly B, Biguet J. Interaction of chloroquine with ferriprotophorphyrin IX. Nuclear magnetic resonance study. Biochimie 1982;64:1015–1025.
135. Fitch CD. Antimalarial schizonticides: ferriprotoporphyrin IX intercalation hypothesis. Parasitol Today 1986;2:330–331.
136. Chou AC, Fitch CD. Control of heme polymerase by chloroquine and other quinoline derivatives. Biochem Biophy Res Commun 1993;195:422–427.
137. Sullivan DJ, Gluzman IY, Russell DG, Goldberg DE. On the molecular mechanism of chloroquine's antimalarial action. Proc Natl Acad Sci USA 1996;93:11,865–11,870.
138. Sullivan DJ, Matile H, Ridley RG, Goldberg DE. A common mechanism for blockade of heme polymerization by antimalarial quinolines. J Biol Chem 1998;273:31,103–31,107.
139. Martiney JA, Cerami A, Slater AF. Inhibition of hemozoin formation in *Plasmodium falciparum* trophozoite extracts by heme analogs: possible implication in the resistance to malaria conferred by the β-thalassemia trait. Mol Med 1996;2:236–246.
140. Atamna H, Krugliak M, Shalmiev G, Deharo E, Pescarmona G, Ginsburg H. Mode of antimalarial effect of methylene blue and some of its analogues on *Plasmodium*

falciparum in culture and their inhibition of *P vinckei petteri* and *P yoelii nigeriensis in vivo*. Biochem Pharmacol 1996;51:693–700.

141. Goldberg DE, Sharma V, Oksman A, Gluzman IY, Wellems TE, Piwnica-Worms D. Probing the chloroquine resistance locus of *Plasmodium falciparum* with a novel class of multidentate metal(III) coordination complexes. J Biol Chem 1997;272:6567–6572.

142. Hawley SR, Bray PG, Mungthin M, Atkinson JD, O'Neill PM, Ward SA. Relationship between antimalarial drug activity, accumulation, and inhibition of heme polymerization in *Plasmodium falciparum in vitro*. Antimicrob Agents Chemother 1998;42:682–686.

143. O'Neill PM, Willock DJ, Hawley SR, Bray PG, Storr RC, Ward SA, et al. Synthesis, antimalarial activity, and molecular modeling of tebuquine analogues. J Med Chem 1997;40:437–448.

144. Meshnick SR. Is haemozoin a target for antimalarial drugs? Ann Trop Med Parasitol 1996;90:367–372.

145. Asawamahasakda W, Ittarat I, Chang CC, McElroy P, Meshnick SR. Effects of antimalarials and protease inhibitors on plasmodial hemozoin production Mol Biochem Parasitol 1994;67:183–191.

146. Famin O, Krugliak M, Ginsburg, H. Kinetics of inhibition of glutathione-mediated degradation of ferriprotoporphyrin IX by antimalarial drugs. Biochem Pharmacol 1999; 58:59–68.

147. Malhotra K, Salmon D, Le Bras J, Vilde JL. Potentiation of chloroquine activity against *Plasmodium falciparum* by the peroxidase-hydrogen peroxide system. Antimicrob Agents Chemother 1990;34:1981–1985.

148. Awasthi YC, Beutler E, Srivastava SK. Purification and properties of human erythrocyte glutathione peroxidase. J Biol Chem 1975;250:5144–5149.

149. Mueller S, Riedel HD, Stremmel, W. Direct evidence for catalase as the predominant H_2O_2-removing enzyme in human erythrocytes. Blood 1997;90:4973–4978.

150. Brown SB, Dean TC, Jones P. Catalatic activity of iron(3)-centred catalysts. Role of dimerization in the catalytic action of ferrihaems. Biochem J 1970;117:741–744.

151. Ribeiro MCA, Augusto O, Ferreira AMC. Inhibitory effect of chloroquine on the peroxidase activity of ferriprotoporphyrin IX. J Chem Soc Dalton Trans 1995;3759–3766.

152. Gluzman IY, Francis SE, Oksman A, Smith CE, Duffin KL, Goldberg DE. Order and specificity of the *Plasmodium falciparum* hemoglobin degradation pathway. J Clin Invest 1994;93:1602–1608.

153. Lee P, Ye Z, Van Dyke K, Kirk RG. X-ray microanalysis of *Plasmodium falciparum* and infected red blood cells: effects of qinghaosu and chloroquine on potassium, sodium, and phosphorus composition. Am J Trop Med Hyg 1988;39:157–165.

154. Orjih AU, Banyal HS, Chelvi R, Fitch CD. Hemin lyses malarial parasites. Science 1981;214:667–669.

155. Chou AC, Fitch CD. Mechanism of hemolysis induced by ferriprotoporphyrin IX. J Clin Invest 1981;68:672–677.

156. Zhang Y, Hempelmann E. Lysis of malarial parasites and erythrocytes by ferriprotoporphyrin IX chloroquine and the inhibition of this effect by proteins. Biochem Pharmacol 1987;36,1267–1273.

157. Meshnick SR, Chang KP, Cerami A. Heme lysis of the bloodstream forms of *Trypanosoma brucei*. Biochem Pharmacol 1977;26:1923–1928.

158. Tappel AL. The mechanism of oxidation of unsaturated fatty acids by hematin compounds. Arch Biochem Biophys 1953;44:378–395.

159. Atamna H, Ginsburg H. The malaria parasite supplies glutathione to its host cell—investigation of glutathione transport and metabolism in human erythrocytes infected with *Plasmodium falciparum*. Eur J Biochem 1997;250:670–679.

160. Clark IA, Hunt NH, Cowden WB, Maxwell LE, Mackie EJ. Radical-mediated damage to parasites and erythrocytes in *Plasmodium vinckei* infected mice after injection of t-butyl hydroperoxide. Clin Exp Immunol 1984;56:524–530.

161. Buffinton GD, Hunt NH, Cowden WB, Clark IA. Detection of short-chain carbonyl products of lipid peroxidation from malaria-parasite (*Plasmodium vinckei*)-infected red blood cells exposed to oxidative stress. Biochem J 1988;249:63–68.

162. Ginsburg H, Demel RA. Interactions of hemin, antimalarial drugs and hemin–antimalarial complexes with phospholipid monolayers. Chem Phys Lipids 1984;35:331–347.

163. Sugioka Y, Suzuki M. The chemical basis for the ferriprotoporphyrin IX–chloroquine complex induced lipid peroxidation. Biochim Biophys Acta 1991;1074:19–24.

164. Martin SK, Oduola AMJ, Milhous WK. Reversal of chloroquine resistance in *Plasmodium falciparum* by verapamil. Science 1987;235:899–901.

165. Martin SK. Chloroquine-resistant *Plasmodium falciparum* and the MDR phenotype. Parasitol Today 1993;9:278–280.

166. Riordan JR, Deuchars K, Kartner N, Alon N, Trent J, Ling V. Amplification of P-glycoprotein genes in multidrug-resistant mammalian cell lines. Nature 1985;316:817–819.

167. Foote SJ, Thompson JK, Cowman AF, Kemp DJ. Amplification of the multidrug resistance gene in some chloroquine-resistant isolates of *P falciparum*. Cell 1989;57:921–930.

168. Foote SJ, Kyle DE, Martin RK, Oduola AMJ, Forsyth K, Kemp DJ, et al. Several alleles of the multidrug-resistance gene are closely linked to chloroquine resistance in *Plasmodium falciparum*. Nature 1990;345:255–258.

169. Wilson CM, Volkman SK, Thaithong S, Martin RK, Kyle DE, Milhous WK, et al. Amplification of *pfmdr1* associated with mefloquine and halofantrine resistance in *P falciparum* from Thailand. Mol Biochem Parasitol 1993;57:151–160.

170. Reed MB, Saliba KJ, Caruna SR, Kirk K, Cowman AF. Pgh1 modulates sensitivity and resistance to multiple antimalarials in *Plasmodium falciparum*. Nature 2000;403:906–909.

171. Su X, Kirkman LA, Fujioka H, Wellems TE. Complex polymorphisms in an approximately 330 kDa protein are linked to chloroquine-resistant *P falciparum* in Southeast Asia and Africa. Cell 1997;91:593–603.

172. Wellems TE, Panton LJ, Gluzman IY, do Rosario VE, Gwadz RW, Walker-Jonah A, et al. Chloroquine resistance not linked to mdr-like genes in a *Plasmodium falciparum* cross. Nature 1990;345:253–255.

173. Bray PG, Hawley SR, Ward SA. 4-Aminoquinoline resistance of *Plasmodium falciparum*: insights from the study of amodiaquine uptake. Mol Pharmacol 1996;50:1551–1558.

174. Bray PG, Hawley SR, Mungthin M, Ward SA. Physicochemical properties correlated with drug resistance and the reversal of drug resistance in *Plasmodium falciparum*. Mol Pharmacol 1996;50:1559–1566.

175. Ginsburg H, Stein WD. Kinetic modelling of chloroquine uptake by malaria-infected erythrocytes. Assessment of the factors that may determine drug resistance. Biochem Pharmacol 1991;41:1463–1470.

176. Bray PG, Boulter MK, Ritchie GY, Howells RE, Ward SA. Relationship of global chloroquine transport and reversal of resistance in *Plasmodium falciparum*. Mol Biochem Parasitol 1994;63:87–94.

177. Mohrle JJ, Zhao Y, Wernli B, Franklin RM, Kappes B. Molecular cloning, characterization and localization of PfPK4, an eIF-2alpha kinase-related enzyme from the malarial parasite *Plasmodium falciparum*. Biochem J 1997;328:677–687.

177a. Ursos LM, Dzekunov SM, Roepe PD. The effects of chloroquine and verapamil on digestive vacuolar pH of *P. falciparum* either sensitive or resistant to chloroquine. Mol Biochem Parasitol 2000;110:125–134.

178. Foley M, Tilley L. Quinoline antimalarials: mechanisms of action and resistance and prospects for new agents. Pharmacol Ther 1998;79:55–87.

179. Mahoney J, Eaton JW. Chloroquine resistant malaria: association with enhanced Plasmodial protease activity. Biochem Biophys Res Commun 1981;100:1266–1271.

180. Bhatia A, Charet P. Action of chloroquine on glutathione metabolism in erythrocytes parasitized by *Plasmodium berghei*. Ann Parasitol Hum Comp 1984;59:317–320.

181. Berger BJ, Martiney J, Slater AFG, Fairlamb AH, Cerami A. Chloroquine resistance is not associated with drug metabolism in *Plasmodium falciparum*. J Parasitol 1995;81:1004–1008.

182. Sahini VE, Dumitrescu M, Volanschi E, Birla L, Diaconu C. Spectral and interferometrical study of the interaction of haemin with glutathione. Biophys Chem 1996;8:245–253.

183. Vander Jagt DL, Hunsaker LA, Garcia KB, Royer RE. Isolation and characterization of the multiple glutathione S-transferases from human liver. Evidence for unique heme-binding sites. J Biol Chem 1985;260:11,603–11,610.

184. Caccuri AM, Aceto A, Piemonte F, Di Ilio C, Rosato N, Federici G. Interaction of hemin with placental glutathione transferase. Eur J Biochem 1990;189:493–497.

185. Mannervik B, Alin P, Guthenberg C, Jensson H, Tahir MK, Warholm M, et al. Identification of three classes of cytosolic glutathione transferase common to several mammalian species: correlation between structural data and enzymatic properties. Proc Natl Acad Sci USA 1985;82:7202–7206.

186. Alin P, Danielson UH, Mannervik B. 4-Hydroxyalk-2-enals are substrates for glutathione transferase. FEBS Lett 1985;179:267–270.

187. Bruns CM, Hubatsch I, Ridderstrom M, Mannervik B, Tainer JA. Human glutathione transferase A4-4 crystal structures and mutagenesis reveal the basis of high catalytic efficiency with toxic lipid peroxidation products. J Mol Biol 1999;288:427–439.

188. Kanner J, German JB, Kinsella JE. Initiation of lipid peroxidation in biological systems. Crit Rev Food Sci Nutr 1987;25:317–364.

189. Deslauriers R, Butler K, Smith IC. Oxidant stress in malaria as probed by stable nitroxide radicals in erythrocytes infected with *Plasmodium berghei*. The effects of primaquine and chloroquine. Biochim Biophys Acta 1987;931:267–275.

190. Aft RL, Mueller GC. Degradation and covalent cross-linking of glutathione reductase by hemin. Life Sci 1985;36:2153–2161.

191. Muller, M,, Meijer C, Zaman GJ, Borst P, Scheper RJ, Mulder NH, et al. Overexpression of the gene encoding the multidrug resistance-associated protein results in increased ATP-dependent glutathione S-conjugate transport Proc Natl Acad Sci USA 1994;91:13,033–13,037.

192. Stieger B, Meier PJ. Bile acid and xenobiotic transporters in liver. Curr Opin Cell Biol 1998;10:462–467.

193. Greenwood, D. Conflicts of interest: the genesis of synthetic antimalarial agents in peace and war. J Antimicrob Chemother 1995;36:857–872.

194. Peters, W. (ed.) Chemotherapy and Drug Resistance in Malaria. London: Academic, 1987.

195. Hofheinz W, Merkli, B. Quinine and quinine analogues. In Peters W, Richards WHG (eds). Antimalarial Drugs II. Berlin: Springer Verlag, 1984, pp. 61–81.

196. Trenholme CM, Williams RL, Desjardins RE, Frischer H, Carson PE, Rieckmann KH, et al. Mefloquine (WR 142,490) in the treatment of human malaria. Science 1975;190:792–794.

197. Palmer KJ, Holliday SM, Brogden RN. Mefloquine. A review of its antimalarial activity, pharmacokinetic properties and therapeutic efficacy. Drugs 1993;45:430–475.

198. Colwell WT, Brown V, Christie P, Lange J, Yamamoto K, Henery DW. Antimalarial arylaminopropanols. J Med Chem 1972;15:771–774.

199. Bryson HM, Goa KL. Halofantrine. A review of its antimalarial activity, pharmacokinetic properties and therapeutic potential. Drugs 1992;43:236–258.

200. Matson PA, Luby SP, Redd SC, Rolka HR, Meriwether RA. Cardiac effects of standard-dose halofantrine therapy. Am J Trop Med Hyg 1996;54:229–231.

201. Olliaro PL, Trigg PI. Status of antimalarial drugs under development. Bull WHO 1995;73:565–571.

202. Vennerstrom JL, Ellis WY, Ager AL, Andersen SL, Gerena L, Milhous WK. Bisquinolines: *N*,*N*-bis(7-chloroquinolin-4-yl)alkanediamines with potential against chloroquine-resistant malaria. J Med Chem 1992;35:2129–2134.

203. Ridley RG, Matile H, Jaquet C, Dorn A, Hofheinz W, Leupin W, et al. Antimalarial activity of the bisquinoline trans-N1,N2-bis (7-chloroquinolin-4-yl)cyclohexane-1,2-diamine: comparison of two stereoisomers and detailed evaluation of the S,S enantiomer, Ro 47–7737. Antimicrob Agents Chemother 1997;41:677–686.

204. Ridley RG, Hofheinz W, Matile H, Jaquet C, Dorn A, Masciadri R, et al. 4-Aminoquinoline analogs of chloroquine with shortened side chains retain activity against chloroquine-resistant *Plasmodium falciparum*. Antimicrob Agents Chemother 1996;40:1846–1854.

205. De D, Krogstad FM, Cogswell FB, Krogstad DJ. Aminoquinolines that circumvent resistance in *Plasmodium falciparum in vitro*. Am J Trop Med Hyg 1996;55:579–583.

206. Ekweozor C, Aderounmu AF, Sodeinde O. Comparison of the relative *in vitro* activity of chloroquine and amodiaquine against chloroquine-sensitive strains of *P falciparum*. Ann Trop Med Parasitol 1987;81:95–99.

207. Churchill FC, Patchen LC, Campbell CC, Schwartz IK, Nguyen-Dinh P, Dickinson CM. Amodiaquine as a prodrug: importance of metabolite(s) in the antimalarial effect of amodiaquine in humans. Life Sci 1985;36:53–62.

208. Fitch CD. Chloroquine-resistant *Plasmodium falciparum*: difference in handling of ^{14}C-amodiaquin and ^{14}C-chloroquine. Antimicrob Agents Chemother 1973;3:545–548.

209. Blauer, G. Interaction of ferriprotoporphyrin IX with the antimalarials amodiaquine and halofantrine. Biochem Int 1988;17:729–734.

210. Slater AFG. Chloroquine: mechanism of drug action and resistance in *Plasmodium falciparum*. Pharmacol Ther 1993;57:203–235.

211. Mungthin M, Bray PG, Ridley RG, Ward SA. Central role of hemoglobin degradation in mechanisms of action of 4-aminoquinolines, quinoline methanols, and phenanthrene methanols. Antimicrob Agents Chemother 1998;42:2973–2977.

212. Bjorkman A, Phillips-Howard PA. Drug-resistant malaria: mechanisms of development and inferences for malaria control. Trans R Soc Trop Med Hyg 1990;84:323–324.

213. Elueze EI, Croft SL, Warhurst DC. Activity of pyronaridine and mepacrine against twelve strains of *Plasmodium falciparum in vitro*. J Antimicrob Chemother 1996;37:511–518.

214. Pradines B, Tall A, Parzy D, Spiegel A, Fusai T, Hienne R, et al. In-vitro activity of pyronaridine and amodiaquine against African isolates (Senegal) of *Plasmodium falciparum* in comparison with standard antimalarial agents. J Antimicrob Chemother 1998;42:333–339.

215. Vennerstrom JL. Bisquinolines and processes for their production and use to treat malaria. US Patent 5,510,356 (1996).

216. Ismail FM, Dascombe MJ, Carr P, North SE. An exploration of the structure–activity relationships of 4-aminoquinolines: novel antimalarials with activity in-vivo J Pharm Pharmacol 1996;48:841–850.

217. Raynes K, Galatis D, Cowman AF, Tilley L, Deady LW. Synthesis and activity of some antimalarial bisquinolines. J Med Chem 1995;38:204–206.

218. Cowman AF, Deady LW, Deharo E, Desneves J, Tilley L. Synthesis and activity of some antimalarial bisquinolinemethanols. Aust J Chem 1997;50:1091–1096.

219. Basco LK, Andersen SL, Milhous WK, Le Bras J, Vennerstrom JL. *In vitro* activity of bisquinoline WR268,668 against African clones and isolates of *Plasmodium falciparum*. Am J Trop Med Hyg 1994;50:200–205.

220. Thompson PE, Werbel LM. Quinine and related alkaloids. In: DeStevens G (ed.). Antimalarial Agents: Chemistry and Pharmacology. New York: Academic, 1972.

221. Barennes H, Pussard E, Mahaman Sani A, Clavier F, Kahiatani F, Granic G, et al. Efficacy and pharmacokinetics of a new intrarectal quinine formulation in children with *Plasmodium falciparum* malaria. Br J Clin Pharmacol 1996;41:389–395.

222. Kremsner PG, Luty AJF, Granger W. Combination chemotherapy for *Plasmodium falciparum* malaria. Parasitol Today 1997;13:167–168.

223. Karbwang J, White NJ. Clinical pharmacokinetics of mefloquine. Clin Pharmacokinet 1990;19:264–279.

224. Mu JY, Israili ZH, Dayton PG. Studies of the disposition and metabolism of mefloquine HCl (WR 142:490), a quinolinemethanol antimalarial, in the rat. Limited studies with an analog, WR 30,090. Drug Metab Dispos 1975;3:198–210.

225. Desneves J, Thorn G, Berman A, Galatis D, La Greca N, Sinding J, et al. Photoaffinity labelling of mefloquine-binding proteins in human serum, uninfected erythrocytes and *Plasmodium falciparum*-infected erythrocytes. Mol Biochem Parasitol 1996;82:181–194.

226. Grellier P, Rigomier D, Clavey V, Fruchart, J-C, Schrevel J. Lipid traffic between high density lipoproteins and *Plasmodium falciparum*-infected red blood cells. J Cell Biol 1991;112:267–277.

227. Berman A, Shearing LN, Ng KF, Jinsart W, Foley M, Tilley L. Photoaffinity labelling of *Plasmodium falciparum* proteins involved in phospholipid transport. Mol Biochem Parasitol 1994;67:235–243.

228. Chevli R, Fitch CD. The antimalarial drug mefloquine binds to membrane phospholipids. Antimicrob Agents Chemother 1982;21:581–586.

229. San George RC, Nagel RL, Farby ME. On the mechanism of the red-cell accumulation of mefloquine, an antimalarial drug. Biochim Biophys Acta 1984;803:174–181.

230. Schwartz DE, Eckert G, Hartmann D, Weber B, Richard-Lenoble D, Ekue JM, et al. Single dose kinetics of mefloquine in man. Plasma levels of the unchanged drug and of one of its metabolites. Chemotherapy 1982;28:70–84.

231. Fitch CD, Chan RL, Chevli R. Chloroquine resistance in malaria: accessibility of drug receptors to mefloquine. Antimicrob Agents Chemother 1979;15:258–62.

232. Vanderkooi G, Prapunwattana P, Yuthavong Y. Evidence for electrogenic accumulation of mefloquine by malarial parasites. Biochem Pharmacol 1988;37:3623–3631.

233. Yuthavong Y, Panijpan B, Ruenwongsa P, Sirawaraporn W. Biochemical aspects of drug action and resistance in malaria parasites. Southeast Asian J Trop Med Public Health 1985;16:459–472.

234. Perrin DD. Dissociation Constants of Organic Bases in Aqueous Solution. London: Butterworth, 1965, p. 531.

235. Strube RE. The search for new antimalarial drugs. J Trop Med Hyg 1975;78:171–185.

236. Peters W, Howells RE, Portus J, Robinson BL, Thomas S, Warhurst DC. The chemotherapy of rodent malaria, XXVII. Studies on mefloquine (WR 142,490). Ann Trop Med Parasitol 1977;71:407–418.

237. Cowman AF, Galatis D, Thompson JK. Selection for mefloquine resistance in *Plasmodium falciparum* is linked to amplification of the *pfmdr1* gene and cross-resistance to halofantrine and quinine. Proc Natl Acad Sci USA 1994;91:1143–1147.

238. Stahel E, Druilhe P, Gentilini M. Antagonism of chloroquine with other antimalarials. Trans R Soc Trop Med Hyg 1988;82:221.

239. Schmidt LH, Crosby R, Rasco J, Vaughan D. Antimalarial activities of various 4-quinolinemethanols with special attention to WR-142,490 (mefloquine). Antimicrob Agents Chemother 1978;13:1011–1030.

240. Schmidt LH, Crosby R, Rasco J, Vaughan D. Antimalarial activities of the 4-quinolinemethanols WR-184,806 and WR-226,253. Antimicrob Agents Chemother 1978;14:680–689.

241. Geary TG, Bonanni LC, Jensen JB, Ginsburg H. Effects of combinations of quinoline-containing antimalarials on *Plasmodium falciparum* in culture. Ann Trop Med Parasitol 1986;80:285–291.

242. Jacobs GH, Aikawa M, Milhous WK, Rabbege JR. An ultrastructural study of the effects of mefloquine on malaria parasites. Am J Trop Med Hyg 1987;36:9–14.

243. Olliaro PL, Castelli F, Caligaris S, Druilhe P, Carosi G. Ultrastructure of *Plasmodium falciparum in vitro* II. Morphological patterns of different quinolines effects. Microbiologica 1989;12:15–28.

244. Dutta P, Fitch CD. Diverse membrane-active agents modify the hemolytic response to ferriprotoporphyrin IX. J Pharmacol Exp Ther 1983;225:729–734.

245. Meshnick SR. Why does quinine still work after 350 years of use? Parasitol Today 1997;13:89–90.
246. Kain KC. Chemotherapy and prevention of drug-resistant malaria. Wilderness Environ Med 1995;6:307–324.
247. Watt G, Loesuttivibool L, Shanks GD, Bordreau EF, Brown AE, Pavanand K, et al. Quinine with tetracycline for the treatment of drug-resistant *falciparum* malaria in Thailand. Am J Trop Med Hyg 1992;47:108–111.
248. Giboda M, Denis MB. Response of Kampuchean strains of *Plasmodium falciparum* to antimalarials: *in vivo* assessment of quinine and quinine plus tetracycline; multiple drug resistance *in vitro*. J Trop Med Hyg 1988;91:205–211.
249. Boudreau EF, Webster HK, Pavanand K, Thosingha L. Type II mefloquine resistance in Thailand. Lancet 1982;2:1335.
250. White NJ. Mefloquine in the prophylaxis and treatment of falciparum malaria. Br Med J 1994;308:286–287.
251. Price RN, Nosten F, Luxemburger C, Kham A, Brockman A, Chongsuphajaisiddhi T, et al. Artesunate versus artemether in combination with mefloquine for the treatment of multidrug-resistant falciparum malaria. Trans R Soc Trop Med Hyg 1995;89:523–527.
252. McGready R, Cho T, Hkirijaroen L, Simpson J, Chongsuphajaisiddhi T, White NJ, et al. Quinine and mefloquine in the treatment of multidrug-resistant *Plasmodium falciparum* malaria in pregnancy. Ann Trop Med Parasitol 1998;92:643–653.
253. Peters W, Robinson BL. The chemotherapy of rodent malaria. XLVI. Reversal of mefloquine resistance in rodent *Plasmodium*. Ann Trop Med Parasitol 1991;85:5–10.
254. Oduola AMJ, Omitowoju GO, Gerena L, Kyle DE, Milhous WK, Sowunmi A, et al. Reversal of mefloquine resistance with penfluridol in isolates of *Plasmodium falciparum* from south-west Nigeria. Trans R Soc Trop Med Hyg 1992;87:81–83.
255. Peel SA, Merritt SC, Handy J, Baric RS. Derivation of highly mefloquine-resistant lines from *Plasmodium falciparum in vitro*. Am J Trop Med Hyg 1993;48:385–397.
256. Wilson CM, Serrano AE, Wasley A, Bogenschutz MP, Shankar AH, Wirth DF. Amplification of a gene related to mammalian *mdr* genes in drug-resistant *Plasmodium falciparum*. Science 1989;244:1184–1186.
257. Peel SA, Bright P, Yount B, Handy J, Baric RS. A strong association between mefloquine and halofantrine resistance and amplification, overexpression, and mutation in the P-glycoprotein gene homolog (*pfmdr*) of *Plasmodium falciparum in vitro* Am J Trop Med Hyg 1994;51:648–658.
258. Cowman AF, Karcz S, Galatis D, Culvenor JG. A P-glycoprotein homolog of *Plasmodium falciparum* is localized on the digestive vacuole. J Cell Biol 1991;113:1033–1042.
259. Basco LK, Le Bras J, Rhoades Z, Wilson CM. Analysis of *pfmdr1* and drug susceptibility in fresh isolates of *Plasmodium falciparum* from subsaharan Africa. Mol Biochem Parasitol 1995;74:157–166.
260. Lim AS, Galatis D, Cowman AF. *Plasmodium falciparum*: amplification and overexpression of *pfmdr1* is not necessary for increased mefloquine resistance. Exp Parasitol 1996;83:295–303.
261. Riffkin C, Chung R, Wall D, Zalcberg JR, Cowman AF, Foley M, et al. Modulation of the function of human MDR1 P-glycoprotein by the antimalarial drug mefloquine Biochem Pharmacol 1996;52:1545–1552.
262. Karcz SR, Galatis D, Cowman AF. Nucleotide binding properties of a P-glycoprotein homologue from *Plasmodium falciparum*. Mol Biochem Parasitol. 58 1993;269–276.
263. Olliaro PL, Yuthavong Y. An overview of chemotherapeutic targets for antimalarial drug discovery. Pharmacol Ther 1999;81:91–110.
264. Vippagunta SR, Dorn A, Matile, H. Bhattacharjee AK, Karle JM, Ellis WY, et al. Vennerstrom JL. Structural specificity of chloroquine-hematin binding related to inhibition of hematin polymerisation and parasite growth. J Med Chem 1999;42:4630–4639.

265. Egan TJ, Hunter R, Kaschula CH, Marques HM, Misplon A, Walden J. Structure–function relationships in aminoquinolines: effect of amino and chloro groups on quinoline–hematin complex formation, inhibition of beta-hematin formation and antiplasmodial activity. J Med Chem 2000;43:283–291.

266. Vennerstrom JL, Ager AL. Jr, Dorn A, Andersen SL, Gerena L, Ridley RG, Milhous WK. Bisquinolines. 2. Antimalarial *N,N*-bis(7-chloroquinolin-4-yl)heteroalkanedia-mines. J Med Chem 1998;41:4360–4364.

267. Basilico N, Monti D, Olliaro P, Taramelli D. Non-iron porphyrins inhibit β-haematin (malaria pigment) polymerisation. FEBS Lett 1997;409:297–299.

268. Ignatushchenko MV, Winter RW, Bachinger HP, Hinrichs DJ, Riscoe MK. Xanthones as antimalarial agents; studies of a possible mode of action. FEBS Lett 1997;409:67–73.

269. Vennerstrom JL, Nuzum EO, Miller RE, Dorn A, Gerena L, Dande PA, et al. 8-Amino-quinolines active against blood stage *Plasmodium falciparum in vitro* inhibit hematin polymerization. Antimicrob Agents Chemother 1999;43:598–602.

270. Pandey AV, Tekwani BL, Singh RL, Chauhan VS. Artemisinin, an endoperoxide anti-malarial, disrupts the hemoglobin catabolism and heme detoxification systems in ma-larial parasite. J Biol Chem 1999;274:19,383–19,388.

271. Färber PM, Becker K, Müller S, Schirmer RH, Franklin RM. Molecular cloning and characterization of a putative glutathione reductase gene, the PfGR2 gene, from *Plasmo-dium falciparum*. Eur J Biochem 1996;239:655–661.

272. Becker K, Färber PM, von der Lieth CW, Müller S. Glutathione reductase and thioredoxin. In Stevenson KJ, Massey V, Williams C.H (eds). Flavins and Flavoproteins XII. Univer-sity Press, Calgary, 1997, pp. 13–22.

273. Müller S, Becker K, Bergmann B, Schirmer RH, Walter RD. *Plasmodium falciparum* glu-tathione reductase exhibits sequence similarities with the human host enzyme in the core structure but differs at the ligand-binding sites. Mol Biochem Parasitol 1995;74:11–18.

274. Becker K, Müller S, Keese MA, Walter RD, Schirmer RH. A glutathione reductase-like flavoenzyme of the malaria parasite *Plasmodium falciparum*: structural considerations based on the DNA sequence. Biochem Soc Trans 1996;24:67–72.

275. Gilberger TW, Färber PM, Becker K, Schirmer RH, Walter RD. Recombinant putative glutathione reductase from *Plasmodium falciparum* exhibits thioredoxin reductase activ-ity. Mol Biochem Parasitol 1996;80:215–219.

276. Birago C, Pace T, Picci L, Pizzi E, Scotti R, Ponzi M. The putative gene for the first enzyme of glutathione biosynthesis in *Plasmodium berghei* and *Plasmodium falciparum*. Mol Biochem Parasitol 1999;99:33–40.

277. Färber PM, Arscott LD, Williams, CH Jr, Becker K, Schirmer RH. Recombinant *Plas-modium falciparum* glutathione reductase is inhibited by the antimalarial dye methylene blue. FEBS Lett 1998;422:311–314.

278. Ursos LM, Dzekunov SM, Roepe PD. The effects of chloroquine and verapanil on diges-tive vacuolar pH of *P. falciparum* either sensitive or resistant to chloroquine. Mol Biochem Parasitol 2000;110:125–134.

7

8-Aminoquinolines

Ralf P. Brueckner, Colin Ohrt, J. Kevin Baird, and Wilbur K. Milhous

INTRODUCTION

The 8-aminoquinolines emerged during the 20th century as the only family of antimalarial compounds with activity against multiple life-cycle stages of the plasmodia that infect humans. Primaquine, the lone representative of 8-aminoquinolines among licensed antimalarials, has been in use for over 50 yr. It remains the only drug licensed for the prevention of malaria relapse (i.e., killing liver stages of the parasite). Primaquine also kills asexual blood stages and sterilizes the sexual-stage gametocytes. Thus, primaquine can prevent infection or relapse, cure disease, and prevent transmission of the infection. This broad range of activities represents the promise held in this family of compounds. A new 8-aminoquinoline, tafenoquine (WR 238605), is now in clinical trials and may revolutionize the prevention of malaria in travelers. Moreover, tafenoquine may provide an urgently needed weapon to combat epidemic malaria with a single regimen of therapy. The factor that most jeopardizes such utility is another trait shared by many 8-aminoquinolines, hemolytic toxicity in people lacking glucose-6-phosphate dehydrogenase (G6PD). G6PD deficiency is one of the most common genetic abnormalities in human beings, and it is especially common where malaria is or has been endemic. The challenge for pharmacologists, biochemists, and parasitologists is separating the therapeutic properties of 8-aminoquinolines from hemolytic toxicity. This chapter will summarize knowledge regarding mechanisms of therapeutic and toxic activities and point out areas where further investigation may lead to advances in our understanding of these mechanisms.

The history of 8-aminoquinolines for malaria began over 100 yr ago when Paul Ehrlich, the "father of chemotherapy," observed selective uptake and staining of tissues by dyes such as methylene blue (1,2). He hypothesized that such selectivity was the result of the existence of specific receptors to which the dye binds and that one could affect parasites residing within those tissues by targeting these receptors. Ehrlich discovered that methylene blue had antimalarial activity, leading to the development of the 8-aminoquinolines. German synthetic chemists developed pamaquine (plasmochin, plasmoquine), the first 8-aminoquinoline for malaria, during the 1920s (Fig. 1). Pamaquine had less activity against falciparum malaria and greater toxicity than expected, but it was effective in preventing relapse caused by vivax malaria and as a transmission-blocking drug.

From: *Antimalarial Chemotherapy: Mechanisms of Action, Resistance, and New Directions in Drug Discovery*
Edited by: P. J. Rosenthal © Humana Press Inc., Totowa, NJ

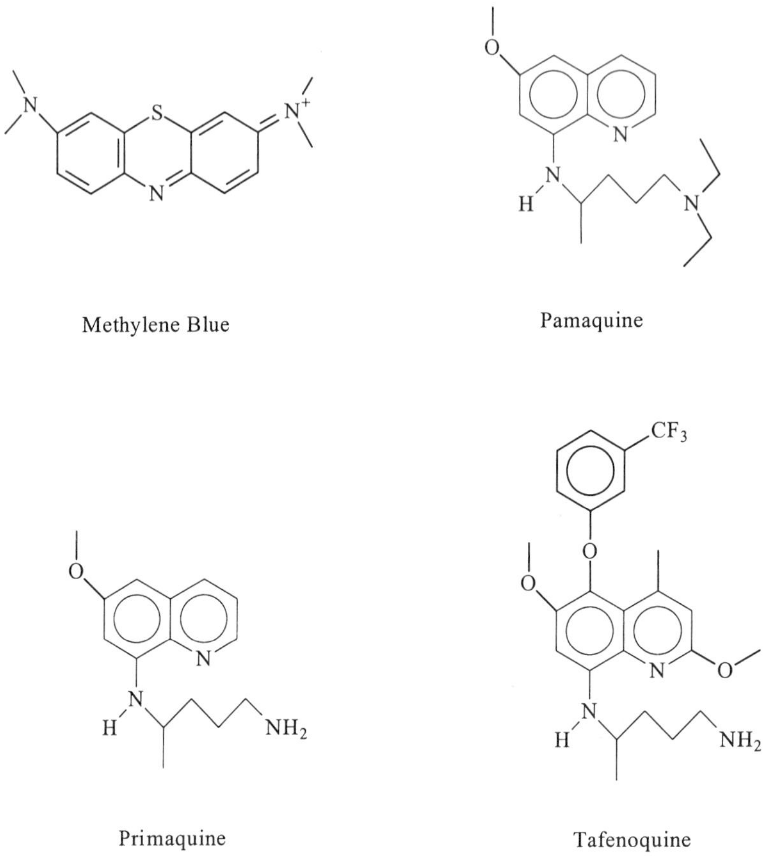

Fig. 1. Antimalarial 8-aminoquinolines and methylene blue. Primaquine has only a side-chain modification from pamaquine, whereas tafenoquine retains the primaquine side chain, but has ring substitutions.

Not until the second World War were efforts renewed to synthesize and systematically evaluate other 8-aminoquinolines. The malaria problem was recognized as a strategic threat to US forces deployed to some of the most malarious areas of the world *(3)*. Extensive research resulted in the discovery of primaquine (Fig. 1). This drug was widely used by United Nations forces deployed to Korea beginning in 1950, where endemic vivax malaria infected many thousands of troops.

Primaquine remains the standard by which other 8-aminoquinolines are compared. Successfully used for the radical cure of vivax malaria since the late 1940s, primaquine remains the only drug approved for this indication. However, like most drugs, it presents disadvantages and limitations. Primaquine has a narrow therapeutic window and can cause side effects at the higher doses sometimes needed to effect cure. Therapeutic doses often produce gastrointestinal discomfort unless taken with food. More importantly, primaquine induces acute intravascular hemolysis in people with an inborn deficiency of G6PD. The relatively short half-life (4–6 h) of primaquine requires daily administration for 14 d to achieve cure. This regimen often results in poor compliance and therapeutic failure. Military conflicts engaging US forces in Korea and Vietnam prompted reinvigoration of synthesis and screening efforts to develop a drug with the therapeutic properties of primaquine but with a longer half-life and better safety margin.

The Vietnam War, in conjunction with the emergence of chloroquine-resistant *Plasmodium falciparum* in Southeast Asia, provided a major impetus for antimalarial drug development, including the effort to improve upon primaquine. The Walter Reed Army Institute of Research (WRAIR), in collaboration with many other groups, led the effort to synthesize and screen many thousands of 8-aminoquinolines to understand the structure–activity relationships driving the therapeutic and toxic properties among the substituents on the core 8-aminoquinoline framework *(4,5)*. It was found that an appropriate substituent at the 2-position resulted in a small improvement in efficacy with decreased general systemic toxicity (Fig. 1). A methyl group at the 4-position increased therapeutic activity, but at the expense of greater toxicity in multiple-dose studies. A phenoxy group at the 5-position decreased toxicity while maintaining or improving activity. Subsequent efforts then focused on synthesis of derivatives having combinations of substitutions at these apparent key positions. It was anticipated that such a derivative would have increased antimalarial activity and less toxicity.

This synthetic effort produced the compounds WR 225448 and tafenoquine (WR 238605) in 1975 and 1979, respectively. WR 225448 is like primaquine but with a methyl group at the 4-position and a trifluoromethyl-phenoxy substituent at the 5-position. Tafenoquine has an additional methoxy substituent at the 2-position (Fig. 1). In addition to effects on activity and toxicity, the 5-position substituent probably provides both an electron-withdrawing effect and hindrance to the oxidative metabolism of the other substituents (W Ellis, personal communication). These features may explain the relatively long elimination half-life of tafenoquine. Tafenoquine was ultimately selected over WR 225448 on the weight of superior therapeutic activity in monkey malaria models and because it produced less methemoglobinemia in dogs. It was hoped that less hemoglobin oxidation would translate into less hemolytic activity.

Nonclinical pharmacology studies found tafenoquine to be generally less toxic than primaquine *(6)*, with a longer half-life *(7)*. Target organs included the liver, blood, and lungs, similar to other 8-aminoquinolines. However, the specific issue of relative hemolytic toxicity in G6PD-deficient humans could not be assessed reliably in vitro or by using animal models. The results of these nonclinical findings suggested therapeutic utility and an exemption for an Investigational New Drug (IND) was filed with the US Food and Drug Administration (FDA) in 1991. Clinical studies in humans began in 1992. Initial safety and pharmacokinetic studies in humans found that tafenoquine, like most other 8-aminoquinolines, caused gastrointestinal disturbances (nausea, cramping, and diarrhea) when administered fasting. These studies also confirmed that the drug had a half-life of 2–3 wk, approximately 50 times longer than primaquine *(6)*.

MECHANISMS OF ACTION AND TOXICITY

The mechanisms of therapeutic action and toxicity of 8-aminoquinolines remain incompletely understood despite five decades of clinical experience with primaquine. The 8-aminoquinolines, unlike other families of antimalarial compounds, seem to adversely affect all stages of the malaria parasite. Hemolysis in G6PD-deficient individuals and gastrointestinal intolerance are the principal toxicities of clinical importance. The full potential of the 8-aminoquinolines, with their extraordinary therapeutic range and properties, has yet to be delivered. A safe and well-tolerated drug that attacks all parasite stages at once would revolutionize the clinical management and control of malaria. The 8-aminoquinolines, more than any other known family of compounds, offer that promise.

Efficacy

Clinical malaria begins when merozoites burst from infected hepatocytes into the bloodstream and invade red blood cells (Chapter 1, Fig. 3). In most instances of primary infection, the merozoites originate from primary tissue schizonts. When the merozoites come from secondary tissue schizonts originating from quiescent stages of *P. vivax* or *P. ovale* called hypnozoites, the onset of parasitemia and clinical symptoms is called a relapse. 8-Aminoquinolines kill tissue schizonts and hypnozoites and thus prevent clinical malaria from either primary infection or relapse.

In the prevention and treatment of malaria, the timing of drug administration in relation to infection largely defines its application. Causal prophylactic drugs kill liver-stage parasites and, thus, need only be taken during exposure to infective mosquitoes. These tissue schizonticides prevent the development or release of merozoites from the liver and, thus, block infection of erythrocytes. Drugs that kill parasites after invasion of red blood cells are called blood schizonticides, and when taken during a period of potential exposure, they are called suppressive prophylactics. Therapy with a tissue schizonticide after a primary clinical episode is termed antirelapse therapy. Presumptive therapy with a tissue schizonticide after exposure is called terminal prophylaxis. Drugs that kill the sexual blood stages (gametocytes) or prevent the development of sporozoites in mosquitoes are termed transmission-blocking agents (gametocyctocidal or sporontocidal therapies, respectively). Overall, the plasmodial life cycle presents many potential targets for antimalarial drug activity.

8-Aminoquinolines exert activity against all stages of the parasite. Primaquine kills blood stages of *P. vivax* (8,9). However, it is the metabolically inactive stages of plasmodia (i.e., mature gametocytes of *P. falciparum* and hypnozoites of *P. vivax*) that exhibit exquisite sensitivity to this compound. The mechanisms of action remain poorly understood, but ultrastructural studies in a variety of microorganisms provide clues. Ultrastructural observations suggest that membranes, especially of the inner mitochondrion, are targeted by 8-aminoquinolines *(10–16)*. Primaquine-treated exoerythrocytic schizonts, gametocytes, and blood-stage trophozoites exhibit membrane abnormalities. The accumulation of radiolabeled primaquine in mitochondria temporally coincided with the appearance of mitochondrial swelling in the tissue stages of *P. fallax (17)*. Furthermore, mitochondrial proliferation in the face of exposure to primaquine appeared to enhance survival of blood stages *(18,19)*. In a yeast system, primaquine prevented growth during developmental events that required functional mitochondria *(20)*.

Metabolically senescent stages of plasmodia are especially sensitive to 8-aminoquinolones. This stage specificity may correlate with the inability of mitochondria to proliferate during particular developmental events. Alternatively, the lack of mechanisms needed to eliminate primaquine or one of its metabolites, or stage-specific inability to cope with oxidative stress may account for this specificity.

Other antimalarial drugs cause morphologic changes and physiologic alterations in plasmodial mitochondria. Those reported to cause ultrastructural changes include artemisinin derivatives *(21,22)*, clindamycin *(23)*, the napthoquinone menoctone *(18)*, and a floxacrine analog *(24)*. Atovaquone, another napthoquinone, acts on mitochondria by inhibiting mitochondrial electron transport *(25)* and collapsing mitochondrial membrane potential *(26)* (Chapter 11). The primary site of action of atovaquone was identified as the cytochrome-*bc*1 complex *(27)*. Mitochondrial protein synthesis inhibitors (e.g., tetracycline, erythromycin) also have antimalarial activity *(28,29)* (Chapter 15).

Interactions between several antimalarial drugs affecting mitochondria have been assessed. Mirincamycin, a compound related to clindamycin, enhanced the radical curative activity of primaquine against *P. cynomolgi* in monkeys *(24)*. Azithromycin was synergistic with primaquine and tafenoquine against *P. falciparum* in vitro (C. Ohrt, unpublished data). Napthoquinones have been reported to be synergistic with 8-aminoquinolines against tissue, but not blood stages of malaria parasites *(24)*. Interactions between drugs with other mechanisms have also been reviewed *(30)*.

The mitochondrial function of plasmodia is incompletely understood *(31)*. Functional mitochondria and an electron transport system are critical for parasite survival *(32)*. Major functions of electron transport in plasmodial mitochondria are believed to be involved in dihydroorotate dehydrogenase, a critical enzyme in *de novo* pyrimidine biosynthesis *(33)*, and to generate potential across the inner mitochondrial membrane *(26)*. Mitochondria may have many other physiological roles, such as the metabolism of amino acids, lipids, and heme, as well as intracellular Ca^{2+} homeostasis *(34)*. Both mitochondrial and nuclear genomes encode these functions.

Which, if any, mitochondrial processes of plasmodia are affected by the 8-aminoquinolines remains to be elucidated. Based on structural features of Plasmodium cytochrome-*b*, Vaidya and colleagues predicted that this would be the site of action of 8-aminoquinolines *(35)*. However, unlike with atovaquone, dihydroorotate dehydrogenase was not affected by 8-aminoquinolines *(36)*. Some evidence suggests that 8-aminoquinolines may alter calcium homeostasis *(37,38)*, and high concentrations of the drug affect vesicular transport *(39,40)*. Altered DNA binding, inhibition of ATP uptake by RNA, and inhibition of proteolysis have also been cited as potential mechanisms of action *(41)*. Many of these effects occurred only at drug concentrations far above those anticipated with a therapeutic dosing regimen. Importantly, the effect of putative metabolites was usually not assessed.

8-Aminoquinolines may be acting on plasmodial mitochondria through the generation of toxic metabolites, by causing oxidative stress, or by both of these mechanisms. 8-Aminoquinolines appear to be metabolized in mitochondria *(42,43)*. They form substrates for monoamine oxidase *(44)*, a mitochondrial flavoprotein *(45)*, which yields an aldehyde *(44,46)*. The presence of alcohol or aldehyde dehydrogenases determines the subsequent biotransformation of the aldehyde (see the subsection Contribution of Metabolism) *(46)*. Therefore, enzymes present in the cytosol and mitochondria of plasmodia may affect the fate of primaquine and its metabolites. The biotransformation of 8-aminoquinolines by plasmodia has not been studied, nor has the activity of aldehyde metabolites been assessed. However, a pentaquine aldehyde was identified as an active anticoccidial metabolite of pentaquine *(44)*.

8-Aminoquinolines and their hydroxylated metabolites apparently produce reactive intermediates (superoxide anion radicals), similar to those of natural host defenses (Fig. 2). The lethal activity of 8-aminoquinolines may mimic cell-mediated immunity against malaria *(49)*. Pro-oxidant drugs have also been noted to cause mitochondrial swelling

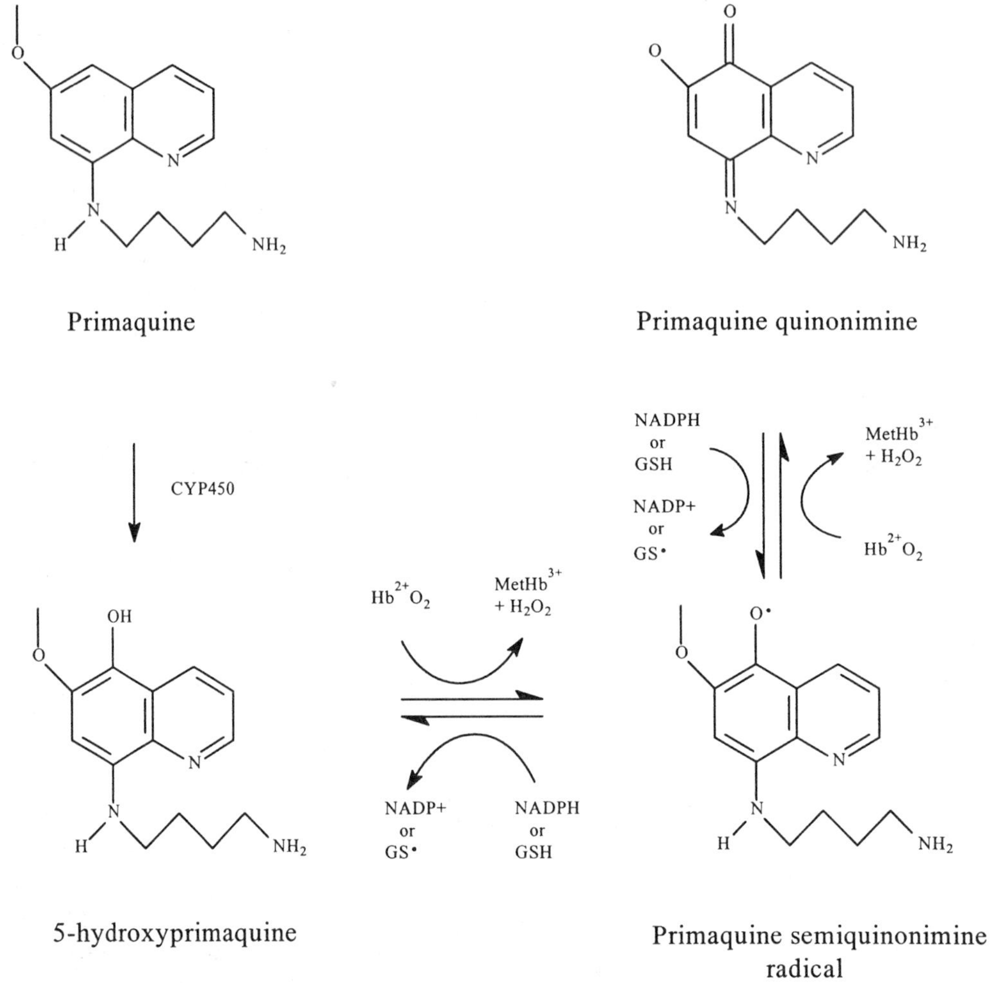

Fig. 2. Proposed pathways for free-radical and hydrogen peroxide production by 8-amino-quinolines. After ring hydroxylation by cytochrome P450, hydroxylated derivatives can participate in pathogenic redox cycling. NADPH is required to regenerate GSH from GSSG (see Fig. 3). H_2O_2 = hydrogen peroxide; Hb = hemoglobin; MetHb = methemoglobin; GSH = reduced glutathione; GSSG = oxidized glutathione. (Adapted from refs. *47* and *48*.)

(50), and reactive oxygen species can cause death in malaria parasites *(49,51)*. On the other hand, an exoerythrocytic *P. berghei* model revealed that superoxide generation by 8-aminoquinolines correlated with methemoglobin formation, but not with antimalarial activity *(10)*. Assessment of the effect of antioxidants on the antimalarial activity of 8-aminoquinolines may shed light on the relative importance of oxidizing radicals in the mechanism of action of these compounds.

Managing oxidant stress is especially important for the survival of plasmodia during specific developmental events. Through digestion of host hemoglobin during the trophozoite and early schizont stages, the parasite and the infected red blood cells face extraordinary oxidative stress. The digestion process generates superoxide, hydrogen peroxide, and hydroxyl radicals *(52,53)*. Plasmodium species have G6PD *(54)* and produce their own glutathione *(55)* to reduce oxidizing agents. A recently reported possible mechanism of action of primaquine is inhibition of glutathione *S*-transferase activity *(56)*.

Tafenoquine has blood stage activity against *P. falciparum* in vitro at concentrations achieved clinically, whereas primaquine does not. Tafenoquine was recently shown to inhibit hematin polymerization more potently than chloroquine, whereas primaquine showed no activity *(57)*. Tafenoquine-induced inhibition of this process may account for its more potent blood schizonticidal activity.

The mode of action of methylene blue analogs, the antimalarials from which 8-amino-quinolines were derived, has been reassessed *(58)*. Methylene blue has a shared mechanism of action with primaquine (i.e., direct stimulation of the erythrocytic hexose–mono-phosphate shunt [HMS]), probably via NADPH oxidation. For methylene blue analogs, the ability to complex with heme, but not HMS activation, correlated with antimalarial activity.

A major constraint of studying the antiparasitic activity of 8-aminoquinolines against tissue schizonts and hypnozoites has been the difficulty of establishing an in vitro culture system for the exoerythrocytic stages of *P. falciparum* and *P. vivax*. In vitro systems used to date do not accurately predict tissue schizonticidal activity. Data from animals models are often difficult to interpret because of interspecies differences in drug metabolism, as well as the inability to separate exoerythrocytic from blood-stage activity of compounds with long half-lives. The developers of 8-aminoquinolines have mostly relied upon *P. cynomolgi* in rhesus monkeys to ascertain antiparasitic activity among drug candidates. Activity in this model has a good correlation with activity against human *P. vivax* infection.

Toxicity

Hemolytic Anemia

The most important toxicity problem linked to 8-aminoquinolines is hemolysis in G6PD-deficient individuals. The mechanism of 8-aminoquinoline-induced hemolysis in these people is not understood. Conceptually, the separation of antimalarial activity from hemolytic toxicity seems likely: if the site of the antimalarial action of 8-amino-quinolines is mitochondria, then because erythrocytes lack mitochondria, the problem of hemolysis would appear separable. Thus, it is critically important to understand the molecular events that mediate the destruction of G6PD-deficient red blood cells by 8-aminoquinolines.

It has been long believed that free-radical production mediates hemolysis in G6PD-deficient red blood cells. However, other mechanisms appear to be involved, and none are established with certainty as the basis of toxicity. Many drugs and infections cause hemolysis in G6PD-deficient individuals *(59)*. Primaquine caused less hemolysis in normal red blood cells than dapsone, but the converse was true in G6PD-deficient subjects *(60)*. These differences suggest the possibility of different mechanisms of drug-induced hemolysis, or simply different dose-response characteristics in normal versus deficient cells.

Many disease states, from Alzheimer's disease to malaria, include damage to membranes and subcellular organelles by free radicals *(61,62)*. A number of important antioxidant systems require NADPH. In both the human erythrocyte and the malaria parasite, the HMS (Fig. 3) is required for detoxification of free radicals through the production of NADPH *(63)*. G6PD, the rate-limiting enzyme in this shunt, is the only source of electrons for the reduction of $NADP^+$ in erythrocytes. Glutathione peroxidase and catalase have each been reported to detoxify about half of the generated hydrogen peroxide in erythrocytes *(64)*. Both of these systems are NADPH dependent *(65,66)*. The erythrocytes of G6PD-deficient individuals produce less NADPH than those of normal individuals and, therefore, may be more susceptible to injury from oxidizing agents *(67)*.

The oxidation of NADPH to reduce oxidized glutathione (via glutathione reductase), free radicals, or methylene blue diminishes the NADPH- to $NADP^+$-ratio, and this directly stimulates the HMS. Primaquine (and especially some of its metabolites) accelerate the HMS through a methylene-blue-like mechanism *(67–69)*. However, methylene blue stimulates the HMS independently of glutathione by directly oxidizing NADPH, whereas primaquine appears to act by both consumption of glutathione and direct oxidation of NADPH *(67,70,71)*.

Several authors have suggested that hemolysis induced by primaquine appears to be mediated by activated oxygen *(72,73)*. The fact that clinically relevant hemolysis follows the administration of 8-aminoquinolines in individuals with genetic deficiencies affecting the detoxification of reactive oxygen species (G6PD, 6-phosphogluconate dehydrogenase, glutathione reductase, glutathione peroxidase, and glutathione synthetase; Fig. 3) *(30,60,74)* supports this hypothesis. Each of these genetic defects affects pathways for the reduction of glutathione or detoxification of oxygen radicals by glutathione.

Under some conditions, primaquine and its hydroxylated metabolites auto-oxidize, generating H_2O2, superoxide, and hydroxyl radicals *(73,75–77)*. However, in some of these reports, high concentrations of primaquine were used. The generation of superoxide by primaquine metabolites may be catalyzed by iron *(10,75)*. In a characterization of the intermediates and products during oxidation and redox cycling of three of primaquine's hydroxylated metabolites, formation of hydrogen peroxide, quinoneimine products (Fig. 2), drug-derived radicals, and hydroxyl radicals were demonstrated. Hydrogen peroxide was suggested to be the primary toxic product *(76,78)*.

However, another series of experiments indicated that oxidative injury to the red blood cell may not be the basis of primaquine-induced hemolysis in G6PD-deficient red blood cells *(68,69)*. The red blood cell possesses a proteolytic pathway that disassembles proteins irreversibly damaged by oxidation *(79)*. The activity of this proteolytic pathway was used to gage oxidative injury in normal red blood cells treated with nitrite, primaquine metabolites, or methylene blue in the context of HMS stimulation. Whereas exceeding the saturation potential of HMS activity by nitrite activated the proteolytic pathway, exerting the same stimulatory potential on the HMS using methylene blue or primaquine metabolites failed to do so. There was no evidence of oxidative injury in association with potent stimulation of the HMS by primaquine. Primaquine metabolites or methylene blue had no direct inhibitory effect on the proteolytic pathway. Stimulation of the HMS by highly reactive 5-hydroxy primaquine metabolites was not associated with an oxidative challenge to erythrocyte protein. It was speculated that NADPH-driven redox equilibrium between oxidized and reduced species of primaquine metabolites in G6PD-deficient red blood cells would strongly favor the oxidized species. Predominance of an oxidized species of a primaquine metabolite (i.e., a

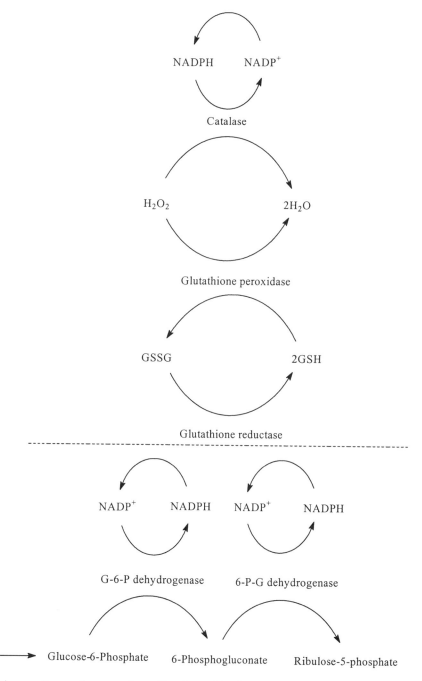

Fig. 3. Pathways for erythrocyte detoxification of hydrogen peroxide. Note NADPH and therefore, G6PD dependence. The HMS or pentose phosphate pathway is below the dotted line.

quinoneimine; Fig. 2) might lead to specific hemolytic events unrelated to oxidative injury (e.g., formation of a heme derivative that is driven from hemoglobin into membranes), similar to the process of phenylhydrazine-induced hemolysis in rats *(80,81)*. This is also an attractive hypothesis for the primaquine-induced hemolysis because it explains the apparent paradox, reported by some investigators, of G6PD-deficient people being less likely to exhibit methemoglobinemia. Limited redox recycling of primaquine may limit the generation of oxygen radicals that generate methemoglobin. Moreover, it largely disposes of the difficulty of explaining massive oxidative injury to red blood cells in the face of the relatively small oxidizing potential produced by a therapeutic dose of primaquine.

The effect of antioxidants on 8-aminoquinoline-induced toxicity has been studied. Tea polyphenols protected erythrocytes from primaquine-induced lysis in vitro (82). They also protected cells and membranes against H_2O_2-induced lipid peroxidation. A superoxide scavenger was shown to block primaquine-induced hemolysis in a dose-dependent manner, but it enhanced the oxidation of oxyhemoglobin to methemoglobin (83). On the other hand, the antioxidant rutin did not prevent primaquine-induced hemolysis but did protect against hemoglobin oxidation (84). Three antioxidants from traditional Chinese medicine were found to inhibit the oxidizing activity of 5,6-dihydroxy-8-aminoquinoline in an in vitro model (85). Understanding the effects of antioxidants may lead to improved understanding of the mechanisms of activity and toxicity of 8-aminoquinolines. Clinical use of antioxidants might mitigate the hemolytic toxicity of primaquine, but such treatments might alter antimalarial activity as well (86).

It has been shown that hemoglobin thiyl radicals, formed as a consequence of dapsone hydroxylamine redox cycling, attack red blood cell membrane skeletal proteins (87,88). A follow-up study illustrated that lipid peroxidation was not involved as an underlying mechanism of dapsone-induced hemolytic anemia (89). However, some evidence supports the role of lipid peroxidation associated with 8-aminoquinoline toxicity (82,85,90,91).

Hemolysis may occur intravascularly (as a result of increased membrane fragility and permeability) or extravascularly (through clearance of damaged cells by the reticuloendothelial system). Primaquine has been reported to both cause membrane fragility (92,93) and altered membrane deformability in erythrocytes (94,95). The G6PD status also affects erythrocyte deformability (96).

In vitro surrogate markers and in vivo animal models are often used to assess the hemolytic toxicity of compounds. The problem with the use of such markers was exemplified by a recent study (90). The (–) enantiomer of primaquine produced more methemoglobin and a greater decrease in reduced glutathione than the (+) enantiomer, whereas the (+) enantiomer caused a greater release of free hemoglobin. Reduced glutathione concentration, methemoglobin levels, Heinz body formation, and release of hemoglobin are often used as correlates of hemolytic toxicity in vitro. However, it is unclear how well any of these markers predict clinical toxicity. Furthermore, static in vitro systems often poorly predict in vivo hemolytic potential of drugs (97). Moreover, because hemolysis in vivo does not become apparent for 1–3 d following 8-aminoquinoline consumption (30), prolonged in vitro incubations may be necessary to reproduce it. Finally, many drugs require metabolic activation before they become hemolytic. Animal studies partially address this problem but may be difficult to interpret because models of human G6PD deficiency are of limited value and animals often metabolize drugs differently than do humans.

Attempts have been made to develop better models to identify the hemolytic potential of drugs (98). A test that incubates phenobarbital-induced microsomes with drugs and G6PD-deficient red blood cells has been described (99–101). Using residual glutathione as a marker, all nonhemolytic compounds were correctly identified. Most, but not all, hemolytic compounds were also correctly classified. This model may be helpful in classifying a new drug candidate as potentially hemolytic, but it may not as reliably identify nonhemolytic drugs. G6PD gene expression following exposure of hepatocytes to new drug candidates might prove to be a more predictive and manageable model. Assessment of G6PD gene expression has been reported in a number of studies *(102–104)*.

Both enantiomers of primaquine *(105)* and tafenoquine (D. Kyle, unpublished observations) have been shown to have similar levels of antimalarial activity. It remains unknown if hemolytic toxicity could be reduced through the development of a single enantiomer. In in vitro and in animal models, the (+) and (–) enantiomers of primaquine appear to have differential toxicity. However, depending on the end point, neither enantiomer is consistently less toxic. Stereoselective elimination of primaquine has also been reported *(43,106)*. The enantiomers of tafenoquine have not yet been evaluated for toxicity.

Methemoglobinemia

8-Aminoquinolines cause methemoglobinemia, but this rarely causes symptoms. Methemoglobin (ferrihemoglobin, hemiglobin) is formed when ferrous iron (Fe^{2+}) of hemoglobin is oxidized to the ferric (Fe^{3+}) state. It is incapable of reversibly binding to oxygen. Methemoglobinemia occurs when the capacity of the methemoglobin reducing system is overwhelmed. NADH methemoglobin reductase has been reported to be responsible for most methemoglobin reduction in red blood cells *(107)*. Congenital deficiency of this enzyme increases the risk for drug-induced methemoglobinemia *(108)*. A second mechanism of methemoglobin reduction is an NADPH-dependent process *(45,107)*. It was considered a reserve system *(107)*, but it is now viewed as functional only in the presence of an artificial carrier (e.g., methylene blue) *(45)*. Glutathione and ascorbic acid are also considered to be reserve systems for methemoglobin reduction *(107)*.

Many drugs, including 8-aminoquinolines, cause methemoglobinemia *(109)*. A good correlation was found between primaquine metabolite-mediated superoxide generation and methemoglobin production *(10)*. Paradoxically, primaquine has been reported to cause more methemoglobinemia in normal individuals than in those with G6PD deficiency *(110,111)*.

At high doses, methylene blue causes methemoglobinemia. However, at pharmacologic doses, it is the treatment of choice for symptomatic methemoglobinemia. Methylene blue functions as a completely reversible redox catalyst. Because of the requirement for NADPH, methylene blue for the treatment of methemoglobinemia is ineffective in G6PD-deficient individuals *(112)*.

Methemoglobin-forming agents may or may not be potent hemolytic agents. However, most drugs that produce hemolytic anemia in G6PD-deficient red blood cells also produce some degree of methemoglobinemia in G6PD normal red blood cells *(47)*.

Contribution of Metabolism

The putative metabolites of primaquine are more toxic than the parent compound. Despite extensive research, no metabolite has been unequivocally linked to any specific toxic effect. The metabolism of 8-aminoquinolones is difficult to study because of the instability of the intermediates and their amphoteric properties *(113,114)*. Radiolabeled drug in humans has been used to elucidate the metabolites generated in vivo.

Recent work has shed new light on the P450-independent metabolism of this class of compounds and suggests that G6PD-linked metabolism or detoxification may play a role in toxicity.

Studies of the metabolism of 8-aminoquinolines in nonhuman systems have contributed to our understanding. As early as 1962, it was hypothesized that primaquine toxicity was mediated by a hydroxylated metabolite forming a quinone capable of redox cycling *(76)*. Hydroxylated derivatives were identified in dog urine following the administration of radioactive primaquine *(115)*. The 5-hydroxy metabolite could form a quinoneimine. In a follow-up study, a quinoneimine was isolated from mouse liver microsomes in which the 8-amino side chain cyclized to produce a third ring system *(116)*. Hydroxylated metabolites were also identified in rats and rhesus monkeys *(47)*. Hydroxylation may be an essential step to hemolytic toxicity *(117)*. Hydroxylated metabolite(s) of primaquine probably contribute to hemolytic toxicity, but none have yet been identified in humans *(76,118)*. Metabolism to the relatively inert carboxylated species of primaquine represents the only unambiguous metabolic pathway of primaquine known in humans *(119,120)*. A growing body of evidence suggests that this metabolite is produced in erythrocytes.

Mihaly and colleagues first described the carboxylic acid derivative of primaquine as the main metabolite *(119)*. Following [^{14}C]-primaquine administration to human volunteers, primaquine accounted for only 2% of the total area under the curve (AUC), whereas the carboxy metabolite accounted for 55%. Over 143 h, 64% of the radioactivity was recovered in the urine, almost all of it being in the form of unidentified metabolites. Therefore, the carboxy metabolite probably undergoes further biotransformation. The metabolism of primaquine is expected to be complex because it contains several metabolically labile constituent groups. Likewise, the structure of tafenoquine suggests that it will undergo even more complex metabolism than primaquine, and initial studies bear this out.

Metabolism independent of cytochrome P450 apparently plays a role in primaquine clearance. The side chain of primaquine undergoes biotransformation to primaquine–aldehyde in cell-free media containing an oxidase (Fig. 4) *(46)*. Primaquine–aldehyde is then converted to carboxyprimaquine by an aldehyde dehydrogenase. Alternatively, alcohol dehydrogenase may convert primaquine to primaquine alcohol. 8-Aminoquinoline oxidases exist in some cell types, but their range of distribution among eukaryotes is poorly defined. These enzyme systems likely generate pentaquine–aldehyde from pentaquine, which is active against coccidia *(44)*. An extended incubation with hamster liver microsomes revealed conversion of primaquine alcohol to carboxyprimaquine to a lactam, all independent of cytochrome P450 *(121)*. The same investigators found that an NADPH-generating system (NADP, glucose-6-phosphate, and G6PD) diminished the production of several metabolites and apparently inhibited the metabolism of primaquine. These data suggest that the cellular location of alcohol and aldehyde dehydrogenases, as well as cofactors of the NADPH-generating system, may influence the toxicity of 8-aminoquinolines.

Erythrocytes play an important role in the metabolism of some xenobiotics. Metabolic degradation of primaquine in the erythrocyte had been proposed as early as 1966 *(93)*. Primaquine-induced osmotic fragility required glucose. Paradoxically, primaquine increased osmotic fragility in G6PD-deficient red blood cells much less than in normal

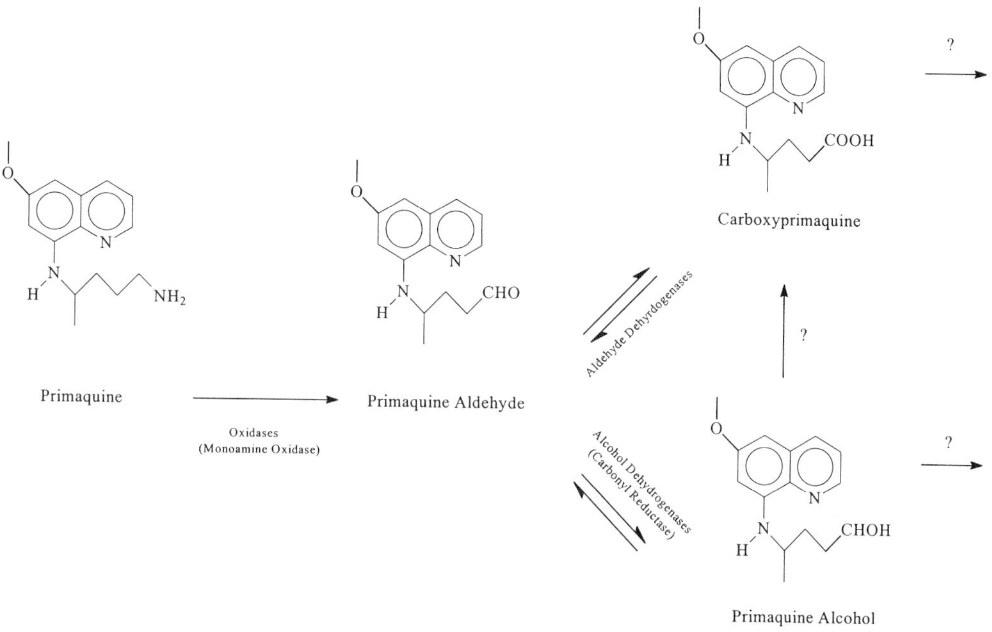

Fig. 4. Proposed pathways for side-chain metabolism of primaquine. Carboxyprimaquine is the main metabolite found in humans. Monoamine oxidase is located in mitochondria. Aldehydes are generally toxic. (Adapted from ref. *46*).

cells. HMS shunt-mediated metabolism of primaquine within the red blood cell was proposed. Human erythroleukemic cells metabolized primaquine predominately to carboxyprimaquine (see the next section) *(122)*. In monkeys, primaquine appeared to be metabolized within erythrocytes: 40% of dosed radioactive primaquine appeared in red blood cells within 4 h, mostly as metabolites *(47)*. Cyclophosphamide may undergo metabolism in erythrocytes through the same pathways as 8-aminoquinolines *(123)*. Although carboxyprimaquine forms in human liver microsomes and isolated mitochondria *(118,124)* erythrocytes probably contribute an appreciable portion of the total mass of carboxyprimaquine.

Accumulated evidence suggests that G6PD-deficient individuals exhibit restricted extrahepatic metabolism of some xenobiotics *(71,125–127)*. G6PD-deficient human lymphocytes were less able than normal cells to metabolize benzopyrene to toxic metabolites. G6PD deficiency restricted the metabolism of daunorubicin to its main metabolite (daunorubicinol) in erythrocytes, thus revealing HMS dehydrogenase activity control of carbonyl-reductase-dependent biotransformation. Moreover, primaquine–aldehyde competed with daunorubicin as a substrate for carbonyl reductase. In another study, primaquine conversion to carboxyprimaquine by human erythroleukemic cells was inhibited by the glutathione reductase inhibitor 1,3-bis-(2-chloroethyl)-nitrosourea (BCNU) *(122)*. This led to a progressive and striking accumulation of an unidentified metabolite. It has been suggested that primaquine-induced hemolysis is caused by NADPH-dependent drug elimination *(70)*. Taken together, these findings suggest that G6PD-deficiency-restricted metabolism may cause the accumulation of a toxic intermediate of primaquine metabolism in erythrocytes.

PROPHYLAXIS

Primaquine

Primaquine prevents malaria by killing parasites soon after they invade hepatocytes. Although primaquine is not yet labeled for this indication, good prophylactic efficacy and tolerance have both been demonstrated in experimental challenge and field trials against *P. falciparum* and *P. vivax* (128–133). A single 30- or 45-mg dose (all doses refer to the base) of primaquine taken the day before, the day of, or the day after experimental challenge with sporozoites did not prevent falciparum malaria (128,132). However, when the same dose was taken 48–72 h after challenge, protection was complete (128,132). When the dose was delayed to beyond 72 h after challenge, protection disappeared. Thus, a dose of primaquine taken about 48 h after inoculation with sporozoites kills developing hepatocyte forms of the parasite, but the developing parasite is only sensitive to the effects of the drug during a relatively narrow time frame. Under conditions of natural exposure, the moment of inoculation is rarely known, so a daily dosing regimen is necessary to prevent malaria. When a 30-mg dose was taken according to a standard dosing regimen for the week before challenge, the day of challenge, and the week following challenge, protection was complete against *P. falciparum* ($n = 8$) and *P. vivax* ($n = 10$). Protection dropped to 67% and 80%, respectively, when 15 mg was administered by this regimen. A daily regimen of 30 mg primaquine base taken by 43 nonimmune adults for 1 yr was 92% efficacious (90% against *P. vivax* and 94% against *P. falciparum*) in a randomized, placebo-controlled trial in hyperendemic Irian Jaya, Indonesia (131). An alternate-day regimen was only 80% efficacious in the same region (74% against *P. falciparum* and 90% against *P. vivax*) (130). In Kenya, an alternate-day regimen had no protective efficacy (133). These studies demonstrate the necessity of a daily 30-mg dose for effective prophylaxis with primaquine. Although a 30-mg dose may cause gastrointestinal upset when taken on an empty stomach (134), the regimen is well tolerated when taken with food (130,131,133,134). The duration of postexposure dosing with primaquine for causal prophylaxis is not known, but the available data suggest that 1 or 2 d may suffice.

Tafenoquine

In vitro and in vivo animal efficacy testing demonstrated that tafenoquine had promising causal prophylactic activity. Moreover, tafenoquine had 5-fold to 15-fold better in vitro blood schizonticidal activity against *P. falciparum* than primaquine. The in vitro activity of tafenoquine against multidrug-resistant falciparum parasites was severalfold greater than against sensitive parasites. This combination of causal and blood-stage activity led to the investigation of tafenoquine for prophylaxis.

The first human efficacy study of tafenoquine found that a single 600-mg oral dose could protect nonimmune volunteers from challenge with *P. falciparum* by infected mosquitoes (135). This and subsequent studies led to a large-scale field study in semi-immune individuals living in a holoendemic area of eastern Africa. Tafenoquine, when given as a 3-d loading regimen followed by weekly administration of 200 or 400 mg for 14 wk, successfully protected 95% of individuals (D. Shanks, unpublished data). In the same study, a 3-d 400-mg loading regimen alone protected individuals for over 60 d in this high-transmission area, where the infection rate in those receiving placebo was over 80%. These regimens were well tolerated when taken with food, but the 400-mg regimen resulted in clinically significant hemolytic reactions in two G6PD-deficient individuals who were inadvertently enrolled. If confirmed in nonimmune individuals, the 3-d regimen can be effectively used as a short-term malaria "vaccine" for travelers and military personnel deployed to endemic areas for 1–2 mo. The utility of a weekly prophylactic regimen was further investigated in a dose-ranging study in Ghana, where 100 and 200 mg weekly also protected individuals living in a high-transmission area (B. Hale, personal communication). Tafenoquine's long half-life prompted an additional study in Thailand, where multidrug-resistant parasites are of particular concern. In that study, 500 mg of tafenoquine was administered monthly and was found to be protective (D. Walsh, personal communication).

Both tafenoquine and primaquine are efficacious for malaria prophylaxis, for radical cure of *P. vivax*, and, in theory, for malaria control. Each carries a unique set of advantages and disadvantages. Both 8-aminoquinolines can result in hemolysis in G6PD-deficient individuals. Primaquine is the only drug in clinical use that been clearly shown to be causally prophylactic for malaria. As such, it is the only drug available that does not require 4 wk of prophylaxis after leaving a malaria endemic area. This property makes it ideal for travelers exposed for just a short time. The most important disadvantage of primaquine prophylaxis is the requirement for daily dosing. A single missed dose at crucial time may lead to prophylaxis failure. Education and blister packs or pillboxes could improve compliance and improve effectiveness. The US FDA labeling of primaquine for this indication is pending.

A tafenoquine loading dose followed by weekly dosing rapidly achieves and maintains an effective concentration for long periods of time. This enables weekly dosing with relatively constant drug concentrations. It is not yet known if tafenoquine has sufficient causal activity or a long enough half-life such that its use can be discontinued upon leaving a transmission area. Additional studies, including phase III clinical trials in nonimmune individuals, will begin soon.

ANTIRELAPSE THERAPY

Relapse may occur with infections by *P. vivax* or *P. ovale*. The risk and timing of relapse with untreated *P. vivax* infection varies among strains. Relapse occurs more often among tropical versus temperate strains. For example, among 54 patients infected in the tropical Pacific, all relapsed within 3 mo *(136)*. In contrast, only 32% of 1021 patients infected by *P. vivax* in Korea relapsed during more than 4 mo of follow-up *(137–139)*. In subtropical India, 11% of 5750 patients relapsed within 12 mo of follow-up *(140,141)*.

Primaquine

The killing of developing or quiescent liver stages with primaquine represents its primary use over the past 50 yr. The standard regimen for antirelapse therapy, conceived as the most convenient and well-tolerated means of delivering a total adult dose of 210 mg base, is 15 mg daily for 14 d, but many variant regimens exist. Experiments in monkeys conducted during the development of primaquine demonstrated that the total dose rather than dosing regimen determined the efficacy of the drug *(142)*. Sixty milligrams daily for 7 d was as effective as 30 mg daily for 14 d *(143)*. Likewise, 45 mg weekly for 8 wk was as effective as 30 mg daily for 14 d *(110)*. These regimens double the total dose of the standard treatment regimen and either is recommended for the treatment of vivax malaria acquired in Southeast Asia or Oceania where failure of the standard 15-mg primaquine regimen is common *(144)*. The Chesson strain of *P. vivax*, acquired by an American soldier in New Guinea during the Second World War and extensively evaluated during early clinical trials of primaquine, often failed treatment with standard therapy (approx 70% efficacy) *(145)*. A total dose of 420 mg was 100% efficacious against the Chesson strain *(110,129,143)*. The 45-mg weekly dose for 8 wk has also been recommended for treatment of vivax malaria in persons having the African A-variant of G6PD deficiency *(110)*. However, this regimen may not be safe for other, more severe, variants (*see* the "Safety" section).

The frequency of relapse following treatment with 15 mg primaquine daily for 14 d varies by geographic origin of the infection. Relapse after supervised treatment in 141 patients in Thailand was 18% *(8,146)*, whereas fewer than 1% of 941 subjects infected in Korea relapsed *(137,138)*. Patients who acquired vivax malaria in New Guinea and were treated with unsupervised standard primaquine therapy had an 11.7-fold higher risk of relapse compared to patients who acquired vivax malaria elsewhere *(147)*. Supervision of treatment dramatically improved therapeutic effectiveness of primaquine: relapse in 218 US soldiers repatriated from Vietnam and given supervised treatment was just 4% *(148)*, whereas 251 soldiers given unsupervised treatment had an 18% relapse rate *(149,150)*. Failure to comply with prescribed primaquine treatment may be the most frequent cause of relapse. Resistance to the standard primaquine treatment regimen has not been convincingly demonstrated (*see* the "Resistance" section).

Some governments in endemic areas recommend a treatment regimen of 15 mg primaquine daily for just 5 d (e.g., India). Early studies documented substantial declines in the number of clinical cases of malaria when the regimen was broadly applied *(151–153)*. However, no well-controlled trial has ever demonstrated this regimen to be effective. Reports of low relapse rates in areas applying the 5-d regimen often fail to account for similarly low rates among patients in the same area given no primaquine at all (i.e., the efficacy of the regimen is at most 50% and may be close to 0%) *(154)*. Experimental challenge trials using this regimen support this conclusion *(155,156)*.

Tafenoquine

Tafenoquine had substantial activity against the liver stage of vivax malaria in initial animal models, and initially entered the WRAIR antimalarial drug development program as the long-sought replacement for primaquine. Nonclinical studies demonstrated activity that was sevenfold greater than primaquine in the rhesus monkey. A drug with a shorter dosing regimen than primaquine may substantially improve effectiveness by making compliance easier. Shorter treatment regimens of tafenoquine (i.e., 300 mg daily for 1 wk, or even 500 mg as a single dose) have been efficacious for the radical cure of *P. vivax* in Thailand *(157)*. However, because of tafenoquine's long half-life and the lack of an in vitro liver-stage model for vivax malaria, it is not possible to tell how much of its improved efficacy profile observed in vivo is the result of a greater intrinsic potency versus a greater (or more consistent) period of drug exposure.

TERMINAL PROPHYLAXIS

Primaquine

Some health care providers prescribe a standard regimen of primaquine treatment following possible exposure to *P. vivax* or *P. ovale*. "Terminal prophylaxis" presumably eliminates liver stages, thus reducing the probability of relapse following 4 wk of postexposure suppressive prophylaxis. One study in Thailand found a high risk of *P. vivax* following treatment of falciparum malaria with a blood schizonticide *(158)*. Thus, treatment of patients who have falciparum malaria with standard primaquine antirelapse therapy, in addition to their blood schizonticide therapy, may reduce the risk of relapse from vivax or ovale malaria.

Tafenoquine

Rieckmann and colleagues are presently evaluating the use of a 3-d tafenoquine regimen (500 mg daily) in Papua New Guinea for terminal prophylaxis and comparing it to a 14-d primaquine eradication course (22.5 mg daily). Preliminary results indicate that the 3-d tafenoquine regimen is comparable to, but may not be superior to, primaquine in eradicating primaquine-refractory hypnozoites of *P. vivax*. However, the acceptability of the 3-d regimen is substantially greater than the 14-d primaquine regimen.

TRANSMISSION BLOCKING

Primaquine

Primaquine has gametocytocidal and sporontocidal properties after a single dose when persons have circulating mature gametocytes *(159–161)*. Although the effect of primaquine on malaria control has not been rigorously evaluated, the World Health Organization has recommended single-dose primaquine to sterilize gametocytes. Specifically, this recommendation stated that primaquine may be considered at the initiation of treatment of *P. falciparum* where reintroduction of the infection is a concern for epidemic control *(162)*. Weekly administration of primaquine in combination with a long-acting blood schizonticide should block malaria transmission *(2)*.

Tafenoquine

Tafenoquine has activity against sporozoites and gametocytes, also making it a candidate as a transmission-blocking drug (D. Kyle, personal communication). There have been no clinical studies conducted to evaluate the transmission-blocking potential of tafenoquine, although nonclinical work suggests that it may be possible to impact transmission within defined areas. Because of its long half-life, tafenoquine has enormous potential as an agent of malaria control. Because humans are the reservoir for this disease, if an isolated population were to be treated, the impact upon malaria transmission should be immediate and dramatic. Before this approach can be implemented, however, a regimen tolerable to people with G6PD deficiency needs to be developed. Alternatively, measures to minimize any potential errors in identification of G6PD-deficient individuals would need to be used.

RESISTANCE

A complex, multifactorial interaction among the parasite, the environment, and the host contribute to resistance to antimalarials. These factors include genetic mutation(s) required by the parasite to confer resistance, the stability of the mutation(s), the drug's mechanism of action and pharmacokinetics, the transmission intensity, whether combination treatment is used, the host's immunity, and drug misuse/noncompliance issues. Induced resistance of blood-stage *P. vivax* parasites to primaquine was unequivocally demonstrated in experimentally infected humans *(9)*. However, resistance to primaquine in liver-stage parasites has not been demonstrated in any animal model, and no compelling demonstration of therapeutic failure has been reported. The mechanisms of resistance to 8-aminoquinolines by blood-stage parasites are not understood. Mitochondrial proliferation has been observed in blood-stage parasites resistant to the lethal effects of 8-aminoquinolines in animal models *(13)*.

Primaquine

Clinical resistance to primaquine has not been documented, even though it has been the only drug available for antirelapse therapy for the past 50 yr *(163)*. Several studies from Thailand have documented failure of the standard regimen of primaquine, but these infections may represent Chesson-strain-like tolerance (rather than an emerging resistance problem). Although many reports described instances of relapse following primaquine treatment, none adequately addressed potential confounding by either reinfection or, more often, failure to comply with prescribed therapy. Another confounding factor is resistance to chloroquine by blood stages of *P. vivax (164,165)*. A recurrence of parasitemia after treatment with chloroquine and primaquine may represent inadequate compliance to the treatment regimen, poor absorption, abnormal metabolism of drug, reinfection, recrudescence of a chloroquine-resistant strain, or relapse of a primaquine-resistant strain. The practical and technical difficulties of sorting out these confounding factors may explain the lack of confirmed reports of resistance. On the other hand, resistance to primaquine in liver stages may not exist.

The most common flaw among published reports of primaquine resistance is the failure to directly observe therapy. Another important confounder in assessing the possibility of resistance is chloroquine therapy. Chloroquine has a long half-life, which can suppress relapse of chloroquine-sensitive strains for 4–5 wk. The use of quinine, rather than chloroquine, for blood schizonticidal therapy may radically improve the sensitivity of studies intended to assess potential resistance to primaquine. This approach solves two important problems: (1) avoiding suppression of relapse by primaquine-resistant but chloroquine-sensitive strains during the critical first month following treatment and (2) precluding confounding of the evaluation by recrudescence of chloroquine-resistant strains. When subjects are infected with the blood stage of the Chesson and other strains of *P. vivax*, where relapse by hypnozoites is not possible, quinine was found to have blood schizoiticidal activity *(166)*. However, among 333 subjects infected in the tropical Pacific, 59% relapsed during the month following treatment with quinine alone *(165)*. The median day of relapse was d 23 after initiating quinine therapy of the primary parasitemia. In contrast, among 256 subjects in parallel studies treated with chloroquine, none relapsed before d 35, and most still had not relapsed by d 60. Chloroquine eliminates parasitemia originating from relapse for a period of approx 1 mo *(165)*. Ideally, primaquine should be administered simultaneously with quinine or chloroquine because these drugs dramatically improve the tissue schizonticidal activity of primaquine *(167)*.

Tafenoquine

Tafenoquine, with its long half-life, theoretically has the risk of inducing resistance to both *P. vivax* and *P. falciparum* blood stages, as well as to *P. vivax* hypnozoites. The rapid demise of Fansidar® (sulfadoxine-pyrimethamine) and mefloquine in areas of widespread use may have been related to their long half-lives. If tafenoquine is used in endemic areas to radically cure *P. vivax* infection, patients will be exposed subsequently to *P. falciparum* and *P. vivax* reinfections while partially suppressive drug concentrations are present. This could result in the development of resistance to tafenoquine and, potentially to primaquine as well. Factors relating to the development of resistance to 8-aminoquinolines should be determined and must be considered when tafenoquine is used. Of note, tafenoquine is more active in vitro against multidrug-resistant *P. falciparum* patient isolates (W. Milhous, unpublished observations), suggesting that it is not cross-resistant with drugs such as halofantrine and mefloquine. This phenomenon may prove helpful to understanding the mechanisms of multiple-drug resistance in malaria.

The use of active drug combinations reduces the likelihood of emergence of resistant isolates. In addition, 8-aminoquinolines kill gametocytes. However, the gametocytes present at the time of initial treatment are not those of greatest concern for preventing the spread of drug-resistant malaria. It is the gametocytes that arise from late treatment failures that are the likely pool for transmission of drug-resistant malaria. These gametocytes usually develop between 14 and 60 d following treatment. It is unknown if tafenoquine, even with its long half-life, would prevent the emergence and spread of drug resistance if coadministered with *P. falciparum* treatment regimens. A concern with this approach would be induction of parasite resistance to 8-aminoquinolines. If tafenoquine is to be coadministered with other drugs, carefully conducted trials of its safety and effectiveness will be indicated, as well as rigorous monitoring for the development of resistance.

SAFETY

Common side effects of 8-aminoquinolines are gastrointestinal. However, with primaquine prophylaxis, the need to withdraw patients for gastrointestinal symptoms appears to be <2% *(131,168)*. Nausea, vomiting, anorexia and diarrhea occur with an incidence of <5%. Tafenoquine has similar gastrointestinal side effects. These effects are greatly decreased when the 8-aminoquinoloines are given with food.

The potentially life-threatening adverse effects from this class of compounds are hemolysis in G6PD-deficient individuals and, very rarely, methemoglobinemia in individuals deficient in methemoglobin reductase. G6PD deficiency, which affects about 400 million people worldwide, is the most common human enzymopathy *(58,169)*. This condition was discovered in the 1950s as the explanation for why certain individuals developed hemolysis following the administration of primaquine *(170)*. In the African phenotype (GdA⁻), only erythrocytes (and possibly hepatocytes) have lowered G6PD enzyme activity *(71)*. This is not the case for the more severe deficiencies, where the enzyme activity is decreased in all tissues. In areas where malaria has been prevalent, G6PD deficient alleles have reached high frequencies (1–50%) *(171)*, suggesting a selective advantage against malaria infection *(172)*. The frequency of G6PD deficiency varies by geographic region and by ethnic group. Reported frequencies of this deficiency are as follows: 2–16% in southern China, 1–7% in southern Italy, 26% in parts of Africa, and 70% among Kurdish Jews *(169)*. A sporadic X-linked form of G6PD deficiency occurs at very low frequencies anywhere in the world. This form usually presents with a more severe phenotype: chronic nonspherocytic hemolytic anemia.

The risk of hemolysis with primaquine has been well established. Studies in humans with mild forms of G6PD deficiency are difficult to conduct. Although few deaths have been reported from primaquine-induced hemolysis, there are many reports of severe adverse events *(173–177)*. The only data currently available for tafenoquine is from two A⁻ Kenyan women who accidentally received 400 mg daily for 3 d (D. Shanks, unpublished data). One study subject required transfusion, and both showed a greater hemolytic response than that seen with 30 mg of daily primaquine in A⁻ African-American males *(110)*. Despite tafenoquine's long-half life and the continued presence of drug in the blood for weeks, spontaneous recovery occurred in the nontransfused individual. Similar recoveries were seen with continued dosing of primaquine in prior studies *(110)*. This recovery reflects a vigorous reticulocyte response following the loss of older red blood cells, which are more deficient in G6PD and more prone to hemolysis.

The risk of complications with G6PD deficiency can be reduced through patient education and screening. If using these compounds for malaria prophylaxis, screening is essential and starting drug dosing several days before departure would allow the detection of any adverse events while the individual is still close to readily available medical care. Although the sensitivity and specificity of currently available G6PD screens is high in hemizygous males and homozygous females, they are less sensitive for heterozygous women. Hemolytic events should not be fatal in such individuals. However, G6PD-deficient people missed due to test failure, human error, or failure to screen could lead to mortality. A point-of-care G6PD test (dipstick) could be developed that would assist care providers in prescribing these drugs more safely.

Methemoglobinemia does not cause symptoms at levels below 15% of total hemoglobin *(108)*. Higher methemoglobin levels have not been seen with the doses of primaquine or tafenoquine used clinically. However, administering an 8-aminoquinoline to an individual with a very rare mutation of the methemoglobin reductase gene could cause symptomatic methemoglobinemia.

CONCLUSION: THE FUTURE OF 8-AMINOQUINOLINES

Primaquine has been and will continue to be important for the treatment and prevention of malaria for the foreseeable future. Tafenoquine will hopefully undergo phase III clinical studies leading to FDA approval and marketing within the next few years. The immediate hope is that it will offer safer, more convenient, and effective protection against malaria in travelers, and it may ultimately have an important role in therapy as well. A single-dosing regimen providing complete protection for short-term exposure would revolutionize malaria chemotherapy for travelers. The brightest hope for this family of drugs is their spectrum of activity across the developmental stages of plasmodia. This property may be exploited to develop intervention strategies that arrest epidemic malaria and break the cycle of transmission within defined foci. The future of 8-aminoquinolines depends in part on whether parasite resistance to this class of drugs develops and on whether an 8-aminoquinoline analog can be developed that retains broad-spectrum activity, yet has less propensity for hemolysis in G6PD-deficient individuals. This will require better methods to evaluate the hemolytic potential of drugs, a better understanding of the metabolism and mechanisms of action of 8-amino-quinolines, and collaboration between biochemists, synthetic chemists, computational chemists, parasitologists, pharmacologists, and clinicians.

ACKNOWLEDGMENTS

We thank Jonathan Vennerstrom, Jean Karle, and Apurba Bhattacharjee for their assistance and advice. We also express gratitude to Patricia Lee for technical assistance with preparing this chapter.

REFERENCES

1. Greenwood D. Conflicts of interest: the genesis of synthetic antimalarial agents in peace and war. J Antimicrob Chemother 1995;36(5):857–872.
2. Carson P. 8-Aminoquinolines In Peters W, Richards WHG (eds)., Antimalarial Drugs II. New York: Springer-Verlag, 1984, pp. 83–121.
3. Beadle C, Hoffman SL. History of malaria in the United States Naval Forces at war: World War I through the Vietnam conflict. Clin Infect Dis 1993;16(2):320–329.
4. Nodiff EA, Chatterjee S, Musallam HA. Antimalarial activity of the 8-aminoquinolines. In Ellis GP and West GB (eds.), Progress in Medicinal Chemistry Amsterdam: Elsevier Science, 1991, vol. 28, pp. 1–40.
5. Sweeney T. 8-Aminoquinolines. In Peters W. and Richards WHG (eds.), Antimalarial Drugs II. New York: Springer-Verlag, 1984, pp. 325–342.
6. Brueckner RP, Lasseter KC, Lin ET, Schuster BG. First-time-in-humans safety and pharmacokinetics of WR 238605, a new antimalarial. Am J Trop Med Hyg 1998;58(5):645–649.
7. Brueckner RP, Fleckenstein, L. Simultaneous modeling of the pharmacokinetics and methemoglobin pharmacodynamics of an 8-aminoquinoline candidate antimalarial (WR 238605). Pharm Res 1991;8(12):1505–1510.
8. Pukrittayakamee S, Vanijanonta S, Chantra A, Clemens R, White NJ. Blood stage antimalarial efficacy of primaquine in *Plasmodium vivax* malaria. J Infect Dis 1994;169(4): 932–935.
9. Arnold J, Alvinig AS, Clayman CB. Induced primaquine resistance in vivax malaria. Trans R Soc Trop Med Hyg 1961;55(4):345–350.
10. Bates MD, Meshnick SR, Sigler CI, Leland P, Hollingdale MR. *In vitro* effects of primaquine and primaquine metabolites on exoerythrocytic stages of *Plasmodium berghei*. Am J Trop Med Hyg 1990;42(6):532–537.
11. Lanners HN. Effect of the 8-aminoquinoline primaquine on culture-derived gametocytes of the malaria parasite *Plasmodium falciparum*. Parasitol Res 1991;77(6):478–481.
12. Boulard Y, Landau I, Miltgen F, Ellis DS, Peters W. The chemotherapy of rodent malaria, XXXIV. Causal prophylaxis Part III: Ultrastructural changes induced in exo-erythrocytic schizonts of *Plasmodium yoelii yoelii* by primaquine. Ann Trop Med Parasitol 1983; 77(6):555–568.
13. Warhurst DC. Why are primaquine and other 8-aminoquinolines particularly effective against the mature gametocytes and the hypnozoites of malaria? Ann Trop Med Parasitol 1984;78(2):165.
14. Peters W, Ellis D, Boulard Y, Landau I. The chemotherapy of rodent malaria XXXVI. Part IV. The activity of a new 8-aminoquinoline, WR 225,448:against exo-erythrocytic schizonts of *Plasmodium yoelii yoelii*. Ann Trop Med Parasitol 1984;78(5):467–478.
15. Goheen MP, Bartlett MS, Queener SF, Smith JW. The effect of primaquine on the ultrastructural morphology of *Pneumocystis carinii*. J Protozool 1991;38(6):164S-165S.

16. Goheen MP, Bartlett MS, Shaw MM, Queener SF, Smith JW. Effects of 8-amino-quinolines on the ultrastructural morphology of *Pneumocystis carinii*. Int J Exp Pathol 1993;74(4):379–387.

17. Aikawa M, Beaudoin RL. *Plasmodium fallax*: high-resolution autoradiography of exoerythrocytic stages treated with Primaquine *in vitro*. Exp Parasitol 1970;27(3):454–463.

18. Howells RE, Peters W, Fullard J. The chemotherapy of rodent malaria. 13. Fine structural changes observed in the erythrocytic stages of *Plasmodium berghei berghei* following exposure to primaquine and menoctone. Ann Trop Med Parasitol 1970;64(2):203–207.

19. Peters W, Irare SG, Ellis DS, Warhurst DC, Robinson BL. The chemotherapy of rodent malaria, XXXVIII. Studies on the activity of three new antimalarials (WR 194,965:WR 228,258 and WR 225,448) against rodent and human malaria parasites (*Plasmodium berghei* and *P. falciparum*). Ann Trop Med Parasitol 1984;78(6):567–579.

20. Rotman, A. Genetics of a primaquin-resistant yeast. J Gen Microbiol 1975;89(1):1–10.

21. Jiang JB, Jacobs G, Liang DS, Aikawa, M. Qinghaosu-induced changes in the morphology of *Plasmodium inui*. Am J Trop Med Hyg 1985;34(3):424–428.

22. Kawai S, Kano S, Suzuki, M. Morphologic effects of artemether on *Plasmodium falciparum* in *Aotus trivirgatus*. Am J Trop Med Hyg 1993;49(6):812–818.

23. Powers KG, Aikawa M, Nugent KM. *Plasmodium knowlesi*: morphology and course of infection in rhesus monkeys treated with clindamycin and its *N*-demethyl-4'-pentyl analog. Exp Parasitol 1976;40(1):13–24.

24. Peters, W., 2nd (ed) Chemotherapy and Drug Resistance in Malaria. Orlando, FL: Academic, 1987.

25. Srivastava IK, Vaidya AB. A mechanism for the synergistic antimalarial action of atovaquone and proguanil. Antimicrob Agents Chemother 1999;43(6):1334–1339.

26. Srivastava IK, Rottenberg H, Vaidya AB. Atovaquone, a broad spectrum antiparasitic drug, collapses mitochondrial membrane potential in a malarial parasite. J Biol Chem 1997;272(7):3961–3966.

27. Fry M, Pudney M. Site of action of the antimalarial hydroxynaphthoquinone, 2-[*trans*-4-(4'-chlorophenyl)cyclohexyl]-3-hydroxy-1,4-naphthoquinone (566C80). Biochem Pharmacol 1992;43(7):1545–1553.

28. Geary TG, Jensen JB. Effects of antibiotics on *Plasmodium falciparum in vitro*. Am J Trop Med Hyg 1983;32(2):221–225.

29. Kiatfuengfoo R, Suthiphongchai T, Prapunwattana P, Yuthavong Y. Mitochondria as the site of action of tetracycline on *Plasmodium falciparum*. Mol Biochem Parasitol 1989;34(2):109–115.

30. Carson PE, Hohl R, Nora MV, Parkhurst GW, Ahmad T, Scanlan S, et al. Toxicology of the 8-aminoquinolines and genetic factors associated with their toxicity in man. Bull WHO 1981;59(3):427–437.

31. Fry M, Beesley JE. Mitochondria of mammalian *Plasmodium* spp. Parasitology 1991;102(Pt1):17–26.

32. Ginsburg H, Divo AA, Geary TG, Boland MT, Jensen JB. Effects of mitochondrial inhibitors on intraerythrocytic *Plasmodium falciparum* in *in vitro* cultures. J Protozool 1986;33(1):121–125.

33. Prapunwattana P, O'Sullivan WJ, Yuthavong, Y. Depression of *Plasmodium falciparum* dihydroorotate dehydrogenase activity in *in vitro* culture by tetracycline. Mol Biochem Parasitol 1988;27(2–3):119–124.

34. Alberts, B., 3rd (ed). Molecular Biology of the Cell. New York: Garland, 1994.

35. Vaidya AB, Lashgari MS, Pologe LG, Morrisey J. Structural features of Plasmodium cytochrome b that may underlie susceptibility to 8-aminoquinolines and hydroxynaphthoquinones. Mol Biochem Parasitol 1993;58(1):33–42.

36. Ittarat I, Asawamahasakda W, Meshnick SR. The effects of antimalarials on the *Plasmodium falciparum* dihydroorotate dehydrogenase. Exp Parasitol 1994;79(1):50–56.

37. Vuist WM, Feijge MA, Heemskerk JW. Kinetics of store-operated Ca^{2+} influx evoked by endomembrane Ca^{2+}-ATPase inhibitors in human platelets. Prostaglandins Leukot Essential Fatty Acids 1997;57(4–5):447–450.

38. Barry SR, Bernal J. Antimalarial drugs inhibit calcium-dependent backward swimming and calcium currents in *Paramecium calkinsi*. J Comp Physiol [A] 1993;172(4):457–466.

39. Somasundaram B, Norman JC, Mahaut-Smith MP. Primaquine, an inhibitor of vesicular transport, blocks the calcium-release-activated current in rat megakaryocytes. Biochem J 1995;309(Pt 3):725–729.

40. Hiebsch RR, Raub TJ, Wattenberg BW. Primaquine blocks transport by inhibiting the formation of functional transport vesicles. Studies in a cell-free assay of protein transport through the Golgi apparatus. J Biol Chem 1991;266(30):20,323–20,328.

41. Grewal RS. Pharmacology of 8-aminoquinolines. Bull WHO 1981;59(3):397–406.

42. Ni YC, Xu YQ, Wang MJ. Rat liver microsomal and mitochondrial metabolism of primaquine *in vitro*. Chung Kuo Yao Li Hsueh Pao 1992;13(5):431–435.

43. Baker JK, McChesney JD. Differential metabolism of the enantiomers of primaquine. J Pharm Sci 1988;77(5):380–382.

44. Armer RE, Barlow JS, Dutton CJ, Greenway DH, Greenwood SD, Lad N, et al. 8-Aminoquinolines as anticoccidials—II. Bioorg Med Chem Lett 1998;8(12):1487–1492.

45. Casarett LJ, Klaassen CD, Amdur MO, Doull J., (eds). Casarett and Doull's Toxicology: The Basic Science of Poisons. New York: McGraw-Hill Health Professions, 1996.

46. Frischer H, Mellovitz RL, Ahmad T, Nora MV. The conversion of primaquine into primaquine–aldehyde, primaquine–alcohol, and carboxyprimaquine, a major plasma metabolite. J Lab Clin Med 1991;117(6):468–476.

47. Fletcher KA, Barton PF, Kelly JA. Studies on the mechanisms of oxidation in the erythrocyte by metabolites of primaquine. Biochem Pharmacol 1988;37(13):2683–2690.

48. Vasquez-Vivar J, Augusto O. Oxidative activity of primaquine metabolites on rat erythrocytes *in vitro* and *in vivo*. Biochem Pharmacol 1994;47(2):309–316.

49. Clark IA, Butcher GA, Buffinton GD, Hunt NH, Cowden WB. Toxicity of certain products of lipid peroxidation to the human malaria parasite *Plasmodium falciparum*. Biochem Pharmacol 1987;36(4):543–546.

50. Reichman N, Porteous CM, Murphy MP. Cyclosporin A blocks 6-hydroxydopamine-induced efflux of Ca^{2+} from mitochondria without inactivating the mitochondrial inner-membrane pore. Biochem J 1994;297(Pt 1):151–155.

51. Dockrell HM, Playfair JH. Killing of blood-stage murine malaria parasites by hydrogen peroxide. Infect Immun 1983;39(1):456–459.

52. Friedman MJ. Oxidant damage mediates variant red cell resistance to malaria. Nature 1979;280(5719):245–247.

53. Vennerstrom JL, Eaton JW. Oxidants, oxidant drugs, and malaria. J Med Chem 1988;31(7):1269–1277.

54. Cappadoro M, Giribaldi G, O'Brien E, Turrini F, Mannu F, Ulliers D, et al. Early phagocytosis of glucose-6-phosphate dehydrogenase (G6PD)-deficient erythrocytes parasitized by *Plasmodium falciparum* may explain malaria protection in G6PD deficiency. Blood 1998;92(7):2527–2534.

55. Atamna H, Ginsburg H. The malaria parasite supplies glutathione to its host cell—investigation of glutathione transport and metabolism in human erythrocytes infected with *Plasmodium falciparum*. Eur J Biochem 1997;250(3):670–679.

56. Srivastava P, Puri SK, Kamboj KK, Pandey VC. Glutathione-S-transferase activity in malarial parasites. Trop Med Int Health 1999;4(4):251–254.

57. Vennerstrom JL, Nuzum EO, Miller RE, Dorn A, Gerena L, Dande PA, et al. 8-Aminoquinolines active against blood stage *Plasmodium falciparum in vitro* inhibit hematin polymerization. Antimicrob Agents Chemother 1999;43(3):598–602.

58. Atamna H, Krugliak M, Shalmiev G, Deharo E, Pescarmona G, Ginsburg H. Mode of antimalarial effect of methylene blue and some of its analogues on *Plasmodium falciparum* in culture and their inhibition of *P. vinckei petteri* and *P. yoelii nigeriensis in vivo*. Biochem Pharmacol 1996;51(5):693–700.

59. Beutler, E. G6PD deficiency. Blood 1994;84(11):3613–3636.

60. Degowin RL, Eppes RB, Powell RD, Carson PE. The haemolytic effects of diaphenyl-sulfone (DDS) in normal subjects and in those with glucose-6-phosphate-dehydrogenase deficiency. Bull WHO 1966;35(2):165–179.

61. Knight JA. Free radicals: their history and current status in aging and disease. Ann Clin Lab Sci 1998;28(6):331–346.

62. Beal MF. Mitochondria, free radicals, and neurodegeneration. Curr Opin Neurobiol 1996;6(5):661–666.

63. Atamna H, Pascarmona G, Ginsburg H. Hexose-monophosphate shunt activity in intact *Plasmodium falciparum*-infected erythrocytes and in free parasites. Mol Biochem Parasitol 1994;67(1):79–89.

64. Gaetani GF, Kirkman HN, Mangerini R, Ferraris AM. Importance of catalase in the disposal of hydrogen peroxide within human erythrocytes. Blood 1994;84(1):325–330.

65. Kirkman HN, Rolfo M, Ferraris AM, Gaetani GF. Mechanisms of protection of catalase by NADPH. Kinetics and stoichiometry. J Biol Chem 1999;274(20):13,908–13,914.

66. Scott MD, Zuo L, Lubin BH, Chiu DT. NADPH, not glutathione, status modulates oxidant sensitivity in normal and glucose-6-phosphate dehydrogenase-deficient erythrocytes. Blood 1991;77(9):2059–2064.

67. Deslauriers R, Butler K, Smith IC. Oxidant stress in malaria as probed by stable nitroxide radicals in erythrocytes infected with *Plasmodium berghei*. The effects of primaquine and chloroquine. Biochim Biophys Acta 1987;931(3):267–275.

68. Baird JK, Davidson DE, Jr, Decker-Jackson JE. Oxidative activity of hydroxylated pri-maquine analogs. Non-toxicity to glucose-6-phosphate dehydrogenase-deficient human red blood cells *in vitro*. Biochem Pharmacol 1986;35(7):1091–1098.

69. Baird JK, McCormick GJ, Canfield CJ. Effects of nine synthetic putative metabolites of primaquine on activity of the hexose monophosphate shunt in intact human red blood cells *in vitro*. Biochem Pharmacol 1986;35(7):1099–1106.

70. Hohl RJ, Kennedy EJ, Frischer H. Defenses against oxidation in human erythrocytes: role of glutathione reductase in the activation of glucose decarboxylation by hemolytic drugs. J Lab Clin Med 1991;117(4):325–331.

71. Amitai Y, Bhooma T, Frischer H. Glucose-6-phosphate dehydrogenase deficiency severely restricts the biotransformation of daunorubicin in human erythrocytes. J Lab Clin Med 1996;127(6):588–598.

72. Cohen G, Hochstein P. Generation of hydrogen peroxide in erythrocytes by hemolytic agents. Biochemistry 1963;3:901–903.

73. Summerfield M, Tudhope GR. Studies with primaquine *in vitro*: superoxide radical for-mation and oxidation of haemoglobin. Br J Clin Pharmacol 1978;6(4):319–323.

74. Frischer H, Ahmad T. Consequences of erythrocytic glutathione reductase deficiency. J Lab Clin Med 1987;109(5):583–588.

75. Vasquez-Vivar J, Augusto O. ESR detection of free radical intermediates during autoxi-dation of 5-hydroxyprimaquine. Free Radic Res Commun 1990;9(3–6):383–389.

76. Vasquez-Vivar J, Augusto O. Hydroxylated metabolites of the antimalarial drug primaquine. Oxidation and redox cycling. J Biol Chem 1992;267(10):6848–6854.

77. Kelman SN, Sullivan SG, Stern A. Primaquine-mediated oxidative metabolism in the human red cell. Lack of dependence on oxyhemoglobin, H_2O_2 formation, or glutathione turnover. Biochem Pharmacol 1982;31(14):2409–2414.

78. Silva JM, O'Brien PJ. Primaquine-induced oxidative stress in isolated hepatocytes as a result of reductive activation. Adv Exp Med Biol 1991;283:359–363.

79. Goldberg AL, Boches FS. Oxidized proteins in erythrocytes are rapidly degraded by the adenosine triphosphate-dependent proteolytic system. Science 1982;215(4536):1107–1109.

80. Itano HA, Matteson JL. Mechanism of initial reaction of phenylhydrazine with oxyhemoglobin and effect of ring substitutions on the biomolecular rate constant of this reaction. Biochemistry 1982;21(10):2421–2426.

81. Itano HA, Hirota K, Hosokawa K. Mechanism of induction of haemolytic anaemia by phenylhydrazine. Nature 1975;256(5519):665–667.

82. Grinberg LN, Newmark H, Kitrossky N, Rahamim E, Chevion M, Rachmilewitz EA. Protective effects of tea polyphenols against oxidative damage to red blood cells. Biochem Pharmacol 1997;54(9):973–978.

83. Grinberg LN, Samuni A. Nitroxide stable radical prevents primaquine-induced lysis of red blood cell. Biochim Biophys Acta 1994;1201(2):284–248.

84. Grinberg LN, Rachmilewitz EA, Newmark H. Protective effects of rutin against hemoglobin oxidation. Biochem Pharmacol 1994;48(4):643–649.

85. Hong YL, Pan HZ, Scott MD, Meshnick SR. Activated oxygen generation by a primaquine metabolite: inhibition by antioxidants derived from Chinese herbal remedies. Free Radic Biol Med 1992;12(3):213–218.

86. Senok AC, Nelson EA, Li K, Oppenheimer SJ. Thalassaemia trait, red blood cell age and oxidant stress: effects on *Plasmodium falciparum* growth and sensitivity to artemisinin. Trans R Soc Trop Med Hyg 1997;91(5):585–589.

87. Bradshaw TP, McMillan DC, Crouch RK, Jollow DJ. Formation of free radicals and protein mixed disulfides in rat red cells exposed to dapsone hydroxylamine. Free Radic Biol Med 1997;22(7):1183–1193.

88. Jollow DJ, Bradshaw TP, McMillan DC. Dapsone-induced hemolytic anemia. Drug Metab Rev 1995;27(1–2):107–124.

899. McMillan DC, Jensen CB, Jollow DJ. Role of lipid peroxidation in dapsone-induced hemolytic anemia. J Pharmacol Exp Ther 1998;287(3):868–876.

90. Agarwal S, Gupta UR, Daniel CS, Gupta RC, Anand N, Agarwal SS. Susceptibility of glucose-6-phosphate dehydrogenase deficient red cells to primaquine, primaquine enantiomers, and its two putative metabolites. II. Effect on red blood cell membrane, lipid peroxidation, MC-540 staining, and scanning electron microscopic studies. Biochem Pharmacol 1991;41(1):17–21.

91. Magwere T, Naik YS, Hasler JA. Primaquine alters antioxidant enzyme profiles in rat liver and kidney. Free Radic Res 1997;27(2):173–179.

92. Miller A, Smith HC. The *in vitro* effect of primaquine on red cell phospholipid metabolism. J Lab Clin Med 1976;88(3):462–468.

93. George JN, O'Brien RL, Pollack S, Crosby WH. Studies of *in vitro* primaquine hemolysis: substrate requirement for erythrocyte membrane damage. J Clin Invest 1966;45(8):1280–1289.

94. Chasis JA, Schrier SL. Membrane deformability and the capacity for shape change in the erythrocyte. Blood 1989;74(7):2562–2568.

95. Thompson SF, Fraser IM, Strother A, Bull BS. Change of deformability and Heinz body formation in G6PD-deficient erythrocytes treated with 5-hydroxy-6-desmethylprimaquine. Blood Cells 1989;15(2):443–452.

96. Johnson RM, Panchoosingh H, Goyette G, Jr, Ravindranath Y. Increased erythrocyte deformability in fetal erythropoiesis and in erythrocytes deficient in glucose-6-phosphate dehydrogenase and other glycolytic enzymes. Pediatr Res 1999;45(1):106–113.

97. Krzyzaniak JF, Alvarez Nunez FA, Raymond DM, Yalkowsky SH. Lysis of human red blood cells. 4. Comparison of *in vitro* and *in vivo* hemolysis data. J Pharm Sci 1997;86(11):1215–1217.

98. Horton HM, Calabrese EJ. Predictive models for human glucose-6-phosphate dehydrogenase deficiency. Drug Metab Rev 1986;17(3–4):261–281.

99. Bashan N, Peleg N, Moses SW. Attempts to predict the hemolytic potential of drugs in glucose-6-phosphate dehydrogenase deficiency of the Mediterranean type by an *in vitro* test. Isr J Med Sci 1988;24(1):61–64.

100. Bloom KE, Brewer GJ, Magon AM, Wetterstroem N. Microsomal incubation test of potentially hemolytic drugs for glucose-6-phosphate dehydrogenase deficiency. Clin Pharmacol Ther 1983;33(4):403–409.

101. Magon A, Leipzig RM, Bloom K, Brewer GJ. Pharmacogenetic interactions in G6PD deficiency and development of an *in vitro* test to predict a drug's hemolytic potential. Prog Clin Biol Res 1981;55:709–724.

102. Tsukamoto N, Chen J, Yoshida A. Enhanced expressions of glucose-6-phosphate dehydrogenase and cytosolic aldehyde dehydrogenase and elevation of reduced glutathione level in cyclophosphamide-resistant human leukemia cells. Blood Cells Mol Dis 1998;24(2):231–238.

103. Ursini MV, Parrella A, Rosa G, Salzano S, Martini G. Enhanced expression of glucose-6-phosphate dehydrogenase in human cells sustaining oxidative stress. Biochem J 1997;323(Pt 3):801–806.

104. Tian WN, Braunstein LD, Apse K, Pang J, Rose M, Tian X, et al. Importance of glucose-6-phosphate dehydrogenase activity in cell death. Am J Physiol 1999;276(5 Pt 1):C1121–C1131.

105. Schmidt LH, Alexander S, Allen L, Rasco J. Comparison of the curative antimalarial activities and toxicities of primaquine and its d and l isomers. Antimicrob Agents Chemother 1977;12(1):51–60.

106. Nicholl DD, Edwards G, Ward SA, Orme ML, Breckenridge AM. The disposition of primaquine in the isolated perfused rat liver. Stereoselective formation of the carboxylic acid metabolite. Biochem Pharmacol 1987;36(20):3365–3369.

107. Jaffe ER. Metabolic processes involved in the formation and reduction of methemoglobin in human erythrocytes. In Bishop C, Surgenor D (eds.), The Red Blood Cell. New York: Academic, 1964, pp. 397–422.

108. Hall AH, Kulig KW, Rumack BH. Drug- and chemical-induced methaemoglobinaemia. Clinical features and management. Med Toxicol 1986;1(4):253–260.

109. Coleman MD, Coleman NA. Drug-induced methaemoglobinaemia. Treatment issues. Drug Safety 1996;14(6):394–405.

110. Alving AS, Johnson CF, Tarlov AR, Brewer GJ, Kellermeyer RW, Carson PE. Mitigation of the haemolytic effect of primaquine and enhancement of its action against exoerythrocytic forms of the Chesson strain of *Plasmodium vivax* by intermittent regimens of drug administraton. Bull WHO 1960;22:621–631.

111. Clyde DF. Clinical problems associated with the use of primaquine as a tissue schizontocidal and gametocytocidal drug. Bull WHO 1981;59(3):391–395.

112. Rosen PJ, Johnson C, McGehee WG, Beutler E. Failure of methylene blue treatment in toxic methemoglobinemia. Association with glucose-6-phosphate dehydrogenase deficiency. Ann Intern Med 1971;75(1):83–86.

113. Idowu OR, Peggins JO, Brewer TG, Kelley C. Metabolism of a candidate 8-aminoquinoline antimalarial agent, WR 238605:by rat liver microsomes. Drug Metab Dispos 1995;23(1):1–17.

114. Idowu OR, Peggins JO, Brewer TG. Side-chain hydroxylation in the metabolism of 8-aminoquinoline antiparasitic agents. Drug Metab Dispos 1995;23(1):18–27.

115. Strother A, Fraser IM, Allahyari R, Tilton BE. Metabolism of 8-aminoquinoline antimalarial agents. Bull WHO 1981;59(3):413–425.

116. Strother A, Allahyari R, Buchholz J, Fraser IM, Tilton BE. *In vitro* metabolism of the antimalarial agent primaquine by mouse liver enzymes and identification of a methemoglobin-forming metabolite. Drug Metab Dispos 1984;12(1):35–44.

117. Magon AM, Leipzig RM, Zannoni VG, Brewer GJ. Interactions of glucose-6-phosphate dehydrogenase deficiency with drug acetylation and hydroxylation reactions. J Lab Clin Med 1981;97(6):764–770.

118. Bangchang KN, Karbwang J, Back DJ. Primaquine metabolism by human liver microsomes: effect of other antimalarial drugs. Biochem Pharmacol 1992;44(3):587–590.

119. Mihaly GW, Ward SA, Edwards G, Orme ML, Breckenridge AM. Pharmacokinetics of primaquine in man: identification of the carboxylic acid derivative as a major plasma metabolite. Br J Clin Pharmacol 1984;17(4):441–446.

120. Dua VK, Kar PK, Sarin R, Sharma VP. High-performance liquid chromatographic determination of primaquine and carboxyprimaquine concentrations in plasma and blood cells in *Plasmodium vivax* malaria cases following chronic dosage with primaquine. J Chromatogr B Biomed Appl 1996;675(1):93–98.

121. Abu-El-Haj S, Allahyari R, Chavez E, Fraser IM, Strother A. Effects of an NADPH-generating system on primaquine degradation by hamster liver fractions. Xenobiotica 1988;18(10):1165–1178.

122. Frischer H, Ahmad T, Nora MV, Carson PE, Sivarajan M, Mellovitz R, et al. Biotransformation of primaquine *in vitro* with human K562 and bone marrow cells. J Lab Clin Med 1987;109(4):414–421.

123. Dockham PA, Sreerama L, Sladek NE. Relative contribution of human erythrocyte aldehyde dehydrogenase to the systemic detoxification of the oxazaphosphorines. Drug Metab Dispos 1997;25(12):1436–1441.

124. Baker JK, Yarber RH, Nanayakkara NP, McChesney JD, Homo F, Landau I. Effect of aliphatic side-chain substituents on the antimalarial activity and on the metabolism of primaquine studied using mitochondria and microsome preparations. Pharm Res 1990;7(1):91–95.

125. Feo F, Pirisi L, Pascale R, Daino L, Frassetto S, Zanetti S, Garcea R. Modulatory mechanisms of chemical carcinogenesis: the role of the NADPH pool in the benzo(a)pyrene activation. Toxicol Pathol 1984;12(3):261–268.

126. Feo F, Ruggiu ME, Lenzerini L, Garcea R, Daino L, Frassetto S, et al. Benzo(a)pyrene metabolism by lymphocytes from normal individuals and individuals carrying the Mediterranean variant of glucose-6-phosphate dehydrogenase. Int J Cancer 1987; 39(5):560–564.

127. Efferth T, Fabry U, Glatte P, Osieka R. Increased induction of apoptosis in mononuclear cells of a glucose-6- phosphate dehydrogenase deficient patient. J Mol Med 1995;73(1):47–49.

128. Arnold J, Alving AS, Hockwald RS, Clayman CB, Dern RJ, Beutler E, et al. The antimalarial action of primaquine against the blood and tissue stages of falciparum malaria (Panama, P-F-6 strain). J Lab Clin Med 1955;46(3):391–397.

129. Arnold J, Alving AS, Hockwald RS, Clayman CB, Dern RJ, Beutler E, et al. The effect of continuous and intermittent primaquine therapy on the relapse rate of Chesson strain vivax malaria. J Lab Clin Med 1954;44(3):429–438.

130. Baird JK, Fryauff DJ, Basri H, Bangs MJ, Subianto B, Wiady I, et al. Primaquine for prophylaxis against malaria among nonimmune transmigrants in Irian Jaya, Indonesia. Am J Trop Med Hyg 1995;52(6):479–484.

131. Fryauff D, Baird J, Basri H, Sumawinata I, Purnomo, RT, Ohrt C, et al. Randomised placebo-controlled trial of primaquine for prophalaxis of falciparum and vivax malaria. Lancet 1995;346:1190–1193.

132. Powell RD, Brewer GJ. Effects of pyrimethamine, chlorguanide, and primaquine against exoerythrocytic forms of a strain of chloroquine-resistant *Plasmodium falciparum* from Thailand. Am J Trop Med Hyg 1967;16(6):693–698.

133. Weiss WR, Oloo AJ, Johnson A, Koech D, Hoffman SL. Daily primaquine is effective for prophylaxis against falciparum malaria in Kenya: comparison with mefloquine, doxycycline, and chloroquine plus proguanil. J Infect Dis 1995;171(6):1569–1575.

134. Clayman C, Arnold J, Hockwald R, Yount E Jr, Edgecomb J, Alving A. Toxicity of primaquine in Caucasians. JAMA 1952;149:1563–1568.

135. Brueckner RP, Coster T, Wesche DL, Shmuklarsky M, Schuster BG. Prophylaxis of *Plasmodium falciparum* infection in a human challenge model with WR 238605:a new 8-aminoquinoline antimalarial. Antimicrob Agents Chemother 1998;42(5):1293–1294.

136. Most H, London IM, Kane CA, Lavietes PH, Schroeder EF, Hayman JM Jr. Landmark article July 20:1946: Chloroquine for treatment of acute attacks of vivax malaria. JAMA 1984;251(18):2415–2419.

137. Alving A, Hankey D, Coatney G, Jones Jr R, Coker W, Garrison P, et al. Korean vivax malaria. II. Curative treatment with pamaquine and primaquine. Am J Trop Med Hyg 1953;6:970–976.

138. Hankey D, Jones Jr, R., Coatney G, Alving A, Coker W, Garrision P, et al. Korean vivax malaria. I. Natural history and response to chloroquine. Am J Trop Med Hyg 1952;6:958–969.

139. Coatney G, Alving A, Jones Jr., R., Hankey D, Robinson D, Garrison P, et al. Korean vivax malaria. V. Cure of the infection by primaquine administered during long-term latency. Am J Trop Med Hyg 1952;6:985–988.

140. Adak T, Sharma VP, Orlov VS. Studies on the *Plasmodium vivax* relapse pattern in Delhi, India. Am J Trop Med Hyg 1998;59(1):175–179.

141. Singh N, Mishra AK, Sharma VP. Radical treatment of vivax malaria in Madhya Pradesh, India. Indian J Malariol 1990;27(1):55–56.

142. Schmidt LH, Fradkin R, Vaughan D, Rasco J. Radical cure of infections with *Plasmodium cynomolgi*: a function of total 8-aminoquinoline dose. Am J Trop Med Hyg 1977;26(6 Pt 1):1116–1128.

143. Clyde DF, McCarthy VC. Radical cure of Chesson strain vivax malaria in man by 7:not 14:days of treatment with primaquine. Am J Trop Med Hyg 1977;26(3):562–563.

144. Bruce-Chwatt L. (ed). Chemotherapy of Malaria, Vol. 27. Geneva: World Health Organization, 1981.

145. Edgecomb J, Arnold J, Yount E Jr, Alving A, Eichelberger L. Primaquine, SN-13272, a new curative agent in vivax malaria: a preliminary report. Nat Malaria Soc 1950;9:285–357.

146. Bunnag D, Karbwang J, Thanavibul A, Chittamas S, Ratanapongse Y, Chalermrut K, et al. High dose of primaquine in primaquine resistant vivax malaria. Trans R Soc Trop Med Hyg 1994;88(2):218–219.

147. Jelinek T, Nothdurft HD, Von Sonnenburg F, Loscher T. Long-term efficacy of primaquine in the treatment of vivax malaria in nonimmune travelers. Am J Trop Med Hyg 1995;52(4):322–324.

148. Kaplan MH, Bernstein LS. Improved therapy for Vietnam acquired vivax malaria. Mil Med 1974;141(6):444–448.

149. Martelo OJ, Smoller M, Saladin TA. Malaria in American soldiers. Arch Intern Med 1969;123(4):383–387.

150. Fisher GU, Gordon MP, Lobel HO, Runcik K. Malaria in soldiers returning from Vietnam. Epidemiologic, therapeutic, and clinical studies. Am J Trop Med Hyg 1970;19(1):27–39.

151. Singh J, Ray A, Misra B, Nair C. Antirelapse treatment with primaquine and pyrimethamine. Indian J Malariol 1954;8:127–136.

152. Basavaraj, H. (1960) Observations on the treatment of 678 malaria cases with primaquine in an area free from malaria transmission in Mysore State, India. Indian J Malariol 14:269–281.

153. Cedillos RA, Warren M, Jeffery GM. Field evaluation of primaquine in the control of *Plasmodium vivax*. Am J Trop Med Hyg 1978;27(3):466–472.

154. Baird JK. Primaquine as anti-relapse therapy for *Plasmodium vivax* [letter; comment]. Trans R Soc Trop Med Hyg 1998;92(6):687.

155. Contacos PG, Coatney GR, Collins WE, Briesch PE, Jeter MH. Five day primaquine therapy—an evaluation of radical curative activity against vivax malaria infection. Am J Trop Med Hyg 1973;22(6):693–695.

156. Miller LH, Wyler DJ, Glew RH, Collins WE, Contacos PG. Sensitivity of four Central American strains of *Plasmodium vivax* to primaquine. Am J Trop Med Hyg 1974;23(2):309–310.

157. Walsh DS, Looareesuwan S, Wilairatana P, Heppner Jr, DG, Tang DB, Brewer TG, et al. Randomized dose-ranging study of the safety and efficacy of WR 238605 (tafenoquine)

in the prevention of relapse of *Plasmodium vivax* malaria in Thailand. J Infect Dis 1999;180(4):1282–1287.

158. Looareesuwan S, White NJ, Chittamas S, Bunnag D, Harinasuta T. High rate of *Plasmodium vivax* relapse following treatment of falciparum malaria in Thailand. Lancet 1987;2(8567):1052–1055.

159. Walker AJ. Potentialities of monthly doses of Camoquin and a gametocidal drug in malaria control. Trans R Soc Trop Med Hyg 1955;49:351–355.

160. Jeffery GM, Young MD, Eyles DE. The treatment of *Plasmodium falciparum* infection with chloroquine, with a note on infectivity of mosquitoes of primaquine- and pyrimthamine-treated cases. Am J Trop Med Hyg 1956;64:1–11.

161. Rieckmann KH, McNamara JV, Kass L, Powell RD. Gametocytocidal and sporontocidal effects of primaquine upon two strains of *Plasmodium falciparum*. Mil Med 1969; 134(10):802–819.

162. WHO. Practical Chemotherapy of Malaria. Geneva: World Health Organization, 1990.

163. Collins WE, Jeffery GM. Primaquine resistance in *Plasmodium vivax*. Am J Trop Med Hyg 1996;55(3):243–249.

164. Murphy GS, Basri H, Purnomo, Andersen EM, Bangs MJ, Mount DL, et al. Vivax malaria resistant to treatment and prophylaxis with chloroquine. Lancet 1993;341(8837):96–100.

165. Baird JK, Leksana B, Masbar S, Fryauff DJ, Sutanihardja MA, Suradi, et al. Diagnosis of resistance to chloroquine by *Plasmodium vivax*: timing of recurrence and whole blood chloroquine levels. Am J Trop Med Hyg 1997;56(6):621–626.

166. Wiselogle, F. A Survey of Antimalarial Drugs 1941–1946. Ann Arbor, MI: Edwards, 1946.

167. Alving AS, Arnold J, Hockwald RS, Clayman CB, Dern RJ, Beutler E, et al. Potentialtion of the curative action of primaquine in vivax malaria by quinine and chloroquine. J Lab Clin Med 1955;46(2):301–306.

168. Soto J, Toledo J, Rodriquez M, Sanchez J, Herrera R, Padilla J, et al. Primaquine prophylaxis against malaria in nonimmune Colombian soldiers: efficacy and toxicity. A randomized, double-blind, placebo-controlled trial. Ann Intern Med 1998;129(3):241–244.

169. Mason PJ. New insights into G6PD deficiency. Br J Haematol 1996;94(4):585–591.

170. Carson P, Flanagan C, Ickes C, Alving A. Enzymatic deficiency in primaquine sensitive erythrocytes. Science 1956;124:484–485.

171. Vulliamy T, Mason P, Luzzatto, L. The molecular basis of glucose-6-phosphate dehydrogenase deficiency. Trends Genet 1992;8(4):138–143.

172. Ruwende C, Khoo SC, Snow RW, Yates SN, Kwiatkowski D, Gupta S, et al. Natural selection of hemi- and heterozygotes for G6PD deficiency in Africa by resistance to severe malaria. Nature 1995;376(6537):246–249.

173. Sarkar S, Prakash D, Marwaha RK, Garewal G, Kumar L, Singhi S, Walia BN. Acute intravascular haemolysis in glucose-6-phosphate dehydrogenase deficiency. Ann Trop Paediatr 1993;13(4):391–394.

174. Choudhry VP, Ghafary A, Zaher M, Qureshi MA, Fazel I, Ghani, R. Drug-induced haemolysis and renal failure in children with glucose-6- phosphate dehydrogenase deficiency in Afghanistan. Ann Trop Paediatr 1990;10(4):335–338.

175. Chugh KS, Singhal PC, Sharma BK, Mahakur AC, Pal Y, Datta BN, et al. Acute renal failure due to intravascular hemolysis in the North Indian patients. Am J Med Sci 1977;274(2):139–146.

176. Karwacki JJ, Shanks GD, Kummalue T, Watanasook C. Primaquine induced hemolysis in a Thai soldier. Southeast Asian J Trop Med Public Health 1989;20(4):555–556.

177. Bouma MJ, Goris M, Akhtar T, Khan N, Kita E. Prevalence and clinical presentation of glucose-6-phosphate dehydrogenase deficiency in Pakistani Pathan and Afghan refugee communities in Pakistan; implications for the use of primaquine in regional malaria control programmes. Trans R Soc Trop Med Hyg 1995;89(1):62–64.

Mechanisms of Quinoline Resistance

Grant Dorsey, David A. Fidock, Thomas E. Wellems, and Philip J. Rosenthal

INTRODUCTION

For decades, the 4-aminoquinoline chloroquine (CQ) was the mainstay for the prevention and treatment of malaria because of its low cost, safety, and efficacy. However, CQ-resistant *Plasmodium falciparum* has now been reported from almost every malaria endemic country, and this drug can no longer be considered appropriate for the treatment of malaria in many areas *(1)*. Reports of CQ-resistant *P. vivax* also have begun to emerge from Asia and South America *(2)*. In response to the problem of CQ resistance, the quinolinemethanol mefloquine has been widely deployed and used for the prevention and treatment of malaria in areas where CQ is no longer effective. However, resistance to this drug has emerged in many malarious regions *(3–8)*. Although the older quinolinemethanols quinine and quinidine remain useful in areas of CQ and mefloquine resistance, these drugs have been losing efficacy, and cases of cross-resistance among the different quinolines have been described *(9–16)*.

The impact of resistance to CQ and other quinoline antimalarials is measured not only by the reduction in their efficacy but also by the increasing necessity to rely on the more expensive and more toxic current alternatives. Strains of *P. falciparum* from Cambodia and Thailand exist that are resistant to all available antimalarials except the artemisinin compounds *(1)*. Given the great success of the quinolines prior to the emergence of resistance, strategies to develop new antimalarials should include new agents that act upon the target of these drugs as well as chemosensitizers that can reverse the resistance phenotype. A better understanding of underlying mechanisms of quinoline resistance should assist these strategies. This chapter reviews current understanding and controversies regarding the mechanisms of resistance to the quinoline antimalarials, with a focus on *P. falciparum* and the most widely used drugs of this class.

MECHANISM(S) OF CHLOROQUINE RESISTANCE

Introduction

Despite massive drug pressure following its introduction in the 1940s, the resistance of *P. falciparum* to CQ was not recognized until the late 1950s, when treatment failures were reported from distinct foci in Southeast Asia and South America *(17)*. Resistance

From: *Antimalarial Chemotherapy: Mechanisms of Action, Resistance, and New Directions in Drug Discovery*
Edited by: P. J. Rosenthal © Humana Press Inc., Totowa, NJ

has steadily spread from these two foci and now is established in almost all malarious areas around the world *(1)*. The emergence of CQ resistance only after many years of widespread CQ use suggests that multiple mutations are required to produce the CQ resistance phenotype *(18)*. It is now generally agreed that CQ acts by disrupting the detoxification of heme in the parasite food vacuole (*see* Chapter 6). The mechanism of resistance to CQ is more controversial. From a biochemical standpoint, CQ-resistant parasites have been found to accumulate less CQ compared to CQ-sensitive parasites *(19–23)*. This difference can be modified by a number of chemosensitizing agents such as the Ca^+ channel blocker verapamil *(24)*. Recent work has attempted to investigate the problem from a genetic standpoint, with the goal of identifying genes that encode proteins that play a role in CQ resistance *(25–27)*.

Chloroquine Resistance and Drug Accumulation

It has been suggested that the accumulation of CQ in the *P. falciparum* food vacuole, which underlies the action of the drug, is related to the binding of CQ to free heme (Chapter 6). Once in the food vacuole, CQ appears to form complexes with heme in its hematin (μ-oxodimer) form and interrupt the normal polymerization of heme as it is released upon hemoglobin digestion. These CQ-hematin complexes are thought to engender parasite toxicity (Chapter 6).

Mechanisms of CQ resistance among different *Plasmodium* species may vary. In murine parasites, such as *P. berghei*, CQ resistance is associated with a decrease in the formation of hemozoin (pigment), which consists of polymerized (and thus detoxified) heme particles *(28)*. However, there are no clear differences in the quantity of hemozoin in CQ-resistant and CQ-sensitive *P. falciparum (29)*.

A number of hypotheses have been proposed to explain differences in CQ accumulation between resistant and sensitive parasites. One theory is that decreased accumulation is the result of increased CQ efflux from CQ-resistant parasites, which actively remove the drug from its site of action *(22,30)*. This theory was supported by data suggesting that CQ-resistant parasites released preaccumulated CQ almost 50 times faster than CQ-sensitive isolates *(30,31)*. These results were considered consistent with the finding that verapamil partially reversed resistance and reduced the apparent rate of drug efflux from CQ-resistant parasites *(30,32)*. CQ resistance was therefore proposed to involve a mechanism analogous to that mediated by P-glycoprotein molecules in mammalian tumor cells (discussed in more detail below) *(32)*. More recent reports, however, found that CQ efflux rates in CQ-resistant and CQ-sensitive strains are similar and that the decreased steady-state levels of CQ in resistant strains are the result of a diminished level of accumulation rather than a drug export mechanism *(23,33–35)*.

Several hypotheses incorporate the concept that decreased CQ accumulation can be the result of diminished drug accumulation. The uptake of diprotic CQ in acid food vacuoles because of a weak-base ion-trapping mechanism is predicted by the Henderson–Hasselbach equation *(21,36,37)*. Increases in vacuolar pH could thus explain decreased accumulation of CQ in resistant parasites *(34,38)*. An increase in vacuolar pH of 0.5 pH units was proposed to be sufficient to decrease CQ accumulation by 10-fold *(35)*. Reports of increased vacuolar pH have been explained by a weakened proton pump, which was thought to be consistent with results showing CQ-resistant parasites to be more susceptible than CQ-sensitive parasites to the proton-pump inhibitor bafilomycin A1 *(23)*. Other studies that used populations of parasites for pH measurements did not detect differences in vacuolar pH between CQ-sensitive and CQ-resistant parasites, however *(37)*. Also, the genes for two of the subunits of the plasmodial (H^+) ATPase have been sequenced and no mutations were found to account for CQ resistance *(39,40)*.

The recent development of sensitive pH-calibrated methods on individual parasitized erythrocytes now indicate that the food vacuole pH is actually *decreased* in CQ-resistant parasites by 0.3–0.5 pH units relative to CQ-sensitive parasites. This was determined using sensitive "thin layer" single-cell photometric analysis of parasites maintained in O_2/CO_2-balanced physiological conditions and using dyes that selectively localize to the cytoplasmic or vacuolar compartments *(41)*. These results appear paradoxical if vacuolar CQ accumulation were explained only by weak-base trapping. However, CQ accumulation in the food vacuole is known to be additionally driven by binding to soluble heme *(19,42)*. Given that there is a steep effect of pH on the conversion of soluble heme to insoluble hemozoin and that the formation of hemozoin is much more efficient at the lower food vacuole pH values of CQ-resistant parasites, then vacuolar acidification would leave significantly less free heme available for the formation of toxic complexes with CQ *(41)*. The result would be reduced CQ accumulation in CQ-resistant parasites, consistent with experimental data showing a reduction in high-affinity drug receptor sites *(19,41,42)*.

Some reports of CQ uptake and activity have suggested that differences in drug accumulation between CQ-sensitive and CQ-resistant parasites are proportionally less than differences in drug susceptibility *(9)*. For instance, parasites demonstrating a fourfold to fivefold difference in CQ accumulation were found to exhibit a 10-fold to 20-fold difference in susceptibility *(9)*. These data provide evidence that, in addition to the alterations in drug accumulation, CQ resistance may be mediated by a reduction in target-site sensitivity or accessibility. Reduced accumulation and activity of CQ in resistant parasites could therefore be the result of alterations in the binding of CQ to heme within the parasite food vacuole, in addition to changes in the transport of CQ across the parasite plasma membrane. In kinetic studies *(42)*, the major difference between susceptible and resistant strains was in the K_d for saturable CQ binding, and the saturable component of CQ accumulation was found to be responsible for the antimalarial activity of the drug. Furthermore, protease inhibitors that blocked hemoglobin digestion and heme release inhibited this saturable component of CQ accumulation, so that the specific activity of CQ was attributed to CQ–heme binding *(42)*. As CQ resistance was associated with a reduced apparent affinity of CQ–heme binding rather than changes in the capacity for CQ to bind heme, it was proposed that the underlying mechanism of resistance is the result of a reduction in the accessibility of free heme.

Alternative explanations for the decreased concentration of CQ in resistant parasites involve loss or alteration of a protein involved in CQ uptake *(43)* or loss or alteration of an intracellular "receptor" *(42,44,45)*. It has been suggested that CQ uptake could be facilitated by a Na^+/H^+ exchanger and that alterations in this exchanger may mediate CQ resistance *(46)*. This proposal was based on the observation that inhibitors of Na^+/H^+ exchange competitively inhibited CQ uptake and that the kinetics of uptake differed between resistant and sensitive strains *(46)*. The Na^+/H^+ proposal invoked kinetics that were measured using intact parasites and, therefore, could have reflected binding of

CQ to another receptor *(47)*. Recent evidence that the specific CQ accumulation phenotypes of CQ-resistant and CQ-sensitive parasites were preserved in sodium-free medium argue against direct involvement of an Na^+/H^+ exchanger in drug transport and CQ resistance *(42)*. In addition, the suggestion that the *cg2* gene, which is associated with CQ resistance (see the next subsection), might encode a Na^+/H^+ exchanger *(48)* was not consistent with analysis of the predicted sequence of CG2 *(49)*. However, available data do not rule out the possibility that an Na^+/H^+ exchanger is indirectly involved in modulating CQ accumulation through alterations in the pH gradient across parasite membranes *(24)*.

The Reversal of CQ Resistance by Chemosensitizing Agents

The activity of CQ against resistant parasites can be enhanced by a number of compounds, including verapamil, desipramine, and chlorpheniramine *(32,50,51)*. The mechanisms of action of these chemosensitizing (CQ resistance "reversal") agents are unclear, although many of these compounds appear to work by enhancing the accumulation of CQ *(52)*. Studies using radiolabeled drug have shown that verapamil significantly increases the steady-state accumulation of CQ in CQ-resistant parasites *(30,33,53–55)*. This CQ accumulation in resistant parasites in the presence of verapamil is still substantially lower than that in susceptible parasites with or without verapamil *(30,33,35,51,53)*. In addition, the effect of verapamil on CQ accumulation at therapeutic concentrations is very small relative to the drug's effect on parasite sensitivity to CQ *(33)*. The lack of a unifying hypothesis to account for both CQ resistance and resistance reversal has led to the proposal that these phenomena may be the result of more than one mechanism *(33,35,46)*. Recent work suggesting that CQ resistance is the result of alterations in the binding of CQ to heme offers evidence that the reversing effect of verapamil is caused by an increase in the apparent affinity of CQ–heme binding *(42)*. Thus, verapamil may reverse CQ resistance by altering CQ–heme affinity and affecting CQ accumulation. Whether other chemosensitizing agents reverse CQ resistance by mechanisms other than the inhibition of CQ accumulation is uncertain.

Evaluation of the Proposed Role for a P-Glycoprotein in Chloroquine Resistance

The observations that CQ-resistant parasites accumulate less CQ than sensitive parasites and that verapamil can modulate this process suggested similarities with the multidrug-resistant (MDR) phenotype of mammalian tumor cells *(32)*. MDR is thought to be caused by the overexpression of an ATP-dependent drug transporter known as P-glycoprotein *(56)*, which is postulated to confer resistance by promoting the efflux of a wide range of cytotoxic drugs out of tumor cells *(57)*. Two MDR gene homologs, designated *pfmdr-1 (58,59)* and *pfmdr-2 (60,61)* have been identified in *P. falciparum*. The *pfmdr-1* gene product, P-glycoprotein homolog-1 (Pgh-1), has a structure shared by many members of the MDR family, with 12 transmembrane regions and 2 nucleotide binding sites *(62)*. The *pfmdr-2* gene predicts a protein more closely related to a mediator of cadmium resistance in yeast *(60,61)*, and little evidence exists to suggests that it plays a role in CQ resistance.

Pgh-1 is localized on the membrane of the parasite food vacuole and has been suggested to have a role in drug transport *(62)*. Although initial studies attempted to correlate the CQ resistance phenotype with *pfmdr-1* gene amplification or mutations

(63), analysis of a genetic cross between CQ-resistant and CQ-sensitive clones of *P. falciparum* showed that this gene did not map with the CQ-resistance determinant and thus could not account for resistance *(25)*. Recent data have also shown that amplification of the *pfmdr-1* gene is not associated with CQ resistance *(15,64)*. In fact, *deamplification* has been associated with increased CQ resistance in vitro *(65–67)*. In population surveys of CQ-resistant strains, different *pfmdr-1* haplotypes were identified from Old and New World malarious regions, including an allele with an Asn to Tyr codon change at position 86 (N86Y; K1 allele) and alleles with codon changes at positions 184, 1034, 1042, and 1246 (7G8 allele) *(63)*. Subsequent studies using field isolates identified some associations between *pfmdr-1* point mutations and *in vivo* or in vitro CQ resistance, but many exceptions, in which CQ resistance could not be attributed to *pfmdr-1* mutations, were also seen (Table 1) *(15,68–76)*. Thus, alterations in *pfmdr-1* copy number or sequence have not generally predicted resistance or sensitivity in field isolates.

Most investigators now believe that alterations in the *pfmdr-1* gene are not primarily responsible for the CQ-resistance phenotype. However, it remains possible that *pfmdr-1* may act as a modulator of CQ resistance or as a factor that affects the fitness of physiologically altered CQ-resistant parasites. Studies in Chinese hamster ovary cells transfected with *pfmdr-1* demonstrated incorporation of Pgh-1 into lysosomes, a decrease in lysosomal pH, and an increased sensitivity to CQ *(78,79)*. Furthermore, when cells were transfected with a *pfmdr-1* gene with mutations previously linked to CQ resistance, the lysosomal pH was not increased and there was no change in CQ sensitivity *(78)*. The extracellular CQ concentrations that affect lysosomal pH in CHO cells, however, are much higher than those that affect heme polymerization in *P. falciparum*. Nevertheless, these data have been taken to suggest that *pfmdr-1* can indirectly enhance CQ accumulation by modulating food vacuole pH, perhaps via an effect on chloride transport, as has been demonstrated for other members of the P-glycoprotein family *(80)*. Transfection of a CQ-sensitive parasite line with *pfmdr-1* from CQ-resistant parasites containing three point mutations had no effect on parasite sensitivity to CQ. However, mutations in Pgh-1 can modulate the response of *P. falciparum* already resistant to CQ *(81)*. Recent studies provided evidence that replacement of the mutant *pfmdr-1* with the wild-type sequence in resistant parasites decreased the CQ median inhibitory concentration (IC_{50}) from high (350 nM) to moderate (204 nM) levels. This replacement was associated with a proportional increase in saturable, steady-state accumulation of CQ and with blunting of the CQ resistance reversal effect of verapamil.

A Genetic Approach to Understanding CQ Resistance

A laboratory cross between CQ-resistant (Dd2, Indochina) and CQ-sensitive (HB3, Honduras) parasites was employed as an alternative approach to understanding the mechanism of CQ resistance *(25)*. Linkage analysis showed that the CQ-resistance determinant in progeny clones mapped to a single locus within a 36-kilobase (kb) region of chromosome 7 that did not contain the *pfmdr-1* gene *(26,82)*. No intermediate drug sensitivity was seen in any of the progenies, arguing against independent effects of polymorphisms in two or more unlinked genes contributing to the inheritance of CQ resistance *(26)*. Additionally, no other chromosome segments mapped perfectly with CQ resistance in a comprehensive search of a detailed genetic map constructed from 35

Table 1
Field Studies of *pfmdr-1* Mutations and Chloroquine Resistance

Study site (ref.)	Patient population (n)	*pfmdr-1* Mutations	Phenotypic correlate[a]	Results
Sudan 1992 (76)	Unspecified (13)	N86Y, D1246Y	In vitro test	No association
Thailand 1993 (15)	Unspecified (11)	N86Y, N1042D, D1246Y	In vitro test	No association
France 1995 (75)	Travelers from Africa (51)	N86Y, N1042D, D1246Y	In vitro test	Positive association (86Y mutation only)
Cambodia 1996 (74)	Symptomatic malaria (10)	N86Y, N1042D, D1246Y	In vitro test	No association
Cameroon 1997 (73)	Uncomplicated malaria (40)	N86Y	14-d in vivo test, RI–RIII vs S	No association
Gambia 1997 (71)	Uncomplicated malaria (children) (40)	N86Y	28-d in vivo test, (RII–RIII vs RI)	Positive association
Gambia 1997 (68)	Uncomplicated malaria (children) (31)	N86Y	In vitro test	Positive association
Gabon 1998 (69)	Uncomplicated malaria (children) (15)	N86Y, D1246Y	In vitro test	No association
Cameroon 1998 (72)	Uncomplicated malaria (children) (102)	N86Y	In vitro test	No association
Thailand 1999 (77)	Unspecified (11)	N86Y, Y184F, N1042D, D1246Y	In vitro test	No association
Irian Jaya 1999 (70)	Asymptomatic volunteers (124)	N86Y, D1246Y	28-d in vivo test, RI–RIII vs S	Positive association for both mutations

[a] In vivo drug responses are described by standard WHO terminology for sensitivity (S) and resistance (RI–RIII), based on the persistence of parasitemia after treatment.

158

independent recombinant progenies *(83)*. Sequence analysis of the 36-kb segment initially identified eight potential genes, and one of these genes, *cg2*, contained a complex set of polymorphisms that strongly correlated with the CQ resistance phenotype in Old World parasite lines. Twenty CQ-resistant parasite clones from Asia and Africa contained an identical set of polymorphisms of the Dd2-type, and 21 CQ-sensitive clones were highly heterogeneous. However, an exception was found with the Sudan 106/1 clone that contained the Dd2-type *cg2* sequence and yet was CQ sensitive *(26)*. Subsequent evaluations of field isolates also found strong association of *cg2* polymorphisms with CQ resistance; however, additional exceptions were identified (Table 2) *(84–87)*. Recently, genetic modification of the *cg2* sequence in CQ-resistant parasites, leading to introduction of polymorphisms associated with CQ sensitivity, did not result in any change in the verapamil-reversible CQ-resistance phenotype. These data provided conclusive evidence that the Dd2 set of mutations present in cg2 was not necessary for CQ resistance *(88)*.

Further investigation of the 36-kb segment that segregated with CQ resistance in the genetic cross revealed the presence of a cryptic gene, *pfcrt*, whose coding sequence was contained within 13 exons *(27)*. The 424-amino-acid-translated product, PfCRT, contains 10 predicted transmembrane domains and has been localized to the food vacuole. Sequence comparisons revealed eight codons that differed between the CQ-resistant and CQ-sensitive clones in the genetic cross. These amino acid substitutions occur within or near predicted transmembrane segments, and six involve changes in charge or hydrophilicity. Sequence analysis of laboratory-adapted Old World isolates demonstrated a clear association between *pfcrt* mutations and CQ resistance. CQ-Resistant isolates from Asia and Africa consistently showed seven of the mutations found in codons of the Dd2 allele (M74I, N75E, K76T, A220S, Q271E, N326S, and R371I) with or without the eighth Dd2 mutation, I356T. Although the sets of mutations in the Old and New World alleles could be clearly distinguished, all shared two mutations (K76T and A220S) that likely underpin a common molecular mechanism of CQ resistance. Episomal transformation of CQ-sensitive parasites with constructs expressing CQ-resistant forms of PfCRT resulted in the transfected lines tolerating CQ concentrations that are lethal to CQ-sensitive parasites and exhibiting verapamil-reversible IC_{90} values only observed in naturally CQ-resistant lines. The dose-response curves were unusually flat, however—an effect that presumably resulted at least in part from the coexpression of the episomal and endogenous chromosomal forms of the *pfcrt* gene. These experiments represent the first successful production of a CQ-resistant line from a CQ-sensitive line in the laboratory, with the verapamil-reversible phenotype directly attributable to the presence of the episomes expressing CQ-resistant forms of PfCRT.

One of the recipients used in these episomal transformation experiments was the Sudan 106/1 line, which had proved to be an exception to the association between the preliminary candidate gene *cg2* and CQ resistance *(26)*. This line is categorically of the CQ-sensitive phenotype not chemosensitized by the presence of verapamil. The *pfcrt* allele in 106/1 carries all of the *pfcrt* mutations associated with Old World CQ resistance except for the K76T codon change, consistent with a central role for this codon in CQ resistance. During transformation experiments with 106/1, a mutant line was selected that lost the episomes but had nevertheless acquired a highly CQ-resistant phenotype. This line

Table 2
Field Studies of *cg2* Polymorphisms and Chloroquine Resistance

Study site (ref.)	Patient population (*n*)	*cg2* Polymorphisms	Phenotypic correlate	Results
Nigeria 1999 (87)	Asymptomatic malaria (children) (39)	G281A, K repeat	In vivo and in vitro	Positive correlation both alone and in combination
Cameroon 1999 (85)	Asymptomatic malaria (children) (24)	12-point mutations, K, Ω, and poly-N repeats	In vivo and in vitro	Positive correlation for 12-point mutations, K and Ω repeats
France 1999 (84)	Travelers, mostly from Africa (99)	K and Ω repeats	In vitro	Positive correlation for both repeats
Cameroon 1999 (86)	Asymptomatic malaria (75)	Ω repeats	In vivo and in vitro	Positive correlation

was found to have a new mutation, K76I, in the 106/1 *pfcrt* allele already harboring the other mutations associated with CQ resistance. Association between CQ resistance and the K76I mutation was confirmed by episomal transformation experiments *(27)*.

Whereas genetic studies indicate a primary role for the identified *pfcrt* mutations in CQ resistance as measured in vitro, the role of these mutations in clinical CQ resistance remains under evaluation. In studies in Mali, the baseline prevalence of the PfCRT K76T mutation was 39%, and this mutation was seen in all infections that occurred within 2 wk following CQ treatment *(89)*. Mutations in *pfmdr-1* showed a lower degree of selection by CQ treatment and were less strongly associated with clinical resistance. In a study in Uganda, all CQ-resistant infections were caused by isolates containing the *pfcrt* K76T mutation (G Dorsey, unpublished data). In both Mali and Uganda, some infections that cleared with CQ treatment also carried the K76T mutation, indicating an in vitro CQ-resistant phenotype. Indeed, in Uganda, where the incidence of malaria and the prevalence of CQ resistance are both higher than in Mali, the K76T *pfcrt* mutation was found in all of 114 tested isolates that caused infections with a range of in vivo CQ sensitivity (36% showing complete clearance after CQ treatment in a 14-d clinical study). For none of the eight identified *pfcrt* mutations or two *pfmdr-1* mutations (N86Y, D1246Y) did the presence or absence of mutations predict whether an infection would clear after CQ treatment. Thus, it appears that, at least in highly malarious areas, where individuals have significant antimalarial immunity, key *pfcrt* mutations are likely necessary for clinical CQ resistance, but other factors are also involved in CQ treatment outcomes. These results point to the importance of host immunity as well as the parasite drug-resistance phenotype in the response of malaria infections to treatment *(68)*.

MECHANISMS OF RESISTANCE TO OTHER 4-AMINOQUINOLINES

The 4-aminoquinoline amodiaquine (AQ) has close structural similarity to CQ (*see* Chapter 13). In vitro and in vivo cross-resistance between these two drugs has been documented in some studies *(90–92)*, whereas other studies did not show consistent cross-resistance *(93)*. In a meta-analysis of clinical trials comparing the two drugs, AQ had significantly better efficacy, even in areas with a high incidence of CQ resistance *(94)*.

Kinetic studies have suggested that AQ may be subject to the same resistance mechanism as CQ, as certain CQ-resistant parasites displayed significantly reduced accumulation of AQ *(9)*. The reduction of drug accumulation in CQ-resistant parasites was less pronounced for AQ than for CQ *(9)*. Differences in the accumulation and antimalarial efficacy of CQ and AQ may be the result of physiochemical differences between the compounds, including the greater lipophilicity of AQ *(95)*. Similarly, other close analogs of CQ with alterations in side-chain length retained activity against CQ-resistant *P. falciparum (96,97)*. Chemosensitizing agents such as verapamil and desipramine failed to enhance the activity of these CQ analogs against CQ-resistant parasites *(96,97)*. These data suggest that the mechanism of CQ resistance may be highly dependent on drug structure, consistent with the involvement of a specific transporter/permease or a specific food vacuole target such as drug–heme binding *(47)*. Further work into the structure–activity relationships of CQ analogs should aid in elaborating the mechanism of CQ resistance and the biochemical basis of circumventing resistance (*see* Chapter 13).

IN VIVO EFFICACY OF CHLOROQUINE RESISTANCE REVERSAL AGENTS

Given the observation that a number of agents can reverse resistance to CQ in vitro, several studies have investigated the potential of combining these agents with CQ for the treatment of malaria. This strategy could provide a means of extending the utility of CQ in areas where resistance has emerged while avoiding the use of more expensive and potentially toxic antimalarials. Although verapamil has been the CQ resistance reversal agent most widely studied in vitro, concerns about toxicity have precluded its investigation in vivo *(98)*. Early in vivo studies combining CQ with the tricyclic antidepressant desipramine and the antihistamine cyproheptadine failed to show any treatment benefit *(99,100)*. With desipramine, this lack of effect may have been the result of extensive binding to plasma proteins *(101)*. In the first *in vivo* study to document the efficacy of reversal agents, investigators reported the clearance of CQ-resistant *P. falciparum* in an Aotus monkey treated with CQ combined with chlorpromazine or prochlorperazine *(102)*.

Recently, investigators in Nigeria have reported a number of studies examining the efficacy of CQ plus chlorpheniramine, a histamine H1 receptor antagonist. Chlorpheniramine is relatively inexpensive, has limited toxicity, and has been widely used to treat CQ-induced pruritus in Africans, although its efficacy for this symptom is debatable *(103)*. When administered to children with uncomplicated malaria, the combination of CQ plus chlorpheniramine was more efficacious than either CQ alone or sulfadoxine–pyrimethamine, as efficacious as halofantrine, and almost as efficacious as mefloquine (Table 3) *(104–108)*. In these studies, 81–98% of patients treated with CQ/chlorpheniramine cleared their parasitemia after 14 d. In addition, the combination was found to be safe and well tolerated, although chlorpheniramine must be given three times a day over a 7-d period. The mechanism by which chlorpheniramine enhances the activity of CQ remains unclear *(106)*. In a recent detailed pharmacokinetic study, peak whole-blood CQ concentrations and the area under the first-moment drug concentration–time curve were significantly increased by chlorpheniramine *(109)*. This result suggests that increasing the uptake and/or concentration of CQ enhances CQ efficacy. Studies of CQ/CQ-resistance reversal agent combinations are needed in other patient populations to further test the potential of this approach to the treatment of uncomplicated malaria.

MECHANISMS OF RESISTANCE TO MEFLOQUINE, QUININE, AND HALOFANTRINE

Introduction

The quinolinemethanol antimalarials, quinine and mefloquine, and halofantrine, a related phenanthrene methanol, are important drugs for the prevention and treatment of malaria in areas of CQ resistance. Although these drugs remain effective in most parts of the world, their efficacy has begun to diminish in some areas and resistance is now widespread in parts of Southeast Asia. In contrast to the relatively slow emergence of CQ resistance, mefloquine resistance was reported within a few years after its introduction *(3)*. Over 50% of clinical infections are now resistant in parts of Southeast Asia, where this drug has been widely used to treat CQ-resistant malaria *(110,111)*. Decreased sensitivity to quinine was reported as early as 1910 *(112)*, but this drug

Table 3
In vivo Studies of Chloroquine Plus Chlorpheniramine

Patient population	Study design	In vivo results	
		CQ plus chlorpheniramine	Comparison group
Uncomplicated malaria (children) (104)	CQ/chlorpheniramine (n = 48) vs CQ alone (n = 49); 14 d	85% S, 4% RI, 10% RII	76% S, 2% RI, 18% RII, 4% RIII
Uncomplicated malaria (children) (106)	CQ/chlorpheniramine (n = 48) vs CQ alone (n = 48; 14 d	98% S, 2% RI	69% S, 21% RI, 4% RII, 6% RIII
Children with parasitological failure after CQ treatment (105)	CQ/chlorpheniramine (n = 21) vs mefloquine (n = 20); 14 d	81% S, 19% RI	100% S
Uncomplicated malaria (children) (107)	CQ/chlorpheniramine (n = 50) vs pyrimethamine/sulfadoxine (n = 50); 14 d	96% S, 4% RI (100% S in patients failing SP)	60% S, 18% RI, 16% RII, 6% RIII
Uncomplicated malaria (children) (108)	CQ/chlorpheniramine (n = 50) vs halofantrine (n = 50); 14 d	96% S, 4% RI	96% S, 4% RI

Note: Drug responses are described by standard WHO terminology for sensitivity (S) and resistance (RI–RIII), based on the persistence of parasitemia after treatment.

retained efficacy in the field for many years. Presently, as with mefloquine, over 50% of *P. falciparum* infections demonstrate some resistance to quinine in areas of Southeast Asia *(113)*. The reports of cross-resistance among mefloquine, quinine, and halofantrine suggest a common mechanism of resistance. Indeed, intrinsic resistance to mefloquine (seen prior to its introduction) and rapidly emerging resistance to this drug have been observed in areas with pre-existing quinine resistance *(3,114,115)*.

P-Glycoprotein, PfCRT and Mefloquine, Quinine, and Halofantrine Resistance

Following the identification of the MDR gene homolog, *pfmdr-1*, a number of studies have investigated its role in resistance to the quinolinemethanol-related compounds. Similar to the mechanism of MDR in tumor cells, resistance to mefloquine, halofantrine, and, to a lesser extent, quinine, may in certain cases be associated with gene amplification and overexpression of Pgh-1. In experiments with *P. falciparum*, stepwise selection for increased mefloquine resistance resulted in amplification and overexpression of *pfmdr-1 (59,65–67)*. Concomitant increases in halofantrine and quinine resistance developed in vitro with the increase in mefloquine resistance *(65,67)*. These results suggested an MDR phenotype for the quinolinemethanol-related compounds. Some studies with field isolates have also demonstrated an association between *pfmdr-1* gene amplification and mefloquine resistance *(15,74,75,77,116,117)*. However, this association was not absolute, suggesting that additional mechanisms for mefloquine resistance must exist (Table 4). That mechanisms other than overexpression of *pfmdr-1* are involved in resistance to quinolinemethanol-related compounds is supported by examples of the selection of parasites with increased resistance to mefloquine and halofantrine that do not have increases in the *pfmdr-1* copy number or expression *(118,119)*.

Studies of *pfmdr-1* sequence polymorphisms and resistance to quinolinemethanol-related compounds have produced mixed results. Parasite lines selected for increased resistance to mefloquine and halofantrine did not show changes in the sequence of *pfmdr-1 (65,67,118,119)*. Several field studies have failed to find a clear association between *pfmdr-1* allelic variation and susceptibility to mefloquine, halofantrine, and quinine *(15,74,75,77,116)*. In one study of Thai field isolates, the presence of the wild-type N86 allele was, in fact, associated with higher mefloquine IC_{50}'s *(117)*. This result suggests a discordance between resistance to mefloquine and CQ, as the mutant Y86 allele is, in some cases, associated with CQ resistance *(63)*. Recently, investigators used plasmid constructs containing allelic variants of the *pfmdr-1* gene to directly measure the effect of introduction or removal of mutations on drug susceptibility in selected CQ-sensitive (wild-type) and CQ-resistant (mutant) parasites. Replacement of the wild-type *pfmdr-1* with an allele containing three point mutations (C1034, D1042, Y1246) decreased the in vitro quinine susceptibility of a quinine-sensitive isolate *(81)*. Removal of the same mutations from the mutant allele resulted in reversion of the quinine response to the more sensitive level. Conversely, insertion of these mutations resulted in increased sensitivity to mefloquine and halofantrine, whereas removal of the mutations decreased sensitivity. These data suggest an additional level of complexity in the role of *pfmdr-1* in mediating resistance to the quinolinemethanol-related compounds.

The mechanism by which Pgh-1 may affect response to the quinolinemethanol-related compounds remains unclear. In some isolates, resistance to mefloquine can be reversed by penfluridol, but not by compounds that reverse resistance to CQ *(120,121)*.

Table 4
Field Studies of *pfmdr-1* Copy Number and Mefloquine Resistance

Study site (ref.)	In vitro sensitivity testing[a]	Results
Thailand 1993 *(15)*	10 of 11 isolates resistant to mefloquine	All 10 resistant isolates had gene amplification; one sensitive isolate had single gene copy
Africa 1995 *(75)*	5 of 15 isolates resistant to mefloquine	No association between gene amplification and drug susceptibility
Cambodia 1996 *(74)*	2 of 10 isolates resistant to mefloquine	No evidence of gene amplification in any of the isolates
Brazil 1998 *(116)*	26 isolates all sensitive to mefloquine	11 of 26 sensitive isolates were analyzed and contained only one gene copy
Thailand 1999 *(77)*	64 isolates all resistant to mefloquine	Among isolates with moderate to high mefloquine resistance; 40 of 62 had gene amplification
Thailand 1999 *(117)*	54 isolates: median $IC_{50} = 41$ ng/mL (5–183)	Increased copy number correlated significantly with increased mefloquine IC_{50} ($p = 0.006$)

[a]Studies differ in methodology for drug susceptibility.

Efflux studies in *P. falciparum* with mefloquine, halofantrine, and quinine have been hampered by the lipophilic nature of these compounds *(15)*. Mefloquine has been reported to interact with high affinity with human P-glycoprotein, supporting its role as a substrate for Pgh-1-mediated drug transport *(57)*. As the binding site of Pgh-1 is predicted to be located on the interior of the food vacuole membrane, genetic changes leading to enhanced activity (e.g., overexpression or mutations) might be expected to increase rather than decrease the concentration of drug in the food vacuole. Thus, the site of quinolinemethanol action may be outside the food vacuole or in the food vacuole membrane *(24)*. It is also possible that Pgh-1 itself is a target of action of the quinolinemethanol compounds or in an indirect way affects the accumulation of drug within the food vacuole *(65)*.

Altered susceptibilities to multiple drugs were also detected in the mutant 106/1 line that was selected for CQ resistance and had undergone the K76I mutation in *pfcrt*. This line displayed a 10-fold reduction in its quinine IC_{50} and a twofold to threefold reduction in the mefloquine and halofantrine IC_{50} values, relative to the parental 106/1 line. An increased susceptibility was also observed for artemisinin, contrasting with a decreased sensitivity to AQ and quinacrine. Thus, it is possible that *pfcrt* mutations can directly or indirectly affect parasite susceptibility to a spectrum of heme-binding antimalarial drugs. This is plausible, given that CQ-resistant parasites harboring mutations in *pfcrt* appear by single-cell photometric analysis to have a more acidic food vacuole with an altered membrane potential *(27)*. Changes in these two parameters could conceivably have very different outcomes in terms of accumulation of different antimalarial drugs and their interactions with heme in the food vacuole. Another interpretation of the findings with the *pfcrt* mutant line is that the altered response to quinine and other drugs is related to changes in expression of other genes in the transformed parasite lines.

SUMMARY

Although our understanding of the mechanisms of resistance to quinoline antimalarials remains incomplete, good progress has been made from both biochemical and genetic standpoints. It now appears that resistance to CQ involves a diminished level of drug uptake into the parasite food vacuole, although enhancement of drug efflux may also play a role. The CQ-resistance phenotype appears to have a high degree of structural specificity, as some CQ analogs offer much improved potency over the parent compound against resistant parasites. These observations are consistent with a role in CQ resistance for specific molecular interactions in drug flux across the food vacuole membrane and/or in heme binding. These interactions may lead to changes in food vacuolar ion conductance and a pH-dependent reduction in the concentration of a soluble receptor for CQ that is most likely free heme.

Recent studies point to a principal role for *pfcrt* mutations in CQ resistance. Although not required, mutations in *pfmdr*-1 may be advantageous to parasites already mutated in the *pfcrt* gene and possessing the CQ-resistant phenotype. It is known that in individuals with antimalarial immunity, infections by parasites with the in vitro CQ-resistance phenotype often clear following CQ treatment, so the presence of *pfcrt* mutations alone cannot predict CQ response in vivo. Clearly, acquired immunity and, likely, other host traits that affect susceptibility to malaria are additional factors that affect the outcome of drug treatment. Whether additional mutations in other parasite genes may also contribute to clinical CQ resistance is unknown.

In contrast to the case with CQ, resistance to mefloquine, quinine, and halofantrine is less well characterized. In some cases, there is good evidence for mediation by amplification and/or polymorphisms in the *pfmdr-1* gene. However, the association between *pfmdr-1* and resistance is incomplete, suggesting roles for other genetic factors, including *pfcrt*.

Quinoline antimalarials have been the mainstay of antimalarial chemotherapy from the time the activity of cinchona bark extracts was first recognized. The spread of resistance threatens the utility of all of the drugs in this class. A better understanding of the mechanisms of resistance to the quinolines may provide insight into the development of novel antimalarials or drug combinations that are able to circumvent resistance.

ACKNOWLEDGMENTS

We thank Steve Ward for valuable comments regarding resistance mechanisms and Chris Plowe for helpful discussions of his recent work, including the sharing of unpublished data.

REFERENCES

1. Barat LM, Bloland PB. Drug resistance among malaria and other parasites. Infect Dis Clin North Am 1997;11:969–987.
2. Whitby, M. Drug resistant *Plasmodium vivax* malaria. J Antimicrob Chemother 1997; 40:749–752.
3. Boudreau EF, Webster HK, Pavanand K, Thosingha, L. Type II mefloquine resistance in Thailand. Lancet 1982;2:1335.
4. Espinal CA, Cortes GT, Guerra P, Arias AE. Sensitivity of *Plasmodium falciparum* to antimalarial drugs in Colombia. Am J Trop Med Hyg 1985;34:675–680.

5. Draper CC, Brubaker G, Geser A, Kilimali VA, Wernsdorfer WH. Serial studies on the evolution of chloroquine resistance in an area of East Africa receiving intermittent malaria chemosuppression. Bull WHO 1985;63:109–118.

6. Raccurt CP, Dumestre-Toulet, V, Abraham, E, Le Bras, M, Brachet-Liermain A, Ripert C. Failure of falciparum malaria prophylaxis by mefloquine in travelers from West Africa. Am J Trop Med Hyg 1991;45:319–324.

7. Looareesuwan S, Viravan C, Vanijanonta, S. Wilairatana P, Suntharasamai P, Charoenlarp P, et al. Randomised trial of artesunate and mefloquine alone and in sequence for acute uncomplicated falciparum malaria. Lancet 1992;339:821–824.

8. White NJ. Mefloquine in the prophlaxis and treatment of falciparum malaria. Br Med J 1994;308:286–287.

9. Bray PG, Hawley SR, Ward SA. 4-Aminoquinoline resistance of *Plasmodium falciparum*: insights from the study of amodiaquine uptake. Mol Pharmacol 1996;50:1551–1558.

10. Churchill FC, Patchen LC, Campbell CC, Schwartz IK, Nguyen-Dinh P, Dickinson CM. Amodiaquine as a prodrug: importance of metabolite(s) in the antimalarial effect of amodiaquine in humans. Life Sci 1985;36:53–62.

11. Elueze EI, Croft SL, Warhurst DC. Activity of pyronaridine and mepacrine against twelve strains of *Plasmodium falciparum* in vitro. J Antimicrob Chemother 1996;37:511–518.

12. Webster HK, Thaithong S, Pavanand K, Yongvanitchit K, Pinswasdi C, Boudreau EF. Cloning and characterization of mefloquine-resistant *Plasmodium falciparum* from Thailand. Am J Trop Med Hyg 1985;34:1022–1027.

13. White NJ. Antimalarial drug resistance: the pace quickens. J Antimicrob Chemother 1992;30:571–585.

14. Wongsrichanalai C, Webster HK, Wimonwattrawatee T, Sookto P, Chuanak N, Thimasarn K, et al. Emergence of multidrug-resistant *Plasmodium falciparum* in Thailand: in vitro tracking. Am J Trop Med Hyg 1992;47:112–116.

15. Wilson CM, Volkman SK, Thaithong S, Martin RK, Kyle DE, Milhous WK, et al. Amplification of *pfmdr 1* associated with mefloquine and halofantrine resistance in *Plasmodium falciparum* from Thailand. Mol Biochem Parasitol 1993;57:151–160.

16. Suebsaeng L, Wernsdorfer WH, Rooney W. Sensitivity to quinine and mefloquine of *Plasmodium falciparum* in Thailand. Bull WHO 1986;64:759–765.

17. Wernsdorfer WH. Epidemiology of drug resistance in malaria. Acta Tropica 1994;56:143–156.

18. O'Neill PM, Bray PG, Hawley SR, Ward SA, Park BK. 4-Aminoquinolines—past, present, and future: a chemical perspective. Pharmacol Ther 1998;77:29–58.

19. Fitch CD. *Plasmodium falciparum* in owl monkeys: drug resistance and chloroquine binding capacity. Science 1970;169:289–290.

20. Fitch CD, Yunis NG, Chevli R, Gonzalez Y. High-affinity accumulation of chloroquine by mouse erythrocytes infected with *Plasmodium berghei*. J Clin Invest 1974;54:24–33.

21. Yayon A, Cabantchik ZI, Ginsburg H. Identification of the acidic compartment of *Plasmodium falciparum*-infected human erythrocytes as the target of the antimalarial drug chloroquine. EMBO J 1984;3:2695–2700.

22. Verdier F, Le Bras J, Clavier F, Hatin I, Blayo MC. Chloroquine uptake by *Plasmodium falciparum*-infected human erythrocytes during in vitro culture and its relationship to chloroquine resistance. Antimicrob Agents Chemother 1985;27:561–564.

23. Bray PG, Howells RE, Ritchie GY, Ward SA. Rapid chloroquine efflux phenotype in both chloroquine-sensitive and chloroquine-resistant *Plasmodium falciparum*. A correlation of chloroquine sensitivity with energy-dependent drug accumulation. Biochem Pharmacol 1992;44:1317–1324.

24. Foley M, Tilley L. Quinoline antimalarials: mechanisms of action and resistance and prospects for new agents. Pharmacol Ther 1998;79:55–87.

25. Wellems TE, Panton LJ, Gluzman IY, do Rosario VE, Gwadz RW, Walker-Jonah A, et al. Chloroquine resistance not linked to mdr-like genes in a *Plasmodium falciparum* cross. Nature 1990;345:253–255.

26. Su X, Kirkman LA, Fujioka H, Wellems TE. Complex polymorphisms in an approximately 330 kDa protein are linked to chloroquine-resistant *P. falciparum* in Southeast Asia and Africa. Cell 1997;91:593–603.

27. Fidock D, Nomura T, Talley A, Cooper R, Dzekunov S, Ferdig M, et al. Mutations in the digestive vacuole transmembrane protein PfCRT confer verapamil-reversible chloroquine resistance to *Plasmodium falciparum*. Cell 2000; in press.

28. Peters, W. Morphological and physiological variations in chloroquine-resistant *Plasmodium berghei*, Vincke and Lips. Ann Soc Belg Med Trop 1965;45:365–376.

29. Krogstad DJ, De, D. Chloroquine: modes of action and resistance and the activity of chloroquine analogs. In: Sherman IW. (ed). Malaria: Parasite Biology, Pathogenesis, and Protection Washington, DC: ASM Press, 1998, pp. 331–339.

30. Krogstad DJ, Gluzman IY, Kyle DE, Oduola AM, Martin SK, Milhous WK, et al. Efflux of chloroquine from *Plasmodium falciparum*: mechanism of chloroquine resistance. Science 1987;238:1283–1285.

31. Vezmar M, Deady LW, Tilley L, Georges E. The quinoline-based drug, *N*-(4-(1-hydroxy-2-(dibutylamino)ethyl) quinolin-8-yl)-4-azidosalicylamide, photoaffinity labels the multidrug resistance protein (MRP) at a biologically relevant site. Biochem Biophys Res Commun 1997;241:104–111.

32. Martin SK, Oduola AM, Milhous WK. Reversal of chloroquine resistance in *Plasmodium falciparum* by verapamil. Science 1987;235:899–901.

33. Bray PG, Boulter MK, Ritchie GY, Howells RE, Ward SA. Relationship of global chloroquine transport and reversal of resistance in *Plasmodium falciparum*. Mol Biochem Parasitol 1994;63:87–94.

34. Geary TG, Divo AD, Jensen JB, Zangwill M, Ginsburg H. Kinetic modelling of the response of *Plasmodium falciparum* to chloroquine and its experimental testing in vitro. Implications for mechanism of action of and resistance to the drug. Biochem Pharmacol 1990;40:685–691.

35. Ginsburg H, Stein WD. Kinetic modelling of chloroquine uptake by malaria-infected erythrocytes. Assessment of the factors that may determine drug resistance. Biochem Pharmacol. 1991;41:1463–1470.

36. Homewood CA, Warhurst DC, Peters W, Baggaley VC. Lysosomes, pH and the antimalarial action of chloroquine. Nature 1972;235:50–52.

37. Krogstad DJ, Schlesinger PH, Gluzman IY. Antimalarials increase vesicle pH in *Plasmodium falciparum*. J Cell Biol 1985;101:2302–2309.

38. Bray PG, Howells RE, Ward SA. Vacuolar acidification and chloroquine sensitivity in *Plasmodium falciparum*. Biochem Pharmacol 1992;43:1219–1227.

39. Karcz SR, Herrmann VR, Cowman AF. Cloning and characterization of a vacuolar ATPase A subunit homologue from *Plasmodium falciparum*. Mol Biochem Parasitol 1993;58:333–844.

40. Karcz SR, Herrmann VR, Trottein F, Cowman AF. Cloning and characterization of the vacuolar ATPase B subunit from *Plasmodium falciparum*. Mol Biochem Parasitol 1994;65:123–133.

41. Dzekunov S, Ursos L, Roepe P. Digestive vacuolar pH of intact intraerythrocytic *P. falciparum* either sensitive or resistant to chloroquine. Mol Biochem Parasitol 2000; 110(1):107–124.

42. Bray PG, Mungthin, M, Ridley RG, Ward SA. Access to hematin: the basis of chloroquine resistance. Mol Pharmacol 1998;54:170–179.

43. Warhurst DC. Antimalarial drugs: mode of action and resistance. J Antimicrob Chemother 18(Suppl B):1986;51–59.

44. Hawley SR, Bray PG, Park BK, Ward SA. Amodiaquine accumulation in *Plasmodium falciparum* as a possible explanation for its superior antimalarial activity over chloroquine. Mol Biochem Parasitol 1996;80:15–25.

45. Chou AC, Chevli R, Fitch CD. Ferriprotoporphyrin IX fulfills the criteria for identification as the chloroquine receptor of malaria parasites. Biochemistry 1980;19:1543–1549.
46. Sanchez CP, Wunsch S, Lanzer M. Identification of a chloroquine importer in *Plasmodium falciparum*. Differences in import kinetics are genetically linked with the chloroquine-resistant phenotype. J Biol Chem 1997;272:2652–2658.
47. Ridley RG. Malaria: dissecting chloroquine resistance. Curr Biol 1998;8:R346–R249.
48. Sanchez CP, Horrocks P, Lanzer M. Is the putative chloroquine resistance mediator CG2 the Na+/H+ exchanger of *Plasmodium falciparum*? Cell 1998;92:601–602.
49. Wellems TE, Wooton JC, Fujioka H, Su XZ, Cooper R, Baruch D, et al. *P. falciparum* CG2, linked to chloroquine resistance, does not resemble Na+/H+ exchangers. Cell 1998;94:285–286.
50. Basco LK, Le Bras, J. In vitro reversal of chloroquine resistance with chlorpheniramine against African isolates of *Plasmodium falciparum*. Jpn J Med Sci Biol 1994;47:59–63.
51. Bitonti AJ, Sjoerdsma A, McCann PP, Kyle DE, Oduola AM, Rossan RN, et al. Reversal of chloroquine resistance in malaria parasite *Plasmodium falciparum* by desipramine. Science 1988;242:1301–1303.
52. Bray PG, Ward SA. A comparison of the phenomenology and genetics of multidrug resistance in cancer cells and quinoline resistance in *Plasmodium falciparum*. Pharmacol Ther 1998;77:1–28.
53. Martiney JA, Cerami A, Slater AF. Verapamil reversal of chloroquine resistance in the malaria parasite *Plasmodium falciparum* is specific for resistant parasites and independent of the weak base effect. J Biol Chem 1995;270:22393–22398.
54. Bayoumi RA, Babiker HA, Arnot DE. Uptake and efflux of chloroquine by chloroquine-resistant *Plasmodium falciparum* clones recently isolated in Africa. Acta Tropica 1994;58:141–149.
55. Walter RD, Seth M, Bhaduri AP. Reversal of chloroquine resistance in *Plasmodium falciparum* by CDR 87/209 and analogues. Trop Med Parasitol 1993;44:5–8.
56. Riordan JR, Deuchars K, Kartner N, Alon N, Trent J, Ling V. Amplification of P-glycoprotein genes in multidrug-resistant mammalian cell lines. Nature 1985;316:817–819.
57. Riffkin CD, Chung R, Wall DM, Zalcberg JR, Cowman AF, Foley M, et al. Modulation of the function of human MDR1 P-glycoprotein by the antimalarial drug mefloquine. Biochem Pharmacol 1996;52:1545–1552.
58. Foote SJ, Thompson JK, Cowman AF, Kemp DJ. Amplification of the multidrug resistance gene in some chloroquine-resistant isolates of *P. falciparum*. Cell 1989;57:921–930.
59. Wilson CM, Serrano AE, Wasley A, Bogenschutz MP, Shankar AH, Wirth DF. Amplification of a gene related to mammalian mdr genes in drug-resistant. *Plasmodium falciparum* Science 1989;244:1184–1186.
60. Rubio JP, Cowman AF. *Plasmodium falciparum*: the *pfmdr2* protein is not overexpressed in chloroquine-resistant isolates of the malaria parasite. Exp Parasitol 1994;79:137–147.
61. Zalis MG, Wilson CM, Zhang Y, Wirth DF. Characterization of the *pfmdr2* gene for *Plasmodium falciparum*. Mol Biochem Parasitol 1994;63:311.
62. Cowman AF, Karcz S, Galatis D, Culvenor JG. A P-glycoprotein homologue of *Plasmodium falciparum* is localized on the digestive vacuole. J Cell Biol 1991;113:1033–1042.
63. Foote SJ, Kyle DE, Martin RK, Oduola AM, Forsyth K, Kemp DJ, et al. Several alleles of the multidrug-resistance gene are closely linked to chloroquine resistance in *Plasmodium falciparum*. Nature 1990;345:255–258.
64. Ekong RM, Robson KJ, Baker DA, and Warhurst DC. Transcripts of the multidrug resistance genes in chloroquine-sensitive and chloroquine-resistant *Plasmodium falciparum*. Parasitology 1993;106:107–115.
65. Cowman AF, Galatis D, Thompson JK. Selection for mefloquine resistance in *Plasmodium falciparum* is linked to amplification of the *pfmdr1* gene and cross-resistance to halofantrine and quinine. Proc Natl Acad Sci USA 1994;91:1143–1147.

66. Barnes DA, Foote SJ, Galatis D, Kemp DJ, Cowman AF. Selection for high-level chloro-quine resistance results in deamplification of the *pfmdr1* gene and increased sensitivity to mefloquine in *Plasmodium falciparum*. Embo J 1992;11:3067–3075.

67. Peel SA, Bright P, Yount B, Handy J, Baric RS. A strong association between mefloquine and halofantrine resistance and amplification, overexpression, and mutation in the P-glycoprotein gene homolog (*pfmdr*) of *Plasmodium falciparum* in vitro. Am J Trop Med Hyg 1994;51:648–658.

68. von Seidlein L, Duraisingh MT, Drakeley CJ, Bailey R, Greenwood BM, Pinder M. Poly-morphism of the Pf*mdr1* gene and chloroquine resistance in *Plasmodium falciparum* in The Gambia. Trans R Soc Trop Med Hyg 1997;91:450–453.

69. Grobusch MP, Adagu IS, Kremsner PG, Warhurst DC. *Plasmodium falciparum*: in vitro chloroquine susceptibility and allele-specific PCR detection of Pf*mdr1* Asn86Tyr poly-morphism in Lambarene, Gabon. Parasitology 1998;116:211–217.

70. Gómez-Saladín E, Fryauff DJ, Taylor WR, Laksana BS. Susanti AI, Purnomo, et al. *Plas-modium falciparum mdr1* mutations and in vivo chloroquine resistance in Indonesia. Am J Trop Med Hyg 1999;61:240–244.

71. Duraisingh MT, Drakeley CJ, Muller O, Bailey R, Snounou G, Targett GA, et al. Evi-dence for selection for the tyrosine-86 allele of the *pfmdr 1* gene of *Plasmodium falciparum* by chloroquine and amodiaquine. Parasitology 1997;114:205–4211.

72. Basco LK, Ringwald, P. Molecular epidemiology of malaria in Yaoundé, Cameroon. III. Analysis of chloroquine resistance and point mutations in the multidrug resistance 1 (*pfmdr 1*) gene of *Plasmodium falciparum*. Am J Trop Med Hyg 1998;59:577–581.

73. Basco LK, Ringwald, P. *pfmdr1* gene mutation and clinical response to chloroquine in Yaoundé, Cameroon. Trans R Soc Trop Med Hyg 1997;91:210–211.

74. Basco LK, de Pecoulas PE, Le Bras J, Wilson CM. *Plasmodium falciparum*: molecular characterization of multidrug-resistant Cambodian isolates. Exp Parasitol 1996;82:97–103.

75. Basco LK, Le Bras J, Rhoades Z, Wilson CM. Analysis of *pfmdr1* and drug susceptibility in fresh isolates of *Plasmodium falciparum* from subsaharan Africa. Mol Biochem Parasitol 1995;74:157–166.

76. Awad-el-Kariem FM, Miles MA, Warhurst DC. Chloroquine-resistant *Plasmodium falciparum* isolates from the Sudan lack two mutations in the *pfmdr1* gene thought to be associated with chloroquine resistance. Trans R Soc Trop Med Hyg 1992;86:587–589.

77. Chaiyaroj SC, Buranakiti A, Angkasekwinai P, Looressuwan S, Cowman AF. Analysis of mefloquine resistance and amplification of *pfmdr1* in multidrug-resistant *Plasmodium falciparum* isolates from Thailand. Am J Trop Med Hyg 1999;61:780–783.

78. van Es HH, Karcz S, Chu F, Cowman AF, Vidal S, Gros P, et al. Expression of the plasmodial *pfmdr1* gene in mammalian cells is associated with increased susceptibility to chloroquine. Mol Cell Biol 1994;14:2419–2428.

79. van Es HH, Renkema, H. Aerts H, Schurr E. Enhanced lysosomal acidification leads to increased chloroquine accumulation in CHO cells expressing the *pfmdr1* gene. Mol Biochem Parasitol 1994;68:209–219.

80. Barasch J, Kiss B, Prince A, Saiman L, Gruenert D, al-Awqati Q. Defective acidification of intracellular organelles in cystic fibrosis. Nature 1991;352:70–73.

81. Reed MB, Saliba KJ, Caruana SR, Kirk K, Cowman AF. Pgh1 modulates sensitivity and resistance to multiple antimalarials in *Plasmodium falciparum*. Nature 2000;403:906–999.

82. Wellems TE, Walker-Jonah A, Panton LJ. Genetic mapping of the chloroquine-resis-tance locus on *Plasmodium falciparum* chromosome. 7 Proc Natl Acad Sci USA 1991;88:3382–3386.

83. Su X, Ferdig MT, Huang Y, Huynh CQ, Liu A, You J, et al. A genetic map and recombi-nation parameters of the human malaria parasite *Plasmodium falciparum*. Science 1999;286:1351–1353.

84. Durand R, Gabbett E, Di Piazza JP, Delabre JF, Le Bras J. Analysis of kappa and omega repeats of the *cg2* gene and chloroquine susceptibility in isolates of *Plasmodium falciparum* from sub-Saharan Africa. Mol Biochem Parasitol 1999;101:185–197.

85. Basco LK, Ringwald, P. Chloroquine resistance in *Plasmodium falciparum* and polymorphism of the CG2 gene. J Infect Dis 1999;180:1979–1986.

86. Basco LK, Ringwald, P. Molecular epidemiology of malaria in Yaounde, Cameroon V. Analysis of the omega repetitive region of the *Plasmodium falciparum* CG2 gene and chloroquine resistance. Am J Trop Med Hyg 1999;61:807–813.

87. Adagu IS, Warhurst DC. Association of *cg2* and *pfmdr1* genotype with chloroquine resistance in field samples of *Plasmodium falciparum* from Nigeria. Parasitol 1999;119:343–348.

88. Fidock D, Nomura T, Cooper R, Su X, Talley A, Wellems TE. Allelic modifications of the *cg2* and cg1 genes do not alter the chloroquine response of drug-resistant *Plasmodium falciparum*. Mol Biochem Parasitol, 2000;110(1)1–10.

89. Djimde A, Doumbo, O, Kayentao K, Duombo S, Diourte Y, Coulibaly D, et al. In vivo chloroquine responses and pfcrt polymorphisms in Bandiagara, Mali. Am J Trop Med Hyg 1999;61(Supp):335–336.

90. Bjorkman, A. and Phillips-Howard PA. The epidemiology of drug-resistant malaria. Trans R Soc Trop Med Hyg 1990;84:177–180.

91. Geary TG, Divo AA, Jensen JB. Activity of quinoline-containing antimalarials against chloroquine-sensitive and -resistant strains of *Plasmodium falciparum* in vitro. Trans R Soc Trop Med Hyg 1987;81:499–503.

92. Scott HV, Tan WL, Barlin GB. Antimalarial activity of Mannich bases derived from 4-(7'-bromo-1',5'-naphthyridin-4'-ylamino)phenol and 4-(7'-trifluoromethylquinolin-4'-ylamino)phenol against *Plasmodium falciparum* in vitro. Ann Trop Med Parasitol 1987;81:85–93.

93. Geary TG, Jensen JB. Lack of cross-resistance to 4-aminoquinolines in chloroquine-resistant *Plasmodium falciparum* in vitro. J Parasitol 1983;69:97–105.

94. Olliaro P, Nevill C, LeBras J, Ringwald P, Mussano P, Garner P, et al. Systematic review of amodiaquine treatment in uncomplicated malaria. Lancet 1996;348:1196–1201.

95. Bray PG, Hawley SR, Mungthin M, and Ward SA. Physicochemical properties correlated with drug resistance and the reversal of drug resistance in *Plasmodium falciparum*. Mol Pharmacol 1996;50:1559–1566.

96. De D, Krogstad FM, Cogswell FB, Krogstad DJ. Aminoquinolines that circumvent resistance in *Plasmodium falciparum* in vitro. Am J Trop Med Hyg 1996;55(6):579–583.

97. Ridley RG, Hofheinz W, Matile H, Jaquet C, Dorn A, Masciadri R, et al. 4-Aminoquinoline analogs of chloroquine with shortened side chains retain activity against chloroquine-resistant *Plasmodium falciparum*. Antimicrob Agents Chemother 1996;40:1846–1854.

98. Watt G, Shanks GD. Reversal of chloroquine-resistant falciparum malaria. Lancet 1990;335:1155.

99. Bjorkman A, Willcox M, Kihamia CM, Mahikwano LF, Howard PA, Hakansson A, et al. Field study of cyproheptadine/chloroquine synergism in falciparum malaria. Lancet 1990;336:59–60.

100. Warsame M, Wernsdorfer WH, Bjorkman A. Lack of effect of desipramine on the response to chloroquine of patients with chloroquine-resistant falciparum malaria. Trans R Soc Trop Med Hyg 1992;86:235–236.

101. Boulter MK, Bray PG, Howells RE, Ward SA. The potential of desipramine to reverse chloroquine resistance of *Plasmodium falciparum* is reduced by its binding to plasma protein. Trans R Soc Trop Med Hyg 1993;87:303.

102. Kyle DE, Milhous WK, Rossan RN. Reversal of *Plasmodium falciparum* resistance to chloroquine in Panamanian Aotus monkeys. Am J Trop Med Hyg 1993;48:126–133.

103. Sowunmi A, Walker O, Salako LA. Pruritus and antimalarial drugs in Africans. Lancet 1989;2:213.

104. Sowunmi A, Oduola AM, Ogundahunsi OA, Falade CO, Gbotosho GO, Salako LA. Enhanced efficacy of chloroquine–chlorpheniramine combination in acute uncomplicated falciparum malaria in children. Trans R Soc Trop Med Hyg 1997;91:63–67.

105. Sowunmi A, Oduola AM. Comparative efficacy of chloroquine/chlorpheniramine combination and mefloquine for the treatment of chloroquine-resistant *Plasmodium falciparum* malaria in Nigerian children. Trans R Soc Trop Med Hyg 1997;91:689–693.

106. Sowunmi A, Oduola AM, Ogundahunsi OA, Salako LA. Enhancement of the antimalarial effect of chloroquine by chloropheniramine in vivo. Trop Med Int Health 1998;3:177–183.

107. Sowunmi A, Oduola AM, Ogundahunsi OA, Salako LA. Comparative efficacy of chloroquine plus chlorpheniramine and pyrimethamine/sulfadoxine in acute uncomplicated falciparum malaria in Nigerian children. Trans R Soc Trop Med Hyg 1998;92:77–81.

108. Sowunmi A, Fehintola FA, Ogundahunsi OA, Oduola AM. Comparative efficacy of chloroquine plus chlorpheniramine and halofantrine in acute uncomplicated falciparum malaria in Nigerian children. Trans R Soc Trop Med Hyg 1998;92:441–445.

109. Okonkwo CA, Coker HA, Agomo PU, Ogunbanwo JA, Mafe AG, Agomo CO, et al. Effect of chlorpheniramine on the pharmacokinetics of and response to chloroquine of Nigerian children with falciparum malaria. Trans R Soc Trop Med Hyg 1999;93:306–311.

110. Nosten F, ter Kuile F, Chongsuphajaisiddhi T, Luxemburger C, Webster HK, Edstein M, et al. Mefloquine-resistant falciparum malaria on the Thai-Burmese border. Lancet 1991;337:1140–1143.

111. Fontanet AL, Johnston DB, Walker AM, Rooney W, Thimasarn K, Sturchler D, et al. High prevalence of mefloquine-resistant falciparum malaria in eastern Thailand. Bull WHO 1993;71:377–383.

112. Bjorkman A, Phillips-Howard PA. Drug-resistant malaria: mechanisms of development and inferences for malaria control. Trans R Soc Trop Med Hyg 1990;84:323–324.

113. Giboda M, Denis MB. Response of Kampuchean strains of *Plasmodium falciparum* to antimalarials: in-vivo assessment of quinine and quinine plus tetracycline; multiple drug resistance in vitro. J Trop Med Hyg 1988;91:205–211.

114. Oduola AM, Sowunmi A, Milhous WK, Kyle DE, Martin RK, Walker O, et al. Innate resistance to new antimalarial drugs in *Plasmodium falciparum* from Nigeria. Trans R Soc Trop Med Hyg 1992;86:123–126.

115. Brasseur P, Kouamouo J, Moyou-Somo R, Druilhe P. Multi-drug resistant falciparum malaria in Cameroon in 1987–1988. II. Mefloquine resistance confirmed in vivo and in vitro and its correlation with quinine resistance. Am J Trop Med Hyg 1992;46:8–14.

116. Zalis MG, Pang L, Silveira MS, Milhous WK, Wirth DF. Characterization of *Plasmodium falciparum* isolated from the Amazon region of Brazil: evidence for quinine resistance. Am J Trop Med Hyg 1998;58:630–637.

117. Price RN, Cassar C, Brockman A, Duraisingh M, van Vugt M, White NJ, et al. The *pfmdr1* gene is associated with a multidrug-resistant phenotype in *Plasmodium falciparum* from the western border of Thailand. Antimicrob Agents Chemother 1999;43:2943–2949.

118. Lim AS, Galatis D, Cowman AF. *Plasmodium falciparum*: amplification and overexpression of *pfmdr1* is not necessary for increased mefloquine resistance. Exp Parasitol 1996;83:295–303.

119. Ritchie GY, Mungthin M, Green JE, Bray PG, Hawley SR, Ward SA. In vitro selection of halofantrine resistance in *Plasmodium falciparum* is not associated with increased expression of Pgh1. Mol Biochem Parasitol 1996;83:35–46.

120. Peters W, Robinson BL. The chemotherapy of rodent malaria. XLVI. Reversal of mefloquine resistance in rodent *Plasmodium*. Ann Trop Med Parasitol 1991;85:5–10.

121. Oduola AM, Omitowoju GO, Gerena L, Kyle DE, Milhous WK. Sowunmi A, et al. Reversal of mefloquine resistance with penfluridol in isolates of *Plasmodium falciparum* from south-west Nigeria. Trans R Soc Trop Med Hyg 1993;87:81–83.

9

Folate Antagonists and Mechanisms of Resistance

Christopher V. Plowe

INTRODUCTION

The antifolates were once thought to be a nearly ideal class of antimalarial agent *(1)*. Antifolate drugs interfere differentially with folate metabolism, an essential parasite pathway that includes enzymes with no human counterparts. They are effective both as prophylactic and therapeutic agents against malaria. However, the antifolates are notoriously quick to fall prey to resistant parasites, and resistance to the commercially available antifolates is now widespread. The most popular formulation, sulfadoxine–pyrimethamine, is no longer recommended for general prophylaxis because of rare but serious cutaneous drug reactions. Are the antifolates a class of antimalarials whose time has come and gone? Most emphatically not, for the following reasons: First, sulfadoxine–pyrimethamine is currently the first-line antimalarial drug in several sub-Saharan African countries where chloroquine resistance is widespread and where other drugs remain far too expensive for general use. Second, several promising new combinations of antifolates that may be less susceptible to parasite resistance and less toxic are in development. Finally, new metabolic pathways that can be targeted with drugs that may behave synergistically with the antifolates have recently been identified in *Plasmodium* species (e.g., the shikimate pathway) *(2)*, and many such discoveries can be anticipated as the malaria-genome-sequencing project proceeds. The antifolate antimalarials will remain in widespread use for the foreseeable future because of a lack of affordable alternatives and will remain one of the major classes of new drugs under development because of their high therapeutic index and their synergy with each other and with other drugs.

This chapter will briefly review the mechanisms of the antifolate antimalarial drugs (dihydrofolate reductase inhibitors, sulfonamides, and sulfones) and will discuss mechanisms of malaria parasite resistance to the individual drugs and drug combinations in use and under development. Distinctions will be made between what is known about mechanisms of in vitro resistance to the individual drugs and what is known, and not known, about the determinants of in vivo resistance to the antifolate drug combinations used for malaria therapy. Despite an increasingly detailed understanding of the molecular basis of resistance to the dihydrofolate reductase inhibitors and sulfa drugs under in vitro conditions, much remains to be learned about the mechanisms of therapeutic failure of antifolate combinations under different epidemiological and immunological conditions in the field.

From: *Antimalarial Chemotherapy: Mechanisms of Action, Resistance, and New Directions in Drug Discovery*
Edited by: P. J. Rosenthal © Humana Press Inc., Totowa, NJ

THE FOLATE BIOSYNTHETIC PATHWAY IN PLASMODIA

Empiric use of antifolates against malaria long predates the demonstration of the folate metabolism pathway in *Plasmodium* species. Sulfonamides were found to be active against primate and bird malarias in the early 1940s *(3,4)* and this activity was found to be reversed by *p*-aminobenzoic acid (*p*ABA) *(5)*, a substrate for dihydropteroate synthase, the enzyme two steps before dihydrofolate reductase in the folate pathway. *De novo* synthesis of folate by malaria parasites was demonstrated over 20 yr ago *(6)*, although subsequent studies have suggested that at least some parasites have the capacity to salvage folate or folate metabolites to supplement *de novo* synthesis *(7)*, a feature that appears to contribute to resistance to the sulfa drugs *(8,9)*. Several recent reviews and an Internet site describe the plasmodial folate pathway in detail and the reader is referred to these comprehensive sources for depictions of the *de novo* and salvage pathways for folate *(10–12)*. Although not all of the enzymes involved in folate metabolism have been identified in plasmodia, this is likely to change as the malaria genome project proceeds. The genes encoding the enzymes in the folate pathway targeted by existing antifolate drugs, dihydrofolate reductase *(13)* and dihydropteroate synthase *(14,15)*, have both been cloned and sequenced, and mutations in these genes have been determined to play a role in resistance to the antifolate drugs.

INHIBITORS OF DIHYDROFOLATE REDUCTASE

The most productive period of antimalarial drug research and development came during World War II, when the Allied Forces found their supply of quinine cut off and mounted an intense effort to identify and design new antimalarial compounds. Among these were the biguanides, including proguanil, and the structurally related pyrimidine derivatives, which were modified to yield pyrimethamine (Fig. 1). Proguanil is cyclized to cycloguanil in the liver, and the mechanism of action of both cycloguanil and pyrimethamine was presumed to be through inhibition of the folate pathway, based on their similar structure to the pyrimidine derivatives and the observation that folate antagonizes their action in vitro. The direct action of these two compounds on malarial dihydrofolate reductase was subsequently demonstrated *(16–18)*.

Discovery of antimalarial activity of the dihydrofolate reductase inhibitors in animal models was quickly followed by human studies, and both proguanil and pyrimethamine were soon used widely for malaria chemoprophylaxis. Unfortunately, resistance arose extremely rapidly in settings where these drugs were widely deployed. Clyde and Shute describe starting monthly pyrimethamine prophylaxis schemes in Tanzanian villages and observing rates of in vivo *Plasmodium falciparum* resistance rise from 0% to 37% in just 5 mo *(19)*. When they moved to a weekly prophylaxis regimen, resistance rose more slowly, but still reached levels of 50–60% within 2 yr. These high rates of resistance were limited to the villages participating in the prophylaxis scheme and those located within 1–2 miles of the prophylaxis villages, but villages more than 2 miles away maintained resistance levels of 0–7%. This very focal and rapid development of antifolate resistance in areas directly under drug pressure led to early suspicions that resistance must be the result of a simple mechanism, such as point mutations in the drug target. Subsequent animal studies showing rapid selection of increasing levels of pyrimethamine resistance *(20,21)* in an apparent stepwise fashion

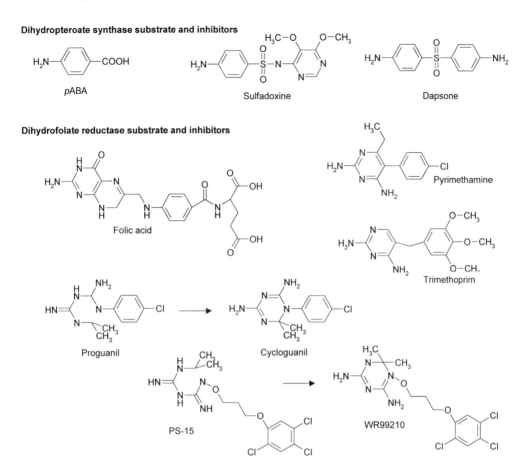

Fig. 1. Natural substrates and drugs inhibiting dihydropteroate synthase and dihydrofolate reductase in *P. falciparum*. Sulfadoxine and dapsone compete with *p*-aminobenzoic acid (*p*ABA) to inhibit dihydropteroate synthase. Pyrimethamine, trimethoprim, cycloguanil (cyclized in the host liver from proguanil), and WR99210 (metabolized from the pro-drug PS-15) inhibit dihydrofolate reductase by competing with dihydrofolic acid.

heightened this suspicion, which was finally confirmed after the gene for dihydrofolate reductase was cloned and sequenced *(13)*. Point mutations conferring specific amino acid alterations in the presumed active-site cavity of dihydrofolate reductase were shown in established culture-adapted parasite lines to be associated with differential resistance to cycloguanil and pyrimethamine *(22–25)*. In contrast to antifolate resistance in bacteria and human cancers, gene amplification does not appear to be a mechanism for such resistance in malaria *(22,23)*.

Plasmodium falciparum dihydrofolate reductase is encoded by a single-copy gene on chromosome 4 that also encodes thymidylate synthase, and the two enzymes form a bifunctional protein *(26,27)*. Although the crystal structure of the *P. falciparum* dihydrofolate reductase has yet to be solved, valuable inferences have been drawn from the derived structures of the enzyme in *Toxoplasma gondii (28)* and *Leishmania major (29)* (Fig. 2), as well as by indirect molecular modeling schemes *(30)*. These inferences, in combination with enzyme kinetic assays of wild-type and mutant malaria

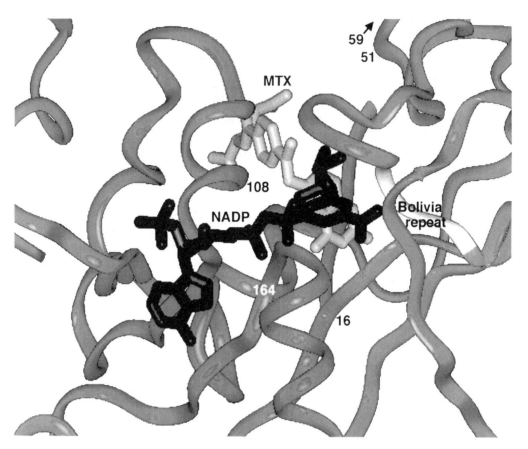

Fig. 2. Ribbon diagram of active site of *P. falciparum* dihydrofolate reductase, showing bound methotrexate (MTX) and NADP, resistance-conferring mutations at labeled amino acids, and the Bolivia repeat mutation. (From ref. *30*.)

dihydrofolate reductase, support the view that nucleotide substitutions found in resistant genotypes alter the enzyme's active-site cavity and result in differential binding affinities for different drugs. These resistance-conferring mutations occur in a stepwise, sequential fashion, with higher levels of in vitro resistance occurring in the presence of multiple mutations. Primary mutations are required for subsequent mutations to be maintained while still preserving enzyme function. Definitive proof that point mutations in dihydrofolate reductase confer resistance to pyrimethamine came from transfection experiments in *P. falciparum*, in which a pyrimethamine-sensitive clone was transformed with mutant dihydrofolate reductase, and the mutant transformants exhibited the predicted levels of pyrimethamine resistance *(31,32)*.

Table 1 summarizes the in vitro resistance of *P. falciparum* dihydrofolate reductase genotypes to pyrimethamine and cycloguanil as well as to two other dihydrofolate reductase inhibitors under development, chlorcycloguanil (the active metabolite of chlorproguanil) and WR99210 (the active metabolite of PS-15). The data shown in Table 1 are from experiments in which naturally occurring and genetically engineered dihydrofolate reductase constructs are used to transform *Saccharomyces cerevisiae* lacking dihydrofolate reductase. This assay in yeast yields relative susceptibilities

Table 1
Naturally Occurring Genotypes of *P. falciparum* Dihydrofolate Reductase and Relative Level of Resistance (IC$_{50}$, 50% inhibitory concentration) Against Dihydrofolate Reductase Inhibitors as Determined in a Yeast Model[a]

Strain source	Amino acid position							Relative IC$_{50}$				Predominant distribution
	16	BR	50	51	59	108	164	PYR	CG	CCG	WR	
3D7 (Wild type)	ala	—	cys	asn	cys	ser	ile	1	1	1	1	W Africa
HB3	ala	—	cys	asn	cys	**ASN**	ile	331	25	26	0.3	W Africa
FCR3	**VAL**	—	cys	asn	cys	**THR**	ile	1.2	829	180	0.8[b]	Rare in nature
It.D12	ala	—	cys	**ILE**	cys	**ASN**	ile	755	146	87	.07	Africa
K1	ala	—	cys	asn	**ARG**	**ASN**	ile	1048	290	108	1.0[b]	Africa
Dd2	ala	—	cys	**ILE**	**ARG**	**ASN**	ile	2371	137	86	1.0[b]	E Africa, SE Asia
Bolivia1	ala	—	cys	**ILE**	cys	**ASN**	**LEU**	9960	1957	596	2.7	S America
Cs1-2	ala	—	cys	asn	**ARG**	**ASN**	**LEU**	6212	ND	1008	ND	S America, SE Asia
V1/S	ala	—	cys	**ILE**	**ARG**	**ASN**	**LEU**	22477	1709	206	1.3	S America, SE Asia
Bolivia2	ala	—	**ARG**	**ILE**	cys	**ASN**	ile	2637	601	325	0.8	S America
Bolivia3	ala	—	**ARG**	**ILE**	cys	**ASN**	**LEU**	20206	6908	722	5.5	S America
Bolivia4	ala	**BR**	cys	**ILE**	cys	**ASN**	**LEU**	6210	622	136	0.7[b]	S America

BR = Bolivia repeat; PYR = pyrimethamine; CG = cycloguanil; CCG = chlorcycloguanil; WR = WR99210.
Mutations are indicated by bold capitals. ND = not done.
[a] The known predominant geographic distribution for each genotype is indicated in the last column.
[b] No significant difference in IC50 from wildtype.

177

similar to those seen in standard in vitro testing in *P. falciparum* and permits the rapid comparison of a wide variety of dihydrofolate reductase genotypes using a large panel of drugs *(33,34)*.

A single point mutation causing a serine to asparagine change at position 108 is linked to pyrimethamine resistance with only a moderate loss of susceptibility to cycloguanil and chlorcycloguanil. The addition of asparagine to isoleucine at codon 51 and/or cysteine to arginine at codon 59 results in higher levels of pyrimethamine resistance, again with only modest effects on cycloguanil and chlorcycloguanil. A serine to threonine mutation at position 108 coupled with an alanine to valine change at position 16 confers resistance to cycloguanil and chlorcycloguanil, with only a moderate loss of susceptibility to pyrimethamine. Finally, an isoleucine to leucine change at position 164 combined with Asn-108 and Ile-51 and/or Arg-59 confers high-level resistance to both pyrimethamine and cycloguanil, with a more modest effect on chlorcycloguanil *(22–25,35)*. An analogous array of point mutations in *P. vivax* dihydrofolate reductase has recently been described *(36)*.

Recombinant *P. falciparum* dihydrofolate reductase enzyme has been expressed in *Escherichia coli* for biochemical and enzyme kinetics studies *(37,38)*. These studies provide a rationale for the specific sequence of accumulation of mutations, based on their effects on drug resistance and enzyme function. Asn-108 occurs first, conferring moderate pyrimethamine resistance at a relatively low cost to enzyme function as measured by k_{cat}/K_m ratios for dihydrofolate. Subsequent mutations at codons 51, 59, and 164 result in lowered binding affinities for pyrimethamine, but come at a cost of up to 40-fold reductions in k_{cat}/K_m ratios for dihydrofolate, suggesting that parasites containing the more highly mutated forms of dihydrofolate reductase might be selected against in the absence of drug pressure.

No dihydrofolate reductase mutations other than these five first discovered to be associated with in vitro resistance were identified in isolates from a wide variety of geographic areas in the approximately 10 yr after the gene was first sequenced in *P. falciparum (23–25,39,40)*. Recently, however, single reports of rare mutations have been made *(41,42)* and two new dihydrofolate reductase mutations were discovered in an area of widespread sulfadoxine–pyrimethamine resistance in Bolivia and found to be common in South America: A cysteine to arginine mutation at codon 50 and a five-amino acid repeat insertion between codons 30 and 31, termed the Bolivia repeat *(29,43)*.

The roles of these newly discovered mutations in antifolate resistance are not yet firmly established, although transfection studies in yeast indicate that the Arg-50 mutation does confer resistance to pyrimethamine and other dihydrofolate reductase inhibitors, whereas the Bolivia repeat does not *(34)*. The association of the Bolivia repeat with other dihyrofolate reductase mutations and its location in the active-site cavity, as well as its high prevalence in a region of the world where clinical pyrimethamine resistance is almost complete and absence in Africa where antifolate resistance is less common *(29)*, argue against the Bolivia repeat being merely a silent mutation. Because the resistance-conferring dihydrofolate reductase mutations diminish dihydrofolate reductase enzyme activity *(38)*, it is plausible that the Bolivia repeat is a compensatory mutation, restoring the efficiency of mutant dihydrofolate reductases. This hypothesis could be tested in enzyme kinetics studies such as those described above.

As shown in Table 1, analysis of all the known dihydrofolate reductase genotypes against a panel of dihydrofolate reductase inhibitors confirms that different specific genotypes are resistant to different drugs. The triple mutant Asn-108/Ile-51/Arg-59, which has emerged in areas in Africa where sulfadoxine-pyrimethamine has begun to fail, has moderate to high-level resistance to pyrimethamine but confers only moderate levels of resistance to both cycloguanil and chlorcycloguanil and no resistance to WR99210. This is consistent with the observation that infections that fail to clear with sulfadoxine–pyrimethamine treatment and harbor this triple mutant can be cleared by a combination of chlorproguanil and dapsone. The addition of the Leu-164 mutation gives rise to a high level of resistance to cycloguanil and chlorcycloguanil as well as pyrimethamine, suggesting that antifolate combinations relying on these drugs may not work in parts of Southeast Asia and South America, where Leu-164 is common *(29,42,43)* and that the arrival of Leu-164 in Africa would signal the end of the utility of proguanil and chlorproguanil there, at least as dihydrofolate reductase inhibitors.

Recent evidence has shown that proguanil does not act solely through metabolism to cycloguanil and inhibition of dihydrofolate reductase, and it is unknown whether the same is true of chlorproguanil. Fidock et al. found that *P. falciparum* transformed with human dihydrofolate reductase was rendered resistant to WR99210 and to cycloguanil, but that susceptibility to proguanil was not affected, implying that proguanil has a site of activity other than dihydrofolate reductase *(44)*. This is consistent with studies showing that the combination of atovaquone and proguanil is active against parasites from areas with high rates of resistance to antifolates *(45)* and that synergy between atovaquone and proguanil relies on the direct action of proguanil at a site other than dihydrofolate reductase *(46)*. These findings illustrate the importance of validating in vivo what we learn about mechanisms of drug resistance in the laboratory. Had it been accepted that proguanil would not work in an area where high rates of the dihydrofolate reductase mutation Leu-164 render cycloguanil useless, a promising new antimalarial combination might never have been found to be highly efficacious in an area of multidrug resistance. The success of clinical trials with atovaquone and proguanil led to renewed efforts to elucidate previously unknown mechanisms of action, providing a good example of research feedback loops between the laboratory and the field.

SULFONAMIDES AND SULFONES

The sulfa drugs were developed and used extensively in the mid-20th century as antibacterial agents, although their antimalarial potential was quickly noted and evaluated *(3,4)*. Development of resistance and relatively poor clinical efficacy as single agents led to the abandonment of sulfas as antimalarials until sulfadoxine was combined with pyrimethamine to form a synergistic antifolate drug combination widely known as Fansidar® (Hoffman-La Roche, Basel) but also manufactured and sold in a variety of other commercial and generic forms. The ability of *p*ABA to antagonize sulfa drugs in vivo *(5,47)* and in vitro *(48)* supported the supposition that they act as *p*ABA analogs, inhibiting dihydropteroate synthase in the parasite folate pathway.

The role of dihydropteroate synthase in sulfa resistance was elucidated following the same pattern described earlier for dihydrofolate reductase, with the cloning of the gene, the identification of point mutations associated with in vitro drug resistance, and detailed characterization of the heterologously expressed wild-type and mutant enzymes.

Like dihydrofolate reductase, dihydropteroate synthase is part of a bifunctional polypeptide, encoded by a gene also encoding dihydro-hydroxymethylpterin pyrophosphokinase, another constitutient of the folate metabolic pathway *(14,15)*. Sequence analysis of the coding regions of dihydropteroate synthase from established parasite cell lines identified a limited number of point mutations, all associated with in vitro resistance to sulfa drugs. The interpretation of in vitro studies of *P. falciparum* resistance to sulfa drugs has been complicated by the need to perform the assays under rigorously standardized, near-zero folate conditions to obtain reproducible results. Under these conditions, the following mutations in dihydropteroate synthase were associated with resistance to sulfadoxine: serine to alanine at codon 436, alanine to glycine at codon 437, lysine to glutamate at codon 540, alanine to glycine at codon 581, and serine to phenylalanine at codon 436 coupled with alanine to either threonine or serine at codon 613 *(8,15)*.

The dihydropteroate synthase mutations were subsequently proven to confer resistance to sulfonamides and sulfones through transfection studies in *P. falciparum (49)*. The Phe-436, Gly-437, Ser-613 triple mutant was the most highly resistant genotype analyzed, with nearly a 1000-fold increase in the median inhibitory concentration (IC_{50}) for sulfadoxine relative to wildtype. This genotype, however, is rare in nature, and the Gly-437, Glu-540, Ala-581 genotype that is prevalent in areas of widespread sulfadoxine–pyrimethamine failure *(29,43)* has not yet been examined in in vitro studies, transfection studies, or enzyme kinetics studies.

The entire dihydro-hydroxymethylpterin pyrophosphokinase–dihydropteroate synthase protein was expressed in *E. coli*, and enzyme kinetics studies performed to investigate the effects of the mutations on enzyme function and on affinity for sulfa drugs *(50)*. The Gly-437 mutation, which is common in epidemiological surveys even in areas of low antifolate resistance *(29,51)*, often as the sole mutation, has little effect on enzyme function. These observations are consistent with Gly-437 being the first dihydropteroate synthase mutation to occur, and then being followed by additional mutations conferring higher levels of resistance, much like the dihydrofolate reductase mutation Asn-108 precedes additional mutations. The measure of catalytic efficiency for the *p*ABA, the k_{cat}/K_m ratio, was found to vary up to ninefold among the enzymes tested, with the wild-type and least mutated enzymes having the best catalytic activity and the enzymes with the lowest binding affinity for the sulfa drugs (i.e., most resistance) having the lowest catalytic activity. This suggests that the mutations in dihydropteroate synthase that confer resistance to the sulfa drugs come at a cost to enzyme function and might be selected against in the absence of drug pressure. The same set of studies showed that the binding-affinity curves for the different enzymes were identical for sulfadoxine, sulfamethoxazole, and dapsone, implying that complete cross-resistance exists among the commonly used sulfonamides and sulfones.

DETERMINANTS OF IN VIVO RESISTANCE TO SULFA–DIHYDROFOLATE REDUCTASE INHIBITOR COMBINATIONS

The above-described studies have provided a detailed understanding of the molecular and biochemical mechanisms of in vitro resistance to the individual dihydrofolate reductase inhibitors and sulfa drugs. Although it seems probable that some degree of resistance to both sulfadoxine and pyrimethamine is necessary for in vivo resistance to both drugs when used in combination, the relative importance of intrinsic parasite resistance to sulfadoxine versus pyrimethamine in causing in vivo sulfadoxine–pyrimethamine failure has not been clearly resolved. Some studies have observed therapeutic success of sulfadoxine–pyrimethamine in the face of in vitro resistance to pyrimethamine, suggesting that sulfadoxine resistance is key to sulfadoxine–pyrimethamine failure, but others have found similar sulfadoxine inhibitory concentrations and differential pyrimethamine susceptibilities among isolates with in vivo sensitive versus resistant phenotypes, suggesting that pyrimethamine resistance is paramount *(52,53)*. In vitro pharmacokinetic studies of the synergistic action of pyrimethamine and sulfadoxine done under physiologic folate and *p*ABA conditions suggested that the in vivo response to sulfadoxine–pyrimethamine may be determined primarily by parasite sensitivity to pyrimethamine *(54)*. However, in vitro experiments under nonphysiological conditions with single drugs may not reflect how parasites respond to drug combinations in human hosts under varying nutritional, pharmacokinetic, and immunological conditions *(55,56)*. The hypothesis that sulfadoxine–pyrimethamine failure is the result of pyrimethamine resistance is therefore not necessarily inconsistent with the in vitro susceptibility, enzyme kinetics, and transfection studies described earlier that clearly demonstrate a role for dihydropteroate synthase mutations in resistance to sulfonamides and sulfones.

It has long been known that folate and *p*ABA antagonize the action of the individual antifolate drugs *(5,24,47,48,57,58)*. When all other conditions are carefully controlled, the addition of low concentrations of folate to in vitro sulfa susceptibility assays has profound antagonistic effects against the sulfa drugs for some but not all parasite isolates *(8)*. This phenomenon, termed the "folate effect," was thought to be of potential importance in resistance to sulfa drugs and sulfa–dihydrofolate reductase inhibitor combinations. The folate effect did not segregate with dihydropteroate synthase genotypes in a genetic cross. Although it was linked to the dihydrofolate reductase gene in the cross progeny, it was not linked with dihydrofolate reductase sequence in other, unrelated parasite lines, suggesting that a gene responsible for the folate effect is located near but not at the dihydrofolate reductase locus on chromosome 4. The exact mechanism or genetic basis of the folate effect is not known at this time, nor is the prevalence of this effect in natural parasite populations. Subsequent studies showed that the folate effect could be completely abolished by the addition of pyrimethamine to assay cultures at concentrations substantially lower than those needed to inhibit dihydrofolate reductase *(9)*. Thus, although the folate effect does appear to affect the action of sulfa drugs as single agents on malaria parasites, it appears to play no role in the acute clinical failure of sulfadoxine–pyrimethamine, the antifolate combination of most public health significance today.

The role of mutations in dihydropteroate synthase for in vivo sulfadoxine–pyrimethamine resistance has been debated in the literature *(59)*. A set of experiments controlling concentrations of sulfadoxine, pyrimethamine, folate, and *p*ABA and using several *P. falciparum* isolates with known dihydrofolate reductase and dihydropteroate synthase genotypes has helped to illuminate this topic *(9)*. Taking into account host differences in elimination times for the two drugs, these experiments support a scenario in which parasites with fewer than the three common dihydrofolate reductase mutations Asn-108, Ile-51, and Arg-59, would be likely to be cleared by sulfadoxine–pyrimethamine irrespective of dihydropteroate synthase genotype. In the presence of the dihydrofolate reductase triple-mutant form, the treatment outcome would depend on

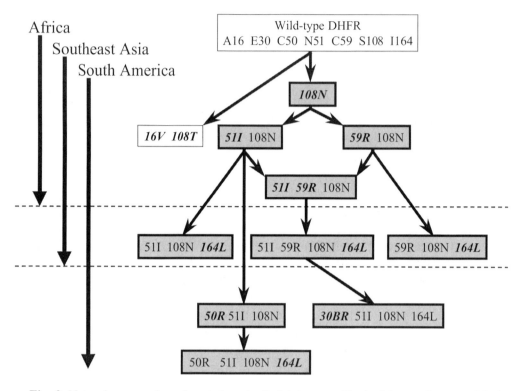

Fig. 3. Natural progression of mutations in *P. falciparum* dihydrofolate reductase with the predominant geographical distribution of mutant genotypes. Single-letter amino acid abbreviations are used throughout, with the exception of "BR" for the Bolivia repeat, a five-amino-acid repetitive insert between codons 30 and 31. Wild type is indicated by an amino acid to the left of the codon number and a mutation by an amino acid to the right of the codon number (e.g., wild-type S108 and mutant 108N). New mutations arising in successive genotypes are indicated by bold italics. Gray boxes indicate the mutations that arise most commonly under drug pressure in vivo.

the dihydropteroate synthase genotype as well as on other factors such as host plasma folate levels and immunity. This model is most consistent with the clinical and epidemiological studies that show an association between the prevalence of mutations in both enzymes with sulfadoxine–pyrimethamine failure rates, and selection for mutations in both enzymes under direct pressure from sulfadoxine–pyrimethamine treatment *(29,42,43,60)*.

Figures 3 and 4 illustrate the order of accumulation of mutations in dihydrofolate reductase and dihydropteroate synthase, respectively, under drug pressure and the predominant geographic distribution of mutant genotypes. The weight of all of the available data from in vitro and epidemiological studies supports the view that in South America, where immunity levels are lower, clinical failure of sulfadoxine–pyrimethamine can be attributed to a genotype comprised of the dihydrofolate reductase mutations Asn-108, with or without Ile-51, accompanied by either Arg-50 or Arg 59, and including Leu-164; and the dihydropteroate synthase mutations Gly-437, Glu-540 and Gly-581. Whether this constellation of mutations results in RI-, RII-, or RIII-level resistance appears to depend on factors other than dihydrofolate reductase and dihydropteroate synthase genotype *(43)*. A "quin-

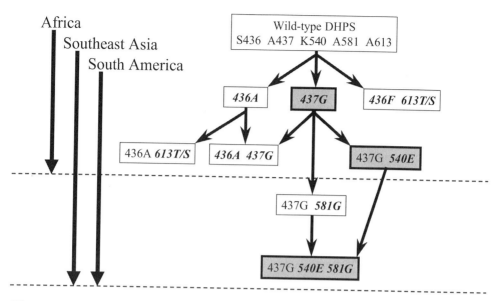

Fig. 4. Natural progression of mutations in *P. falciparum* dihydropteroate synthase with the predominant geographical distribution of mutant genotypes. Single-letter amino acid abbreviations are used throughout. Wild type is indicated by an amino acid to the left of the codon number and a mutation by an amino acid to the right of the codon number (e.g., wild-type A437 and mutant 437G). New mutations arising in successive genotypes are indicated by bold italics. Gray boxes indicate the mutations that arise most commonly under drug pressure in vivo.

tuple mutant" with the dihydrofolate reductase mutations Asn-108, Ile-51, and Arg-59 and dihydropteroate synthase mutations Gly-437 and Glu-540 is probably responsible for the relatively low-level in vivo resistance to sulfadoxine pyrimethamine that is increasingly common in east and central Africa. It is important to note that in Africa, the prevalence of these resistant genotypes exceeds the prevalence of in vivo resistance, indicating that other factors permit many individuals to clear these relatively resistant genotypes, as discussed in the following section.

The dihydrofolate reductase Leu-164 mutation is absent in Africa at the present time, and the dihydropteroate synthase Gly-581 mutation is very rare there, despite several years of widespread pyrimethamine-sulfadoxine use in eastern and southern African countries. Should these two mutations arise and be maintained in the parasite population, high-level resistance to sulfadoxine–pyrimethamine can be expected. The higher level of immunity in most of Africa results in a high proportion of chronic and asymptomatic and, therefore, untreated infections. If the two mutations associated with the highest levels of resistance are sufficiently deleterious to enzyme function, they will be selected against in the absence of drug pressure. It is possible that the amount of drug pressure applied to the total parasite population will be insufficient to permit these particular mutations to arise or persist in Africa. If this hypothesis is correct, antifolates may have a longer useful life in Africa than they have elsewhere.

Relatively little is known about the molecular basis of in vivo resistance to antifolate combinations other than sulfadoxine–pyrimethamine. Both in vitro and clinical studies indicate that chlorproguanil–dapsone is active against the genotypes of sulfadoxine–

pyrimethamine-resistant *P. falciparum* found in Africa *(34,61)*. (W Watkins, personal communication), probably because of chlorcycloguanil's relative ability to inhibit parasites with the pyrimethamine-resistant Asn-108/Ile-51/Arg-59 dihydrofolate reductase genotype common in Africa.

Trimethoprim–sulfamethoxazole, used primarily as an antibacterial agent, has been recommended as empiric treatment for febrile illness in children in areas where malaria is endemic *(62–64)*, and daily prophylaxis with this combination was recently found to reduce morbidity and mortality among HIV-infected persons in an African city *(65,66)*. Pyrimethamine is generally more active against malaria than trimethoprim is, and in vitro studies have found cross-resistance between pyrimethamine, trimethoprim, and related compounds *(67,68)* although cross-resistance between trimethoprim and pyrimethamine may not be complete *(69)*. These earlier studies did not include analysis of the dihydrofolate reductase genotypes of the parasite lines tested, but analysis of dihydrofolate reductase genotypes in yeast suggest that trimethoprim resistance and pyrimethamine resistance are caused by the same sets of mutations (unpublished data). Sulfadoxine and sulfamethoxazole inhibit several dihydropteroate synthase genotypes equally with a K_i correlation coefficient of 1.0, indicating complete cross-resistance between these two drugs *(50)*.

One report found that trimethoprim–sulfamethoxazole had a poor efficacy as a treatment for malaria in Uganda and was selected for an unusual dihydrofolate reductase genotype consisting of wild-type Ser-108 with mutant Ile-51 and Arg-59 *(70)*. However, this genotype has not been found in several large surveys, including in adjacent African countries and areas where trimethoprim–sulfamethoxazole is widely used for bacterial infections *(29,40,42)*, nor has the existence of the Ser-108/Ile-51/ Arg-59 genotype been demonstrated by DNA sequencing. Before instituting policies of widespread trimethoprim–sulfamethoxazole prophylaxis in areas where HIV infection and malaria are both highly prevalent, it will be important to have a clear understanding of the molecular mechanisms of resistance to trimethoprim–sulfamethoxazole in *P. falciparum* and to assess the potential for daily prophylaxis with this combination to select for parasites highly resistant to sulfadoxine–pyrimethamine and other antifolate combinations. On the population level, widespread trimethoprim–sulfamethoxazole prophylaxis could shorten the useful life-span of sulfadoxine–pyrimethamine in areas where it is already in use and introduce antifolate resistance in areas where they are currently being held in reserve. On the individual level, HIV-infected persons receiving daily trimethoprim–sulfamethoxazole prophylaxis who are or become infected with *P. falciparum* may be more likely to fail sulfadoxine–pyrimethamine treatment, with an increased risk of progression to severe disease and death.

OTHER FACTORS CONTRIBUTING TO IN VIVO ANTIFOLATE RESISTANCE

Factors other than decreased affinity of drugs for target enzymes are certain to contribute to the in vivo response to sulfadoxine–pyrimethamine and the other antifolate combinations. As described earlier, folate and *p*ABA antagonize the antifolate drugs in *P. falciparum* cultures *(58)*, and some parasites can use exogenous folate to antagonize the sulfa drugs *(7–9)*. The effects of folate and *p*ABA levels in host serum on the in vivo response to sulfadoxine–pyrimethamine are relatively unstudied, but a higher rate of sulfadoxine–pyrimethamine treatment failures among persons receiving folic acid supplements has been reported *(71)*. Plasma folate determinations in studies of the molecular basis of antifolate resistance in vivo may clarify the role of host folate levels in therapeutic efficacy of the antifolates.

Partial immunity to malaria certainly must contribute to the therapeutic efficacy of all antimalarial drugs, including the antifolates. In areas where malaria is highly endemic, as in much of sub-Saharan Africa, individuals gradually develop partial immunity to malaria disease, although they continue to become infected by the parasite *(72)*. Semi-immune older children or adults can clear low-level resistant infections that immunologically naive infants or young children cannot clear. One small study has shown a strong association between longer histories of exposure to malaria and increased efficacy of sulfadoxine–pyrimethamine *(73)*. Mutations in target enzymes that determine intrinsic resistance will be more tightly correlated with clinical antifolate failure in settings where there is less immunity, such as Southeast Asia and South America, than in Africa *(43,74)*.

Finally, host differences in the ability to absorb or metabolize drugs may contribute to therapeutic efficacy of antifolates. For example, differences in the ability to metabolize the antifolate drug proguanil into its active form, cycloguanil, contribute to the prophylactic efficacy of proguanil *(75)*, and individual differences in the pharmacokinetics of sulfonamides have been suggested to account for some cases sulfadoxine–pyrimethamine failure *(76)*.

SUMMARY AND CONCLUSIONS

The antifolate antimalarial drugs are the only line of defense against chloroquine-resistant malaria in most of the malaria endemic world. Sulfadoxine–pyrimethamine is still used as the first- or second-line drug in much of South America and nearly all of sub-Saharan Africa, where the cost of newer antimalarial drugs precludes their widespread use. Several African countries now rely on sulfadoxine–pyrimethamine as the first-line drug, and when it fails, as it will, there are no affordable alternatives ready to replace it. Several new antifolate drugs and drug combinations are now in development, including atovaquone–proguanil (Malarone®) *(77)*, chlorproguanil (Lapudrine®)–dapsone (LapDap) *(78)*, and PS-15–sulfa combinations *(79)*. Chlorproguanil–dapsone appears to be active against the forms of sulfadoxine–pyrimethamine-resistant *P. falciparum* found in East Africa and is in the late stages of development as an inexpensive alternative to sulfadoxine–pyrimethamine. This antifolate combination also has a short elimination time, which may result in slower selection of resistant genotypes *(80)*. Perhaps even more promising in the long run is the dihydrofolate reductase inhibitor PS-15, the active metabolite of which, WR99210, is effective against even the most highly resistant forms of *P. falciparum (34,79)*. Thus, even if sulfadoxine–pyrimethemine is eventually abandoned because of resistance, understanding the mechanisms of resistance to the antifolate class of antimalarial drugs will be important for developing strategies for deterring the development and slowing the spread of resistance. Continued surveillance for new mutations and assessment of their roles in conferring resistance will be important both for validating molecular methods for surveillance of resistance and for the development of new antifolate drugs and drug combinations designed to overcome antifolate resistance. Close cooperation between field and laboratory researchers will be key to success in these endeavors.

New and not yet fully understood mechanisms of action and resistance have recently been discovered for the antifolate antimalarial drugs *(9,44,46)*, as have new biochemical pathways that provide folate precursors *(2)*. With the malaria genome project well underway *(81)* and renewed efforts to develop new antimalarial drugs in progress *(82,83)*, we can expect that mechanisms of action and mechanisms of resistance of the antifolate antimalarial drugs will continue to be a rapidly evolving field with direct relevance to global public health.

REFERENCES

1. Peters W. Chemotherapy and Drug Resistance in Malaria. New York, Academic, London, 1987.
2. Roberts F, Roberts CW, Johnson JJ, Kyle DE, Krell T, Coggins JR, et al. Evidence for the shikimate pathway in apicomplexan parasites. Nature 1998;393:801–805.
3. Coggeshall LT. The selective action of sulfanilamide on the parasites of experimental malaria in monkeys in vivo and in vitro. J Exp Med 1940;71:13–20.
4. Walker HA, van Dyke HB. Control of malaria infection (*P. lophurae*) in ducks by sulfonamides. Proc Soc Exp Biol Med 1941;48:368–372.
5. Maier J, Riley E. Inhibition of antimalarial action of sulfonamides by p-aminobenzoic acid. Proc Soc Exp Biol Med 1942;50:152–154.
6. Ferone, R. Folate metabolism in malaria. [review]. Bull WHO 1977;55:291–298.
7. Krungkrai J, Webster HK, Yuthavong Y. De novo and salvage biosynthesis of pteroylpentaglutamates in the human malaria parasite, *Plasmodium falciparum*. Mol Biochem Parasitol 1989;32:25–37.
8. Wang P, Read M, Sims PF, Hyde JE. Sulfadoxine resistance in the human malaria parasite *Plasmodium falciparum* is determined by mutations in dihydropteroate synthetase and an additional factor associated with folate utilization. Mol Microbiol 1997;23:979–986.
9. Wang P, Brobey RK, Horii T, Sims PF, Hyde JE. Utilization of exogenous folate in the human malaria parasite *Plasmodium falciparum* and its critical role in antifolate drug synergy. Mol Microbiol 1999;32:1254–1262.
10. Triglia T, Cowman AF. The mechanism of resistance to sulfa drugs in *Plasmodium falciparum*. Drug Resist 1999;2:15–19.
11. Cowman AF. The molecular basis of resistance to the sulfones, sulfonamides, and dihydrofolate reductase inhibitors. In Sherman IW (ed). Malaria: Parasite Biology, Pathogenesis and Protection Washington, DC: ASM, 1998, pp. 317–330.
12. Ginsburg, H. Malaria parasite metabolic pathways: folate biosynthetic pathway. http://sites.huji.ac.il/malaria/maps/folatebiopath.html.
13. Bzik DJ, Li WB, Horii T, Inselburg J. Molecular cloning and sequence analysis of the *Plasmodium falciparum* dihydrofolate reductase–thymidylate synthase gene. Proc Natl Acad Sci USA 1987;84:8360–8364.
14. Triglia T, Cowman AF. Primary structure and expression of the dihydropteroate synthetase gene of *Plasmodium falciparum*. Proc Natl Acad Sci USA 1994;91:7149–7153.
15. Brooks DR, Wang P, Read M, Watkins WM, Sims PF, Hyde JE. Sequence variation of the hydroxymethyldihydropterin pyrophosphokinase: dihydropteroate synthase gene in lines of the human malaria parasite, *Plasmodium falciparum*, with differing resistance to sulfadoxine. Eur J Biochem 1994;224:397–405.
16. Ferone R, Burchall JJ, Hitchings GH. *Plasmodium berghei* dihydrofolate reductase. Isolation, properties, and inhibition by antifolates. Mol Pharmacol 1969;5:49–59.
17. Ferone, R. Dihydrofolate reductase from pyrimethamine-resistant *Plasmodium berghei*. J Biol Chem 1970;245:850–854.
18. McCutchan TF, Welsh JA, Dame JB, Quakyi IA, Graves PM, Drake JC, et al. Mechanism of pyrimethamine resistance in recent isolates of *Plasmodium falciparum*. Antimicrob Agents Chemother 1984;26:656–659.

19. Clyde DF, Shute GT. Resistance of *Plasmodium falciparum* in Tanganyika to pyrimethamine administered at weekly intervals. Trans R Soc Trop Med Hyg 1957;51:505–513.
20. Bishop, A. An analysis of the development of resistance to proguanil and pyrimethamine in *Plasmodium* gallinaceum. Parasitology 1962;52:495–518.
21. Diggens SM, Gutteridge WE, Trigg PI. Altered dihydrofolate reductase associated with a pyrimethamine-resistant *Plasmodium berghei* produced in a single step. Nature 1970;228:579–580.
22. Peterson DS, Walliker D, Wellems TE. Evidence that a point mutation in dihydrofolate reductase–thymidylate synthase confers resistance to pyrimethamine in falciparum malaria. Proc Natl Acad Sci USA 1988;85:9114–9118.
23. Cowman AF, Morry MJ, Biggs BA, Cross GA, Foote SJ. Amino acid changes linked to pyrimethamine resistance in the dihydrofolate reductase–thymidylate synthase gene of *Plasmodium falciparum*. Proc Natl Acad Sci USA 1988;85:9109–9113.
24. Peterson DS, Milhous WK, Wellems TE. Molecular basis of differential resistance to cycloguanil and pyrimethamine in *Plasmodium falciparum* malaria. Proc Natl Acad Sci USA 1990;87:3018–3022.
25. Foote SJ, Galatis D, Cowman AF. Amino acids in the dihydrofolate reductase–thymidylate synthase gene of *Plasmodium falciparum* involved in cycloguanil resistance differ from those involved in pyrimethamine resistance. Proc Natl Acad Sci USA 1990;87:3014–3017.
26. Chen GX, Zolg JW. Purification of the bifunctional thymidylate synthase–dihydrofolate reductase complex from the human malaria parasite *Plasmodium falciparum*. Mol Pharmacol 1987;32:723–730.
27. Snewin VA, England SM, Sims PF, Hyde JE. Characterisation of the dihydrofolate reductase–thymidylate synthetase gene from human malaria parasites highly resistant to pyrimethamine. Gene 1989;76:41–52.
28. Reynolds MG, Roos DS. A biochemical and genetic model for parasite resistance to antifolates. *Toxoplasma gondii* provides insights into pyrimethamine and cycloguanil resistance in *Plasmodium falciparum*. J Biol Chem 1998;273:3461–3469.
29. Plowe CV, Cortese JF, Djimde A, Nwanyanwu OC, Watkins WM, Winstanley PA, et al. Mutations in *Plasmodium falciparum* dihydrofolate reductase and dihydropteroate synthase and epidemiologic patterns of pyrimethamine–sulfadoxine use and resistance. J Infect Dis 1997;176:1590–1596.
30. Warhurst DC. Antimalarial drug discovery: development of inhibitors of dihydrofolate reductase active in drug resistance. Drug Discovery Today 1998;3:538–546.
31. Wu Y, Sifri CD, Lei HH, Su XZ, Wellems TE. Transfection of *Plasmodium falciparum* within human red blood cells. Proc Natl Acad Sci USA 1995;92:973–977.
32. Wu Y, Kirkman LA, Wellems TE. Transformation of *Plasmodium falciparum* malaria parasites by homologous integration of plasmids that confer resistance to pyrimethamine. Proc Natl Acad Sci USA 1996;93:1130–1134.
33. Wooden JM, Hartwell LH, Vasquez B, Sibley CH. Analysis in yeast of antimalaria drugs that target the dihydrofolate reductase of *Plasmodium falciparum*. Mol Biochem Parasitol 1997;85:25–40.
34. Cortese JF, Plowe CV. Antifolate resistance due to new and known *Plasmodium falciparum* dihydrofolate reductase mutants expressed in yeast. Mol Biochem Parasitol 1998;94:205–214.
35. Zolg JW, Plitt JR, Chen GX, Palmer S. Point mutations in the dihydrofolate reductase-thymidylate synthase gene as the molecular basis for pyrimethamine resistance in *Plasmodium falciparum*. Mol Biochem Parasitol 1989;36:253–262.
36. Eldin de Pecoulas P, Tahar R, Ouatas T, Mazabraud A, Basco LK. Sequence variations in the *Plasmodium vivax* dihydrofolate reductase–thymidylate synthase gene and their relationship with pyrimethamine resistance. Mol Biochem Parasitol 1998;92:265–273.
37. Sano G, Morimatsu K, Horii T. Purification and characterization of dihydrofolate reductase of *Plasmodium falciparum* expressed by a synthetic gene in Escherichia coli. Mol Biochem Parasitol 1994;63:265–273.

38. Sirawaraporn W, Sathitkul T, Sirawaraporn R, Yuthavong Y, Santi DV. Antifolate-resistant mutants of *Plasmodium falciparum* dihydrofolate reductase. Proc Natl Acad Sci USA 1997;94:1124–1129.

39. Basco LK, Eldin de Pecoulas P, Wilson CM, Le Bras J, Mazabraud A. Point mutations in the dihydrofolate reductase–thymidylate synthase gene and pyrimethamine and cycloguanil resistance in *Plasmodium falciparum*. Mol Biochem Parasitol 1995;69:135–138.

40. Reeder JC, Rieckmann KH, Genton B, Lorry K, Wines B, Cowman AF. Point mutations in the dihydrofolate reductase and dihydropteroate synthatase genes and *in vitro* susceptibility to pyrimethamine and cycloguanil of *Plasmodium falciparum* isolates from Papua New Guinea. Am J Trop Med Hyg 1996;55:209–213.

41. Zindrou S, Dung NP, Sy ND, Skold O, Swedberg G. *Plasmodium falciparum*: mutation pattern in the dihydrofolate reductase-thymidylate synthase genes of Vietnamese isolates, a novel mutation, and coexistence of two clones in a Thai patient. Exp Parasitol 1996;84:56–64.

42. Wang P, Lee CS, Bayoumi R, Djimde A, Doumbo O, Swedberg G, et al. Resistance to antifolates in *Plasmodium falciparum* monitored by sequence analysis of dihydropteroate synthetase and dihydrofolate reductase alleles in a large number of field samples of diverse origins. Mol Biochem Parasitol 1997;89:161–177.

43. Kublin JG, Witzig RS, Shankar AH, Zurita JQ, Gilman RH, Guarda JA, et al. Molecular assays for surveillance of antifolate-resistant malaria. Lancet 1998;351:1629–1630.

44. Fidock DA, Wellems TE. Transformation with human dihydrofolate reductase renders malaria parasites insensitive to WR99210 but does not affect the intrinsic activity of proguanil. Proc Natl Acad Sci USA 1997;94:10,931–10,936.

45. de Alencar FE, Cerutti C, Jr., Durlacher RR, Boulos M, Alves FP, Milhous W, et al. Atovaquone and proguanil for the treatment of malaria in Brazil. J Infect Dis 1997;175:1544–1547.

46. Srivastava IK, Vaidya AB. A mechanism for the synergistic antimalarial action of atovaquone and proguanil. Antimicrob Agents Chemother 1999;43:1334–1339.

47. Thurston JP. The chemotherapy of *Plasmodium berghei*. II. Antagonism of the action of drugs. Parasitol 1954;44:90–110.

48. Watkins WM, Sixsmith DG, Chulay JD, Spencer HC. Antagonism of sulfadoxine and pyrimethamine antimalarial activity in vitro by p-aminobenzoic acid, p-aminobenzoylglutamic acid and folic acid. Mol Biochem Parasitol 1985;14:55–61.

49. Triglia T, Wang P, Sims PG, Hyde JE, Cowman AF. Allelic exchange at the endogenous genomic locus in *Plasmodium falciparum* proves the role of dihyropteroate synthase in sulfadoxine-resistant malaria. EMBO J 1998;17:3807–3815.

50. Triglia T, Menting JGT, Wilson C, Cowman AF. Mutations in dihydropteroate synthase are responsible for sulfone and sulfonamide resistance in *Plasmodium falciparum*. Proc Natl Acad Sci USA 1997;94:13944–13949.

51. Diourte Y, Djimde A, Doumbo OK, Sagara I, Coulibaly A, Dicko A, et al. Pyrimethamine–sulfadoxine efficacy and selection for mutations in *Plasmodium falciparum* dihydrofolate reductase and dihydropteroate synthase in Mali. Am J Trop Med Hyg 1999;60:475–478.

52. Nguyen-Dinh P, Spencer HC, Chemangey-Masaba S, Churchill FC. Susceptibility of *Plasmodium falciparum* to pyrimethamine and sulfadoxine/pyrimethamine in Kisumu, Kenya. Lancet 1982;1:823–825.

53. Schapira A, Bygbjerg IC, Jepsen S, Flachs H, Bentzon MW. The susceptibility of *Plasmodium falciparum* to sulfadoxine and pyrimethamine: correlation of in vivo and in vitro results. Am J Trop Med Hyg 1986;35:239–245.

54. Watkins WM, Mberu EK, Winstanley PA, Plowe CV. The efficacy of antifolate antimalarial combinations in Africa: a predictive model based on pharmadocynamic and pharmacokinetic analyses. [review]. Parasitol Today 1997;13:459–464.

55. Watkins WM, Mberu EK, Winstanley PA, Plowe CV. More on "the efficacy of antifolate antimalarial combinations in Africa." Parasitol Today 1999;15:131–132.

56. Sims P, Wang P, Hyde JE. Selection and synergy in *Plasmodium falciparum*. Parasitol Today 1999;15:132–134.

57. Rollo IM. The mode of action of sulphonamides, proguanil and pryimethamine on *Plasmodium gallinaceum*. Br J Pharmacol 1955;10:208–214.

58. Chulay JD, Watkins WM, Sixsmith DG. Synergistic antimalarial activity of pyrimethamine and sulfadoxine against *Plasmodium falciparum* in vitro. Am J Trop Med Hyg 1984;33:325–330.

59. Sims P, Wang P, Hyde JE. On "The efficacy of antifolate antimalarial combinations in Africa." Parasitol Today 1998;14:136–137.

60. Curtis J, Duraisingh MT, Warhurst DC. *In vivo* selection for a specific genotype of dihydropteroate synthetase of *Plasmodium falciparum* by pyrimethamine–sulfadoxine but not chlorproguanil–dapsone treatment. J Infect Dis 1998;177:1429–1433.

61. Nzila-Mounda A, Mberu EK, Sibley CH, Plowe CV, Winstanley PA, Watkins WM. Kenyan *Plasmodium falciparum* field isolates: correlation between pyrimethamine and chlorcycloguanil activity in vitro and point mutations in the dihydrofolate reductase domain. Antimicrob Agents Chemother 1998;42:164–169.

62. Bloland PB, Redd SC, Kazembe P, Tembenu R, Wirima JJ, Campbell CC. Co-trimoxazole for childhood febrile illness in malaria-endemic regions. Lancet 1991;337:518–520.

63. Ronn AM, Msangeni HA, Mhina J, Wernsdorfer WH, Bygbjerg IC. High level of resistance of *Plasmodium falciparum* to sulfadoxine- pyrimethamine in children in Tanzania. Trans R Soc Trop Med Hyg 1996;90:179–181.

64. Sheng WD, Jiddawi MS, Hong XQ, Abdulla SM. Treatment of chloroquine-resistant malaria using pyrimethamine in combination with berberine, tetracycline or cotrimoxazole. East Afr Med J 1997;74:283–284.

65. Anglaret X, Chene G, Attia A, Toure S, Lafont S, Combe P, et al. Early chemoprophylaxis with trimethoprim–sulphamethoxazole for HIV-1- infected adults in Abidjan, Cote d'Ivoire: a randomised trial. Lancet 1999;353:1463–1468.

66. Wiktor SZ, Sassan-Morokro M, Grant AD, Abouya L, Karon JM, Maurice C, et al. Efficacy of trimethoprim–sulphamethoxazole prophylaxis to decrease morbidity and mortality in HIV-1-infected patients with tuberculosis in Abidjan, Cote d'Ivoire: a randomised controlled trial. Lancet 1999;353:1469–1475.

67. Basco LK, Le Bras J. In vitro sensitivity of *Plasmodium falciparum* to anti-folinic agents (trimethoprim, pyrimethamine, cycloguanil): a study of 29 African strains. Bull Soc Pathol Exot 1997;90:90–93.

68. Walter RD, Bergmann B, Kansy M, Wiese M, Seydel JK. Pyrimethamin-resistant *Plasmodium falciparum* lack cross-resistance to methotrexate and 2,4-diamino-5-(substituted benzyl) pyrimidines. Parasitol Res 1991;77:346–350.

69. Petersen, E. In vitro susceptibility of *Plasmodium falciparum* malaria to pyrimethamine, sulfadoxine, trimethoprim and sulfamethoxazole, singly and in combination. Trans R Soc Trop Med Hyg 1987;81:238–241.

70. Jelinek T, Kilian AH, Curtis J, Duraisingh MT, Kabagambe G, von Sonnenburg F, et al. *Plasmodium falciparum*: selection of serine 108 of dihydrofolate reductase during treatment of uncomplicated malaria with co-trimoxazole in Ugandan children. Am J Trop Med Hyg 1999;61:125–130.

71. van Hensbroek MB, Morris-Jones S, Meisner S, Jaffar S, Bayo L, Dackour R, et al. Iron, but not folic acid, combined with effective antimalarial therapy promotes haematological recovery in African children after acute falciparum malaria. Trans R Soc Trop Med Hyg 1995;89:672–676.

72. Marsh, K. Malaria—a neglected disease? [review]. Parasitology 1992;104(Suppl):S53–S69.

73. Baird JK, Basri H, Jones TR, Purnomo, Bangs MJ, Ritonga A. Resistance to antimalarials by *Plasmodium falciparum* in Arso PIR, Irian Jaya, Indonesia. Am J Trop Med Hyg 1991;44:640–644.

74. Plowe CV, Kublin JG, Doumbo OK. P-falciparum dihydrofolate reductase and dihydro-pteroate synthase mutations: epidemiology and role in clinical resistance to antifolates. [review]. Drug Resist 1998;1:389–396.

75. Watkins WM, Mberu EK, Nevill CG, Ward SA, Breckenridge AM, Koech DK. Variability in the metabolism of proguanil to the active metabolite cycloguanil in healthy Kenyan adults. Trans R Soc Trop Med Hyg 1990;84:492–495.

76. Anonymous. Advances in Malaria Chemotherapy. World Health Organization Technical Report Series No. 711. Geneva, World Health Organization, 1984, p. 29

77. Radloff PD, Philipps J, Nkeyi M, Hutchinson D, Kremsner PG. Atovaquone and proguanil for *Plasmodium falciparum* malaria. Lancet 1996;347:1511–1514.

78. Amukoye E, Winstanley PA, Watkins WM, Snow RW, Hatcher J, Mosobo M, et al. Chlorproguanil–dapsone: an effective treatment for uncomplicated falciparum malaria. Antimicrob Agents Chemother 1997;41:2261–2264.

79. Rieckmann KH, Yeo AE, Edstein MD. Activity of PS-15 and its metabolite, WR99210, against *Plasmodium falciparum* in an in vivo–in vitro model. Trans R Soc Trop Med Hyg 1996;90:568–571.

80. Watkins WM, Mosobo M. Treatment of *Plasmodium falciparum* malaria with pyrimetha-mine–sulfadoxine: selective pressure for resistance is a function of long elimination half-life. Trans R Soc Trop Med Hyg 1993;87:75–78.

81. Bowman S, Lawson D, Basham D, Brown D, Chillingworth T, Churcher CM, et al. The complete nucleotide sequence of chromosome 3 of *Plasmodium falciparum*. Nature 1999;400:532–538.

82. Kaiser, J. Raising the stakes in the race for new malaria drugs. [news]. Science 1998;281:1930.

83. Butler, D. Malaria research deal seeks to make up for industry's retreat. [news]. Nature 1998;395:417–418

10

Artemisinin and Its Derivatives

Steven R. Meshnick

INTRODUCTION

Artemisinin and its derivatives are endoperoxide-containing natural products that are being used widely as antimalarials in many parts of the world. The most commonly used artemisinin derivatives are artesunate, artemether, arteether, and dihydro-artemisinin (Fig. 1). Artelinic acid (Fig. 1) *(1)* is currently in preclinical development. A variety of newer artemisinin derivatives have been synthesized and tested; these are reviewed in Chapter 16. This chapter will review recent progress in understanding the pharmacology and mechanisms of action of the artemisinin derivatives that are currently in clinical use. The reader is referred to an excellent recent supplement to *Medicine Tropicale* (Vol. 58, Supplement 3, 1998) for a collection of detailed review articles on all aspects of these drugs.

Artemisia annua—sweet wormwood or qinghao—has been used by Chinese herbal medicine practitioners for about 2000 yr to treat hemorrhoids and fever. Patients were told to "take a handful of sweet wormwood, soak it in a sheng (approx 1 L) of water, squeeze out the juice and drink it all" *(2)*. The active ingredient of this herb—artemisinin (qinghaosu)—was discovered in 1972 by a group of Chinese scientists *(3)*. A series of articles published in 1982 presented a large body of in vitro, animal, and clinical data on artemisinin as well as artemether and artesunate *(4–9)*.

Artemisinin derivatives were used widely in China by the 1980s. Western interest in these agents began to grow as multidrug-resistant *Plasmodium falciparum* strains began to spread, especially in Southeast Asia. By the early 1990s, artemisinin derivatives were being widely used in Thailand, Burma, and Vietnam. Several artemisinin derivatives are now being developed and/or marketed by Western pharmaceutical companies, including Rhone-Poulenc (artemether) *(10)*, Novartis (artemether plus benflumetol) *(11)*, and Sanofi Winthrop (artesunate) *(12)*. The results of all clinical studies using artemisinin derivatives to treat both complicated and uncomplicated malaria have been compiled into two reviews in the Cochrane Library *(13,14)*

MECHANISM OF ACTION OF ARTEMISININ

The mechanism of action of artemisinin has recently been reviewed *(15–18)*. There is a general consensus that the killing action of artemisinin involves an iron-catalyzed

From: *Antimalarial Chemotherapy: Mechanisms of Action, Resistance, and New Directions in Drug Discovery*
Edited by: P. J. Rosenthal © Humana Press Inc., Totowa, NJ

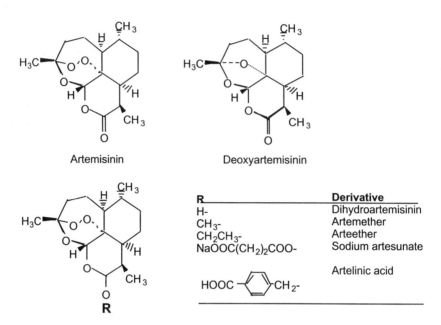

Fig. 1. Structures of artemisinin and derivatives.

decomposition of artemisinin into free radicals (Fig. 2). There are a number of pieces of evidence for this:

1. The endoperoxide bridge is essential for antimalarial activity (19). Derivatives with a single oxygen instead of two, such as deoxartemisinin (Fig. 1), are inactive. Endoperoxides are known to be unstable, especially in the presence of iron, and to breakdown to form free radicals.
2. The malaria parasite is rich in heme-iron, derived from breaking down host cell hemoglobin (20). This could explain why artemisinin is selectively toxic to parasites.
3. Free-radical scavengers inhibit artemisinin's antimalarial activity, whereas other free radical generators promote it (21–23).
4. Artemisinin treatment of membranes and infected and uninfected erythrocytes generates typical free-radical-damage end products such as thiobarbituric-reacting substances and oxidized thiols (21–28).
5. Iron catalysis of the irreversible decomposition of artemisinin has been demonstrated by cyclic voltammetry (29), and iron-catalyzed artemisinin-derived free radicals have been detected by electron paramagnetic resonance spectroscopy (25,30).
6. Iron chelators antagonize the antimalarial and acute toxic effects of the drug (25).
7. Structure–activity relationship studies showed a high correlation between antimalarial activities and heme binding (31), and that the predicted pharmacophore (drug receptor) resembles heme (32).
8. Artemisinin and its derivatives are inactive against the RC strain of *Plasmodium berghei* (33) and the related intraerthrocytic apicomplexan parasite, Babesia microti (34), which lack hemozoin.

Recently, an alternate mechanism for activation of artemisinin was proposed which is not free radical dependent (35).

Artemisinin does not act like a typical oxidant drug (29). First, unlike most other oxidant drugs, artemisinin cannot be cyclically oxidized and reduced. Therefore, only one free radical can result from one drug molecule. Second, all of the oxidant end

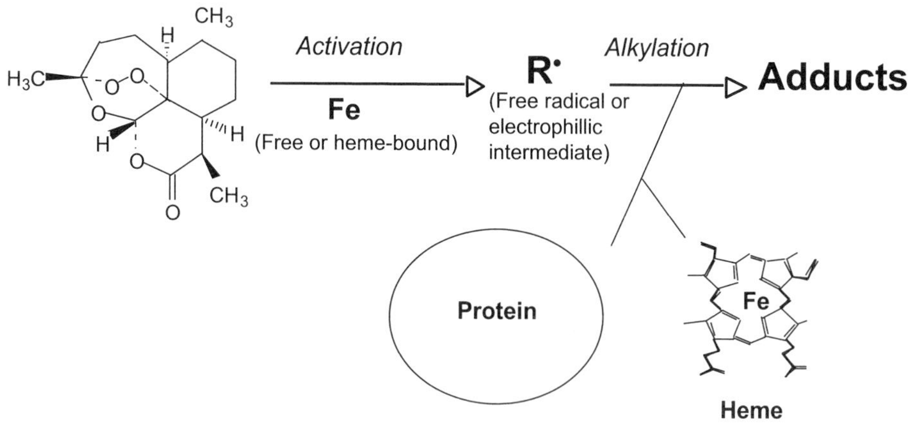

Fig. 2. Postulated mechanism of action of artemisinin.

products observed experimentally, were only observed at very high drug concentrations (>100 μM), but the drug is effective at concentrations at least 1000-fold lower. Accordingly, it was suggested that the artemisinin-derived free radical may damage specific targets, rather than cause promiscuous damage like other oxidant drugs *(36)*.

But what are the specific targets of artemisinin-derived free radicals? One possibility is heme. Artemisinin forms covalent bonds with heme when incubated in a cell-free solution and these same artemisinin–heme adducts appear to form in artemisinin-treated parasites *(37)*. The structure of an artemisinin–porphyrin adduct has recently been elucidated *(38)* as has an artemisinin-induced oxidation product of the porphyrin ring *(39)*.

The modification of heme by artemisinin could kill the parasite in several ways. First, artemisinin or its heme adduct might be able to inhibit hemozoin biosynthesis or cause hemozoin degradation. At high micromolar concentrations, artemisinin inhibits hemoglobin digestion by malaria parasites and inhibits hemozoin formation in cell-free conditions *(40)*. However, artemisinin treatment caused no change in the hemozoin content of *P. falciparum* cultures *(41)*, suggesting that heme metabolism might not be the major intracellular target.

Artemisinin also forms covalent adducts with protein, but not with DNA *(42,43)*. Protein alkylation is heme-dependent, and covalent bonds form with protein preferentially to heme. This was demonstrated by analyzing the reaction products of dihydroartemisinin plus hemoglobin and of dihydroartemisinin plus globin (the protein portion of hemoglobin). Dihydroartemisinin reacted rapidly with hemoglobin but not with globin. When the heme and globin moieties of the modified hemoglobin were separated, 80% of the dihydroartemisinin was attached to the protein (globin) portion and only a small amount was attached to the heme *(43)*. Thus, heme is necessary for the activation of artemisinin into an alkylating agent which preferentially attacks proteins.

Unlike classical oxidant drugs that involve oxygen free radicals, artemisinin's mechanism depends on the formation of carbon-centered free radicals. Posner and colleagues *(44)* first showed that the iron-mediated decomposition of artemisinin in solution involved the formation of a carbon-centered free radical that was necessary for antimalarial activity; this was later confirmed by other laboratories *(45–47)*. Robert and Meunier *(38)* showed that the alkylation of porphyrins was also depended on the formation of a carbon-centered free radical.

The alkylation of specific malaria proteins by artemisinin has been demonstrated *(48)*. When *P. falciparum*-infected erythrocytes were incubated with radiolabeled artemisinin derivatives, six specific malaria proteins were labeled. These are not highly abundant proteins, suggesting that they react selectively with the drug. Protein alkylation could mediate the killing action of artemisinin derivatives because it occurred at therapeutic concentrations of drug and because the same proteins were alkylated by three different active derivatives. Furthermore, no proteins were alkylated in uninfected red cells or in infected red cells exposed to a 20-fold excess of radiolabeled inactive deoxyarteether.

One of the major alkylation targets is the malarial translationally controlled tumor protein (TCTP) *(49)*, a protein whose function is unknown. Recently, recombinant TCTP has been found to bind heme *(49)*. Also, immunofluorescence and immunoelectron microscopy studies show that some of the malarial TCTP is present in the food vacuole membranes, where it is in proximity to the heme-rich food vacuole *(50)*. Thus, it is likely that the reaction between artemisinin and TCTP occurs because of an association between TCTP and heme. However, the reaction between artemisinin and TCTP or other malaria proteins may be adventitious and not mediate the killing action of the drug.

Another reason for the selective toxicity of artemisinin derivatives to malaria parasites is that the parasites accumulate far more drug than host cells *(25,51,52)*. Artemisinin appears to get into the malaria parasite through a tubovesicular network that connects the membrane surrounding the parasite to the periphery of the red cell *(53)*.

TOXICITY

Adverse effects are rare in patients treated with artemisinin derivatives. In a prospective study of over 3500 patients in Thailand, there was no evidence for serious adverse effects *(54)*. Artemisinin derivatives also appear to be safe for pregnant women *(55)*.

In several animal studies however, artemisinin derivatives have been clearly shown to cause neurotoxicity at high doses (reviewed in ref. *56*; *see also* ref. *57*). There have been two case reports of patients suffering neurological problems after receiving artemisinin treatments *(58,59)*. However, the neurological problems in these two isolated cases may have been unrelated to their treatment. In light of the very large number of patients treated safely with artemisinin, neurotoxic adverse effects, if they occur, are quite rare *(60)*.

In vitro, artemisinin is toxic to neuronal cells by a mechanism that may be similar to its antimalarial mechanism. Heme potentiates the toxicity of artemisinin derivatives to neuronal cells in vitro *(61)*. There is also evidence that the drug binds to protein in these cells *(62,63)*.

DRUG RESISTANCE

There have been no clinical reports of artemisinin resistance. Recently, two *P. falciparum*-infected patients were found to fail supervised artesunate therapy, but parasites from these patients appear to be sensitive to artemisinin in vitro *(64)*. One reason for absence of resistance might be that the drug has a gametocytocidal effect in vivo *(65,66)*. Thus, parasites in patients treated with artemisinin derivatives might be much less likely to infect mosquitoes and be spread to other patients. Second, artemisinin derivatives are now frequently used in combination with other antimalarials such as mefloquine *(67)* or benflumetol (lumefantrine) *(68–70)*. Combination chemotherapy tends to delay the onset of resistance.

Artemisinin-resistant strains of *P. falciparum (71)* and *P. yoelii (72)* have been obtained in the laboratory. Various clinical isolates and lab strains of *P. falciparum* have been found to vary in sensitivities to artemisinin in vitro (reviewed in ref. *73*; *see also* refs. *74* and *75*). There is no evidence that this variation in sensitivity is associated with clinical resistance. Interestingly, strains that are resistant to mefloquine tend to be less sensitive to artemisinin, suggesting some overlap in mechanisms *(73,75)*. This may somehow be related to the observation that these two drugs are synergistic *(76,77)*.

We have recently undertaken studies to determine the mechanism of resistance of the artemisinin-resistant strain of *P. yoelii (78)*. The resistant strain (ART) is fourfold resistant compared to the wild-type (NS) strain and reverts back to sensitive unless it is kept under drug pressure. We investigated whether resistance was the result of diminished drug accumulation or to alteration in the drug target TCTP. ART strains accumulated about half as much drug as the NS strain. In addition, the ART strain expressed 2.5 times as much TCTP as the NS strain. Whereas the increased expression of TCTP lends credence to the possibility that it is involved in the drug's mechanism of action, artemisinin resistance appears to be multifactorial.

PHARMACOLOGY

Artemisinin derivatives are administered by various routes (reviewed in refs. *79* and *80*). Artemisinin, dihydroartemisinin, artesunate, and artemether can be administered orally. Artemether and arteether can be administered intramuscularly in oil. Suppository formulations of artemisinin and artesunate have also been used. For severe malaria intravenous artesunate is used. Artesunate, artemether, and arteether are metabolized in vivo into dihydroartemisinin, which appears to be the main biologically active form of the drugs.

It is technically quite challenging to measure serum levels of artemisinin derivatives. The best method is high-performance liquid-chromatography (HPLC) electrochemical detection *(81)*. A much simpler way to measure serum levels is by bioassay, but this method does not distinguish between active metabolites *(82,83)*. Artemisinin derivatives, in general, have relatively short half-lives ranging from under 1 h to 11 h (reviewed in ref. *84*).

Artemisinin derivatives have shorter parasite clearance times than any other antimalarial (reviewed in refs. *13* and *14*). Artemisinin derivatives are most effective against late ring to early trophozoite stages *(85)*. Because multiple stages may coexist within a single host and because artemisinin derivatives have such short half-lives, short treatment regimens with artemisinin derivatives will not clear all the parasites. This explains why artemisinin monotherapy protocols have high recrudescence rates unless the drug is given for 7 d or more. For this reason, it is currently recommended that artemisinin derivatives be used in conjunction with other antimalarials with longer half-lives such as mefloquine or beflumetol *(86)*. In most of these protocols, artemisinin derivatives are administered in the first day or two and cause a rapid decrease in parasite biomass. Mefloquine or benflumitol are coadministered because they maintain therapeutic blood concentrations for several days and can destroy the few remaining parasites that escaped killing by the artemisinin derivative. A second advantage of combining artemisinin with other antimalarials is that it will delay the appearance of resistance.

CLINICAL STUDIES

Although there have been a number of studies evaluating artemisinin derivatives used alone in the treatment of malaria (reviewed in ref. *15*), monotherapy has been generally associated with unacceptably high recrudescence rates. Thus, a consensus has developed that artemisinin derivatives are most appropriately used in combinations with other drugs.

Artemisinin derivatives are most clearly valuable in the treatment of severe malaria. Their efficacy in severe malaria may be a result of their rapid action; patients treated with these drugs rapidly defervesce, clear parasitemias, and recover from coma *(87,88)*. Intramuscular injections of artemether or artesunate, intravenous injections of artesunate, and artesunate rectal suppositories have all proven to be effective *(14,15)*. In a meta-analysis of studies comparing artemisinin derivatives and quinine, the artemisinin derivatives (especially artesunate) were more effective at preventing mortality *(14)*. Thus, artemisinin derivatives are recommended for the treatment of severe malaria in areas of quinine resistance and may be useful in other areas as well.

The use of artemisinin derivatives in the treatment of uncomplicated malaria is somewhat more controversial. Combinations of artesunate plus mefloquine or artemether plus benflumitol are effective and particularly useful in Southeast Asia, where there is widespread resistance to chloroquine and antifolates, and partial resistance to mefloquine *(69)*. Conversely, other drugs, such as sulfadoxine/pyrimethamine, are still effective in subsaharan Africa. It has been suggested that the introduction of artemisinin derivatives here should be delayed, because there are still questions about toxicity and because the early and unnecessary introduction of artemisinin derivatives in Africa might lead to earlier development of artemisinin resistance *(89)*. However, current evidence suggests that antifolate resistance will soon be a major problem in Africa and that there is a need to develop artemisinin combinations which will be effective in this region *(90)*.

CONCLUSION

Over the past decade, we have learned a great deal about the mechanisms of action of, and resistance to, classical antimalarials such as chloroquine, mefloquine, and Fansidar. Unfortunately, many of these insights have occurred after the drugs have started to lose efficacy because of drug resistance. With the artemisinin derivatives, we have the opportunity to obtain these insights while the drugs are still quite active, and thus, perhaps, use this information to prolong their effective life-spans.

REFERENCES

1. Li QG, Peggins JO, Lin AJ, Masonic KJ, Trotman KM, Brewer TG. Pharmacology and toxicology of artelinic acid: preclinical investigations on pharmacokinetics, metabolism, protein and red blood cell binding, and acute and anorectic toxicities. Trans R Soc Trop Med Hyg 1998;92:332–340.
2. Klayman DL. Qinghaosu (artemisinin): an antimalarial drug from China. Science 1985;228:1049–1055.
3. Lusha, X. A new drug for malaria. China Reconstructs 1979;28:48–49.
4. China Cooperative Research Group. The chemistry and synthesis of qinghaosu derivatives. China Cooperative Research Group on qinghaosu and its derivatives as antimalarials. J Tradit Chin Med 1982;2:9–16.

5. China Cooperative Research Group. Clinical studies on the treatment of malaria with qinghaosu and its derivatives. China Cooperative Research Group on qinghaosu and its derivatives as antimalarials. J Tradit Chin Med 1982;2:45–50.

6. China Cooperative Research Group. Studies on the toxicity of qinghaosu and its derivatives. China Cooperative Research Group on qinghaosu and its derivatives as antimalarials. J Tradit Chin Med 1982;2:31–38.

7. China Cooperative Research Group. Chemical studies on qinghaosu (artemisinine). China Cooperative Research Group on qinghaosu and its derivatives as antimalarials. J Tradit Chin Med 1982;2:3–8.

8. China Cooperative Research Group. Metabolism and pharmacokinetics of qinghaosu and its derivatives. China Cooperative Research Group on qinghaosu and its derivatives as antimalarials. J Tradit Chin Med 1982;2:25–30.

9. China Cooperative Research Group. Antimalarial efficacy and mode of action of qinghaosu and its derivatives in experimental models. China Cooperative Research Group on qinghaosu and its derivatives as antimalarials. J Tradit Chin Med 1982;2:17–24.

10. Helenport JP, Roche G. What have been the strategies for the registration, positioning and control of medical information for intramuscular artemether? Med Trop (Marseille) 1998;58:73–76.

11. Skelton-Stroud P, Mull R. Positioning, labelling, and medical information control of co-artemether tablets (CPG 56697): a fixed novel combination of artemether and benflumetol. Novartis Co-Artemether International Development Team. Med Trop (Marseille) 1998;58: 77–81.

12. Moneton P, Ducret JP. Positioning, labelling and control of medical information: artesunate strategy and Arsumax development story. Med Trop (Marseille) 1998;58:70–72.

13. McIntosh H, Olliaro P. (1999) Artemisinin derivatives for treating uncomplicated malaria. Cochrane Database Systemativ Reviews, No. 4. www.cochrane.org.

14. McIntosh H, Olliaro P. (1999) Artemisinin derivatives for treating severe malaria. Cochrane Database Systemativ Reviews, No. 4. www.cochrane.org.

15. Meshnick SR, Taylor TE, Kamchonwongpaisan S. Artemisinin and the antimalarial endoperoxides: from herbal remedy to targeted chemotherapy. Microbiol Rev 1996;60:301–315.

16. Cumming JN, Ploypradith P, Posner GH. Antimalarial activity of artemisinin (qinghaosu) and related trioxanes: mechanism(s) of action. Adv Pharmacol 1997;37:253–297.

17. Robert A, Meunier B. Is alkylation the main mechanism of action of the antimalarial drug artemisinin? Chem Soc Rev 1998;27:273–279.

18. Meshnick SR. Artemisinin antimalarials: mechanisms of action and resistance. Med Trop (Marseille) 1998;58:13–17.

19. Brossi A, Venugopalan B, Dominguez L, Gerpe HJ, Yeh JL. Flippen-Anderson, Buchs P,et al. Arteether, a new antimalarial drug: synthesis and antimalarial properties. J Med Chem 1988;31:645–650.

20. Rosenthal PJ, Meshnick SR. Hemoglobin catabolism and iron utilization by malaria parasites. Mol Biochem Parasitol 1996;83:131–139.

21. Meshnick SR, Tsang TW, Lin FB, Pan HZ, Chang CN, Kuypers F, et al. Activated oxygen mediates the antimalarial activity of qinghaosu. Prog Clin Biol Res 1989;313:95–104.

22. Levander OA, Ager AL Jr, Morris VC, May RG. Qinghaosu, dietary vitamin E, selenium, and cod-liver oil: effect on the susceptibility of mice to the malarial parasite Plasmodium yoelii. Am J Clin Nutr 1989;50:346–352.

23. Krungkrai SR, Yuthavong Y. The antimalarial action on *Plasmodium falciparum* of qinghaosu and artesunate in combination with agents which modulate oxidant stress. Trans R Soc Trop Med Hyg 1987;81:710–714.

24. Meshnick SR, Thomas A, Ranz A. Xu CM, Pan HZ. Artemisinin (qinghaosu): the role of intracellular hemin in its mechanism of antimalarial action. Mol Biochem Parasitol 1991;49:181–189.

25. Meshnick SR, Yang YZ, Lima V, Kuypers F, Kamchonwongpaisan S, Yuthavong Y. Iron-dependent free radical generation from the antimalarial agent artemisinin (qinghaosu). Antimicrob Agents Chemother 1993;37:1108–1114.
26. Scott MD, Meshnick SR, Williams RA, Chiu DT, Pan HC, Lubin BH, et al. Qinghaosu-mediated oxidation in normal and abnormal erythrocytes. J Lab Clin Med 1989;114:401–406.
27. Wei N, Sadrzadeh SM. Enhancement of hemin-induced membrane damage by artemisinin. Biochem Pharmacol 1994;48:737–741.
28. Berman PA, Adams PA. Artemisinin enhances heme-catalysed oxidation of lipid membranes. Free Radical Biol Med 1997;22:1283–1288.
29. Zhang F, Gosser DK Jr, Meshnick SR. Hemin-catalyzed decomposition of artemisinin (qinghaosu). Biochem Pharmacol 1992;43:1805–1809.
30. Butler AR, Gilbert BC, Hulme P, Irvine LR, Renton L, Whitwood AC. EPR evidence for the involvement of free radicals in the iron-catalysed decomposition of qinghaosu (artemisinin) and some derivatives; antimalarial action of some polycyclic endoperoxides. Free Radical Res 1998;28:471–476.
31. Paitayatat S, Tarnchompoo B, Thebtaranonth Y, Yuthavong Y. Correlation of antimalarial activity of artemisinin derivatives with binding affinity with ferroprotoporphyrin IX. J Med Chem 1997;40:633–638.
32. Woolfrey JR, Avery MA, Doweyko AM. Comparison of 3D quantitative structure-activity relationship methods: analysis of the in vitro antimalarial activity of 154 artemisinin analogues by hypothetical active-site lattice and comparative molecular field analysis. J Comput Aided Mol Des 1998;12:165–181.
33. Peters W, Li ZL. Robinson BL, Warhurst DC. The chemotherapy of rodent malaria, XL. The action of artemisinin and related sesquiterpenes. Ann Trop Med Parasitol 1986;80:483–489.
34. Wittner M, Lederman J, Tanowitz HB, Rosenbaum GS, Weiss LM. Atovaquone in the treatment of Babesia microti infections in hamsters. Am J Trop Med Hyg 1996;55:219–222.
35. Haynes RK, Pai HHO, Voerste A. Ring opening of artemisinin (qinghaosu) and dihydro-artemisinin and interception of the open hydroperoxides with formation of N-oxides—a chemical model for antimalarial mode of action. Tetrahedron Lett 1999;40:15–18.
36. Meshnick SR. Free radicals and antioxidants. Lancet 1994;344:1441–1442.
37. Hong YL, Yang YZ, Meshnick SR. The interaction of artemisinin with malarial hemozoin. Mol Biochem Parasitol 1994;63:121–128.
38. Robert A, Meunier B. Characterization of the first covalent adduct between artemisinin and a heme model. J Am Chem Soc 1997;119:5968–5969.
39. Bharel S, Vishwakarma RA, Jain SK. Artemisinin mediated alteration of haemin to a delta-meso oxidation product: relevance to mechanism of action. J Chem Soc Perkin Trans 1998;1:2163–2166.
40. Pandey AV, Tekwani BL, Singh RL, Chauhan VS. Artemisinin, an endoperoxide antimalarial, disrupts the hemoglobin catabolism and heme detoxification systems in malarial parasite. J Biol Chem 1999;274:19,383–19,388.
41. Asawamahasakda W, Ittarat I. Chang CC, McElroy P, Meshnick SR. Effects of antimalarials and protease inhibitors on plasmodial hemozoin production. Mol Biochem Parasitol 1994;67:183–191.
42. Yang YZ, Asawamahasakda W, Meshnick SR. Alkylation of human albumin by the antimalarial artemisinin. Biochem Pharmacol 1993;46:336–339.
44. Posner GH, Oh CH, Wang D, Gerena L, Milhous WK, Meshnick SR, et al. Mechanism-based design, synthesis, and in vitro antimalarial testing of new 4-methylated trioxanes structurally related to artemisinin: the importance of a carbon-centered radical for antimalarial activity. J Med Chem 1994;37:1256–1258.
45. Haynes RK, Vonwiller SC. The behaviour of quinghaosu (artemisinin) in the presence of heme iron(II) and (III). Tetrahedron Lett 1996;37:253–260.

46. Jefford CW, Favarger F, Vicente M, and Jacquier Y. The decomposition of cis-fused cyclopenteno-1,2,4-trioxanes induced by ferrous salts and some oxophilic reagents. Helv. Chim. Acta 1995;78:452–458.

47. O'Neill PM, Bishop LP, Searle NL, Maggs JL, Ward SA, Bray PG, et al. The biomimetic iron-mediated degradation of arteflene (Ro-42-1611), an endoperoxide antimalarial—implications for the mechanism of antimalarial activity. Tetrahedron Lett 1997;38:4263–4266.

48. Asawamahasakda W, Ittarat I, Pu YM, Ziffer H, Meshnick SR. Reaction of antimalarial endoperoxides with specific parasite proteins. Antimicrob Agents Chemother 1994;38:1854–1858.

49. Bhisutthibhan J, Pan XQ, Hossler PA, Walker DJ, Yowell CA, Carlton J, et al. The *Plasmodium falciparum* translationally controlled tumor protein homolog and its reaction with the antimalarial drug artemisinin. J Biol Chem 1998;273:16,192–16,198.

50. Bhisutthibhan J, Philbert MA, Fujioka M, Aikawa M, Meshnick SR. The *Plasmodium falciparum* translationally controlled tumor protein: Subcellular localization and calcium binding. Eur. J. Cell Biology 1999;78:665–670.

51. Gu HM, Warhurst DC, Peters W. Uptake of [3H] dihydroartemisinine by erythrocytes infected with *Plasmodium falciparum* in vitro. Trans R Soc Trop Med Hyg 1984;78:265–270.

52. Kamchonwongpaisan S, Chandrangam G, Avery MA, Yuthavong Y. Resistance to artemisinin of malaria parasites (*Plasmodium falciparum*) infecting alpha-thalassemic erythrocytes in vitro. Competition in drug accumulation with uninfected erythrocytes. J Clin Invest 1994;93:467–473.

53. Akompong T, VanWye J, Ghori N, Haldar K. Artemisinin and its derivatives are transported by a vacuolar-network of *Plasmodium falciparum* and their anti-malarial activities are additive with toxic sphingolipid analogues that block the network. Mol Biochem Parasitol 1999;101:71–79.

54. Price R, van Vugt M, Phaipun L, Luxemburger C, Simpson J, McGready R, et al. Adverse effects in patients with acute falciparum malaria treated with artemisinin derivatives. Am J Trop Med Hyg 1999;60:547–555.

55. McGready R, Cho T, Cho JJ, Simpson JA, Luxemburger C, Dubowitz L, et al. Artemisinin derivatives in the treatment of falciparum malaria in pregnancy. Trans R Soc Trop Med Hyg 1998;92:430–433.

56. Brewer TG, Genovese RF, Newman DB, Li Q. Factors relating to neurotoxicity of artemisinin antimalarial drugs "listening to arteether." Med Trop (Marseille) 1998;58:22–27.

57. Nontprasert A, Nosten-Bertrand M, Pukrittayakamee S, Vanijanonta S, Angus BJ, White NJ. Assessment of the neurotoxicity of parenteral artemisinin derivatives in mice. Am J Trop Med Hyg 1998;59:519–522.

58. Elias Z, Bonnet E, Marchou B, Massip P. Neurotoxicity of artemisinin: possible counseling and treatment of side effects. Clin Infect Dis 1999;28:1330–1331.

59. Miller LG, Panosian CB. Ataxia and slurred speech after artesunate treatment for falciparum malaria. N Engl J Med 1997;336:1328.

60. Dayan AD. Neurotoxicity and artemisinin compounds do the observations in animals justify limitation of clinical use? Med Trop (Marseille) 1998;58:32–37.

61. Fishwick J, McLean WG, Edwards G, Ward SA. The toxicity of artemisinin and related compounds on neuronal and glial cells in culture. Chem Biol Interact 1995;96:263–271.

62. Kamchonwongpaisan S, McKeever P, Hossler P, Ziffer H, Meshnick SR. Artemisinin neurotoxicity: neuropathology in rats and mechanistic studies in vitro. Am J Trop Med Hyg 1997;56:7–12.

63. Fishwick J, Edwards G, Ward SA, McLean WG. Binding of dihydroartemisinin to differentiating neuroblastoma cells and rat cortical homogenate. Neurotoxicology 1998;19:405–412.

64. Luxemburger C, Brockman A, Silamut K, Nosten F, van Vugt M, Gimenez F, et al. Two patients with falciparum malaria and poor in vivo responses to artesunate. Trans R Soc Trop Med Hyg 1998;92:668–669.

65. Kumar N, Zheng H. Stage-specific gametocytocidal effect in vitro of the antimalaria drug qinghaosu on *Plasmodium falciparum*. Parasitol Res 1990;76:214–218.

66. Price RN, Nosten F, Luxemburger C, ter Kuile FO, Paiphun L, Chongsuphajaisiddhi T, et al. Effects of artemisinin derivatives on malaria transmissibility. Lancet 1996;347:1654–1658.

67. Nosten F, Hien TT, White NJ. Use of artemisinin derivatives for the control of malaria. Med Trop (Marseille) 1998;58:45–49.

68. Vugt MV, Wilairatana P, Gemperli B, Gathmann I, Phaipun L, Brockman A, et al. Efficacy of six doses of artemether-lumefantrine (benflumetol) in multidrug-resistant *Plasmodium falciparum* malaria. Am J Trop Med Hyg 1999;60:936–942.

69. van Vugt M, Brockman A, Gemperli B, Luxemburger C, Gathmann I, Royce C, Slight T, Looareesuwan S, White NJ, Nosten F. Randomized comparison of artemether–benflumetol and artesunate–mefloquine in treatment of multidrug-resistant falciparum malaria. Antimicrob Agents Chemother 1998;42:135–139.

70. von Seidlein L, Bojang K, Jones P, Jaffar S, Pinder M, Obaro S, et al. A randomized controlled trial of artemether/benflumetol, a new antimalarial and pyrimethamine/sulfadoxine in the treatment of uncomplicated falciparum malaria in African children. Am J Trop Med Hyg 1998;58:638–644.

71. Inselburg, J. Induction and isolation of artemisinine-resistant mutants of *Plasmodium falciparum*. Am J Trop Med Hyg 1985;34:417–418.

72. Peters W, Robinson BL. The chemotherapy of rodent malaria. LVI. Studies on the development of resistance to natural and synthetic endoperoxides. Ann Trop Med Parasitol 1999;93:325–339.

73. Le Bras J. In vitro susceptibility of African *Plasmodium falciparum* isolates to dihydroartemisinin and the risk factors for resistance to qinghaosu. Med Trop (Marseille) 1998; 58:18–21.

74. Wongsrichanalai C, Nguyen TD, Trieu NT, Wimonwattrawatee T, Sookto P, Heppner DG, et al. In vitro susceptibility of *Plasmodium falciparum* isolates in Vietnam to artemisinin derivatives and other antimalarials. Acta Trop 1997;63:151–158.

75. Wongsrichanalai C, Wimonwattrawatee T, Sookto P, Laboonchai A, Heppner DG, Kyle DE, et al. In vitro sensitivity of *Plasmodium falciparum* to artesunate in Thailand. Bull WHO 1999;77:392–398.

76. Chawira AN, Warhurst DC, Robinson BL, Peters W. The effect of combinations of qinghaosu (artemisinin) with standard antimalarial drugs in the suppressive treatment of malaria in mice. Trans R Soc Trop Med Hyg 1987;81:554–558.

77. Ekong R, Warhurst DC. Synergism between arteether and mefloquine or quinine in a multidrug-resistant strain of *Plasmodium falciparum* in vitro. Trans R Soc Trop Med Hyg 1990;84:757–758.

78. Walker DJ, Pitsch JL, Peng MM, Robinson BL, Peters W, Bhisutthibhan J, et al. Mechanisms of artemisinin resistance in the rodent malaria pathogen plasmodium yoelii. Antimicrob Agents Chemother 2000;44:344–347.

79. McIntosh HM, Olliaro P. Treatment of severe malaria with artemisinin derivatives. A systematic review of randomised controlled trials. Med Trop (Marseille) 1998;58:61–62.

80. McIntosh HM, Olliaro P. Treatment of uncomplicated malaria with artemisinin derivatives. A systematic review of randomised controlled trials. Med Trop (Marseille) 1998;58:57–58.

81. Melendez V, Peggins JO, Brewer TG, Theoharides AD. Determination of the antimalarial arteether and its deethylated metabolite dihydroartemisinin in plasma by high-performance liquid chromatography with reductive electrochemical detection. J Pharm Sci 1991;80:132–138.

82. Li X, Rieckmann K. A bioassay for derivatives of qinghaosu (artemisinin). Trop Med Parasitol 1992;43:195–196.

83. Teja-Isavadharm P, Nosten F, Kyle DE, Luxemburger C, Ter Kuile F, Peggins JO, et al. Comparative bioavailability of oral, rectal, and intramuscular artemether in healthy subjects: use of simultaneous measurement by high performance liquid chromatography and bioassay. Br J Clin Pharmacol 1996;42:599–604.

85. ter Kuile F, White NJ, Holloway P, Pasvol G, Krishna S. *Plasmodium falciparum*: in vitro studies of the pharmacodynamic properties of drugs used for the treatment of severe malaria. Exp Parasitol 1993;76:85–95.

86. White NJ. Qinghaosu in combinations. Med Trop (Marseille) 1998;58:85–88.

87. White NJ, Olliaro P. Artemisinin and derivatives in the treatment of uncomplicated malaria. Med Trop (Marseille) 1998;58:54–56.

88. Boele van Hensbroek M. The role of the qinghaosu derivatives in the treatment of severe malaria. Med Trop (Marseille) 1998;58:59–60.

89. Anonymous. The Role of Artemisinin and Its Derivatives in the Current Treatment of Malaria (1994–1995). WHO/MAL/94.1067. Geneva: World Health Organization, 1994.

90. White NJ, Nosten F, Looareesuwan S, Watkins WM, Marsh K, Snow RW, et al. Averting a malaria disaster. Lancet 1999;353:1965–1967.

11

Atovaquone–Proguanil Combination

Akhil B. Vaidya

INTRODUCTION

Development of an atovaquone–proguanil combination, trademarked Malarone, during the 1990s has been a major step in addressing the need for antimalarial drugs with targets different from those of agents for which resistance is already rampant in the field *(1)*. Atovaquone affects parasite mitochondrial functions in a selective manner *(2,3)* and, thus, constitutes an entirely new class of antimicrobial agents. While atovaquone as a single agent has been used for treating *Pneumocystis carinii* pneumonia and toxoplasmosis in immunodeficient patients *(4,5)*, it met with unacceptable rates of treatment failure when used against malaria *(6,7)*. The inclusion of proguanil as a synergistic agent with atovaquone appears to have overcome the high rate of treatment failure, and the resulting drug, Malarone, has been approved for treatment of falciparum malaria in more than 30 countries. This chapter aims to provide a perspective on the development of this new drug and its clinical efficacy. Furthermore, recent studies on mechanisms of action as well as resistance to this drug will be discussed. It is important to note that the atovaquone–proguanil combination may be one of the few antimalarials for which significant details of drug action and resistance are available *before* its widespread introduction. This information may prove useful in devising strategies for drug usage as well as in the development of the next generation of antimalarials with mitochondrion-specific modes of action.

DEVELOPMENT OF ATOVAQUONE

Atovaquone is a naphthoquinone belonging to a family of compounds that have been investigated as antimalarials for over 50 yr. Early investigations on naphthoquinones as antimalarials have been previously reviewed in some detail elsewhere *(8,9)*. Hooker *(10)* was the first to recognize the presence of naphthoquinones in plant extracts and to synthesize lapachol, a 2-alkylnaphthoquinone, in 1936. Efforts to find substitutes for quinine during World War II included investigations on naphthoquinones, and hydrolapachol *(see* Fig. 1 for structures) was found to have antimalarial activity. This led to collaborative efforts between academic and industrial scientists, resulting in synthesis of hundreds of hydrolapachol analogs and their testing as antimalarials in a duck malaria model *(11)*. The most promising compound to emerge from this early study, lapinone, was found to be effective in treating vivax malaria but needed to be

From: *Antimalarial Chemotherapy: Mechanisms of Action, Resistance, and New Directions in Drug Discovery*
Edited by: P. J. Rosenthal © Humana Press Inc., Totowa, NJ

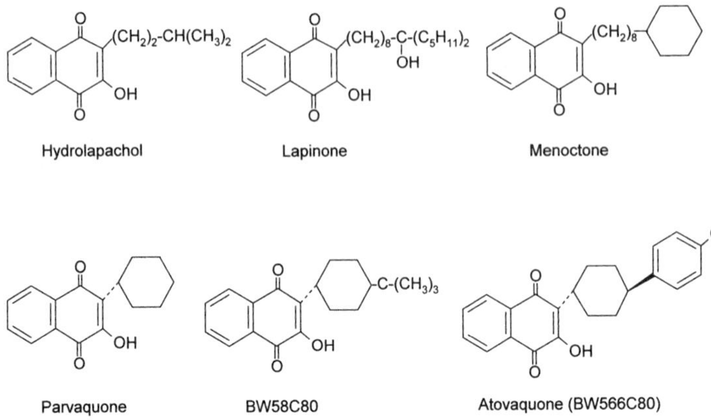

Fig. 1. Structure of hydroxynaphthoquinones investigated as antimalarials.

given parenterally in large doses *(12)*. The advent of chloroquine as an inexpensive orally available antimalarial at about the same time diminished interest in developing hydroxynaphthoquinones as antimalarials. In the 1960s, coinciding with the emergence of chloroquine resistance, there was a renewed interest in naphthoquinones as antimalarials *(8,13,14)*. One compound, menoctone, was chosen for clinical testing but proved to be disappointing against malaria *(15)*. Menoctone, however, was effective against *Theileria parva* infection in cattle *(16)*, which then led to extensive structure–activity studies. Parvaquone was identified as an effective and economic antitheilerial agent from these investigations with about a 90% cure rate in field studies *(17)*. Modifications of the cyclohexyl moiety of parvaquone were extensively investigated and found to have broad-spectrum antiparasitic activities *(18)*. One such compound, BW58C80, was tested in humans but found to be rapidly converted to an inactive red-colored metabolite that was secreted in the urine and, thus, was dropped from further development *(1)*. Modification of the 4'-position of the cyclohexyl ring by a chlorophenyl moiety resulted in compound 566C80, which was metabolically stable and had broad-spectrum activity against a number of eukaryotic pathogens, including malaria parasites *(1)*. The compound 566C80 was named atovaquone and has been registered as Mepron.

ATOVAQUONE AS AN ANTIMALARIAL

Cultured *Plasmodium falciparum* isolates from different parts of the world were inhibited by atovaquone at low nanomolar concentrations (median inhibitory concentration [IC_{50}] 0.7–4.3 n*M*) regardless of the relative resistance of the isolates to other antimalarials *(1)*. Oral doses of the drug to Aotus monkeys infected with *P. falciparum* and mice infected with *P. yoelii* and *P. berghei* were highly effective in curing malaria infection *(1)*. Following a phase I evaluation of toxicity, a single dose of 500 mg atovaquone was given to patients with *P. falciparum* malaria in the United Kingdom and was found to give prompt clinical response with removal of asexual parasites from the blood smears *(6)*. Most of these patients, however, developed recrudescent malaria *(6)*. In larger studies done in Thailand *(7)* as well as in Zambia (reviewed in ref. *19*), atovaquone was tested as a single agent in varying doses for its ability to cure uncomplicated *P. falciparum* malaria. Although the drug resulted in rapid parasite and fever clearance, the overall cure rate *(66%)* was disappointingly inadequate *(7,19)*. Paired parasites from several recrudescing patients were cultured to assess sensitivity to atovaquone *(7)*. Although all of the parasites isolated upon admission of the patients were sensitive to atovaquone with an IC_{50} of about 3.3 ng/mL, the paired recrudescent parasites showed high levels of resistance (IC_{50} of >3000 ng/mL). These observations suggested rapid emergence of atovaquone-resistant parasites in about one-third of the patients given atovaquone as a single agent. Clearly, atovaquone as a stand-alone antimalarial drug was judged unacceptable. In this regard, it is of interest to note that the drug failure in *P. carinii* pneumonia treated with atovaquone alone does not appear to be as high as in case of malaria.

It was also noted that atovaquone-resistant *P. falciparum* readily arose in parasite cultures even when treated at doses up to 100 n*M* *(20)*. Rathod et al. *(21)*, in a seminal observation, subsequently showed that *P. falciparum* isolates from certain parts of the world (especially from Southeast Asia) developed atovaquone resistance at 1000-fold higher frequency than parasites from some other areas (e.g., Central America). The biological basis for such differences is not understood but clearly has far-reaching implications for strategies to control malaria. Rathod et al. *(21)* also examined the frequency of resistance emergence against an unrelated antimalarial compound, 5-fluoroorotate, and found that one strain (3D7) had a high-frequency drug-resistance phenotype against atovaquone but not against 5-fluoroorotate. This suggests that more than one mechanism for the high-frequency drug-resistance phenotype may be operational among the parasite populations. Possible explanations for the high frequency of atovaquone resistance emergence will be described in a later section of this chapter.

IN VITRO SYNERGY BETWEEN ATOVAQUONE AND PROGUANIL

The problem of rapid resistance development to atovaquone when used as a single agent necessitated a search for a partner drug that could synergize with atovaquone and reduce the chances of resistance development. Because existing antimalarials could be investigated and deployed more easily, the focus of a detailed in vitro study was on such compounds *(22)*. As can be expected, certain drugs had additive effects, whereas others had antagonistic effects *(22)*. A few drugs had clear synergistic activity, and the highest synergistic action was seen with proguanil when tested against three different *P. falciparum* isolates *(22)*. Proguanil has been used as an antimalarial for almost 50 yr, has a very favorable safety record, and can be produced inexpensively. It has been known for a long time that proguanil needs to be metabolized to an active compound, cycloguanil, for its antimalarial action *(23,24)*; proguanil on its own has antimalarial activity in vitro at 10,000-fold higher concentrations than cycloguanil *(25)*, concentrations that cannot be achieved in vivo. Cycloguanil inhibits parasite dihydrofolate reductase (DHFR) preferentially and interferes with the folate-dependent metabolism of the parasites, particularly thymidine synthesis. When cycloguanil was tested with atovaquone, it failed to synergize in any significant manner *(22)*. Furthermore, other parasite DHFR inhibitors, pyrimethamine and WR99210, also failed to have synergy with atovaquone *(22)*. It is also of interest to note that as part of a clinical study to evaluate atovaquone in combination with other antimalarials, proguanil alone was also tested in 18 patients from Thailand *(7)* in doses as high as 1 g/d for 3 d; in more than

90% of the patients, proguanil alone failed to clear the parasites. The failure of proguanil as a single agent in Thailand was likely the result of a widespread presence of cycloguanil-resistant parasites, although direct testing for drug resistance in this cohort of patients was not conducted. Thus, the remarkable synergy by proguanil was apparently independent of its antifolate activity. A mechanism explaining this synergy has recently been proposed *(26)* and will be described in a later section.

CLINICAL STUDIES WITH THE ATOVAQUONE–PROGUANIL COMBINATION

Between 1990 and 1996, a total of 12 clinical studies were conducted to evaluate atovaquone alone or in combination with other antimalarials, mainly proguanil *(6,7,27–35)*. These studies have been extensively reviewed *(19,27)*. Although the studies focused almost exclusively on uncomplicated falciparum malaria, enrolling 1395 patients, a few non-falciparum-malaria patients were also included. In a series of uncontrolled dose-ranging studies done in Thailand, tetracycline, doxycycline, pyrimethamine, and proguanil were investigated in combination with atovaquone *(7)*. Atovaquone plus pyrimethamine gave a cure rate of 75% and thus was inadequate for treating falciparum malaria in Thailand. Tetracycline and doxycycline in combination with atovaquone gave 100% and 91% cure rates, respectively, and could be considered adequate. However, these antibiotics are not recommended for use in children. Proguanil in combination with atovaquone gave an acceptably high rate of cure even at the lower doses tested *(7)*. The optimal dose for adults was 1000 mg atovaquone combined with 400 mg proguanil given daily for 5 d. The cure rate with this dose was 100%.

Based on the above-cited dose-searching trials, the atovaquone–proguanil combination was investigated in several randomized controlled trials with or without comparator drugs *(7,19,27–35)*. The atovaquone–proguanil combination had highly favorable effects in these trials. For example, in four such controlled studies, atovaquone–proguanil had cure rates ranging from 98% to 100% compared to 8% or 30% for chloroquine alone, 87% for chloroquine combined with pyrimethamine–sulfadoxine, 86% for mefloquine, and 81% for amodiaquine. Overall, 521 patients were treated with the atovaquone–proguanil combination in these trials and compared with 474 patients treated with the comparator drugs *(19)*. Seven of the atovaquone–proguanil-treated patients and 64 of the comparator-drug-treated patients developed recrudescent malaria. Most of the apparent recrudescent cases in atovaquone–proguanil-treated cohorts were believed to be the result of reinfections and not true treatment failures. Thus, atovaquone–proguanil is an effective therapy for multidrug-resistant falciparum malaria in all parts of the world where clinical trials have been conducted.

A limited number of clinical studies have also examined the efficacy of the atovaquone–proguanil combination for the treatment of non-falciparum malaria *(19)*. The results show that the combination works well for vivax malaria and for a limited number of *P. malariae* and *P. ovale* infections as well. Although the atovaquone–proguanil combination appears to be effective against gametocytes, recurrence of vivax malaria in a large proportion of patients suggests that the drug is not effective against the hypnozoites of these parasites *(19)*. A recent study combining atovaquone–proguanil with primaquine shows favorable outcome in treating recurrent vivax malaria *(36)*.

The atovaquone–proguanil combination was also evaluated in clinical studies for prophylaxis of malaria *(37,38)*. In placebo-controlled trials, 250 mg atovaquone and 100 mg proguanil were administered daily for 10–12 wk to examine their efficacy as causal prophylactics against falciparum malaria. The combination was 98% effective in preventing parasitemia compared to the placebo. In a study involving volunteers challenged with infected mosquito bites, atovaquone by itself was also found to have activity against the liver stages of *P. falciparum (39)*. These studies support a fixed-dose combination of atovaquone and proguanil for a highly effective prophylaxis regimen against falciparum malaria.

MECHANISM OF ATOVAQUONE ACTION

Studies conducted as early as the 1940s suggested that hydroxynaphthoquinones inhibited mitochondrial respiration *(40,41)*. These investigations, however, were done in heterologous mitochondria from yeast or mammalian tissues. Thus, the results, although suggestive of mitochondria as targets for hydroxynaphthoquinones, could not explain the apparent selective toxicity and therapeutic value of these compounds. Fry and Beesley *(42)* were the first to report successful isolation of malaria parasite mitochondria for biochemical studies in 1991; although, these mitochondria did not seem to be well-coupled *(42)*. Using the isolated organelles from *P. falciparum* and *P. yoelii*, Fry and Pudney *(2)* showed that atovaquone inhibited the bc_1 complex with IC_{50} of approx 10^{-9} M, whereas the mammalian bc_1 complex was inhibited with the IC_{50} of approx 5×10^{-7} M. These results for the first time suggested that the selective toxicity of an antimalarial hydroxynaphthoquinone was the result of the preferential inhibition of the parasite mitochondrial electron transfer chain.

Mitochondrial functions in malaria parasites were shrouded in a bit of mystery for many years. Lack of a complete citric acid cycle and an acristate morphology of the blood-stage mitochondria seemed to diminish their significance in many investigators' views. Gutteridge et al. *(43)*, however, pointed out early that at least one critical enzyme in the obligatory pyrimidine biosynthesis pathway, dihydroorotate dehydrogenase (DHOD), required functional mitochondrial electron transport chain for disposing the electrons generated in the process. As reviewed elsewhere *(44)*, in addition to DHOD, many critical physiological processes are also likely to be relegated to the parasite mitochondria. Because the 6-kb mitochondrial genome in malaria parasites is the smallest such molecule known—encoding only three proteins *(45–48)*—hundreds of other mitochondrial proteins required to maintain functional mitochondria will need to be encoded in the nucleus, translated by the cytoplasmic ribosomes, and imported into mitochondria. In addition to the proteins, malarial mitochondrial will also need to import the entire set of tRNAs necessary for translation of the three essential electron transport proteins encoded by the mitochondrial genome. An extensive system of metabolite transport molecules will also be necessary for mitochondrial functioning in malaria parasites. A continuing survey of the released genomic sequences from the Malaria Genome Project consortium clearly supports this view; at this early stage at least 100 putative mitochondrially targeted proteins can be surmised by sequence analysis (A. Vaidya, unpublished data). However, isolation of biochemically active mitochondria from malaria parasites in sufficient quantity and quality remains a major challenge.

The difficulties associated with isolating biochemically active mitochondria from malarial parasites necessitated alternative approaches to investigate mitochondrial physiology. The key function of mitochondria is to generate an electrochemical gradient across the inner membrane, which is then used as an energy source for the myriad of synthetic and transport activities associated with mitochondria. Thus, the electropotential across the mitochondrial inner membrane, called $\Delta\psi_m$, is an excellent surrogate for assessing the general physiological state of mitochondria. For this purpose, a flow cytometric assay to measure $\Delta\psi_m$ in intact, live malaria parasites was developed *(3)*. This assay uses very low concentrations (2 nM) of a lipophilic cationic fluorescent dye, 3,3'-dihexyloxacarbocyanine iodide (DiOC$_6$), as a probe in conjunction with flow cytometry to assess $\Delta\psi_m$. At 2 nM concentration, DiOC$_6$ rapidly partitions into energized mitochondria within the live parasites without perturbing the parasite mitochondrial physiology and remains partitioned in the mitochondria for an extended period. The partitioning is dependent on the maintenance of $\Delta\psi_m$ because inclusion of carbonyl cyanide *m*-chlorophenyl hydrazine (CCCP), a protonophore, abolishes the probe accumulation *(3)*. Thus, this assay permitted analysis of the effect of various compounds on the mitochondrial physiology of live, intact parasites. The usual mitochondrial electron transfer chain inhibitors, myxothiazol, antimycin, and cyanide, collapsed the parasite $\Delta\psi_m$ in a dose-dependent manner *(3)*. Rotenone, a complex I inhibitor, did not affect $\Delta\psi_m$ as expected because of the absence of this complex in the parasite mitochondria. Atovaquone collapsed $\Delta\psi_m$ in a dose-dependent manner with an EC$_{50}$ of about 15 nM *(3)*. Inhibition of mitochondrial electron transport by these compounds, as judged by parasite respiration, correlated with their effects on $\Delta\psi_m$. Other antimalarial drugs, such as chloroquine and tetracycline, did not affect parasite mitochondrial physiology under these conditions. Atovaquone did not have any significant effect on the $\Delta\psi_m$ of mammalian cells, again confirming its selective activity against parasite mitochondria *(3)*.

In multicellular organisms collapsed the $\Delta\psi_m$ has profound effects on cellular physiology. The collapsed $\Delta\psi_m$ could be a cause or a consequence of mitochondrial permeability transition, in which a large pore forms within the mitochondrial inner membrane, resulting in the release of solutes up to 1500 Daltons in size from the mitochondrial matrix (reviewed in refs. *49–52*). In mammalian cells, this also leads to the release of proteins present within the intermembrane space, most notably the cytochrome-*c* *(53)*, which participate in triggering the caspases cascade that leads to apoptosis. Thus, a large body of evidence accumulated over the last few years shows that mitochondrial permeability transition is a central step in the activation of the programmed cell death pathway *(51)*. Although analogous apoptosis pathways have not been detected in unicellular organisms, programmed cell death has been hinted at in some species *(54–58)*. It is conceivable that a programmed cell death pathway would be evolutionarily selected for in unicellular organisms inasmuch as it may provide a measure of protection for the neighboring members of the species when a cell undergoes death. It clearly would be of interest to investigate such pathways especially in parasitic pathogens.

As for the malaria parasites with atovaquone-mediated $\Delta\psi_m$ collapse, the demise may occur through the disruption of several processes. Lack of pyrimidine synthesis because of inhibition of dihydroorotate dehydrogenase, a critical enzyme in the essential *de novo* pyrimidine biosynthesis, is one such process *(43,59)*. In addition, all metabolite and protein transport across the inner membrane will cease in parasites with collapsed $\Delta\psi_m$, the net result being a major disruption of the parasite metabolism. Parasite death, thus, could ensue because of such disruption; the form of death, however, remains unclear. Do parasites lyse, being unable maintain homeostasis, in a manner similar to necrotic cell death? Or, do they undergo an ordered dismantling of their macromolecular organization in a manner similar to apoptosis? Although we do not have much information about these processes, morphological observations of "crisis forms" of parasites are suggestive of an orderly demise. If correct, an understanding of the death process could prove quite useful.

A MECHANISM FOR ATOVAQUONE–PROGUANIL SYNERGY

The success of proguanil as a synergistic agent was somewhat surprising because resistance to proguanil alone was quite common in parts of the world where the combination was tested in clinical trials *(7)*. Further, the antimalarial activity of proguanil is mediated by cycloguanil, a parasite DHFR inhibitor that is a metabolite of cytochrome P450-mediated cyclization of proguanil *(23,24,60)*. Although approx 20–30% of the Asian and African population are deficient for the P450 isoform believed to carry out this metabolic activation *(61,62)*, the atovaquone–proguanil combination was quite effective in these populations. Thus, there was a suspicion that proguanil acted as the pro-drug to provide synergy to atovaquone rather than as its metabolite cycloguanil.

To assess its effect on mitochondrial physiology, proguanil was tested alone and in combination with atovaquone for its effect on parasite $\Delta\psi_m$ as well as on electron transport *(26)*. At pharmacologically relevant concentrations, proguanil by itself had no appreciable effect on parasite $\Delta\psi_m$ or respiration *(26)*. However, it significantly enhanced atovaquone-mediated $\Delta\psi_m$ collapse at micromolar concentrations *(26)*. This enhancing effect was mediated by the pro-drug itself because neither cycloguanil nor pyrimethamine (another parasite DHFR inhibitor) were able to affect atovaquone-mediated $\Delta\psi_m$ collapse *(26)*. Proguanil-mediated enhancement was specific for atovaquone because effects of other inhibitors of mitochondrial electron transport such as myxothiazol and antimycin were not altered by inclusion of proguanil. It was rather surprising that proguanil did not enhance the ability of atovaquone to inhibit parasite electron transport *(26)*. Thus, the synergy between atovaquone and proguanil appears to be mediated by the enhancement of $\Delta\psi_m$ collapse at a lower concentration of atovaquone.

It appears quite clear that proguanil acts to enhance the atovaquone effect as a biguanide, rather than as its metabolite cycloguanil *(26)*. Biguanides have a long history of being used as agents that affect cellular physiology *(63)*. Drugs such as metformin are currently used as hypoglycemic agents for the treatment of insulin-independent diabetes *(64)*. It was initially suggested that these compounds are uncouplers of oxidative phosphorylation *(65)*; however, the uncoupling effect is seen at millimolar concentrations, which are pharmacologically not relevant. Pharmacokinetic studies have shown that proguanil concentrations required for the enhancement of atovaquone activity are achieved in an adult within 3.5 h after an oral dose of 200 mg *(66,67)*. Hence, the dose of the atovaquone–proguanil combination recommended for treating adults (1000 mg atovaquone and 400 mg proguanil per day for 3 d) should be sufficient to achieve the effective concentrations in plasma for its optimal antimalarial activity.

The molecular basis for the proguanil enhancement is unclear. The fact that proguanil did not enhance the atovaquone-mediated electron transport inhibition suggests that the mitochondrial depolarization activity of atovaquone could be uncoupled from its electron transport inhibition effect. Some in vitro studies have suggested that proguanil may have intrinsic activity independent of its metabolic activation and DHFR inhibition *(25,68)*. Indeed, at concentrations higher than 12 μM, proguanil does seem to have an effect on $\Delta\psi_m$ in malaria parasites *(26)*, although specificity of this effect is unclear because a number of compounds can affect mitochondrial physiology at high concentrations. The concentrations of proguanil used in studies suggesting intrinsic activity *(68)* were significantly higher (IC$_{50}$ of 50–75 μM) than those achieved in vivo. Thus, the relevance of the intrinsic in vitro activity of proguanil to the clinical situation remains unclear. In contrast, the synergistic activity of proguanil in experiments described by Srivastava and Vaidya *(26)* was observed at pharmacologically achievable drug concentrations. Nevertheless, it would be important to determine whether similar mechanisms apply to both the intrinsic in vitro activity and the atovaquone synergy shown by proguanil.

RESISTANT MUTANTS DEFINE THE ATOVAQUONE-BINDING REGION

When atovaquone is used as a single agent, resistant malaria parasites arose quickly, as described earlier. A study of such mutants could give insights into the molecular basis for drug action. Based on sequence analyses of the mitochondrially encoded cytochrome-*b* of malaria parasites, it was suggested previously that certain unique structural features of the parasite protein may underlie the remarkably selective antiparasite activity of the effective hydroxynaphthoquinones *(46)*. To examine this further, a series of atovaquone-resistant *P. yoelii* parasites were derived by suboptimal treatment of infected mice with atovaquone *(69)*. Resistance in this rodent malaria system arose in a single step and quite readily, consistent with the observation of 30% recrudescence during the clinical trials when atovaquone was used as a single agent. A total of nine independent mutants were derived through this regimen *(69)*.

The atovaquone-resistant malaria parasites were also resistant to the collapse of $\Delta\psi_m$ as well as respiration inhibition by atovaquone *(69)*. The IC$_{50}$ ranged approx 1000-fold higher than that for the parental parasites, ranging from 10,000 to 25,000 nM compared to about 15 nM for the parental parasites. Thus, development of atovaquone resistance in malaria parasites is accompanied by concomitant resistance to atovaquone-mediated $\Delta\psi_m$ collapse and electron transport inhibition. The $\Delta\psi_m$ in the resistant parasites in the presence of myxothiazol, a standard cytochrome-*bc*$_1$ complex inhibitor, was also examined. The EC$_{50}$ for myxothiazol in the parental parasites is about 180 nM, and in the resistant parasites the EC$_{50}$ values increased only twofold to fourfold. Hence, the level of cross-resistance for this inhibitor appeared to be at a much lower level than for atovaquone *(69)*.

It was of interest to see if proguanil could continue to have synergism even in atovaquone-resistant parasites. For atovaquone-resistant parasites, inclusion of proguanil did not affect the $\Delta\psi_m$ collapse profile for atovaquone *(69)*. This suggests that inclusion of proguanil will have no synergism with atovaquone once atovaquone resistance has emerged.

The foregoing observations strongly suggest the possibility of structural changes within the atovaquone-binding site in malaria parasites. In a number of different organisms, essentially all naturally arising mutants resistant to inhibitors of the cytochrome-

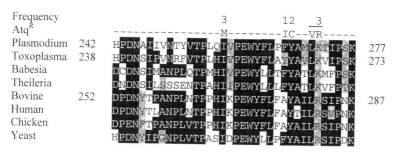

Fig. 2. Alignment of the e–f loop of the cytochrome *b* from eight different organisms. Amino acids conserved in 50% or more of the organisms are shaded in negative contrast for identity and in gray for conservative changes. Positions of conserved residues in which alterations are known to confer resistance to atovaquone in *P. yoelii* (Atq^R) are indicated. Concurrent mutations required for Atq^R in *Plasmodium* are marked with an overline. Numbers in the first line indicate the frequency of each amino acid changes in nine independent resistant parasite lines *(69)*.

bc$_1$ complex carry mutations in the cytochrome-*b* gene *(70)*. Hence, the cytochrome-*b* genes of the 6-kb mitochondrial genome from each of the nine independent atovaquone-resistant *P. yoelii* lines were examined. Mutations leading to amino acid changes were seen to cluster around a region of the ubiquinol oxidation (Q$_o$) site. As summarized in Fig. 2, three independent atovaquone-resistant lines had identical two-base-pair changes resulting in L271V and K272R mutations. Three others had identical one-base-pair changes resulting in a I258M mutation; two lines had a one-base-pair change giving a Y268C mutation; and one had a single change resulting in a F267I mutation. For one of the atovaquone-resistant lines, the entire mtDNA was cloned and completely sequenced. This sequence revealed total identity with the parental mtDNA except for the two base-pair mutations in the cytochrome-*b* gene noted *(69)*. Mutations in the vicinity of the Q$_o$ site of cytochrome-*b* have also been reported in clinical isolates of *P. carinii* from two out of four patients who failed atovaquone prophylaxis *(71)*, as well as in *P. berghei* subjected to an in vivo atovaquone escalation regimen *(72)*. Although no biochemical studies on mitochondrial functions in these apparently atovaquone-resistant organisms were carried out *(71,72)*, the location of the mutations are consistent with the findings in *P. yoelii* described here *(69)*.

Inhibitors of the cytochrome-*bc*$_1$ complex are believed to act mainly as ubiquinone–ubiquinol antagonists by interfering with ubiquinol oxidation or ubiquinone reduction steps of the proton-motive Q cycle *(73)*. Crystallographic evidence has now localized myxothiazol, stigmatellin, and antimycin to sites that correspond very well with the locations of the mutations, providing resistance in various systems *(74–77)*. Atovaquone-resistance mutations also localized to the general vicinity of the ubiquinol oxidation region of cytochrome-*b*. They mapped within a highly conserved 15-amino-acid region within the e–f loop of this subunit *(69)*, which contains the universal PEWY sequence found in all cytochrome-*b*. Of the five amino acid changes conferring atovaquone resistance, three (I258, Y268, and L271) involved residues that are absolutely conserved in all cytochrome-*b*, whereas the other two (F267 and K272) involved residues that differed between the parasite and vertebrate proteins.

In the cavity defined by the atovaquone-resistance-associated mutations, two amino acid residues that bear different side chains in the parasite and vertebrate cytochrome-

b seem to acquire a special significance as to the selectivity of atovaquone binding. These are F267 and K272 in malaria parasites corresponding to A278 and R283 in the chicken and human. These positions are also conserved in *Toxoplasma* and *Theileria* cytochrome-*b* (in *Toxoplasma,* there is a tyrosine instead of phenylalanine at position 267). Hence, it can be suggested that an aromatic side chain at position 267 in combination with lysine at 272 is required for sensitivity to atovaquone. If so, then in the vertebrate cytochrome-*b,* alanine at position 278 in combination with the larger arginine at position 283 would appear to be responsible for resistance to atovaquone. This would then explain the selective toxicity of atovaquone toward parasites without affecting the vertebrate mitochondrial functions. Consistent with this proposal is the observation that other atovaquone-resistance-associated amino acid changes also alter subtly the hydrophobicity or volume of this cavity at absolutely conserved positions *(69).* These changes may greatly diminish the accessibility and/or affinity of atovaquone for this cavity without significantly affecting that of ubiquinol and effective electron transfer to the iron–sulfur protein. For efficient electron transport, ubiquinone has to move in and out of the catalytic sites of the bc_1 complex. The flexible polyisoprenyl side chain at the 2-carbon position could aid this movement, whereas the relatively inflexible cyclohexyl–chlorophenyl side chain at the 2 position in atovaquone may hinder it by possibly interacting directly with the resistance-associated residues of cytochrome-*b.*

INVOLVEMENT OF ATOVAQUONE IN RESISTANCE EMERGENCE: A HYPOTHESIS

The rapid emergence of atovaquone-resistant parasites through mutations within the parasite mtDNA appears quite paradoxical at first: The 6-kb mtDNA is extremely well conserved. Among mtDNA from five divergent *Plasmodium* species that have been sequenced, there is about 90% sequence identity. The remarkable conservation of the sequence can be exemplified by the observation that two geographically distant *P. falciparum* isolates differ at only one nucleotide position out of 5966 bases *(78).* Yet, the resistance mutations arise quickly and spread through the entire parasite population in an individual. I wish to propose that the mechanism of atovaquone action is closely tied to the mechanism of rapid resistance emergence and that inclusion of proguanil is able to mitigate this situation. The hypothesis is schematically summarized in Fig. 3.

The mode of mtDNA replication in malaria parasites requires extensive gene conversion and recombination among the multiple copies present in each mitochondrion *(79).* This mode of replication, which is dramatically different from host mtDNA replication, results in extensive copy correction of the genome and in the high degree of sequence conservation. Atovaquone as a single agent inhibits electron transport and collapses mitochondrial membrane potential at similar concentrations *(3).* This leads to the formation of reactive oxygen species (ROS), which act as locally active mutagens. Advantageous mutations will be selected and spread through the population by the copy-

---

Fig. 3. A hypothesis to explain the rapid emergence of atovaquone resistance in malaria parasites. **(A)** A model for mitochondrial DNA replication as proposed by Preiser et al. *(79).* The 6-kb mtDNA in malaria parasites is tandemly arrayed *(80),* and electron microscopic as

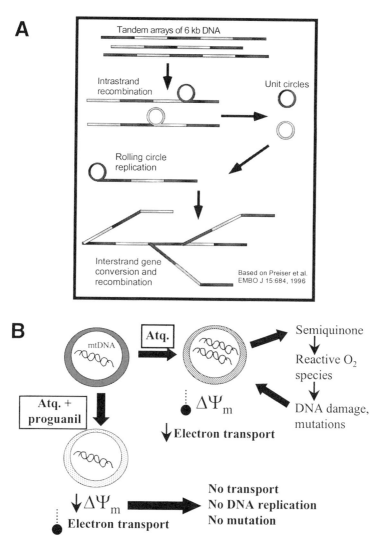

(**Fig. 3.** *continued*) well as gel mobility data *(79)* suggest that a unit-length mtDNA is likely released from the tandem array through *intrastran*d recombination and is circularized. The unit-length circle replicated through the rolling circle mode, generating the tandem arrays. The tandem arrays appear to undergo extensive *interstran*d gene conversion and recombination. This would result in copy correction such that a "master copy" sequence will prevail in the parasite population. Any advantageous mutation in the mtDNA will similarly be propagated through the population because the mutated sequence will be preferred as the "master copy." (**B**) Mitochondrial membrane potential in the presence of atovaquone alone or in combination with proguanil. Atovaquone alone will inhibit electron transport at the cytochrome-bc_1 complex level, generating semiquinone, which will give rise to reactive oxygen species. These will act as local DNA damaging agents causing mtDNA mutations. Continued exposure to the suboptimal atovaquone concentrations will select for those mutations imparting atovaquone resistance. In contrast, when proguanil is included with atovaquone, the $\Delta\psi_m$ collapse precedes electron transport inhibition. Thus, the possibility of ROS-mediated DNA damage is reduced, yet the mitochondrial physiology is severely compromised. Under this condition, parasite demise will occur before accumulation of mtDNA mutations that can provide selective advantage for growth in the presence of atovaquone.

correction mechanism. Proguanil lowers the concentrations at which atovaquone collapses membrane potential without affecting its electron transport inhibition profile *(26)*. Because mitochondrial DNA replication is inhibited in the absence of membrane transport (dependent on $\Delta\psi_m$), mutations cannot arise even in the presence of higher levels of ROS. Thus, inclusion of proguanil will also reduce the chances of mutations arising in mtDNA. Thus, $\Delta\psi_m$ collapse is likely to have a more dire consequence for the parasite compared to electron transport inhibition, and that mtDNA mutations emerge as a consequence of atovaquone mediated ROS accumulation. This proposal would suggest that mtDNA replication and repair are likely to be closely linked to the drug-resistance mechanism.

CONCLUDING REMARKS

Development of the atovaquone–proguanil combination for malaria treatment and prophylaxis has been a major event during the last decade. It is quite likely that this drug will assume an increasingly important role in treating multidrug-resistant malaria and as a causal prophylactic. Although it is the first antimalarial to be developed by the pharmaceutical industry in decades, its general deployment in the field is likely to be guided by caution. The rapidity with which resistance developed against atovaquone when used as a single agent would argue for controlled release of the drug for therapeutic purposes. It is unclear, however, whether such caution is also warranted when considering the atovaquone–proguanil combination. Clinical trials so far have failed to report resistance emergence following the recommended regimen of the combination. Mechanistic studies also seem to suggest a mode of drug action that would limit rapid resistance emergence. The industry's position appears to advance the atovaquone–proguanil combination as a prophylactic with treatment doses to be made available for drug-resistant malaria through a donation program *(81)*. It will be important to have an active postrelease surveillance program to monitor resistance emergence. As mentioned at the beginning of this chapter, this drug is unique because its mode of action and resistance are reasonably well understood before its widespread release.

It should be mentioned that the cost of atovaquone–proguanil at present is very high; this is the major factor for its limited use. It would be important to search for means to bring the cost down. Another area that would require further development concerns formulations of the atovaquone–proguanil combination suitable for patients who are unable to take the medication orally. Parenteral and/or suppository formulations could be highly valuable to treat severe multidrug-resistant malaria. It is tempting to end on a note of hope that the success of this selectively antimitochondrial drug will kindle further interest in research and development involving other compounds with similar mode of action.

ACKNOWLEDGMENTS

I wish to dedicate this chapter to the numerous researchers (now merged, discharged, and/or distributed) at the former Wellcome Research Laboratories and their collaborators whose foresight and perseverance brought forth this new antimalarial to the world from the brink of being dumped as a failure. I thank colleagues in my laboratory, both past and present, for their enthusiastic contributions. Work in my laboratory is supported by a grant from NIH (AI28398), which is gratefully acknowledged.

REFERENCES

1. Hudson AT, Dickins M, Ginger CD, Gutteridge WE, Holdich T, Hutchinson DBA, et al. 566C80: A broad spectrum anti-infective agent with activity against malaria and opportunistic infections in IDS patients. Drugs Exp Clin Res 1991;17:427–435.

2. Fry M, Pudney M. Site of action of the antimalarial hydroxynaphthoquinone, 2-[*trans*-4-(4'-chlorophenyl)cyclohexyl]-3-hydroxy-1,4–naphthoquinone (566C80). Biochem Pharmacol 1992;43:1545–1553.

3. Srivastava IK, Rottenberg H, Vaidya AB. Atovaquone, a broad spectrum antiparasitic drug, collapses mitochondrial membrane potential in a malarial parasite. J Biol Chem 1997;272: 3961–3966.

4. Hughes W, Leoung G, Kramer F, Bozzette SA, Safrin S, Frame P, et al. Comparison of atovaquone (566C80) with trimethoprim-sulfamethoxazole to treat Pneumocystis carinii pneumonia in patients with AIDS. N Engl J Med 1993;328:1521–1527.

5. Kovacs JA. Efficacy of atovaquone in treatment of toxoplasmosis in patients with AIDS. The NIAID–Clinical Center Intramural AIDS Program. Lancet 1992;340:637–638.

6. Chiodini PL, Conlon CP, Hutchinson DB, Farquhar JA, Hall AP, Peto TE. et al. Evaluation of atovaquone in the treatment of patients with uncomplicated *Plasmodium falciparum* malaria. J Antimicrob Chemother 1995;36:1073–1078.

7. Looareesuwan S, Viravan C, Webster HK, Kyle DE, Hutchinson DB, Canfield CJ. Clinical studies of atovaquone, alone or in combination with other antimalarial drugs, for treatment of acute uncomplicated malaria in Thailand. Am J Trop Med Hyg 1996;54:62–66.

8. Porter TH, Folkers, K. Antimetabolites of coenzyme Q: their potential application as antimalarials. Angew Chem (Engl) 1974;13:559–569.

9. Hudson AT. Lapinone, menoctone, hydroxyquinolinequionones and similar structures. In: Peters W, Richards WHG (eds). Handbook of Experimental Pharmacology, Vol 68, Antimalarial Drugs. New York: Springer-Verlag, 1984, pp. 343–361.

10. Hooker SC. Lomatiol. Part II. Its occurrence, constitution, relation to, and conversion into lapachol. Also a synthesis of lapachol. J Am Chem Soc 1936;58:1181–1190.

11. Fieser LF, Berliner E, Bondhus FJ, Chang FC, Dauben WG, Etlinger MG, et al. Naphthoquinone antimalarials. I–XVII. J Am Chem Soc 1948;70:3151–3244.

12. Fawaz G, Haddad FS. The effect of lapinone (M-2350) on *P. vivax* infection in man. Am J Trop Med Hyg 1951;31:569–571.

13. Fieser LF, Schirmer JP, Archer S, Lorenz PR, Pfaffenbach PII. Naphthoquinone antimalarials. XXIX. 2-Hydroxy-3-(ω-cyclohexylalkyl)-1,4-naphthoquinones. J Med Chem 1967;10:513–517.

14. Fieser LF, Nazer MZ, Archer S, Berberian DA, Slighter RG. Naphthoquinone antimalarials. XXX. 2-Hydroxy-3-[ω-(1-adamantyl)alkyl]-1,4-naphthoquinones. J Med Chem 1967; 10:517–521.

15. WHO Chemotherapy of Malaria and Resistance to Antimalarials; Report of a WHO Scientific Group. WHO Tech Rep Ser No. 529, Geneva: World Health Organization, 1973, p. 70.

16. McHardy N, Haigh AJB, Dolan TT. Chemotherapy of *Theileria parva* infection. Nature 1976;261:698–699.

17. McHardy N, Hudson AT, Morgan DWT, Rae DG, Dolan TT. Activity of 10 naphthoquinones, including parvaquone (993C) and menoctone, in cattle artificially infected with *Theileria parva*. Res Vet Sci 1983;35:347–352.

18. Hudson AT, Randall AW, Fry M, Ginger CD, Hill B, Latter VS, et al. Novel anti-malarial hydroxynaphthoquinones with potent broad spectrum anti-protozoal activity. Parasitology 1985;90:45–55.

19. Looareesuwan S, Chulay JD, Canfield CJ, Hutchinson DBA. Malarone (atovaquone and proguanil hydrochloride): a review of its clinical development for treatment of malaria. Am J Trop Med Hyg 1999;60:533–541.

20. Gassis S, Rathod PK. Frequency of drug resistance in *Plasmodium falciparum*: a nonsynergistic combination of 5-fluoroorotate and atovaquone suppresses in vitro resistance. Antimicrob Agents Chemother 1996;40:914–919.

21. Rathod PK, McErlean T, Lee PC. Variations in frequencies of drug resistance in *Plasmodium falciparum*. Proc Natl Acad Sci USA 1997;94:9389–9393.

22. Canfield CJ, Pudney M, Gutteridge WE. Interactions of atovaquone with other antimalarial drugs against *Plasmodium falciparum* in vitro. Exp Parasitol 1995;80:373–381.

23. Carrington HC, Crowther AF, Davey DG, Levi AA, Rose FL. A metabolite of "Paludrine" with high antimalarial activity. Nature 1951;168:1080.

24. Crowther AF, Levi AA. Proguanil-the isolation of a metabolite with high antimalarial activity. Br J Pharmacol 1953;8:93–97.

25. Watkins WM, Sixsmith DG, Chulay JD. The activity of proguanil and its metabolites, cycloguanil and *p*-chlorophenylbiguanide, against *Plasmodium falciparum* in vitro. Ann Trop Med Parasitol 1984;78:273–278.

26. Srivastava IK, Vaidya AB. A Mechanism for the synergistic antimalarial action of atovaquone and proguanil. Antimicrob Agents Chemother 1999;43:1334–1339.

27. Kremsner PG, Looareesuwan S, Chulay JD. Atovaquone and proguanil hydrochloride for treatment of malaria. J Travel Med 1999;6:S18–S20.

28. Radloff PD, Philipps J, Nkeyi M, Hutchinson DBA, Kremsner PG. Atovaquone and proguanil for *Plasmodium falciparum* malaria. Lancet 1996;340:1511–1514.

29. Radloff PD, Philipps J, Nkeyi M, Hutchinson DBA, Kremsner PG. Atovaquone plus proguanil is an effective treatment for *Plasmodium ovale* and *P. malariae* malaria. Trans R Soc Trop Med 1996;90:682.

30. de Alencar FE, Cerutti C Jr, Durlacher RR, Boulos M, Alves FP, Milhous W, et al. Atovaquone and proguanil for the treatment of malaria in Brazil. J Infect Dis 1997;175:1544–1547.

31. Sabchareon A, Attanath P, Phanuaksook P, Chanthavanich P, Poonpanich Y, Mookmanee D, et al. Efficacy and pharmacokinetics of atovaquone and proguanil in children with multidrug-resistant *Plasmodium falciparum* malaria. Trans R Soc Trop Med Hyg 1998;92:201–206.

32. Looareesuwan S, Wilairatana P, Chalermarut K, Rattanapong Y, Canfield CJ, Hutchinson D.B. Efficacy and safety of atovaquone/proguanil compared with mefloquine for treatment of acute *Plasmodium falciparum* malaria in Thailand. Am J Trop Med Hyg 1999;60:526–532.

33. Mulenga M, Sukwa T.Y, Canfield CJ, Hutchinson DB. Atovaquone and proguanil versus pyrimethamine/sulfadoxine for the treatment of acute falciparum malaria in Zambia. Clin Ther 1999;21:841–852.

34. Anabwani G, Canfield CJ, Hutchinson DB. Combination atovaquone and proguanil hydrochloride vs. halofantrine for treatment of acute *Plasmodium falciparum* malaria in children. Pediatr Infect Dis J 1999;18:456–461.

35. Bustos DG, Canfield CJ, Canete-Miguel E, Hutchinson DB. Atovaquone–proguanil compared with chloroquine and chloroquine–sulfadoxine–pyrimethamine for treatment of acute *Plasmodium falciparum* malaria in the Philippines. J Infect Dis 1999;179:1587–1590.

36. Looareesuwan S, Wilairatana P, Glanarongran R, Indravijit KA, Supeeranontha L, Chinnapha S, et al. Atovaquone and proguanil hydrochloride followed by primaquine for treatment of *Plasmodium* vivax malaria in Thailand. Trans R Soc Trop Med Hyg 1999;93:637–640.

37. Shanks GD, Gordon DM, Klotz FW, Aleman GM, Oloo AJ, Sadie D, et al. Efficacy and safety of atovaquone/proguanil as suppressive prophylaxis for *Plasmodium falciparum* malaria. Clin Infect Dis 1998;27:494–499.

38. Shanks GD, Kremsner PG, Sukwa TY, van der Berg JD, Shapiro TA, Scott TR, et al. Atovaquone and proguanil hydrochloride for prophylaxis of malaria. J Travel Med 1999;6:S21–S27.

39. Shapiro TA, Ranasinha CD, Kumar N, Barditch-Crovo P. Prophylactic activity of atovaquone against *Plasmodium falciparum* in humans. Am J Trop Med Hyg 1999;60:831–836.

40. Wendel WB. The influence of naphthoquinones upon the respiratory and carbohydrate metabolism of malarial parasites. Fed Proc 1946;5:406–407.

41. Ball EG, Anfinsen CB, Cooper O. The inhibitory action of naphthoquinones on respiratory processes. J Biol Chem 1947;169:257–270.

42. Fry M, Beesley JE. Mitochondria of mammalian *Plasmodium* species. Parasitology 1991;102:17–26.

43. Gutteridge WE, Dave D, Richards WHG. Conversion of dihydroorotate to orotate in parasitic protozoa. Biochim Biophys Acta 1979;582:390–401.

44. Vaidya AB. Mitochondrial physiology as a target for atovaquone and other antimalarials. In: Sherman IW. (ed). Malaria: Parasite Biology, Pathogenesis, and Protection Washington, DC: ASM, 1998, pp. 355–368.

45. Vaidya AB, Akella R, Suplick, K. Sequences similar to genes for two mitochondrial proteins and portions of ribosomal RNA in tandemly arrayed 6 kilobase pair DNA of a malarial parasite. Mol Biochem Parasitol 1989;35:97–107.

46. Vaidya AB, Lashgari MS, Pologe LG, Morrisey J. Structural features of *Plasmodium* cytochrome b that may underlie susceptibility to 8-aminoquinolines and hydroxnaphthoquinones. Mol Biochem Parasitol 1993;58:33–42.

47. Feagin JE. The extrachromosomal DNAs of apicomplexan parasites. Annu Rev Microbiol 1994;48:81–104.

48. Wilson RJ, Williamson DH. Extrachromosomal DNA in the Apicomplexa. Microbiol Mol Biol Rev 1997;61:1–16.

49. Zoratti M, Szabo I. The mitochondrial permeability transition. Biochim Biophys Acta 1995;1241:139–176.

50. Bernardi P. Mitochondrial transport of cations: channels, exchangers, and permeability transition. Physiol Rev 1999;79:1127–1155.

51. Susin SA, Zamzami N, Kroemer G. Mitochondria as regulators of apoptosis: doubt no more. Biochim Biophys Acta 1998;1366:151–165.

52. Halestrap AP, Connern CP, Griffiths EJ, Kerr PM. Cyclosporin A binding to mitochondrial cyclophilin inhibits the permeability transition pore and protects hearts from ischaemia/reperfusion injury. Mol Cell Biochem 1997;174:167–172.

53. Liu X, Kim CN, Yang J, Jemmerson PL, Wang X. Induction of apoptotic program in cell-free extracts: requirement for dATP and cytochrome c. Cell 1996;86:147–157.

54. Cornillon S, Foa C, Davoust J, Buonavista N, Gross JD, Golstein P. Programmed cell death in Dictyostelium. J Cell Sci 1994;107:2691–2704.

55. Ameisen JC. The origin of programmed cell death. Science 1996;272:1278–1279.

56. Christensen ST, Wheatley DN, Rasmussen MI, Rasmussen L. Mechanisms controlling death, survival and proliferation in a model eukaryote, Tetrahymena thermophila. Cell Death Differ 1995;2:301–308.

57. Welburn SC, Dale C, Ellis D, Beecroft R, Pearson TW. Apoptosis in procyclic Trypanosoma brucei rhodesiense in vitro. Cell Death Differ 1995;2:285–300.

58. Ridgley EL, Xiong ZH, Ruben L. Reactive oxygen species activate a Ca2+-dependent cell death pathway in the unicellular organism Trypanosoma brucei brucei. Biochem J 1999;340:33–40.

59. Hammond DJ, Burchell JR, Pudney M. Inhibition of pyrimidine biosynthesis de novo by 2-(4-*t*-butylcyclohexyl)-3-hydroxy-1,4-napthoquinone in vitro. Mol Biochem Parasitol 1985;14:97–109.

60. Helsby NA, Ward SA, Howell R.E, Breckenridge AM. The pharmacokinetics and activation of proguanil in man: consequences of variability in drug metabolism. Br J Clin Pharmacol 1990;30:287–291.

61. Ward SA, Helsby NA, Skjelbo E, Brosen K, Gram LF, Breckenridge AM. The activation of the biguanide antimalarial proguanil co-segregates with mephenytoin oxidation polymorphism—a panel study. Br Clin J Pharmacol 1991;31:689–692.

62. Helsby NA, Edwards G, Breckenridge AM, Ward SA. The multiple dose pharmacokinetics of proguanil. Br J Clin Pharmacol 1993;35:653–656

63. Schafer, G. Biguanides. A review of history, pharmacodynarmcs and therapy. Diabete Metab 1983;9:148–163.

64. Dunn CJ, Peters DH. Metformin. A review of its pharmacological properties and therapeutic use in non-insulin-dependent diabetes mellitus. Drugs 1995;49:721–749.

65. Schafer, G. Site specific uncoupling and inhibition of oxidative phosphorylation by biguanides. Biochim Biophys Acta 1969;172:334–337.

66. Kusaka MR, Setiabudy R, Chiba K, Ishizaki T. Simultaneous measurements of proguanil and its metabolites in human plasma and urine by reversed-phase high performance liquid chromatography:and its preliminary application in relation to genetically determined S-mephenytoin 4'-hydroxylation status. Am J Trop Med Hyg 1996;54,189–196.

67. Beerahee, M. Clinical pharmacology of atovaquone and proguanil hydrochloride. J Travel Med 1999;6:S13–S17.

68. Fidock DA, Wellems TE. Transformation with human dihydrofolate reductase renders malaria parasites insensitive to WR99210 but does not affect intrinsic activity of proguanil. Proc Natl Acad Sci USA 1997;94:10,931–10,936.

69. Srivastava IK, Morrisey JM, Darrouzet E, Daldal F, Vaidya AB. Resistance mutations reveal the atovaquone-binding domain of cytochrome b in malaria parasites. Mol Microbiol 1999;33:704–711.

70. Brasseur G, Saribas AS, Daldal F. A composition of mutations located in the cytochrome b subunit of the bacterial and mitochondrial bc_1 complex. Biochim Biophys Acta 1996;1275:61–69.

71. Walker DJ, Wakefield AE, Dohn MN, Miller RF, Baughman RP, Hossler PA, et al. Sequence polymorphisms in the Pneumocystis carinii cytochrome b gene and their association with atovaquone prophylaxis failure. J Infect Dis 1998;178:1767–1775.

72. Syafruddin D, Siregar JE, Marzuki S. Mutations in the cytochrome b gene of *Plasmodium berghei* conferring resistance to atovaquone. Mol Biochem Parasitol 1999;104:185–194.

73. Trumpower BL, Gennis RB. Energy transduction by cytochrome complexes in mitochondrial and bacterial respiration: the enzymology of coupling electron transfer reactions to transmembrane proton translocation. Annu Rev Biochem 1994;63:675–716.

74. Xia D, Yu CA, Kim H, Xia JZ, Kachurin AM, Zhang L, et al. Crystal structure of the cytochrome $bc1$ complex from bovine heart mitochondria. Science 1997;277:60–66.

75. Zhang Z, Huang L, Shulmeister VM, Chi YI, Kim KK, Hung LW, et al. Electron transfer by domain movement in cytochrome bc_1. Nature 1998;392:677–684.

76. Iwata S, Lee JW, Okada K, Lee JK, Iwata M, Rasmussen B, et al. Complete structure of the 11-subunit bovine mitochondrial cytochrome $bc1$ complex. Science 1998;281:64–71.

77. Kim H, Xia D, Yu CA, Xia JZ, Kachurin AM, Zhang L, et al. Inhibitor binding changes domain mobility in the iron–sulfur protein of the mitochondrial bc_1 complex from bovine heart. Proc Natl Acad Sci USA 1998;95:8026–8033.

78. McIntosh MT, Srivastava R, Vaidya AB. Divergent evolutionary constraints on mitochondrial and nuclear genomes of malaria parasites Mol Biochem Parasitol 1998;95:69–80.

79. Preiser PR, Wilson, RJM, Moore PW, McCready S, Hajibhageri MAN, Blight KJ, et al. Recombination associated with the replication of malarial mitochondrial DNA. EMBO J 1996;15:684–693.

80. Vaidya AB, Arasu P. Tandemly arranged gene clusters of malarial parasites that are highly conserved and transcribed. Mol Biochem Parasitol 1987;22:249–257.

81. Oyediran ABO, Heisler MH. Malarone donation program. J Travel Med 1999;6:S28–S30.

The Antimalarial Drug Portfolio and Research Pipeline

Piero L. Olliaro and Wilbur K. Milhous

INTRODUCTION

Drugs are the mainstay of malaria case management and prevention and this situation is unlikely to change in the foreseeable future. This chapter intends to give the following:

- A brief overview of the antimalarial drug pipeline, ranging from promising lead compounds to compounds in current use that are still undergoing research.
- A review of 7 specific drugs or drug classes.
- A discussion of the implications of drug discovery and development in view of the needs of malaria treatment and prevention. The broad research agenda should, in principle, investigate both opportunities leading to the next generation of antimalarial drugs (unrelated to existing ones, thus undamaged from cross-resistance) and how the antimalarial drugs we have already developed can be protected from resistance.

There is an ongoing debate as to whether the meager resources allocated for malaria should be used to develop new drugs or to improve access to existing drugs. The problem is that both are needed and are intimately linked. Until and unless drug deployment and use are improved, drugs will not reach the people in need of treatment, or when they do, irrational use and misuse will continue to erode the drugs' potential and create resistance. New drugs are needed, but the prospects are unpromising, mainly because malaria is not considered a profitable market for the pharmaceutical industry. Even when new drugs do become available, they are thrown in the same system that will curtail their life-span.

Antimalarial drug output of the 20th century is summarized in Table 1. Treatment and prevention of malaria still depend mostly on drugs discovered in the first half of the twentieth century or even earlier, as is the case for quinine.

The current portfolio of antimalarial drugs at various stages of research, development, and deployment for treatment and prophylaxis of malaria is summarized in Table 2. Traditional antimalarial drugs in current use are omitted. At first look, the pipeline would seem fairly rich and overall well balanced, with compounds at various stages of development. It is important though at this point to compare what R&D offers or intends to deliver to the essential needs for antimalarial chemotherapy. These are as follows:

- *Uncomplicated falciparum malaria.* Overreliance on the quinoline-type and folate inhibitor families of antimalarials has largely been the cause of the emergence and spread of cross-

From: *Antimalarial Chemotherapy: Mechanisms of Action, Resistance, and New Directions in Drug Discovery*
Edited by: P. J. Rosenthal © Humana Press Inc., Totowa, NJ

Table 1
Antimalarial Drug Output in the 20th Century

Drug	Approximate year in use
Quinine, pamaquine	1830–1930
Mepacrine, chloroquine	1930s
Proguanil, amodiaquine	1940s
Pyrimethamine, primaquine	1950s
Pyrimethamine–sulfa combinations	1960s
Artemisinin	1970s
Artesunate, artemether, pyronaridine, Mefloquine, halofantrine	1980s
Atovaquone–proguanil, artemether–lumefantrine, arteether	1990s

Note: Approximate dates at which drugs were registered or came into use. Registration in the country of origin does not imply wider availability. In the case of artemisinin-type compounds, use was limited to China for a long time; as of today, none of those products has been granted unrestricted marketing authorization by Western drug regulatory agencies, except arteether injectable. Pyronaridine is still registered in China only.

resistance among members of the same family. In general, the problem has been, and continues to be, that deployment is uncontrolled (a drug is put on the market as it becomes available) and exploited to—and sometimes beyond, as is the case for chloroquine—the point that it becomes ineffective. This problem is also compounded with lack of compliance to the prescribed regimen, which is often related to drug cost and inconvenient drug regimens (*see* also Chapter 5).
Protecting current and future drugs against resistance must be the primary objective.
New drugs with novel mechanisms of action to avoid cross-resistance are needed.
These regimens must be affordable and adapted to the conditions of use. For instance, we must consider differences between areas such as Africa and Southeast Asia in terms of specific problems (multidrug resistance in areas of Southeast Asia) and affordable costs.

- *Severe malaria.* Falciparum malaria evolves almost invariably to severe disease if left untreated. The patient eventually develops severe complications and dies if appropriate diagnosis and treatment is not established in time. Treatment is administered parenterally at least until the patient regains consciousness. Quinine and injectable artemisinin derivatives are currently used. A meta-analysis of studies comparing quinine to artemether showed that the two drugs are equivalent in preventing mortality and sequelae (*1,2*). However, quinine efficacy is fading in Thailand.

These and other studies confirm that mortality depends primarily on the delay in establishing the correct therapy; mortality and neurological sequelae are, in practice, relatively frequent despite the establishment of otherwise effective antimalarial therapy.

Thus, the current priority is not a new injectable drug, but rather to develop and implement alternative approaches to prevent progression to severe malaria. Research is also needed to better understand the pathogenesis of severe malaria in view of identifying adjunct treatments (in combination with antimalarial drugs).

HALOFANTRINE AND DESBUTYLHALOFANTRINE

The current formulation of halofantrine hydrochloride is poorly bioavailable (8–12%) and has highly variable pharmacokinetics. Potentially fatal cardiotoxicity has been reported. The two problems are related. Halofantrine produces EKG abnormalities (QTc prolongation) at the currently recommended dose in fasted individuals. Because of variable absorption, the currently recommended treatment probably overdoses the majority of patients to effectively treat all cases. Also, absorption can be improved by using fatty food, but then serum levels are unpredictable and often unacceptably high. High levels carry an increased risk of QTc changes and toxicity. Recent studies suggested that the second dose may be more toxic *(3)*, and confirmed an interaction between halofantrine and mefloquine *(4)*.

Thus, the problem that could not be resolved with halofantrine base has been to improve bioavailability in a predictable manner, limit interindividual and intraindividual variability, and reduce the absolute and total dose given, all to reduce the risk of cardiac adverse events without compromising efficacy. The proposed new formulations that have been identified would increase costs significantly, despite reduction in the cost of active substance (J. Horton, personal communication). A micronized formulation was tested and proved promising but was not further developed *(5)*.

Although cardiac toxicity is apparent with the parent drug, studies performed on isolated perfused animal hearts suggest that the desbutyl metabolite has minimal effect on QTc when compared with halofantrine or quinidine *(6)*. Halofantrine and desbutyl-halofantrine have similar intrinsic activities in vitro *(7)*. Pending the outcome of phase I studies, the metabolite could be a candidate replacement drug for halofantrine for treatment as well as prophylaxis alone or in combination with other drugs.

PYRONARIDINE

Pyronaridine (2-methoxy-7-chloro-10–[3',5'-bis-(pyrrolidinyl-1-methyl)-4'-hydroxy anilino] benzo-[*b*]-1,5-naphthyridine) is a Mannich-base antimalarial that has been synthesized and developed by the Institute of Parasitic Diseases, Academy of Preventive Medicine, Shanghai, China, and has been registered in that country since the 1980s *(8)*. However, none of the formulations studied (enteric-coated [EC] tablet [containing 175 mg of pyronaridine phosphate, corresponding to 100 mg of pyronaridine base]; capsules [100 and 50 mg of pyronaridine base]; and injection [80 mg base in 2 mL]) are registered outside China because of the failure to meet international regulatory standards. Moreover, the high cost-of-goods and the poor bioavailability of the Chinese oral formulations result in treatment costs (reportedly US$ 3–4) that make this drug unaffordable in most of the malarious areas of the world. In the mid-1990s a project was started by the UNDP/WB/WHO Special Programme for Research and Training in Tropical Diseases (TDR) that included a new capsule formulation and the upgrade of the dossier. After initial formulation studies and phase I and IIa trials, the project has not progressed, mostly because of the lack of a commercial partner and GMP material for regulatory studies *(8a)*.

Pyronaridine appears to be the most active compound of the Mannich-base family. An analysis of in vitro data on 798 isolates from various sources showed the following (P. Olliaro and J. Le Bras, unpublished data): (1) insignificant differences in the in vitro responses of parasite strains from Thailand and various African locations; (2) a moderate correlation between the median inhibitory concentrations (IC_{50}'s) to chloroquine and pyronaridine (r^2 ranging from 0.001 to 0.476). The correlation with mefloquine has not been characterized yet.

Pyronaridine is a blood schizontocide; gametocytocidal activity has been reported in vitro but not in vivo *(9)*. Its mechanism of action remains unclear. It is possible that pyronaridine acts via a common mechanism with other 4-aminoquinolines, by interfering with heme metabolism, probably by blocking hemozoin formation. Electron micro-

Table 2
Summary of Antimalarial Drugs in Development

Compounds	Route	Phase	Intended objective	Approach
Chemical modification, optimization of existing compounds				
Artemisinin derivatives				
Newer peroxide-bridge compounds			Improve efficacy; reduce cost-of-goods	Total synthesis
Artelinic acid	po	Phase I	Improve bioavailability	Protection against metabolism
Arteether	im	Registration	A product for Western regulatory authorization	GMP production
Chloroquine analogs	po	Predevelopment to phase I	Restore activity against resistant strains	Modified alkyl side chain of chloroquine; bisquinolines
Proguanil analogues	po		Activity against mutants, better therapeutic index	Synthesis of biguanide pro-drug
Primaquine analogs				
Tafenoquine, CDRI 80/53, newer 8-aminoquinolines	po	Predevelopment to registration	Improve therapeutic index of primaquine; optimize dosing schedule	Longer $t_{1/2}$, improved activity; lower toxicity
Desbutylhalofantrine	po		Avoid halofantrine toxicity; improve bioavailability	Synthesise halofantrine metabolite
Mannich base				
Pyronaridine	po		Improve activity against quinoline-resistant strains	A Mannich-base
Antifolates				
Chlorproguanil+dapsone	po		Activity against pyrimethamine–sulfa resistant strains	Short-lived compounds; relatively non-cross-resistant

222

New Drug Classes			
Atovaquone (plus proguanil)	po	A new target; overcome cross-resistance	A metabolically stable naphthoquinone
Inhibitors of phospholipid metabolism	po	A new target; overcome cross-resistance	
Resistance modifiers	po	Restore activity against resistant strains	Combination of chloroquine with efflux inhibitor
New formulations			
Rectal artesunate	ir	Prevent evolution to severe disease in non-*per-os* patients	A rectal formulation for use where parenteral drugs not available
Drug combinations			
Artemether+lumefantrine	po	Mutual protection	Fast-acting, short-lived drug + slower, longer-acting drug
Artesunate+mefloquine, chloroquine, amodiaquine, pyrimethamine/sulfa, etc.	po	Mutual protection; protect current first-line drugs; delay occurrence of resistance; reduce transmission?	

scopy findings confirm that the parasite digestive system is targeted *(10)*. Initial data suggesting that that the target of pyronaridine and other 9-anilinoacridines was the parasite topoisomerase II *(11)*, have been challenged by further experiments with acridine analogs *(12)*.

Almost all clinical studies published so far have used Chinese enteric-coated tablets. They disolve slowly in vitro (approximately 20% release after 15 h [V. Navaratnam and S. Ismail, personal communication]) and are poorly bioavailable (19 ± 7% as compared to intramuscular injection) with a C_{max} following oral administration of 600 mg 127.5 ng/mL, and the T_{max} of 14 h *(13)*. However, this formulation proved efficacious in Chinese and non-Chinese studies, including two recent trials in adults with uncomplicated falciparum malaria in Cameroon and Thailand *(14,15)*, and one in children in Cameroon *(16)*. In Cameroon, it proved 100% effective in 40 adult patients (at a total dose of 29–34 mg/kg [8 mg/kg in four administrations] over 3 d) and 41 pediatric cases. Chloroquine, used as the comparator drug, was only 44% effective in adults and 40% in children. In Thailand, two pyronaridine regimens (mean total dose 25.6 mg/kg over 3 d and 36.7 mg/kg over 5 d) were compared. The cure rates were 63% and 88%, respectively. Parasite clearance rates were similar in the two studies: 76.8 ± 14.6% in Cameroon; 86.7 ± 24.4% in Thailand, with the high-dose regimen. The different cure rates reported in Cameroon and Thailand may be partly explained by the different duration of follow-up: In the Thai study, 21 of the 22 recrudescent cases on either pyronaridine dosage were registered between d 14 and d 28 *(17)*.

More recently, two capsule strengths, 50 and 100 mg, were formulated at the University Sains Malaysia. The formulated product released 96.76 ± 4.23% and 101.14 ± 5.09, respectively, within 4–6 min, using the standard USP test (V. Navaratnam and S. Ismail, unpublished data). This formulation showed comparable absorption and pharmacokinetic profiles to a pyronaridine solution when administered at 6 mg/kg in a randomized, crossover phase I study. The mean C_{max} was 154.2 ng/mL (solution), 120.4 ng/mL (capsule); the elimination half-life (160.3 h for the solution and 191.2 h for the capsule formulation) appeared to be substantially longer than that reported in earlier studies with Chinese enteric-coated tablets. Drug levels during d 2– 6 ranged between 50 and 60 ng/mL (as compared to IC_{50} <21 nmol/L in field isolates). *(18)*

CHLORPROGUANIL–DAPSONE

This combination (also referred to as Lapdap) is being developed as a sulfadoxine–pyrimethamine (SP) replacement particularly for Africa. Chlorproguanil and dapsone are well-researched and cheap products, so their combination should be marketable at a low price.

Long elimination half-lives (about 100 and 200 h, respectively) are the paradoxical blessing and limitation of SP. On the one hand, the long half-lives are expected to provide a period of chemoprophylaxis after treatment, particularly sought after in high-transmission areas. On the other hand, they also cause the drug to exert strong selection pressure for resistance by specific point mutations in the dihydrofolate reductase (DHFR) and and dihydropteroate synthases (DHPS) genes. Historically, resistance to SP has developed soon after introduction of the drug for routine use. Conversely, a rapidly eliminated combination, like Lapdap (half-lives of 13 and 26 h for chlorproguanil and dapsone, respectively) would have little or no chemoprophylactic effect, but is also expected to be less vulnerable to antifolate resistance. This has been confirmed in the clinical setting *(19)*. Moreover, resistance to DHFR inhibitors is relatively drug-specific. The mutations primarily involved in resistance to chlorcycloguanil (DHFR paired point mutations S108T/A16V, or I164L/S108N) occur at low frequency in Africa whereas those for pyrimethamine (DHFR S108N, N51I, C59R) are common especially in East Africa *(20)*. Although the high prevalence of DHFR mutants containing I164L in Southeast Asia makes Lapdap ineffective in those regions *(21)*, the drug remains effective in treating SP failures in East Africa. However, the question was raised recently as to whether Lapdap's lifespan would already be endangered by current levels of SP resistance in East Africa and whether it should be protected from the time of deployment through a combination with an artemisinin derivative (see next section).

Preliminary work was conducted in the late 1980s in Kenya, suggesting that a single dose of Lapdap (chlorproguanil 1.2 mg/kg, dapsone 2.4 mg/kg) had comparable efficacy to standard SP *(22)*. Those doses were expected to provide plasma levels exceeding inhibitory concentrations for approximately 6 d *(23)*.

A more recent double-blind trial compared one dose of Lapdap (1.2 mg/kg, and 2.4 mg/kg, respectively) followed by placebo on d 1 and 2 (CD1 group), to three doses at 24-h intervals (CD3 group), and to SP (1.25 mg/kg and 25 mg/kg) with placebo on d 1 and 2 (SP group) in symptomatic falciparum malaria. A community control group was employed to estimate the monthly incidence of new parasitemia. All treatment groups were effective in achieving initial clearance of parasites: by d 7, slides were negative in 93.4, 98.0, and 99.3% of groups CD1, CD3, and SP, respectively. However, in comparison with the control group, the relative risk of new parasitemia during follow-up was 2.1, 1.3, and 0.63 for groups CD1, CD3, and SP, respectively *(24)*.

A dose-raising tolerance study in healthy volunteers selected a new dose regimen of 2 mg/kg and 2.4 mg/kg for chlorproguanil and dapsone, respectively, for further clinical testing in an ongoing two-center double-blind trial in Kenya and Malawi. Children with uncomplicated falciparum malaria are being randomized to either three doses of Lapdap or one dose of SP (followed by two doses of placebo); they are reviewed on d 7 to ensure clearance of parasitemia and are then actively followed for 12 mo. The protocol calls for every episode of uncomplicated malaria to be retreated with the study medication. The principal objectives of this ongoing trial are measurement of (1) the annual incidence of clinical malaria and (2) failure of therapy, with each drug regimen (P. Winstanley, personal communication).

THIRD-GENERATION ANTIFOLATE ANTIMALARIAL DRUG COMBINATIONS

Observations on the lack of complete cross-resistance of proguanil analogs and their triazine metabolites have stimulated interest in DHFR inhibitors in combination with DHPS inhibitors for development as third-generation "Fansidar (SP)-like" drugs. In addition, adverse drug reaction registers in Sweden and the United Kingdom *(25)* suggest less risk for severe allergic reactions with companion sulfa drugs, which have elimination half-lives such as dapsone rather than sulfa drugs with long half-lives, such as sulfadoxine. Reports of allergic reactions to SP resulted in withdrawal of recommendations for use in malarial prophylaxis *(26)*. Although a second-generation LapDap combination may present an inexpensive SP replacement drug for treatment in Africa, studies from Thailand continue to suggest poor treatment efficacy against multidrug resistant-strains. Simple *para*-chloro substitutions in chlorproguanil synthesis result in only a threefold increase in intrinsic activity over proguanil or cycloguanil, whereas the more active triazine WR99210 exhibits extraordinary activity against all resistant strains. The development of WR99210 was abandoned because of gastrointestinal intolerance and poor bioavailability, as well as early assumptions made about possible cross-resistance among other antifolates. As methods for elucidating the molecular basis of resistance in DHFR inhibitors evolved, interest peaked with the synthesis of the biguanide pro-drug WR250417 (PS-15) which obviated the problems with bioavailablity. This drug was less toxic and more efficacious that proguanil in vitro and in animal studies *(27)*. Intensified surveillance will determine if new point mutations in DHFR will eventually confer resistance to the active triazines. In the meantime, lead optimization should continue to facilitate selection of more potent and less toxic biguanide "pro-drugs." Drugs may be formulated in combination with dapsone for treatment as well as prophylaxis of multidrug-resistant strains in travelers.

RECTAL ARTESUNATE

Rectal formulations of artemisinin and its derivatives have been used for quite some time *(28)*, albeit, in most cases, their utility has been severely limited by lack of stability in a hot climate. A formulation of artesunate as suspension in soft gelatin capsule for rectal use appears to have advantages over traditional suppositories. Its bioavailability compares well with the oral route, although after oral administration, artesunate was more rapidly absorbed and converted into its bioactive metabolite, dihydroartemisinin *(29)*.

The rectal artesunate formulation has been tested primarily in sequential combination with oral mefloquine for the treatment of (moderately) severe malaria in Thailand *(30,31)*. When the results of two studies are compared (P. Olliaro, S. Looareesuwann, and V. Navaratnam, unpublished data), there appears to be no obvious advantage of intense dosing during the early part of treatment. Four doses within the first 12 h (at start, 4, 8, and 12 h) of treatment and two doses (at start and 12 h) produced comparable reduction of parasitemia and sustained clearance at d 28. The only significant difference was a faster time to parasite clearance with 1600 mg (eight doses of 200 mg over 60 h) than with 1200 mg (six doses). In general, parasite reduction rates were lower than those with oral artesunate for uncomplicated malaria. The apparent difference could be the result of either the different severity of disease or the relative disposition and bioavailability of the rectal and oral formulations.

More recently, attention on rectal artesunate has focused on the potential life-saving benefits of using this formulation in *non per os* malaria patients, where no parenteral administration of antimalarials is possible or safe, to cover a patient en route to hospital. Studies are being conducted to support international registration of the drug for such an indication *(32)*.

ARTELINIC ACID

Artelinic acid is an artemisinin derivative being developed by the Walter Reed Army Institute of Research for oral treatment of uncomplicated malaria *(33)*. The drug has the added advantage that it can also be formulated for intravenous injection to treat severe and complicated disease as a replacement drug for quinidine gluconate. Intravenous quinine is not approved for use in the United States, and there are growing public health concerns about access to quinidine gluconate as its availability dwindles with the introduction of more effective cardioactive drugs. Artelinic acid is more stable than artesunate in solution and is expected to have a longer shelf life. Arlelinic acid is believed to have a lower potential for neurotoxicity than arteether, because it is only partially metabolized to dihydroartemisinin, the putative neurotoxin implicated in neurotoxicity of the arteminsinin class of drugs. Safety profiles and regulatory approval of all artemisinin-type drugs are tainted by reports of dose-dependent brainstem neuropathology in animal models *(34,35)*. A confounder in the development process is that drug-induced neurologic side effects will be difficult to discriminate from those of severe and complicated malaria. Surrogate models could serve to predict relationships between auditory function and drug-induced neuropathology. Auditory discrimination tasks are currently being used to provide for objective behavioral measurements of neurotoxicity and it is hoped that these models will serve as valuable tools for safety assessment of candidate drugs *(36)*.

DRUG COMBINATIONS INCLUDING ARTEMISININ DERIVATIVES

Increasing attention is being given to resistance as the prime determinant of a drug's life span of effective use. Strategies for protecting both the drugs in use and drugs to come against the emergence of resistance are thus becoming of the greatest priority. The emergence of parasite resistance to drugs is almost inevitable, and the factors involved are only partly known *(37)*. Combining drugs is an approach that has been tried traditionally with fixed combinations of antifolates such as pyrimethamine plus sulfadoxine (plus mefloquine) or plus dapsone, and, more recently, with chlorproguanil plus dapsone and with atovaquone plus proguanil. The principle behind the choice of compounds for combinations is that they act synergistically.

More recently, artemisinin-type compounds have been combined with other antimalarial drugs. The rationale for including artemisinin derivatives in the combination is in their advantage in reducing the parasite biomass and gametocyte carriage *(38)*. They reduce *Plasmodium falciparum* biomass by 100,000 fold per asexual life cycle, compared to 100- to 1000-fold for other antimalarial drugs. Thus only the residuum of parasites (maximum of 10^5 parasites) is exposed to the second drug alone, reducing selective pressure for the emergence of resistance. Moreover, they also reduce gametocyte carriage, thus also the selection pressure for the spread of resistance. Irrespective of very short residence times in the organism, artemisinin-type compounds do not need intense schedules of administration. However, when used alone, they should be administered for 7 d, which is obviously impractical. In contrast, 3 d regimens are highly efficacious when combined with other drugs such as mefloquine *(39)*. The introduction of a regimen including artesunate at 4 mg/kg/d for 3 d plus mefloquine at 25 mg/kg in two divided doses on d 1 and 2 in an area where mefloquine resistance averaged 30% has resulted in restored efficacy and reduced transmission *(40,40a)*.

Randomized, placebo-controlled, double-blinded studies are underway to assess the safety and efficacy of combinations of artesunate with one of the currently used antimalarial drugs in large numbers of patients in various epidemiological settings across Africa and elsewhere. The first of these studies compared SP alone to SP combined with either 1-d (4 mg/kg) or 3-d artesunate treatment (total dose 12 mg/kg) in 600 Gambian children under 10 yr of age. Both combination regimens were significantly more effective than single-agent SP in clearing parasites faster and reducing gameto-cyte carriage. However, in this area, where parasites are SP sensitive, only the 3-d regimen proved significantly superior to SP alone (28-d failure rates = 7.3 and 2.1%, respectively) *(41)*.

ARTEMETHER PLUS LUMEFANTRINE

A fixed combination of artemether (20 mg) and lumefantrine (150 mg) has been developed by the Chinese Academy of Medical Sciences and Novartis. As of the end of 1999, it has been registered in Switzerland, the United Kingdom (marketed as Riamet®), and some 16 malaria-endemic countries (as Coartem®) for the treatment of adults and children with acute, uncomplicated malaria. The prices of the two products differ significantly.

The principle of this combination is to combine a rapid-acting, short-lived drug (artemether) with a long-resident drug (lumefantrine $t_{1/2}$ = 40–105 h), thus achieving rapid parasite and fever clearance, protecting either drug against resistance, and preventing recrudescence after artemether therapy. Lumefantrine, previously referred to as benflumetol, is an aryl amino alcohol blood schizonticide that probably acts by inhibiting hemozoin formation.

The product has been tested clinically in a total of approx 1900 patients in 15 clinical trials conducted in China, India, Gambia, Tanzania, Thailand, and Europe. Of these trials, nine were randomized, double-blinded comparisons with chloroquine, SP, quinine, quinine–SP, halofantrine, mefloquine, or artesunate–mefloquine.

Whereas a four-dose regimen produced 28-d cure rates over 95% in areas of known chloroquine resistance, the same regimen was efficacious in only 76.5% of cases in areas of multidrug resistance in Thailand, and was significantly inferior to mefloquine and artesunate–mefloquine. In the same areas, a six-dose regimen gave 28-d cure rates over 97%. Thus, the manufacturer's recommended regimens vary with the immunity of the patients and probability of multidrug-resistant malaria *(41a,b)*.

TAFENOQUINE

Tafenoquine (SB252263 or WR238605) is an 8-aminoquinoline analog of primaquine, a drug with a narrow therapeutic index. The history and rationale of tafenoquine's development *(42)* by the United States Army Medical and Materiel Command along with codevelopment partner Smith Kline Beecham Pharmaceuticals are presented in detail in Chapter 7. Preclinical and clinical evaluations demonstrated that this drug has excellent oral bioavailability and improved efficacy, reduced toxicity, and a better half-life than primaquine. Pharmacokinetic studies demonstrated that tafenoquine has a half-life of 2–3 wk in healthy volunteers. With significant activity against hepatic stages of both *vivax* and *falciparum* malaria, it is expected that long-term dosing in travelers may be discontinued as soon as exposure has ended. This causal prophylactic activity makes the drug unique from other suppressive prophylactic drug regimens. The drug has completed phase II studies in Africa and Thailand and phase III studies are planned.

Interestingly, the blood-stage activity of tafenoquine has been attributed to the inhibition of the putative mode of action of chloroquine hematin. In studies comparing the in vitro activity of chloroquine and 15, 8-aminoquinoline candidate drugs (including tafenoquine and primaquine), tafenoquine was the most active. Although tafenoquine's mechansim of action may be "chloroquine-like," the drug is more active against chloroquine-resistant strains. In defining the structure–activity relationships of various 8-aminoquinoline drugs, tafenoquine exhibited equivalent activity (in vitro IC_{50}- 0.7–1.5 µM) to that of primaquine against chloroquine-susceptible strains, but chloroquine–resistant and multidrug (mefloquine, pyrimethamine)-resistant strains were considerably more susceptible, with IC_{50}'s ranging from 0.06 to 0.3 µM. These observations prompted a retrospective comparison of tafenoquine against mefloquine in strains acquired by the Armed Forced Medical Research Institute in the Medical Sciences in Thailand (unpublished data). Resistance to mefloquine and subsequent cross-resistance to halofantrine in Thailand has been emerging in Thailand since mefloquine's introduction in Indochina (*43*). Evaluation for the cross-resistance of 48 strains collected during the period 1988–1992 demonstrated a correlation ($R^2 = 0.6299$) between mefloquine and halofantrine, but no correlation between tafenoquine and mefloquine, tafenoquine and halofantrine, or tafenoquine and quinine. Accordingly, the "anti-multidrug-resistance" properties of tafenoquine and other 8-aminoquinolines merit special attention for elucidating structure–activity relationships.

CONCLUSIONS

The ever-increasing demand for new antimalarials is primarily driven by the relentless pace at which parasite resistance emerges and spreads. However, the output of new antimalarials will never keep pace with the loss of drugs because of the emergence of resistance. The nature of malaria, its prevalence in the developing world, the lack of financial incentives, and the consequent lack of interest by the Western pharmaceutical industry all call for innovative approaches to develop new affordable drugs and to safeguard the available ones. Several considerations follow.

1. Resistance is the prime determinant of a drug's life-span. Protecting the effective use of a drug must rank number one in priority for research and control programs.
2. Rational deployment when a drug is first introduced for use and sensible prescribing are effective measures of protecting drug efficacy. In analogy with other diseases, "extra mileage" may be obtained from available compounds by utilizing drug combinations and rotating the use of antimalarials.
3. Novelty in chemical structure and mechanisms of action should guide the choice of leads in discovery programs.
4. The time frame from discovery through development, to clinical trials and drug registration is such that most of the compounds currently in the discovery pipeline cannot be expected to be available for general use in the near future. New approaches are needed in developing new drugs for tropical diseases, including both preregistration and postregistration activities. The efficiency of the development process must be improved and cost and times reduced while maintaining a quality standard for the resulting products to withstand international registration.

REFERENCES

1. McIntosh H, Olliaro P. Artemisinin derivatives for treating severe malaria. Cochrane Database Syst Rev 2000;2:cd000527.
2. The Artemether–Quinine Meta-analysis Study Group. A meta-analysis of trials comparing artemether with quinine in the treatment of severe falciparum malaria using individual patient data. Report to TDR and Wellcome Trust, 1999.

3. Touze JE, Bernard J, Keundjian A, Imbert P, Viguier A, Chaudet H, et al. Electrocardio-graphic changes and halofantrine plasma level during acute falciparum malaria.Am J Trop Med Hyg 1996;54:225–228.

4. Nosten F, ter Kuile FO, Luxemburger C, Woodrow C, Kyle DE, Chongsuphajaisiddhi T, et al. Cardiac effects of antimalarial treatment with halofantrine Lancet 1993;341(8852):1054–1056.

5. Ramsay AR, Msaki EP, Kennedy N, Ngowi FI, Gillespie SH. Evaluation of the safety and efficacy of micronized halofantrine in the treatment of semi-immune patients with acute, *Plasmodium falciparum* malaria. Ann Trop Med Parasitol 1996;90(5):461–466.

6. Woosley R, Wesche DL, Schuster BG. Method of treating malaria with desbutylhalo-fantrine. US Patent 5,711,966 (1998).

7. Basco LK, Gillotin C, Gimenez F, Farinotti R, Le Bras J. Antimalarial activity in vitro of the *n*-desbutyl derivative of halofantrine. Tran Roy Soc Trop Med Hyg. 1992;86:12–13.

8. Fu S, Xiao SH. Pyronaridine: a new antimalarial drug. Parasitol Today 1991;7:310–312.

8a. Olliaro P. Pyronaridine development at a standstill: no one prepared to foot the bill? A review of Chinese development and more recent studies. Curr Opin Infect Dis 2000;2(1):71–75.

9. Ringwald P, Meche FS, Basco LK. Short report: effects of pyronaridine on gameto-cytes in patients with acute uncomplicated falciparum malaria. Am J Trop Med Hyg 1999;61(3):446–448.

10. Kawai S, Kano S, Chang C, Suzuki M. The effects of pyronaridine on the morphology of *Plasmodium falciparum* in Aotus trivirgatus. Am J Trop Med Hyg 1996;55(2):223–229.

11. Chavalitshewikoon P, Wilairatana P, Gamage S, Dennis W, Figgit D, Ralph R. Structure–activity relationship and modes of action of 9-anilinoacridines against chloroquine-resistant Plasmodium falciparum *in vitro*. Antimicrob Agents Chemother 1993;37:403–406.

12. Wilairat P, Petmitr P, Pongvilairat G. XIV International Congress for tropical Medicine and Malaria, Nagasaki, 1996.

13. Feng Z, Wu ZF, Wang CY, Jiang NX. Pharmacokinetics of pyronaridine in malaria patients Chung Kuo Yao Li Hsueh Pao 1987;8(6):543–546.

14. Ringwald P, Bickii J, Basco L. Randomised trial of pyronaridine versus choroquine for acute uncomplicated falciparum malaria in Africa. Lancet. 1996;347:24–28.

15. Looareesuwan S, Kyle D, Viravan C, Vanijanta S, Wilairat P, Wernsdorfer W. Clinical study of pyronaridine for the treatment of acute uncomplicated falciparum malaria in Thailand. Am J Trop Med Hyg 1996;54:205–209.

16. Ringwald P, Bickii J, Basco LK. Efficacy of oral pyronaridine for the treatment of acute uncomplicated falciparum malaria in African children. Clin Infect Dis 1998;26(4):946–953.

17. Looareesuwan S, Olliaro P, Kyle D, Wernsdorfer W. Pyronaridine. Lancet 1996;247:1189–1190.

18. Navaratnam V, Looareesuwan S, Ismail S, Jamyaraman SD, Chinwongprom K, Mansor SM, et al. Comparative single-dose pharmacokinetics of pyronaridine solution and a new capsule formulation in healthy normal volunteers (HNVs). Am J Trop Med Hyg 1997; 57(3)(Suppl):104 (abstract).

19. Curtis J, Duraisingh MT, Warhurst DC. In vivo selection for a specific genotype of dihydropteroate synthetase of *Plasmodium falciparum* by pyrimethamine-sulfadoxine but not chlorproguanil–dapsone treatment. J Infect Dis 1998;177(5):1429–1433.

20. Khan B, Omar S, Kanyara JN, Warren-Perry M, Nyalwidhe J, Peterson DS, et al. Antifolate drug resistance and point mutations in *Plasmodium falciparum* in Kenya. Trans R Soc Trop Med Hyg 1997;91(4):456–460.

21. Wilairatana P, Kyle DE, Looareesuwan S, Chinwongprom K, Amradee S, White NJ, et al. Poor efficacy of antimalarial biguanide–dapsone combinations in the treatment of acute, uncom-plicated, falciparum malaria in Thailand. Ann Trop Med Parasitol 1997;91(2):125–132.

22. Watkins WM, Brandling-Bennett AD, Nevill CG, Carter JY, Boriga DA, Howells RE, et al. Chlorproguanil/dapsone for the treatment of non-severe *Plasmodium falciparum* malaria in Kenya: a pilot study. Trans R Soc Trop Med Hyg 1988;82(3):398–403.

23. Winstanley P, Watkins W, Muhia D, Szwandt S, Amukoye E, Marsh K. Chlorproguanil/dapsone for uncomplicated *Plasmodium falciparum* malaria in young children: pharmacokinetics and therapeutic range. Trans R Soc Trop Med Hyg 1997;91(3): 322–3227.

24. Amukoye E, Winstanley PA, Watkins WM, Snow RW, Hatcher J, Mosobo M, et al. Chlorproguanil-dapsone: effective treatment for uncomplicated falciparum malaria. Antimicrob Agents Chemother 1997;41(10):2261–2264.

25. Bjorkman A, Phillips-Howard PA. Adverse reactions to sulfa drugs: implications for malaria chemotherapy. Bull WHO 1991;69:297–304.

26. CDC. Adverse reactions to Fansidar and updated recommendations for its use in the prevention of malaria. MMWR 1985;33:713–714.

27. Canfield CJ, Milhous WK, Ager AL, Rossan RN, Sweeney TR, Lewis NJ, et al. PS-15: a potent, orally active antimalarial from a new class of folic acid antagonists. Am J Trop Med Hyg 1993;49:121–126.

28. Cao XT, Bethell DB, Pham TP, Ta TT, Tran TN, Nguyen TT, et al. Comparison of artemisinin suppositories, intramuscular artesunate and intravenous quinine for the treatment of severe childhood malaria. Trans R Soc Trop Med Hyg 1997;91(3): 335–342.

29. Navaratnam V, Mansor SM, Mordi MN, et al. Comparative pharmacokinetic study of oral and rectal formulations of artesunic acid in healthy volunteers. Eur J Clin Pharmacol 1998;54:411–414.

30. Looareesuwan S, Wilairatana P, Vanijanonta S, Viravan C, Andrial M. Efficacy and tolerability of a sequential, artesunate suppository plus mefloquine, treatment of severe falciparum malaria. Ann Trop Med Parasitol. 1995; 89(5): 469–475.

31. Looareesuwan S, Wilairatana P, Molunto W, Chalermrut K, Olliaro P, Andrial M. A comparative clinical trial of sequential treatments of severe malaria with artesunate suppository followed by mefloquine in Thailand. Am J Trop Med Hyg 1997;57(3):348–353.

32. Gomes M, Olliaro P, Folb P. What role can public health institutions play in drug development for the poor? A case study of artesunate. Med Trop (Marseille) 1998;58(Suppl 3):97–100.

33. Lin AJ, Klayman DL, Milhous WK. Antimalarial activity of new water soluble dihydroartemisinin derivatives. J Med Chem 1987;30:2147–2150.

34. Brewer TG, Grate SJ, Peggins JO, Weina PJ, Peetras BS, Heiffer MH, et al. Fatal neurotoxicity of arteether and artemeter. Am J Trop Med Hyg 1994;5:251–259.

35. Genovese RF, Newman DB, Li Q, Peggin JO, Brewer TG. Dose-dependent brainstem neutopathology following repeated arteether administation in rats. Brain Res Bull 1998;45:199–202.

36. Genovese RF, Newman DB, Petras JM, Brewer TG. Behavioral and neural toxicity of arteether in rats. Pharm Biochem Behav 1998;60:449–458.

37. White NJ, Olliaro P. Strategies for the prevention of antimalarial drug resistance: rationale for combination chemotherapy for malaria. Parasitol Today, 1996;12(19):399–401.

38. White NJ. Preventing antimalarial drug resistance through drug combinations. Drug Resist Updates 1998;1:3–9.

39. McIntosh H, Olliaro P. Artemisinin derivatives for treating uncomplicated malaria. Cochrane Database Syst Rev 2000;2:CD000256.

40. Price, R.N, Nosten F, Luxemburger C, van Vugt M, Phaipun L, Chongsuphajaisiddhi T, et al. Artesunate/mefloquine treatment of multi-drug resistant falciparum malaria. Trans R Soc Trop Med Hyg 1997;91:574–577.

40a. Nosten F, van Vugt M, Price R, Luxemburger C, Thway KL, Brockman A, et al. Effect of artesunate-mefloquine combination of incidence of Plasmodium falciparum malaria and mefloquine resistance in western Thailand: as prospective study. Lancet 2000;356:297–302.

41. von Seidlein L, Milligan P, Bojang K, Anyalebechi C, Gosling R, Coleman R, et al. A randomized, placebo-controlled, double-blind trial of artesunate plus pyrimethamine/sulfadoxine combinations in African children with uncomplicated malaria. The Lancet 2000;355(9201):352–357.

41a. van Vugt M, Brockman A, Gemperli B, Luxemburger C, Gathmann I, Royce C, Slight T, et al. Randomized comparison of artemether-benflumetol and artesunate-mefloquine in treatment of multidrug-resistant falciparum malaria. Antimicrob Agents Chemother 1998;42(1):135–139.

42a. van Vugt M, Wilairatana P, Gemperli B, Gathmann I, Phaipun L, Brockman A, et al. Efficacy of six doses of artemether-lumefantrine (benflumetol) in multi-drug-resistant falciparum malaria. Am J Trop Med Hyg 1999;60(6):936–942.

42. Peters, W. The evolution of tafenoquine—antimalarial for a new millennium. Trans R Soc Med 1999;92:345–352.

43. Wongsrichanalai C, Webster HK, Wimonwattrawatee T, Sookto P, Chuanak N, Thimasarn K, et al. Emergence of multidrug-resistant Plasmodium falciparum in Thailand: in vitro tracking. Am J Trop Med Hyg 1992;47(1):112–116.

III
New Compounds, New Approaches, and New Targets

13

Novel Quinoline Antimalarials

Paul A. Stocks, Kaylene J. Raynes, and Stephen A. Ward

INTRODUCTION

Since the first total synthesis of a quinoline-based antimalarial in the early part of this century, thousands of chemical analogs have been synthesized and screened for biological activity against malaria *(1)*. However, despite the evaluation of such a vast library of potential drug candidates we are still unsure about the essential pharmacophore and our understanding of their mechanisms of action are rudimentary and surrounded in controversy. So, as we move into the 21st century, we find ourselves relying on quinoline-based treatments for malaria that are empirically derived and based on original leads from the 1930s and 1940s. In addition, the emergence of pervasive strains of *Plasmodium falciparum* resistant to quinoline-based drugs has further brought into question the utility of this class of drug as a global solution to malaria infection *(2)*. In defense of this class of drug, it is clear that they target a biological process that is totally unique to the malarial parasite, resulting in selectivity and limited host toxicity. Further, if we look at chloroquine, it is clear that the parasite has found it difficult to acquire resistance to this drug (resistance first reported some 15–20 yr after its introduction into use and following many millions of parasite drug exposures) *(3)*. The degree of in vitro chloroquine resistance appears to peak in the 250- to 300-nM range as reported as early as the mid 1970s, and despite the continued geographical spread of resistant isolates and the continued widespread use of the drug in many parts of the world, the degree of resistance never exceeds these values. This may suggest that the resistance mechanism(s) is already operational at its maximal potential. As with the mechanism of action, mechanisms of resistance are also poorly understood. As such we do not know if it is possible to redesign the molecule to circumvent resistance although the literature suggests this is a possibility, as we will discuss. Despite these reservations, the desperate need for new antimalarials coupled with the historical benefits of the quinolines in terms of selective activity and clinical efficacy (in the absence of resistance), limited host toxicity, ease of use, and affordability have prompted a number of groups to pursue the search for novel quinoline-based antimalarials. In recent years, a number of chemical classes of drugs have been investigated including 8-aminoquinolines, 4-aminoquinolines, bisquinolines, and quinolinemethanols. In many cases, investigators have attempted to apply rational drug design strategies to their programs based on our limited understanding of drug action and resistance. The design of

From: *Antimalarial Chemotherapy: Mechanisms of Action, Resistance, and New Directions in Drug Discovery*
Edited by: P. J. Rosenthal © Humana Press Inc., Totowa, NJ

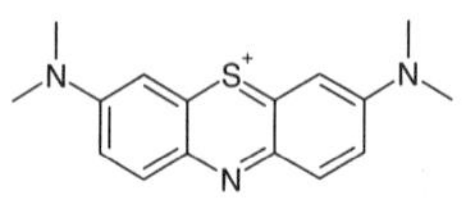

1 methylene blue

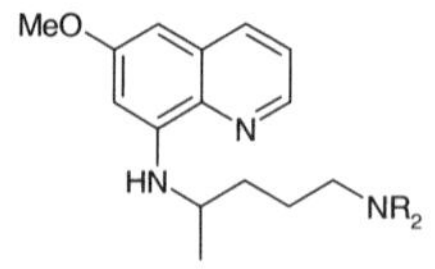

2 R = Et, pamaquine
3 R = H, primaquine

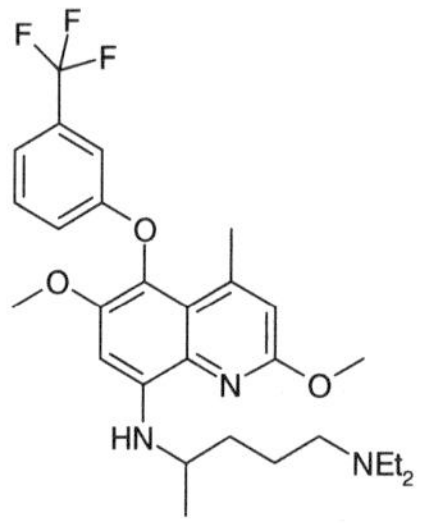

4 tafenoquine

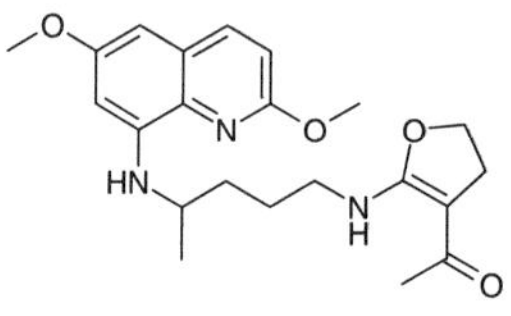

5

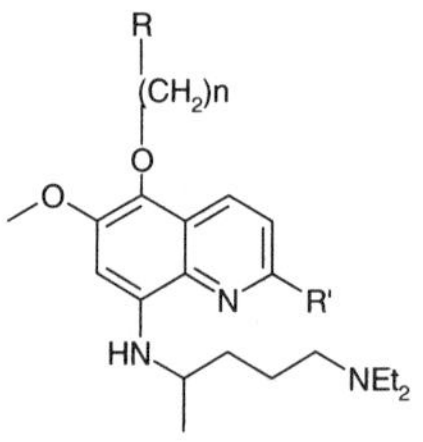

6

Scheme I

aminoquinoline drugs that contain structural features for activity against resistant strains but also functionality to aid in the prevention of toxicity through selective parasite accumulation is one such potentially powerful approach to the generation of compounds that can be used for both malarial prophylaxis and treatment. In this chapter, we will consider recent examples in the development of novel quinoline-based antimalarial drugs that we hope will convince the reader that this class of antimalarial still has a promising future.

8-AMINOQUINOLINES

The development of synthetic quinoline-based antimalarial drugs began with the discovery of the chemotherapeutic effects of methylene blue (**1**) (Scheme I) on human malaria made by Guttman and Ehrlich *(4)*. It was subsequently shown that replacing the methyl group with a basic side chain improved activity. The logical extension of this work was to attach similar basic side chains to a number of unrelated heterocyclic ring systems, including the quinoline ring. This strategy ultimately led to the development of the first synthetic quinoline-based antimalarials, pamaquine (**2**) and primaquine (**3**) in the 1920s *(5)*. Pamaquine (**2**) was shown to be very active, but was later dropped because of unacceptable toxicity. Primaquine (**3**) was synthesized as a less toxic analog and is the standard drug to eradicate liver forms of *Plasmodium vivax* and *P. ovale*; however, the clinical usefulness of this derivative against erythrocytic stages was limited because of poor efficacy and, to a lesser extent, its hematological toxicity *(6)*. The hemotoxicity of primaquine is thought to result from oxidative metabolism to the ring hydroxylated metabolites, 5-hydroxyprimaquine and 5,6-dihydroxylprimaquine. Several attempts have been made to redesign the primaquine molecule to limit the potential for reactive metabolite formation while retaining antiparasitic activity. One such attempt was the fluorination of the parent molecule at the 5-position; unfortunately, this derivative still displayed significant bioactivation in vitro *(7)*.

During the last decade, substantial efforts have been made to identify 8-aminoquinolines that have a better therapeutic indices than that of primaquine **(3)** and that exhibit activity against blood stage parasites at therapeutically achievable concentrations *(8,9)*. From these studies, tafenoquine (etaquine, WR 238605) **(4)** was introduced for development. Initial clinical studies in Thailand have shown that tafenoquine **(4)** is well tolerated, more efficacious, and has a longer half-life than primaquine *(10)*. The compound is also a causal prophylactic agent, preventing the development of malaria parasites in the liver and the consequent development of a blood-stage infection, as well as exerting direct effects against all bloods stages *(11)*. Another 8-aminoquinoline, which has been in preclinical trials, is CDRI 80/53 **(5)**. This derivative differs from primaquine only by the 2,4-dihydrofuran group present in the basic side chain anchored onto the quinoline nucleus in the 8-position. In preclinical studies, this compound displayed comparable activity to primaquine. It is more active than primaquine in rodent and simian models, both as a blood schizonticide and causal prophylactic *(12,13)*. A particularly promising observation is the absence of methaemoglobineamia to date *(14)*.

Over the years, many 8-aminoquinolines have been developed containing various alkoxy and arloxy substituents in the 5-position of the quinoline ring system **(6)** *(15–17)*. When the substituent is a linear unsaturated aliphatic chain ($n = 5$) or a 4',3'-substituted aryl group, activity is preserved. Unfortunately, the inclusion of these chemical entities produces compounds that are cross-resistant with other antimalarials, thereby limiting their therapeutic potential. It is this balance between good activity and limited cross-resistance to other available antimalarials that is proving extremely difficult to achieve. A major limitation to the development of the 8-aminoquinolines is the paucity of information on their true mechanisms of action and toxicity. The observation that the basic 8-aminoquinoline structure can be modified to separate the hematoxicological properties from antiparasitic activity, coupled with the observations of achievable activity against blood-stage parasites, opens the way for the further development of this class of antimalarial. Rational design of these drugs will necessitate further investigations into the fundamental mechanisms behind both activity and toxicity.

4-AMINOQUINOLINES

Currently Used 4-Aminoquinolines: The Starting Points for Chemical Modification

Chloroquine **(7)** (Scheme II), a 4-aminoquinoline, was first synthesized in 1934 and became the most widely used antimalarial drug by the 1940s *(18)*. From a chemical viewpoint, it proved attractive because of its ease of synthesis, its stability and low cost of production. Various mechanisms have been proposed to rationalize the mode of action of chloroquine and the 4-aminoquinolines in general (Chapter 7). It is important

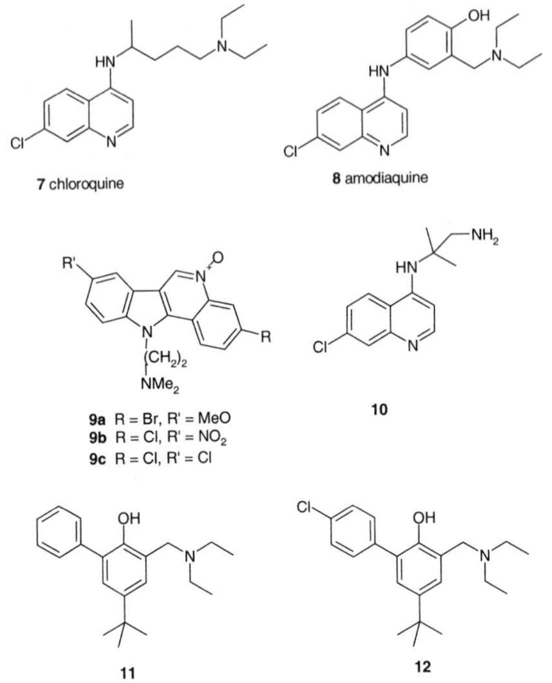

7 chloroquine   **8** amodiaquine

9a R = Br, R' = MeO
9b R = Cl, R' = NO₂
9c R = Cl, R' = Cl

10

11   **12**

Scheme II

at this point to briefly review those aspects of chloroquine action for which there appears to be a consensus opinion, as this knowledge has implications for rational drug design and our understanding of the structure–activity relationship (SAR). Chloroquine accumulates to high concentrations within the parasite *(19)*. It was originally proposed that this accumulation was the result of proton trapping; however, recent data suggest that this may be less important than intraparasitic receptor binding as a mechanism of accumulation *(20)*. All available evidence indicates that this intraparasitic receptor is heme or ferriprotoporphyrin IX *(21)* and availability of heme is essential to the action of all the quinoline antimalarials tested to date other than the 8-aminoquinolines *(20,22)*. Chloroquine is believed to exert its activity by interfering with the heme detoxification processes the parasite uses to eliminate heme following hemoglobin digestion, although the specifics of this are controversial (Chapter 7). This interaction with heme leads to increased levels of heme or heme : drug complex beyond a toxic threshold which then kills the parasite. The critical involvement of this interaction in the mechanism of drug action has a number of implications with respect to the exploitation of this target. An interaction with heme would predict a lack of stereoselectivity in drug action, which is the case. Further, it should be possible to model, using modern computer technologies, the potential drug interactions with heme or its µ-oxo-dimer as a tool to aid rational design. The fact that the use of other surrogate test systems, such as the heme polymerization assay, have failed to show a clear correlation with antimalarial activity may bring into question the quantitative value of this model, as it clearly fails to take into account the amount of drug capable of reaching the target in the physiological setting. These physicochemical parameters are readily incorporated into molecular modeling studies.

The search for novel quinoline-based antimalarials with pharmacological benefits over and above those provided by chloroquine has continued throughout this century with the emergence of chloroquine resistance (Chapter 9) acting as an additional impetus. The chloroquine analog amodiaquine (**8**) was developed in a large-scale screening program, initiated by the US Army at the end of the Second World War *(23,24)*. Amodiaquine, like chloroquine, is a potent blood schizonticide with activity against some chloroquine-resistant strains of *Plasmodia (25)*. It has been used as an alternative to chloroquine for over 40 yr. Amodiaquine differs chemically from chloroquine in that it contains a 4-hydroxyanilino function in its side chain, although it is important to note that amodi-aquine and chloroquine both have four carbon atoms between the secondary and tertiary nitrogens. Molecular modeling studies have indicated that the internitrogen separation between the quinoline nitrogen and the alkylamino nitrogen is approximately 8.3 Å in both chloroquine and amodiaquine *(26)*. The presence of the Mannich alkylamino side chain is vital; removal of this group results in a complete loss of antimalarial activity. However, a recent report indicated the maintenance of significant antimalarial activity in a chloroquine analog lacking the terminal nitrogen, which was replaced with a carbon atom. This seems to question the view that intranitrogen distances are key to the pivotal interaction with heme. These investigators actually showed this analog to interact poorly with heme as a target which may implicate an alternative mechanism of action for this new analog *(27)*.

Early Attempts to Establish 4-Aminoquinoline SAR

Early structure–activity studies with amodiaquine and chloroquine revealed the key role of the 7-position in the quinoline ring. Focusing on amodiaquine, the 7-chloro derivative exhibited the best activity, whereas the introduction of other substituents at this position, including a methoxy, ethoxy, methyl, or bromo, led to a decrease in activity *(28)*. Further studies by Heindel et al. demonstrated that disubstitution of the quinoline ring with differ-ent substituents could improve in vivo activity *(29)*. Preliminary screening demonstrated that substitution with Cl and F at the 7-position improved activity, whereas introduction of a CF_3 at the 7-position decreased antimalarial efficacy in vivo. Attempts to restrict the spatial flexibility of the 4-aminoquinolines resulted in the synthesis of indoloquinoline (**9**) a compound which exhibited poor antimalarial activity in vivo against chloroquine-sensi-tive *P. berghei (30)*. However, related compounds have shown that other analogs contain-ing the indoloquinoline nucleus do have promising activity against Plasmodial strains in vitro *(31)*. Structure–activity studies with these indoloquinolines revealed that the basic side chain as well as the ring N-oxide are critical for activity, as is a bromine or chlorine in position 3 (**9a**). Substitution at positions 7–10 were not essential, although the most potent analog in these studies was the 8-nitro compound (**9b**). Replacement of the 8-methoxyl (**9c**) by Cl also produced high activity in this series. This study confirms the potential of the rigid indoloquinoline nucleus in the design of novel compounds effective as agents for the treat-ment of malaria. Despite considerable efforts in this area and the synthesis of many genera-tions of quinolines, none of these early compounds would appear to have shown enough promise to merit their further.

Structural Modifications Aimed at Circumventing Resistance

As a direct result of chloroquine resistance in *P. falciparum*, a variety of chemical approaches have been used in an attempt to develop more effective agents specifically against resistant parasites. The weight of evidence suggests that chloroquine resistance results from a decrease in the drug concentration achieved at the target site, rather than mutation of the target receptor *(32)*. One very simplistic strategy to increase activity against all parasites involved chemical substitutions specifically designed to prolong the elimination half-life of the drug in the host. For example, in compound **(10)**, a quaternary carbon atom was introduced into the side chain in an attempt to reduce total–body clearance and, hence, prolong the half-life against resistant and sensitive parasites. Compound **10** was active against *P. berghei* in vivo *(33)*. However, this strategy does not get around the problem of treating parasite populations with differential 4-aminoquinoline sensitivity and the reduced rate of elimination may have disadvantages in terms of resistance development.

A more recent advance in the preparation of highly potent 4-aminoquinolines was reported by Werbel et al. in 1986 *(34)*. Modification of the α-(dialkyl amino)-*o*-cresol structure **(11)** led to **(12)**, which was significantly more potent than chloroquine or amodiaquine in both the treatment and prophlyaxis of experimental malaria. Werbel et al. examined a series of hybrid structures of **(12)** compared to amodiaquine in the hope that incorporation of the 7-chloroquinoline moiety would enhance activity further. A quantitative structure–activity relationship (QSAR) study was used to establish the most suitable substituents on the phenyl ring. The *p*-chlorophenyl group conferred maximal potency, with tebuquine **(13)** (Scheme III) achieving complete parasite clearance (using two chloroquine-resistant parasite strains) at doses of 1 or 2 mg/kg in mice. In this model, tebuquine **(13)** was more potent than chloroquine. Tebuquine is highly active against *P. falciparum.* For example we have measured a median inhibitory concentration (IC_{50}) of 0.9 n*M* against a chloroquine-sensitive isolate and 20.8 n*M* against a chloroquine-resistant isolate *(35)*. Based on the understanding that drug accumulation at the site of action is an important parameter, we have hypothesized that this improved activity seen with tebuquine is a function of the a *p*-chlorophenyl substituent in the 5'-position of the side chain, which will increase accumulation by increasing lipid solubility. We have since formally confirmed this relationship *(36)*. On the basis of these very encouraging early results in experimental models of malaria, tebuquine was selected for preclinical toxicology studies prior to evaluation in man. Unfortunately, further development was curtailed after detailed in vitro toxicological studies revealed acute white cell toxicity at high doses. Upon further investigation into the SARs of tebuquine, it was found that insertion of a methylene spacer between the two phenyl rings **(14a)** led to a loss of much of the antimalarial activity, as did a sulfur spacer **(14b)** and a *tert*-butyl group **(15a)** *(37)*. Use of a cyclohexyl group in place of *tert*-butyl **(15b)** restored substantial activity with other straight or branched chains resulting in moderate activity. From this follow-up study, it was apparent that although simple 6-alkyl analogs did retain activity, none of the analogs could match the activity of tebuquine. Because of the toxicological problems associated with this lead compound, further investment in the development of these structures has stopped.

The degree of cross-resistance between 4-aminoquinoline antimalarials varies with structure; for example, highly chloroquine-resistant isolates of *P. falciparum* may show moderate or almost no cross-resistance with amodiaquine or related drugs such as amopyroquine *(38)*. These observations have stimulated further research into drugs containing Mannich side chains. One promising candidate for the treatment of chloroquine-resistant malaria is pyronaridine **(16)**, a drug that was synthesized in China in the

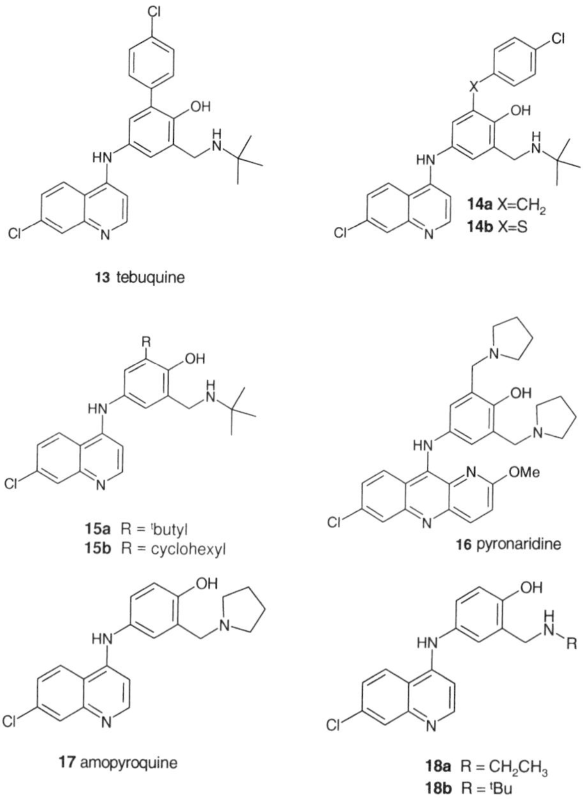

13 tebuquine

14a X=CH$_2$
14b X=S

15a R = ^{t}butyl
15b R = cyclohexyl

16 pyronaridine

17 amopyroquine

18a R = CH$_2$CH$_3$
18b R = ^{t}Bu

Scheme III

early 1970s and is currently being studied in uncomplicated malaria in Africa as monotherapy *(39,40)*. Clinical trials of pyronaridine involving more than 1000 patients have shown high efficacy against *P. falciparum* and *P. vivax* with few side effects *(41)*. This compound is currently used for the treatment of chloroquine-resistant *P. falciparum* in China. The further development of this promising new drug is likely to involve its combination with an artemisinin. An important consideration with this drug is the potential for it to undergo bioactivation to a reactive metabolite in an analogous fashion to amodiaquine, because both compounds retain the conjugated 4-aminophenol moiety.

Amopyroquine *(17)* is another structural analog of amodiaquine in which the diethylamino side chain is replaced with a pyrrolidine group. This replacement results in a drug that is more active than both chloroquine and amodiaquine against both chloroquine-sensitive and chloroquine-resistant strains of *P. falciparum* in vitro *(42)*. Chemically, the pyrrolidino and diethylamino groups are very similar and differences in in vitro activity are difficult to rationalize. However, differences in in vivo activity may reflect differences in their metabolic disposition. Amodiaquine is extensively de-ethylated to desethylamodiaquine **(18a)** and this metabolite is significantly less active than the parent drug molecule against chloroquine-resistant parasites in vitro (i.e., the more water-soluble metabolite shows greater cross resistance with chloroquine that the parent drug molecule) *(43)*. In contrast, the pyrrolidino functionality of amopyroquine is not susceptible to oxidative dealkylation as in amodiaquine. Thus, the activity of amopyroquine against resistant strains in vitro should translate into potent in vivo activity. This difference in metabolism illustrates the importance of studying the activity of 4-amino-quinoline plasma metabolites and their potential implications in the design of novel drugs that have activity against resistant strains. A recent study by Hawley et al. has investigated the replacement of the diethylamino function with an *N-tert* butyl and pyrrolidino function. *N-tert*-butyl amodiaquine (**18b**) was designed on the basis that this drug cannot undergo de-ethylation to metabolites with reduced activity against resistant strains *(44)*. When studied in vitro against four strains of *P. falciparum* (3D7, HB3, K1 and PH3) amopyroquine and *N-tert*-butyl amodiaquine showed greater levels of activity compared with both amodiaquine and desethylamodiaquine against both resistant and sensitive isolates.

Substitution in the 4-Aminophenol Ring

These investigations have been undertaken in an attempt to identify sites of chemical modification that can selectively influence antimalarial activity or the potential toxicity of this chemical moiety. O'Neill et al. have examined the effect of chemical manipulation on the biological activity of tebuquine *(45)*. Utilizing novel chemical methodology, analogs of tebuquine in which the hydroxyl function was absent or substituted with a fluorine atom have been synthesized (**19a,b**) (Scheme IV). The novel compounds were tested against chloroquine-sensitive (HB3) and chloroquine-resistant (K1) strains of *P. falciparum*. Tebuquine was the most potent compound tested, whereas replacement of the hydroxyl function with hydrogen or fluorine resulted in a fourfold loss of activity. However, both of these compounds were more active than chloroquine against a chloroquine-sensitive strain. Molecular modeling studies indicated that tebuquine and the substituted derivatives would have similar and favorable binding interaction energies with heme. The differences in activity were shown to relate to the inferior cellular accumulation of the fluorotebuquine and dehydroxytebuquine analogs.

Further substitutions in the aromatic ring have produced the *bis*-Mannich quinoline antimalarials such as (**20**). These compounds have been reported to exhibit superior activity to chloroquine against both sensitive and resistant strains of *P. falciparum* in vitro *(46,47)*. Rieckmann and colleagues has performed extensive studies on quinoline *bis*-Mannich compounds (**21**) *(48)*. Using the Saimiri bioassay model, ex vivo antimalarial activity of a series of *bis*-Mannichs has been studied against the K1 strain of *P. falciparum*. These compounds were found to be as active as both amodiaquine and pyronaridine in vitro and three to four times more potent than chloroquine. In addition, four of the compounds showed superior activity to chloroquine, amodiaquine, and pyronaridine in serum collected 7 d after initial dosage. Antimalarial activity was absent from serum samples obtained from monkeys receiving either amodiaquine or chloroquine.

The synthesis and biological evaluation of a series of tebuquine analogs bearing various alky groups in place of the 4-chlorophenyl moiety has recently been reported by Raynes et al. *(49)*. All of the derivatives (**22a–g**) inhibited growth of both chloroquine-sensitive (HB3) and the chloroquine-resistant (K1) parasites in vitro. As stated earlier, the replacement of the diethylamino function of amodiaquine with the *N-tert*-butylamino group of the 4'-hydroxyanilino side chain (*tert*-butylamodiaquine) led to a substantial increase in antimalarial activity against both strains. There was a 1.5-fold increase in activity of *tert*-butylamodiaquine against the chloroquine sensitive strain and almost a 4-fold increase in activity against the chloroquine-resistant strain. The

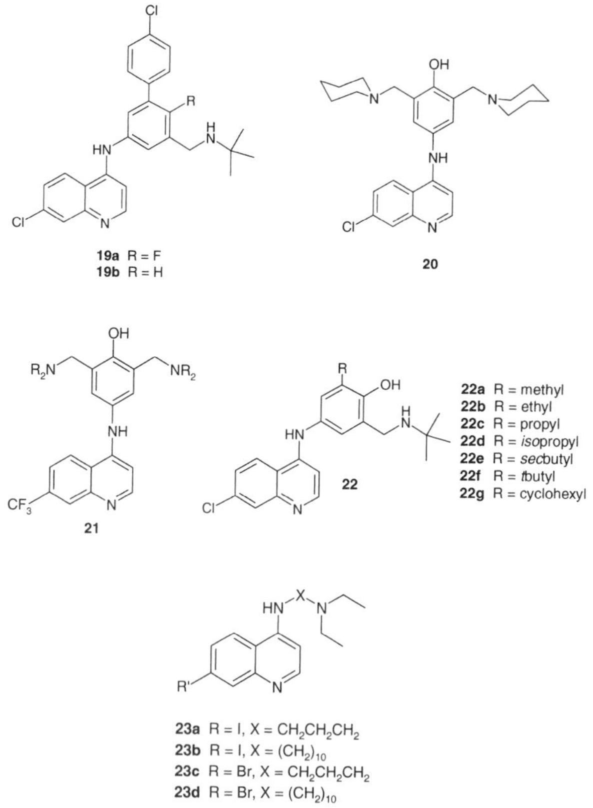

19a R = F
19b R = H

20

21

22

22a R = methyl
22b R = ethyl
22c R = propyl
22d R = isopropyl
22e R = secbutyl
22f R = tbutyl
22g R = cyclohexyl

23a R = I, X = CH₂CH₂CH₂
23b R = I, X = (CH₂)₁₀
23c R = Br, X = CH₂CH₂CH₂
23d R = Br, X = (CH₂)₁₀

Scheme IV

cellular accumulation ratio (CAR) for *tert*-butylamodiaquine was found to be five to nine times greater than amodiaquine in chloroquine-sensitive isolates and twofold to threefold greater than amodiaquine in chloroquine-resistant strains.

A similar decrease in the level of cross-resistance as seen between amodiaquine and *tert*-butylamodiaquine was observed between amodiaquine and these new alkyl derivatives. It was proposed that the shape/length ratio of the 5'-alkyl substituent has a marked effect on drug activity. Activity increased as the length of the alkyl group increased with optimum activity observed with the propyl and isopropyl derivatives. Replacement of the linear alkyl group containing only one branch with a bulkier, nonplanar group such as a *N-tert*-butyl or cyclohexyl substituent markedly reduced the efficacy of the derivatives against both strains compared to amodiaquine or *tert*-butylamodiaquine. All the 5'-alkyl Mannich-base derivatives displayed less cross resistance than amodiaquine, with resistance indices (IC_{50} K1/IC_{50} HB3) between 1.5 and 3.7 compared to 5.3 for amodiaquine. The 5'-propyl–and 5'-isopropyl–substituted derivatives (**22c** and **22d**) were twofold more active than *tert*-butylamodiaquine and 7-fold more active than amodiaquine against the chloroquine-resistant (K1) isolate. The reason for the greater activity for these two derivatives is unknown. However, given the structural similarities between *tert*-butylamodiaquine and the new derivatives, it is probable that the 5'-alkyl derivatives and *tert*-butylamodiaquine accumulate to similar levels in the chloroquine-resistant parasite, resulting in the increased activity.

Short-Chain Chloroquine Analogs

Krogstad et al. has recently synthesized a series of 4-aminoquinoline chloroquine analogs with a range of substituents at the 7-position of the quinoline ring and variable-length diaminoalkyl side chains *(50)*. Data on antimalarial activity suggested that those compounds with diaminoalkyl side chains shorter than four carbons or longer than seven carbons were active against chloroquine-susceptible, chloroquine-resistant, and multiresistant strains of *P. falciparum* in vitro and exhibited no cross-resistance with chloroquine. In support of their argument that they had managed to circumvent the chloroquine-resistance mechanism, none of these more active compounds displayed a verapamil effect in chloroquine-resistant isolates. In contrast, aminoquinolines with intermediate-length side chains of four to six carbons shared cross-resistance with chloroquine. In vitro evaluation of the 7-substituted analogs of these compounds further confirmed the importance of this position in the quinoline ring. Removal of the chlorine atom at the 7-position of the quinoline ring curtailed antimalarial activity and most other substitutions on the ring produced a marked reduction in antiplasmodial activity. However, 7-iodo- and 7-bromo-aminoquinolines with short (2–3 carbon) or long (10–12 carbon) diaminoalkane side chains **(23a–d)** exhibited superior activity to chloroquine against chloroquine-resistant (Indochina I) and chloroquine-susceptible (Haiti 135) *P. falciparum* parasites *(51)*. This structural information was used to develop a hypothetical model of the chloroquine-resistance mechanism based on an interaction between the cationic sites within the drug and a putative drug-resistance protein with two appropriately placed anionic binding sites. In this model, the length of the alkylamino side chain was critical in determining the ability of drug to interact with the "resistance protein."

The superiority of the short chain chloroquine analogs was also proposed by Ridley et al. *(52)*. They carried out extensive studies with more than 130 analogs of chloroquine including many with a shortened alkylamino side-chain. They demonstrated activity against chloroquine-susceptible and resistant strains of *P. falciparum*, the absence of significant cross resistance and activity in vivo in the *P. berghei* model. Four of these compounds, possessing a diethylaminoethyl, diethylaminopropyl, dimethylaminoisopropyl and diethylaminoisopropyl side-chains **(24a–d)** (Scheme V) were selected for further detailed assessment. All four of these compounds showed significantly lower IC_{50}'s against the chloroquine-resistant K1 strain than was observed for chloroquine, although the IC_{50}'s remained twofold to threefold higher than those against the chloroquine-susceptible NF54 strain. When evaluated against 77 *P. falciparum* isolates, there was a strong correlation between the activities of the 4 compounds and that of chloroquine. A major drawback of these analogs was the metabolic lability of the dialkylamino function. From metabolism studies, it was found that all four compounds produced a monodesethylalkyl metabolite and one produced the *bis*-desethylalkyl metabolite. Although the monodesethylalkyl metabolites were as active as the parent compound against chloroquine-susceptible *P. falciparum*, they were significantly less active against chloroquine-resistant strains (i.e., they showed a greater resistance factor than chloroquine itself). As these dealkylated products were likely to be major plasma metabolites, it was suggested that this potential might compromise their clinical utility. These data also argue against the model of resistance proposed by

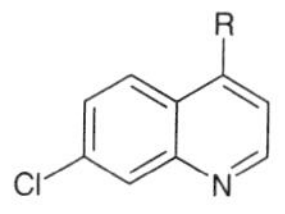

24a R = NHCH$_2$CH$_2$CH$_2$N(C$_2$H$_5$)$_2$
24b R = NHCH$_2$CH$_2$N(C$_2$H$_5$)$_2$
24c R = NHCH(CH$_3$)CH$_2$N(CH$_3$)$_2$
24d R = NHCH(CH$_3$)CH$_2$N(C$_2$H$_5$)$_2$

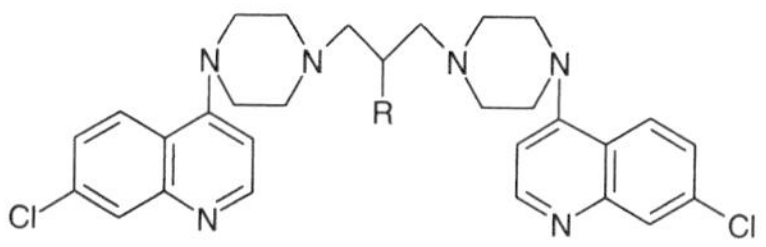

25
R= H piperaquine
R = OH hydroxylpiperquine

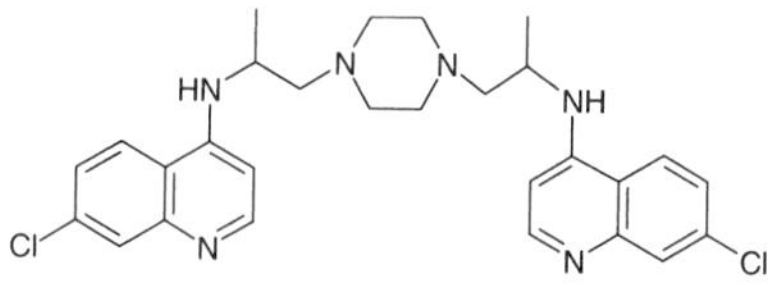

26 dichloroquinazine (12,278RP)

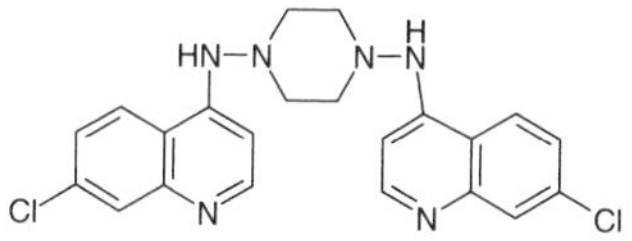

27

Scheme V

Krogstad et al., because these dealkylated metabolites retain the same charge distribution and side-chain length as the parent compound, yet show greater cross-resistance that chloroquine itself.

The development of the Roche analogs as reported by Ridley et al. has been terminated partly because of toxicological problems with some of the more active analogs (*52*). However, Krogstad et al., are continuing with the development of their short-chain compounds and it is hoped that some of these will eventually become available for clinical use.

Although we have not had a new 4-aminoquinoline antimalarial for some 50 yr, there are reasons to continue our efforts in this area. Experience tells us that chloroquine has been the most successful single drug for the treatment and prophylaxis of malaria. Further, the 4-aminoquinolines are easily synthesized and inexpensive to produce, a key consideration for drugs destined for use in those areas of the world where malaria is endemic, and they are generally well tolerated with acceptable toxicity profiles for treatment of the acute infection. What recent structural evaluations have confirmed is that it is possible to produce 4-aminoquinoline analogs with greater antimalarial activity than current drugs and with a reduced cross-resistance pattern to chloroquine. The ability to modify the structure in order to alter toxicological profile and host dispositional characteristics will also prove invaluable in the rational design of the next generation of 4-aminoquinolines. This process will become easier when we fully understand the mechanisms of action and resistance of the 4-aminoquinolines at the cellular, molecular, and chemical levels.

BISQUINOLINES

In the search for quinoline compounds that evade the resistance mechanism, a particularly promising finding was that several bisquinolines are active against chloroquine-resistant strains of malaria parasites *(53–56)*. Bisquinolines, as the name suggests, are compounds that contain two quinoline nuclei combined through an aliphatic or aromatic linker. Early examples of such agents include bis(quinolyl)piperazines, such as piperaquine (**25**), dichloroquinazine (**26**, 12,278RP), and 1,4-*bis*(7-chloro-4-quinolylamino)piperazine) (**27**) *(53–55,57)*. A mixture of dichloroquinazine (12,278RP) and 12,494RP (**28**) (Scheme VI) was shown to be clinically effective against *P. falciparum,* exerting a suppressive effect for up to 3 wk *(58)*. Piperaquine and its analog, hydroxypiperaquine, were shown to be more potent than chloroquine against both chloroquine-sensitive and chloroquine-resistant strains of malaria parasites. Unfortunately, up to 20% cross-resistance with chloroquine against *P. berghei* has been reported for piperaquine and hydroxylpiperaquine *(55)*.

In 1992, interest in the bisquinolines was revived by Vennerstrom and collegues *(56)*. They looked at an alternative series of bisquinolines, including *N,N'-bis*(7-chloroquinolin-4-yl)alkanediamine derivatives and a (±)-*trans-N,N-bis*(7-chloroquinolin-4-yl)cyclohexane-1,2-diamine derivative (WR 268,668) (**29**), because they displayed superior in vitro and in vivo antimalarial activity compared to chloroquine *(56)*. These authors concluded that a linker that exhibited less flexibility compared to an aliphatic bridge enhanced activity. Unfortunately although this derivative displayed good activity against chloroquine-resistant isolates, some cross-resistance was noted, which could be reduced when used in combination with desipramine, confirming that this compound shared the chloroquine-resistance mechanism. It was later found that the S,S-enantiomer of this compound was more active than the racemate against chloroquine-resistant strains, and further pharmacodynamic investigations showed that this derivative exhibited a longer half-life. However, against these positive properties was the observation that this derivative displayed unacceptable phototoxicity that precluded further development *(59)*.

More recently, another series of *N,N'-bis*(quinolin-4-yl)diamine derivatives (**30**) has been evaluated for activity against the malaria parasite. These bisquinoline derivatives displayed good activity against seven chloroquine-resistant strains and five chloroquine-sensitive strains of *P. falciparum,* with cross-resistance indices between 0.9 and 2.8 compared to 8.7 for chloroquine *(60,61)*. This ability of bisquinolines to partially circumvent the parasite's mechanism of resistance inspired additional research into the synthesis of novel bisquinolines. One such approach was reported by Raynes and co-workers, this group synthesized two series of bisquinolines, coupled through a diamide linkage in either the 6- or 8-position of the quinoline ring, while retaining the basic side chain of chloroquine. These derivatives, *N,N'-bis*[4–((4-(diethylamino)-1-methylbutyl)amino)-quinolin-8 or 6-yl]alkanoamide *(31)*, were effective against a chlo-

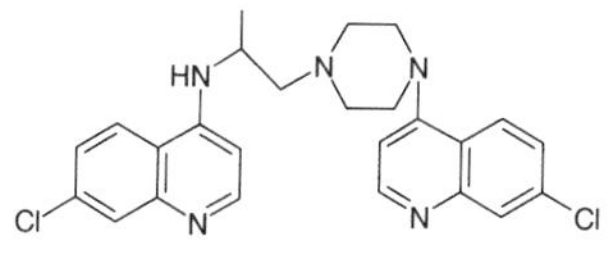

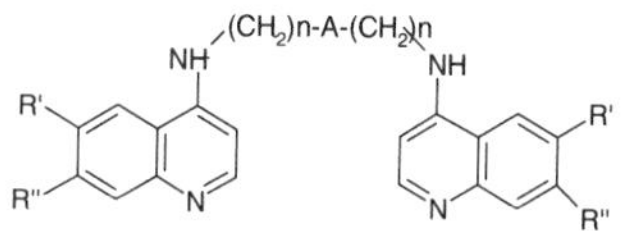

R' = halogen or CF3 and R'' = H or halogen
N,N'bis(quinolin-4-yl)diamine
30

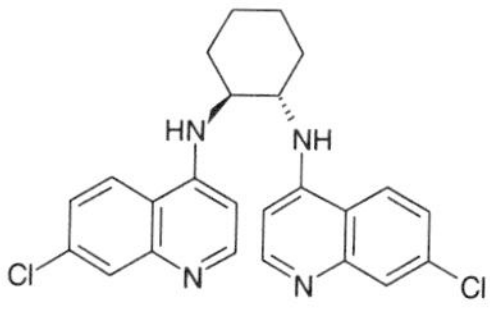

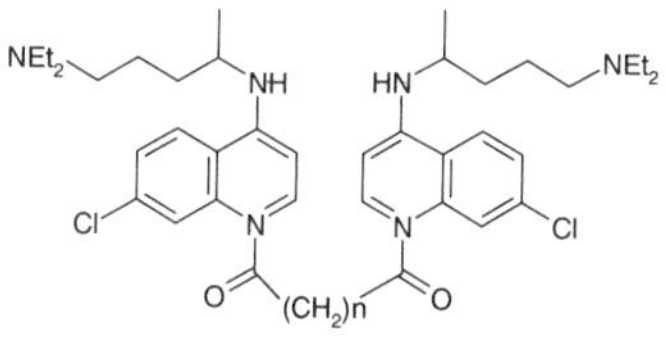

bis-4-aminoquinolines
31

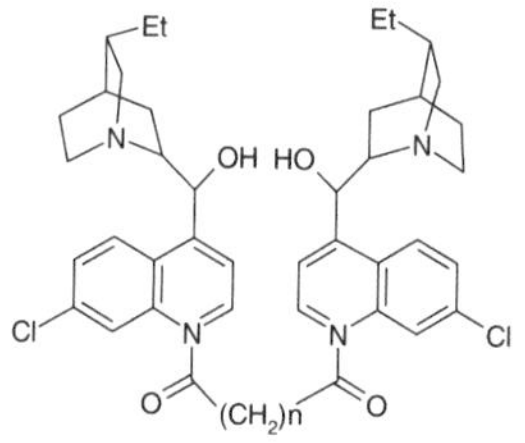

Bis-4-quinolinemethanols
32

Scheme VI

roquine-resistant isolate of *P. falciparum* (FAC8), with resistance indices between 0.7 and 2.2 compared to 10 for chloroquine *(62,63)*. A correlation between activity and heme polymerization was interpreted as suggesting a similar mode of action as chloroquine *(63)*. A further modification in which the quinoline nucleus was linked through a diamide bridge in the 8-position but retained the basic moiety of the cinchona alkaloids afforded a series that displayed excellent activity against both chloroquine- and mefloquine-resistant strains (**32**) *(64)*. Taken all together, these results suggest that the place of attachment of the linker is irrelevant, it can be anchored onto the quinoline nucleus in either the 4-, 6-, or 8-position and still retain activity.

More recently, *N,N-bis*(7-chloroquinolin-4-yl)heteroalkanediamines were shown to be active against *P. falciparum* and *P. berghei* in vivo. Bisquinolines with alkyl ether and piperazine bridges were shown to be substantially more effective than those with alkylamine bridges in vivo, this being attributed to increased water solubility and absorption *(65)*. These authors reported that there was no relationship between the length of the heteroalkane bridge and antimalarial activity. Somewhat surprisingly, no correlation was observed between in vitro and in vivo antimalarial activities, suggesting diminished drug uptake in the in vitro assay. As previously reported *(63)*, a correlation between inhibition of heme polymerization and efficacy was observed *(65)*.

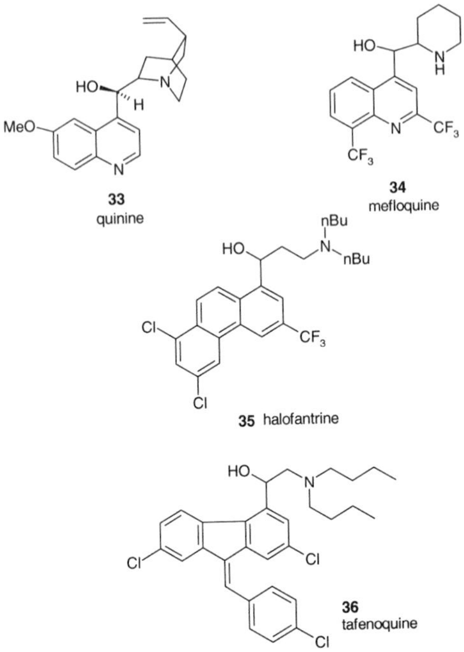

33
quinine

34
mefloquine

35 halofantrine

36
tafenoquine

Scheme VII

QUINOLINEMETHANOLS

Quinine, a cinchona alkaloid, is the original quinoline methanol structure. The first reports of decreased sensitivity to quinine (**33**) (Scheme VII) occurred in Brazil in 1910. However, presumably as a function of the extent of parasite exposure, quinine has retained its efficacy in the field much longer than chloroquine. Nonetheless, reports of quinine resistance are increasing and efficacy with quinine treatment has fallen below 50% in some parts of Southeast Asia (66). In these areas, quinine is now prescribed with tetracycline in an effort to increase cure rates. Despite its historic importance in malaria chemotherapy the exploitation of the quinoline methanol structure was not seriously undertaken until the second half of this century.

In 1963, the Walter Reed Army Institute for Research initiated another large-scale screening of potential antimalarial drugs. By the mid-1980s, some 300,000 compounds had been screened. Only a handful of useful drug candidates emerged from these studies. The most promising group of compounds was the quinolinemethanols, which proved to be potent against both *P. falciparum* and *P. vivax* (67). However, the first-generation compounds produced unacceptable photosensitization (68). Mefloquine (**34**), was subsequently synthesized and shown to have little photosensitizing effect (69). Mefloquine has proved to be effective in antimalarial chemotherapy over the last 15 yr, especially against chloroquine-resistant strains of malaria parasites (70). However, reports of resistance to mefloquine have been increasing since its introduction to the field in the 1980s. In Thailand, where mefloquine has been used extensively, significant mefloquine resistance developed within 5 yr of introduction (71). The use of mefloquine has been associated with adverse neuropsychiatric effects, including anxiety, depression, hallucinations, acute psychosis, and seizures (72).

Recently, Bhattacharjee and Karle investigated the importance of stereoelectronic properties for the activity of the quinolinemethanols *(73)*. It was found that potency related to electronic features such as electrostatic potential, hydrogen bonding ability, and electrophilicity. In addition, the antimalarial activity between mefloquine and its *threo* analog showed an approximate 2.6-fold difference.

As part of the Walter Reed screening program, the quinoline moiety of the quinolinemethanols was replaced by other aromatic groups to form the aryl(amino)carbinols. Of this class of compound, halofantrine, a 9-phenanthrenemethanol, showed the most potency *(74)*. Halofantrine **(35)** has been successfully used in the field to treat chloroquine-resistant strains of *P. falciparum (74–77)*. Lumefantrine **(36)** is a fluorene analog of halofantrine with activity against *P. falciparum (78)*. This compound is one component of the novel antimalarial combination Co-artem. The quinoline methanols and related structures reported above all share the problem of poor and variable bioavailability. These problems coupled with an apparent ease of resistance development may limit future interest in the development of this class of antimalarial drug.

REFERENCES

1. Hofheinz W, Merkli B. Quinine and quinine analogues. In: Peters W, Richards WHG, (eds). Handbook of Experimental Pharmacology, Vol 68/II, Antimalarial Drugs II. New York: Springer-Verlag, 1984, pp. 61–81.
2. Peters W. Drug resistance in malaria parasites of animals and man. Adv Parasitol 1998;41:1–62.
3. Peters W. Chemotherapy and Drug Resistance in Malaria. London: Academic, 1987.
4. Guttman P, Ehrlich P. Uber die wirkung des methyebleu bei malaria. Berl Klin Wochensclir 1891;28:953–956.
5. Geary TG, Divo AA, Jensen JB. Activity of quinoline-containing antimalarials against chloroquine-sensitive and -resistant strains of *Plasmodium falciparum in vitro*. Trans R Soc Trop Med Hyg 1987;81(3):499–503.
6. Carson PE, Hohl R, Nora MV, Parkhurst GW, Ahmad T, Scanlan S, et al. Toxicology of the 8-aminoquinolines and genetic factors associated with their toxicology in man. Bull WHO 1981;59:427–437.
7. O' Neill PM. The effect of chemical substitution on the metabolism and antimalarial activity of amodiaquine and primaquine. PhD thesis, The University of Liverpool, 1995.
8. Nodiff EA, Chatterjee S, Masallani HA. Antimalarial activity of the 8-aminoquinolines. Prog Med Chem 1991;28:1–40.
9. Bhatt BK, Seth M, Bhaduri AP. Recent developments in 8-aminoquinoline antimalarials. Prog Drug Res 1984;28:197–231.
10. Brueckner RP, Lasseter KC, Lin ET, Schuster BG. First-time-in-humans safety and pharmacokinetics of WR 238605: a new antimalarial. Am J Trop Med Hyg 1998;58(5):645–649.
11. Brueckner RP, Coster T, Wesche DL, Shmuklarsky M, Schuster BG. Prophylaxis of *Plasmodium falciparum* infection in a human challenge model with WR 238605, a new 8-aminoquinoline antimalarial. Antimicrob Agents Chemother 1998;42(5):1293–1294.
12. Peters W, Robinson BL, Milhous WK. The chemotherapy of rodent malaria. LI. Studies on a new 8-aminoquinoline, WR 238,605. Ann Trop Med Parasitol 1993;87(6):547–552.
13. de Alencar FE, Cerutti C Jr, Durlacher RR, Boulos M, Alves FP, Milhous W, et al. Atovaquone and proguanil for the treatment of malaria in Brazil. J Infect Dis 1997;175(6):1544–1547.
14. Srivastava P, Pandey VC, Misra AP, Gupta P, Raj K, Bhaduri AP. Potential inhibitors of plasmodial heme oxygenase; an innovative approach for combating chloroquine resistant malaria. Bioorg Med Chem 1998;6(2):181–187.

15. Sweeney TR. Drugs with quinine-like action. In: Peters W, Richards WHG (eds). Antimalarial Drugs II: Current Antimalarials and New Drug Developments. Berlin: Springer-Verlag, 1984, pp. 267–313.
16. Oduola AM, Milhous WK, Weatherly NF, Bowdre JH, Desjardins RE. *Plasmodium falciparum*: induction of resistance to mefloquine in cloned strains by continuous drug exposure *in vitro*. Exp Parasitol 1988;67(2):354–360.
17. Vennerstrom JL, Nuzum EO, Miller RE, Dorn A, Gerena L, Dande PA, Ellis WY, et al. 8-Aminoquinolines active against blood stage *Plasmodium falciparum in vitro* inhibit hematin polymerization. Antimicrob Agents Chemother. 1998;43(3):598–602.
18. Loeb LF, Clarke WM, Coatney GR, Coggeshall LT, Dieuaide FR, Dochez AR, et al. Activity of a new antimalarial agent chloroquine (SN 7618). J Am Med Assoc 1946;130:1069–1070.
19. Bray PG, Hawley SR, Ward SA. 4-Aminoquinoline resistance of *Plasmodium falciparum*: insights from the study of amodiaquine uptake. Mol Pharmacol 1996;50:1551–1558.
20. Bray PG, Raynes KJ, Mungthin M, Ginsburg H, Ward SA. Cellular uptake of chloroquine is dependant on binding to ferriprotoporphyrin IX, is independent of NHE activity in *Plasmodium falciparum*. J Cell Biol. 1999;145(2):363–376.
21. Raynes KJ, Bray PG, Ward SA. Altered binding of chloroquine to ferriprotoporphyrin IX is the basis for chloroquine resistance. Drug Resist Updates 1999;2:97–103.
22. Hawley SR, Bray PG, Mungthin M, Atkinson JD, O'Neill PM, Ward SA. Relationship between antimalarial drug activity, accumulation and inhibition of heme polymerization in *Plasmodium falciparum in vitro*. Antimicrob Agents Chemotherap 1998;42(3):682–686.
23. Ekweozer C, Aderounmu AF, Sodeinde O. Comparison of the relative *in vitro* activity of chloroquine and amodiaquine against chloroquine-sensitive strains of P falciparum. Ann Trop Med Parasitol. 1987;81:95–99.
24. Greenwood D. Conflicts of interest: the genesis of synthetic antimalarial agents in peace and war. J Antimicrob Chemother 1995;36:857–872.
25. Watkins WM, Sixsmith DG, Spencer HG, Boriga DA, Karjuki DM, Kipingor T, et al. Effectiveness of amodiaquine as a treatment for chloroquine-resistant *Plasmodium falciparum* infections in Kenya. Lancet 1984;1:357–359.
26. Koh HL, Go ML, Ngiam TL, Mak JW. Conformational and Structural Features determining *in vitro* antimalarial activity in some indolo[3,2-c.] quinolines, anilinoquinolines and tetrahydroindolo[3,2-d] benzazepeines. Eur J Med Chem 1994;29:107–113.
27. Vippagunta SR, Dorn A, Matile H, Bhattacharjee AK, Karle JM, Ellis WY, et al. Structural specificity of chloroquine–hematin binding related to inhibition of hematin polymerization and parasite growth. J Med Chem 1999;42(22):4630–4639.
28. Heindel ND, Molnar J. Synthesis and antimalarial activity of amodiaquine analogs. J Med Chem 1970;13(1):156–157.
29. Heindel ND, Bechara IS, Ohnmacht CJ, Molnar J, Lemke TF, Kennewell PD. Diaminoquinoline antimalarials. J Med Chem 1969;12(5):797–801.
30. Werbel LM, Kesten SJ, Turner WR. Structure–activity relationships of antimalarial indolo[3,2-c]quinolines [1,2]. Eur J Med Chem 1993;28:837–852.
31. Go ML, Koh, HL, Ngiam TL, Phillipson JD, Kirby GC, O'Neill MJ, et al. Synthesis and *in vitro* antimalarial activity of some indolo[3,2-c]quinolines. Eur J Biochem 1992;27:391–394.
32. Bray PG, Ward SA, Ginsburg H. Na+/H+ antiporter, chloroquine uptake and drug resistance: inconsistencies in a newly proposed model. Parasitol Today 1999;15(9):360–363.
33. Schraufstatler E. Arch Pharmacol (Weinheim) 1965;298:655.
34. Werbel LM, Cook PD, Elslager EF, Hung JH, Johnson JL, Kesten SJ, et al. Synthesis, antimalarial activity, and quantitative structure–activity relationships of tebuquine and a series of related 5-[(7-chloro-4–quinolinyl)amino]-3-[(alkylamino)methyl][1,1'-biphenyl]-2-ols and N-oxides. J Med Chem 1986;29:924–939.
35. O'Neill PM, Willock DJ, Hawley SR, Bray PG, Storr RC, Ward SA, et al. Synthesis, antimalarial activity and molecular modeling of tebuquine analogues. J Med Chem 1997;40:437–448.

36. Bray PG, Hawley SR, Mungthin M, Ward SA. Physicochemical properties correlated with drug resistance and the reversal of drug resistance in P. falciparum. Mol Pharmacol 1996;50:1559–1566.

37. Kesten SJ, Johnson J, Werbel LM. Synthesis and antimalarial effects of 4-[(7-chloro-4-quinolinyl)amino]-2-[(diethylamino)methyl]-6-alkylphenols and their N-oxides. J Med Chem 1987;30:906–911.

38. Ward SA, Bray PG, Mungthin M, Hawley SR. Current views on the mechanisms of resistance to quinoline-containing drugs in *Plasmodium falciparum*. Ann Trop Med Parasitol 1995;89:121–124.

39. Peters W. Pyronaridine against multiresistant *falciparum* malaria. Lancet 1996; 347(9001):625.

40. Ringwald P, Eboumbou EC, Bickii J, Basco LK. *In vitro* activities of pyronaridine, alone and in combination with other antimalarial drugs, against *Plasmodium falciparum*. Antimicrob Agents Chemother 1999;43(6):1525–1527.

41. Ringwald P, Meche FS, Basco LK. Short report: effects of pyronaridine on gametocytes in patients with acute uncomplicated *falciparum* malaria. Am J Trop Med Hyg 1999;61(3):446–448.

42. Peters W, Robinson BL. The Chemotherapy of Rodent Malaria. XLVII. Studies on pyronaridine and other mannich base antimalarials. Ann Trop Med Parasitol 1992;86:455.

43. Ruscoe JE, Jewell H, Maggs JL, O'Neill PM, Storr RC, Ward SA, et al. The effect of chemical substitution on the metabolic activation, metabolic detoxification, and pharmacological activity of amodiaquine in the mouse. J Pharm Exp Ther 1995;273(1):393–404.

44. Hawley SR, Bray PG, O'Neill PM, Naisbitt DJ, Park BK, Ward SA. Manipulation of the N-alkyl substituent in amodiaquine to overcome the verapamil-sensitive chloroquine resistance component. Antimicrob Agents Chemother 1996;40:2345–2349.

45. O' Neill PM, Willock DJ, Hawley SR, Bray PG, Storr RC, Park BK. Synthesis, antimalarial activity and molecular modelling of tebuquine analogues. J Med Chem. 1997;40(4):437.

46. Barlin GB, Ireland SJ, Nguyen TMT, Kotecka B, Rieckmann KH. Potential antimalarials XXI. Mannich base derivatives of 4-[7-chloro (and 7-trifluoromethyl)quinolin-4-ylamino]phenol. Aust J Chem 1994;47:1553–1560.

47. Barlin GB, Nguyen TMT, Kotecka B, Rieckmenn KH. Potential antimalarials XV. Di-mannich bases of 4-[7-chloroquinolin-4-ylamino]phenol and 2-[7-bromo(and trifluormethyl)-1-5-naphthiridin-4-ylamino]phenol. Aust J Chem 1992;45:1651–1662.

48. Kotecka BM, Barlin GB, Edstein MD, Rieckmann KH. New quinoline di-Mannich base compounds with greater antimalarial activity than chloroquine, amodiaquine or pyronaridine. Antimicrob Agents Chemotherap. 1997;41:1369–1374.

49. Raynes KJ, Stocks PA, O'Neill PM, Park BK, Ward SA. New 4-aminoquinolines Mannich base antimalarials I. Effect of an alkyl substituent in the 5'-position of the 4'-hydroxyanilino sidechain. J Med Chem 1999;42:2747–2751.

50. De D, Krogstad FM, Cogswell FB, Krogstad DL. Aminoquinolines that circumvent resistance in *Plasmodium falciparum in vitro*. Am J Trop Med Hyg 1996;55:597–583.

51. De D, Krogstad FM, Byers LD, Krogstad DL. Structure–activity relationships for antiplasmodial activity among 7-substituted 4-aminoquinolines. J Med Chem 1998;41:4918–4926.

52. Ridley RG, Hofheinz W, Matile H, Jaquet C, Dorn A, Masciadri R, et al. 4-Aminoquinoline analogs of chloroquine with shortened side chains retain activity against chloroquine-resistant *Plasmodium falciparum*. Antimicrob Agents Chemotherap 1996;40(8):1846–1854.

53. Li Y, Hu Y, Huang HZ, Zhu DQ, Huang WJ, Wu DL, et al. Hydroxylpiperaquine in the treatment of *falciparum* malaria. Chin Med J 1981;94:301–302.

54. Lin C, Feny-yi Q, Yan-chang Z. Field observations on the antimalarial piperaquine. Chin Med J. 1982;95:281–286.

55. Lin C. Recent studies on the antimalarial efficacy of piperaquine and hydroxyl piperaquine. Chin Med J. 1991;104:161–164.

56. Vennerstrom J, Ellis WY, Ager AL, Anderson SL, Gerena L, Milhous WK. Bisquinolines, N,N'-bis[7–chloroquinoline-4–yl]alkanediamines with potential against chloroquine resistant malaria. J Med Chem 1992;35:2129–2134.

57. Basco LK, Anderson SL, Milhous WK, Vennerstrom J. *In vitro* activity of Bisquinoline WR 268,668 against African clones and isolates of *Plasmodium falciparum*. Am J Trop Med Hyg 1994;50:200–205.

58. Le Bras J, Deloron P, Charmot G. Dichloroquinazine[4-aminoquinoline], effective *in vitro* against chloroquine resistance *Plasmodium falciparum*. Lancet 1983;1:73–74.

59. Ridley RG, Matile H, Jaquet C, Dorn A, Hofheinz W, Luepin W, et al. Antimalarial activity of the bisquinoline trans N,N-Bis[7-chloroquinolin-4-yl]cyclohexan-1,2-diamine: comparison of the two steroisomers and detailed evaluation of the S,S enantiomer, Ro 47–7737. Antimicrob Agents Chemother 1997;41:677–686.

60. Hofheinz W, Leupin W. N,N-Bis[quinolin-4–yl]diamine derivatives, their preparation and their use as antimalarials. Chem Abstr 1996;124:260860f.

61. Hofheinz W, Masciadri R. Bisquinolines for the treatment of malaria. Chem Abstr 1996;124:260861g.

62. Raynes KJ, Galatis D, Cowman AF, Tilley L, Deady LW. Synthesis and activity of some antimalarial bisquinolines. J Med Chem 1995;38:204–206.

63. Raynes KJ, Foley M, Tilley L. Novel bisquinoline antimalarials, antimalarial activity and inhibition of haem polymerization. Mol Biochem Parasitol 1996;52:551–559.

64. Cowman AF, Deady LW, Deharo E, Desevnes J, Tilley L. Synthesis and activity of some antimalarial bisquinoline methanols. Aust J Chem 1997;50:1091–1096.

65. Dorn A, Vippagunta SR, Matile H, Jaquet C, Vennerstrom JL, Ridley RG. An assessment of drug–haematin binding as a mechanism for inhibition of haematin polymerization by quinoline antimalarials. Biochem Pharmacol 1998;55(6):727–36.

66. Watt G, Loesuttivibool L, Shanks GD, Bordreau EF, Brown AE, Pavanand K, et al. Quinine with tetracycline for the treatment of drug-resistant *falciparum* malaria in Thailand. Am J Trop Med Hyg 1992;47:108–111.

67. Hofheinz W, Merkli B. Quinine and quinine analogues. In: Peters W. and Richards WHG. (eds). Antimalarial Drugs II. Berlin: Springer-Verlag, 1984, pp. 61–81.

68. Pullman TNK, Eichelberger L, Alving AS, Jones R, Craige B, and Whorton CM. The use of SN-10,275 in the prophylaxis and treatment of sporozoite-induced vivax malaria (Chesson strain). J Clin Invest 1948;27:12–16.

69. Ohnmacht CJ, Patel AR, Lutz RE, Antimalarials. 7. Bis[trifluoromethyl]-[2-piperidyl]-4-quinolinemethanols. J Med Chem 1971;14:926–928.

70. Palmer KJ, Holliday SM, Brogden RN. Mefloquine. A review of its antimalarial activity, pharmacokinetic properties and therapeutic efficacy. Drugs 1993;45:430–475.

71. Mockenhaupt FP. Mefloquine resistance in *Plasmodium falciparum*. Parasitol Today 1995;11:248–253.

72. Riffkin C, Chung R, Wall D, Zalcberg JR, Cowman AF, Foley M, et al. Modulation of the function of human MDR-1 P-glycoprotein by the antimalarial drug mefloquine. Biochem Pharmacol 1996;52:1545–1552.

73. Bhattacharjee AK, Karle JM. Functional correlation of molecular electronic properties with potency of synthetic carbinolamine antimalarial agents. Bioorg Med Chem 1998;6:1927–1933.

74. Bryson HM, Goa KL. Halofantrine. A review of its antimalarial activity, pharmacokinetic properties and therapeutic potential. Drugs 1992;43:236–258.

75. Ringwald P, Bickii J, Basco LK. *In vitro* activity of antimalarials against clinical isolates of *Plasmodium falciparum* in Yaounde, Cameroon. Am J Trop Med Hyg 1996;55(3):254–258.

76. Falade CO, Salako LA, Sowunmi A, Oduola AM, Larcier P. Comparative efficacy of halofantrine, chloroquine and sulfadoxine–pyrimethamine for treatment of acute uncomplicated *falciparum* malaria in Nigerian children, Ann Trop Med Parasitol 1997;91(1):7–16.

77. Fryauff DJ, Baird JK, Basri H, Wiady I, Purnomo, Bangs MJ, et al. Halofantrine and primaquine for radical cure of malaria in Irian Jaya, Indonesia. Ann Trop Med Parasitol 1997;91(1):7–16.
78. Wernsdorfer WH, Landgraf B, Kilimali VA, Wernsdorfer G. Activity of benflumetol and its enantiomers in fresh isolates of *Plasmodium falciparum* from East Africa. Acta Trop 1998;70(1):9–15.

14

New Antimalarial Trioxanes and Endoperoxides

Gary H. Posner, Mikhail Krasavin, Michael McCutchen, Poonsakdi Ploypradith, John P. Maxwell, Jeffrey S. Elias, and Michael H. Parker

BACKGROUND

Folk medicine is often a rich source of leads for discovery of valuable new drugs *(1)*. Quinine was discovered this way, based on traditional medicinal use of the bark of the Cinchona tree, and the powerful anticancer drug taxol was discovered in Yew trees. Chinese folk medicine has now led to isolation, identification, and clinical use of artemisinin (qinghaosu, **1**) (Scheme I), a sesquiterpene 1,2,4-trioxane lactone, for rapid and effective chemotherapy of individuals infected with *Plasmodium falciparum* malaria parasites *(2)*.

The history of the development of antimalarial endoperoxides (Chapter 2) and drugs of this class that are already available or undergoing clinical testing (Chapter 11) are discussed elsewhere in this volume. Also, several recent reviews of antimalarial chemotherapy using 1,2,4-trioxanes are available *(3–6)*. Additionally, a new monograph on biomedical chemistry has one chapter devoted to the fundamental organic chemistry by which trioxanes kill malaria parasites with special mechanistic focus on carbon-centered free-radical intermediates *(7)*; such mechanistic understanding at the molecular level has allowed rational design of a series of new antimalarial peroxide drug candidates. This chapter will provide a brief summary of the fundamental chemical mechanism by which trioxanes kill malaria parasites and then an update on new, rationally designed, therapeutically promising, antimalarial trioxanes and endoperoxides.

In brief mechanistic summary, we were the first, in 1992, to show that iron(II)-induced reductive cleavage of the peroxide linkage in 1,2,4-trioxanes like artemisinin (**1**) produces carbon-centered free radicals *(8)*. This iron(II)-triggered rupturing of the trioxane O–O bond and formation of C-centered radicals then leads to a cascade of reactions, involving highly electrophilic and alkylating epoxides, as well as strongly oxidizing high-valent iron–oxo intermediates *(9,10)* (Scheme II). Any one or a combination of these reactive intermediates has the potential of killing the malaria parasite by disrupting (i.e., alkylating or oxidizing) some of its vital biomolecules.

From: *Antimalarial Chemotherapy: Mechanisms of Action, Resistance, and New Directions in Drug Discovery*
Edited by: P. J. Rosenthal © Humana Press Inc., Totowa, NJ

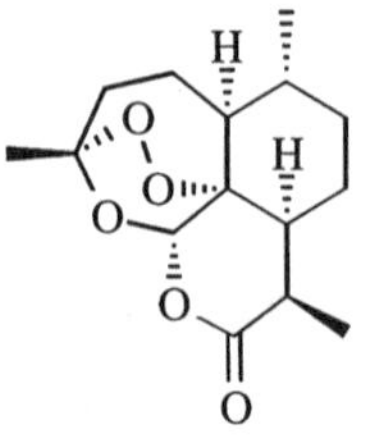

artemisinin
(qinghaosu, **1**)

Scheme I

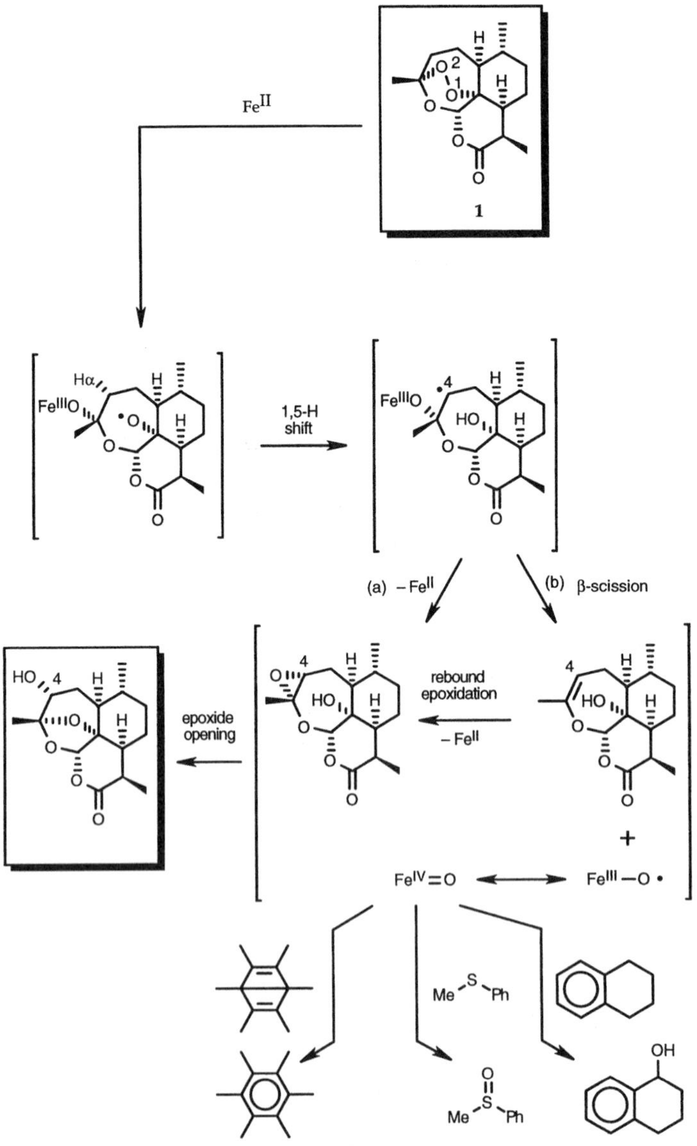

Scheme II

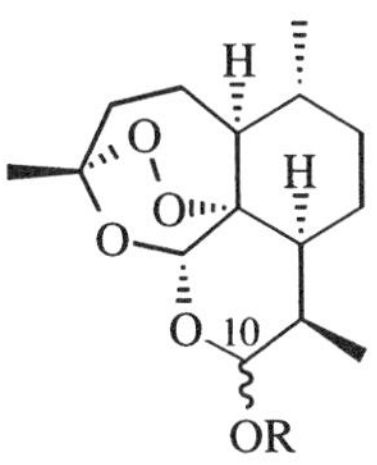

2, R = H, dihydroartemisinin

3, R = Me, artemether

4, R = Et, arteether

5, R = COCH$_2$CH$_2$COONa, sodium artesunate

6, R = CH$_2$—⬡—COONa

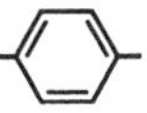

sodium artelinate

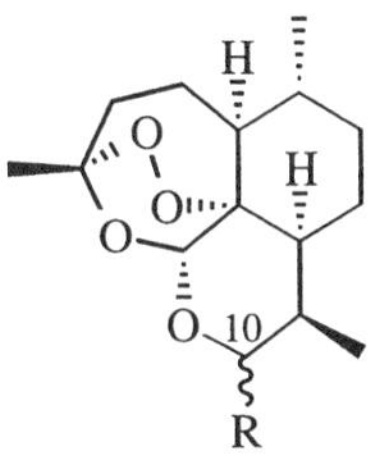

7, R = CF$_3$

8, R = Et

9, R = *n*-Pr

10, R = Ar

Scheme III

NEW TRIOXANES

Artemisinin Derivatives

Because artemisinin does not have good solubility in water or in vegetable oils, organic chemists have reduced its lactone carbonyl group to form the lactol dihydro-artemisinin (DHA, **2**) (Scheme III) *(3–6)*. Derivatization of DHA with methanol or ethanol leads to vegetable oil-soluble artemether (**3**) or arteether (**4**), and derivatization with a carboxyl-bearing carboxylic acid or benzylic alcohol leads to water-soluble artesunate (**5**) or artelinate (**6**) salts, respectively. Each of these derivatives (**3–6**) has been used to cure mammals of their malaria infections *(3–6)*. However, the C-10 acetal functionality in all of these DHA derivatives (**3–6**) is subject to chemical and/or enzymatic hydrolysis, thereby making them pro-drugs of the parent DHA (**2**). Because DHA has some undesirable physiological properties *(3–6)*, however, nonacetal derivatives of DHA have been prepared; these include C-10-CF$_3$ analog **7** *(11)*, C-10–ethyl analog **8** *(12)*, C-10–propyl analog **9** *(13)*, and C-10–aryl and –heteroaryl derivatives **10** *(14–16)*. Generally, these C-10 nonacetal analogs are considerably more hydrolytically stable than artemether (**3**) and arteether (**4**), even in the stomach acid pH range *(17)*. Several of these C-10 nonacetal 10-deoxoartemisinin analogs (e.g., **10**, Ar = 2'-furyl, 5'-methyl-2'-furyl, 5'-ethyl-2'-furyl, 5'-*t*-butyl-2'-furyl, and *N*-methyl-2'-pyrrolyl) are potent antimalarials, with the first two of these furyl derivatives being potent antimalarials even when administered orally to rodents. Preliminary testing for acute toxicity showed the first two furyl analogs to be relatively safe (i.e., at least comparable to artemether) *(16)*.

Another series of C-10 nonacetal derivatives of artemisinin (**1**) has been prepared (Scheme IV) from C-10 unsaturated aldehyde (**11**) *(18)*, itself formed from arte-misinin on gram scale in 69% yield. Without disrupting the chemically delicate peroxide bond in aldehyde (**11**), organometallic reagents converted this aldehyde into

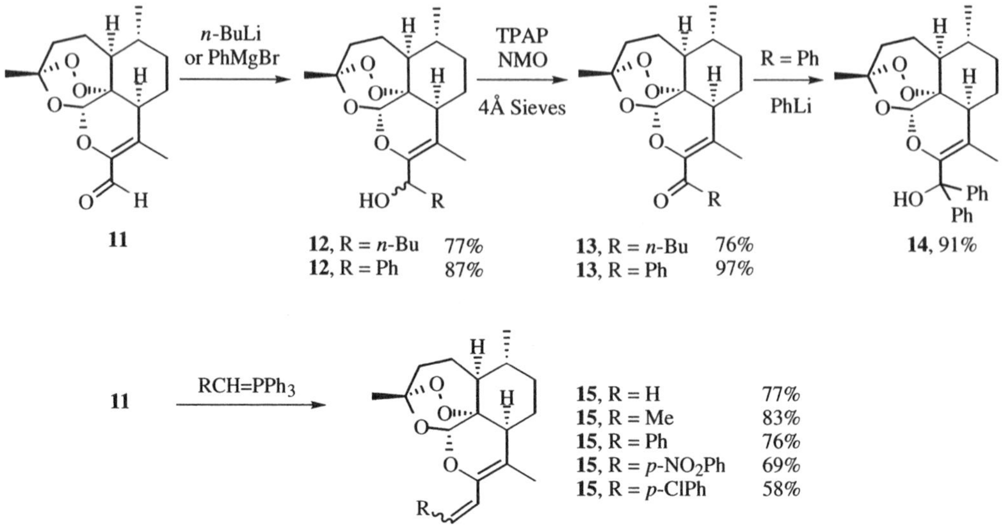

Scheme IV

a series of C-10 nonacetal analogs **12–15** (Scheme IV). These new, enantiomerically pure, semisynthetic analogs range in antimalarial potency between inhibitory concentrations (IC_{50}) of 4.3 and 28 nM, compared to artemisinin with an IC_{50} = 10 nM *(18)*.

Dimers of dihydroartemisinin have been shown in vitro to have some antimalarial activity *(19)*, and more robust C-10 carbon-substituted dimers (**16**) and (**17**) (Scheme V) are potent antimalarials *(20)*. Likewise, some dimers (e.g., **18**) of C-10 nonacetal aldehyde (**11**) also have considerable antimalarial potency *(20)*.

Because all of the new chemical entities (**7–18**) are derived from natural artemisinin, each of these semisynthetic trioxanes is enantiomerically pure. In contrast, structurally simplified trioxanes that are prepared from inexpensive raw materials readily available in bulk from commercial chemical supply companies are usually prepared as racemic mixtures; nevertheless, such synthetic trioxanes often can be synthesized in only a few chemical operations, and the source and purity of the starting raw materials is usually highly reliable. Furthermore, synthetic trioxanes often feature structural units that are not easy to incorporate into semisynthetic artemisinin analogs. Such structural units in synthetic trioxanes often help clarify questions about biological mechanism of action and about structure–activity relationships, ultimately leading to the next generation of medicinal trioxanes.

Structurally Simplified Trioxanes

International research has produced a large number of structurally simplified trioxanes *(3,5,7,12,14)*. This review, however, emphasizes only the three types (**19–21**) (Scheme VI) that are orally efficacious in curing animals having been intentionally infected with malaria parasites. Of the Geneva series of "fenozan" trioxanes, fenozan (**19**) is a particularly potent blood schizontocide effective orally in animals infected with different strains of drug-resistant malaria parasites *(21,22)*. Structurally simplified artemisinin-like trioxane phosphate ester (**20a**) and benzyl ether (**20b**), rationally designed to be

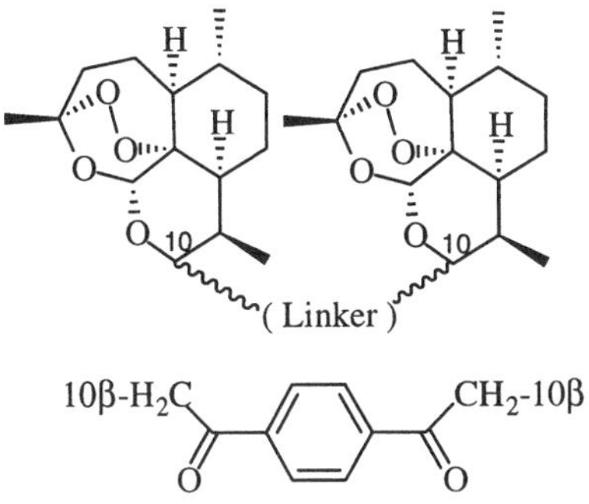

16 (IC$_{50}$ = 1.9 nM)

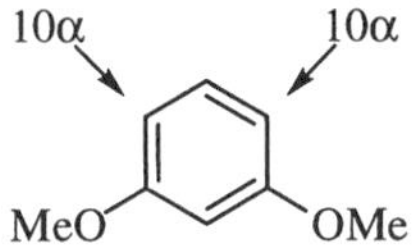

17 (IC$_{50}$ = 1.3 nM)

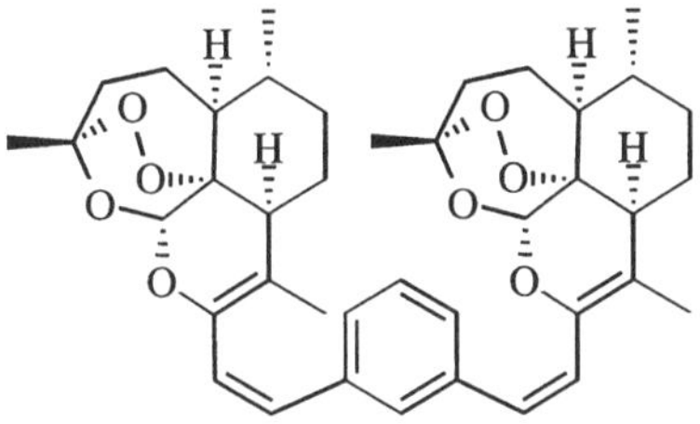

18 (IC$_{50}$ = 18 nM)

Scheme V

hydrolytically more stable than dihydroartemisinin esters and ethers *(23)*, were shown to be as effective as arteether against multidrug-resistant *P. falciparum* in Aotus monkeys *(24)*; this monkey model is considered to be the best primate model for experimental treatment of blood-induced infections of *P. falciparum*. Finally, very simple and easily prepared 3-aryl trioxanes (**21**), designed based on mechanistic understanding at the molecular level, were shown to be as effective as artemisinin in curing malarious rodents *(25)*. It is expected that further preclinical evaluations of one or more of these promising synthetic trioxanes (**19–21**) will produce a lead compound to enter clinical trials.

Recent study at Johns Hopkins University of chemical structure–antimalarial activity relationships in the (**21**) series of synthetic trioxanes has generated diverse new analogs. With the 3-aryl group in trioxanes (**21**) being *p*-biphenyl, *p*-chlorophenyl, or *p*-trifluoromethoxyphenyl, antimalarial potency ranged from about 0.5 to 2 times that of artemisinin. Considerably lower antimalarial activity was observed for trioxane (**21**) with a 3-(*m*-trifluoromethoxy)phenyl group. When the β-methoxy group in trioxane (**21a**) was replaced by a β-benzyloxy or a β-(*p*-fluorobenzyloxy) group, antimalarial potency was not changed significantly compared to that of (**21a**). With the six-

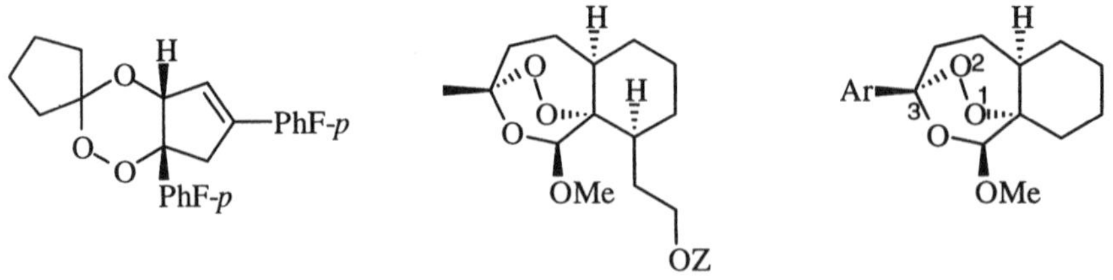

19 (fenozan)
(IC$_{50}$ = 20 nM)

20a, Z = P(OPh)$_2$
(IC$_{50}$ = 4 nM)

20b, Z = CH$_2$Ph
(IC$_{50}$ = 20 nM)

21a, *p*-FPh
(IC$_{50}$ = 30 nM)

21b, *p*-HOCH$_2$Ph
(IC$_{50}$ = 15 nM)

21c, *p*-AcOCH$_2$Ph
(IC$_{50}$ = 20 nM)

Scheme VI

membered carbocyclic ring in trioxane (**21a**) replaced by a seven-membered carbocyclic ring, antimalarial potency decreased sharply. Likewise, reversing the positions of the peroxy and ether groups in trioxane (**21a**) also caused a sharp decrease in antimalarial potency.

Because water solubility is a desirable characteristic of any clinically useful new antimalarial trioxane, trioxane (**21**) with a 3-*p*-carboxyphenyl substituent was prepared at Johns Hopkins University. Like artelinic acid (**6**), this 3-*p*-carboxyphenyl trioxane (**21**) is indeed soluble in water and has good antimalarial efficacy in vivo as well as a good safety profile. Its diverse pharmacological properties are being thoroughly evaluated at this time.

NEW ENDOPEROXIDES

Several endoperoxides such as natural yingzhaosu A (**22**) (Scheme VII) *(26)*, synthetic arteflene (**23**) *(27)*, and synthetic endoperoxide sulfone (**24**) *(28,29)* are potent antimalarials. Their in vitro antimalarial potencies are typically in the 10- to 75-n*M* range, compared to artemisinin having an IC$_{50}$ of 8–10 n*M*. Although yingzhaosu occurs in nature, it is not available in large amounts. Even though arteflene passed successfully through preclinical trials, Hoffmann–La Roche recently decided to discontinue development of this endoperoxide antimalarial in part because of its difficult synthesis (R. Masciadri and C. Hubschwerlen, personal communication). However, very significant advances during 1998 in simplifying laboratory synthesis of such endoperoxides *(29,30)* are now making them much more readily available. Some of these new chemical entities are now under preclinical antimalarial evaluation.

COMBINATION THERAPY

Although peroxidic antimalarial drugs like artemisinin (**1**) and its semisynthetic ether and ester derivatives (**3–6**) are very fast acting, which is crucial for rapid treatment of life-threatening cerebral malaria, they are typically administered for only a few days, and recrudescence of the malaria parasites occurs too often. To overcome this undesir-

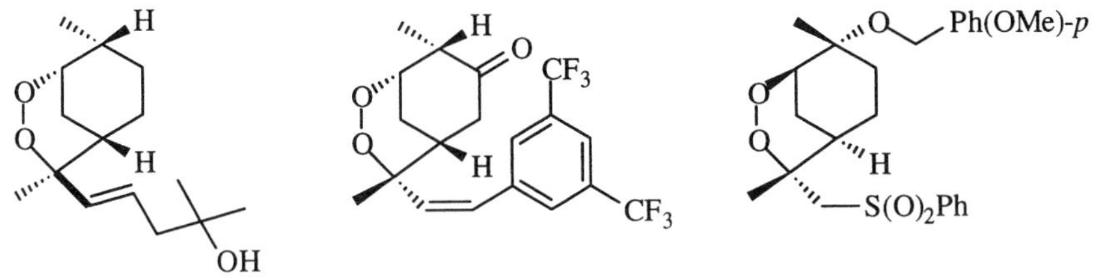

22 (yingzhaosu A)
($IC_{50} = 17$ nM)

23 (arteflene)
($IC_{50} = 71$ nM)

24
($IC_{50} = 14$ nM)

Scheme VII

able feature of short-term malaria chemotherapy with peroxide drugs, treatment with a combination of a peroxide drug plus a longer-lasting antimalarial has been developed. Novartis has developed CGP 56697, combining artemether with the longer-acting antimalarial benflumetol, for safe and effective malaria chemotherapy; in one study reported recently, "no neurologic, cardiac, or other adverse reactions were observed" *(31,32)*. Along similar lines, sequential treatment with artesunate suppositories and then with mefloquine is producing very encouraging preliminary results *(33–36)*. Artemisinin combined with sphingolipid analogs also produces heightened antimalarial responses *(37)*. The practical clinical utility of this type of promising combination antimalarial chemotherapy remains to be established in widespread field tests *(38)*.

CONCLUSIONS

The trioxane and endoperoxide antimalarials described in this chapter represent promising new peroxides that effectively kill *P. falciparum* malaria parasites. The leading members of these peroxidic antimalarials are not only efficacious but relatively safe. Preclinical and then clinical trials should identify peroxide antimalarial drug candidates. Performance of such carefully regulated trials will require considerable financial investment from industrial and/or government sources before a new antimalarial peroxide drug is approved for general use in the United States.

ACKNOWLEDGMENT

The NIH (grant AI-34885) is gratefully thanked for financially supporting our malaria research at Johns Hopkins University.

REFERENCES

1. Swain T (ed). Plants in the Development of Modern Medicine. Cambridge, MA: Harvard University Press, 1972.
2. Klayman DL. Qinghaosu (artemisinin): An antimalarial drug from China. Science 1985;228:1049–1055.
3. Avery MA, Alvim-Gaston M, Woolfrey JR. Synthesis and structure activity relationships of peroxidic antimalarials based on artemisinin. Adv Med Chem 1999;4:125–217.
4. Posner GH. Antimalarial peroxides in the qinghaosu (artemisinin) and yingzhaosu families. Exp Opin Ther Patents 1998;8:1487–1494.
5. Ziffer H, Highet RJ, Klayman DL. Artemisinin: an endoperoxide antimalarial from Artemisia annua L. Prog Chem Org Nat Prod 1997;72:121–214.

6. Haynes RK, Vonwiller SC. From qinghao, marvelous herb of antiquity, to the antimalarial trioxane qinghaosu—and Some Remarkable New Chemistry. Acc Chem Res 1997;30:73–79.

7. Posner GH, Cumming JN, Krasavin M. Carbon-centered radicals and rational design of new antimalarial peroxide drugs. In Biomedical Chemistry: Applying Chemical Principles to the Understanding and Treatment of Disease (Torranoe, PF, ed). New York: Wiley, 2000, pp. 289–309.

8. Posner GH, Oh CH. A regiospecifically oxygen-18 labeled 1,2,4-trioxane: a simple chemical model system to probe the mechanism(s) for the antimalarial activity of artemisinin (qinghaosu). J Am Chem Soc 1992;114:8328–8329.

9. Posner GH, Cumming JN, Ploypradith P, Oh CH. Evidence for Fe(IV)=O in the molecular mechanism of action of the trioxane antimalarial artemisinin. J Am Chem Soc 1995;117: 5885–5886.

10. Kapetanaki S, Varotsis C. Ferryl-oxo heme intermediate in the antimalarial mode of action of artemisinin. FEBS Lett 2000;474:238–241.

11. Abouabdellah A, Bégué J-P, Bonnet-Delpon D, Gantier J-C, Nga TTT, Thac TD. Synthesis and *in vivo* Antimalarial Activity of 12α-Trifluoromethyl-Hydroartemisinin. Bioorg Med Chem Lett 1996;6:2717–2720.

12. Haynes RK, Vonwiller SC. Efficient preparation of novel qinghaosu artemisinin derivatives. Synlett 1992;481–483.

13. Pu YM, Ziffer H. Synthesis and antimalarial activities of 12β-allyldeoxoartemisinin and its derivatives. J Med Chem 1995;38:613–616.

14. Jung M, Lee SA Concise synthesis of novel aromatic analogs of artemisinin. Heterocycles 1997;45:1055–1057.

15. Woo SH, Parker MH, Ploypradith P, Northrop J, Posner GH. Direct conversion of pyranose anomeric OH→F→R in the artemisinin family of antimalarial trioxanes. Tetrahedron Lett 1998;39:1533–1536.

16. Posner GH, Parker MH, Northrop J, Elias JS, Ploypradith P, Xie S, et al. Orally active, hydrolytically stable, semi-synthetic, antimalarial trioxanes in the artemisinin family. J Med Chem 1999;42:300–304.

17. Jung M, Lee S. Stability of acetal and nonacetal-type analogs of artemisinin in simulated stomach acid. Bioorg Med Chem Lett 1998;8:1003–1006.

18. O'Dowd H, Ploypradith P, Xie S, Shapiro TA, Posner GH. Antimalarial artemisinin analogs. synthesis via chemselective C–C bond formation and preliminary biological evaluation. Tetrahedron 1999;55:3625–3636.

19. Beekman AC, Barenstsen ARW, Woerdenbag HJ, Van Uden W, Pras N, Konings AWT, et al. Stereochemistry-dependent cytotoxicity of some artemisinin derivatives. J Nat Prod 1997;60:325–330.

20. Posner GH, Ploypradith P, Parker MH, O'Dowd H, Woo SH, Northrop J, et al. Antimalarial, antiproliferative, and antitumor activities of artemisinin-derived, chemically robust, trioxane dimers. J Med Chem 1999; 42:4275–4280.

21. Peters W, Robinson BL, Tovey G, Rossier JC, Jefford CW. The Chemotherapy of Rodent Malaria. L. The activities of some synthetic 1,2,4-trioxanes against chloroquine-sensitive and chloroquine-resistant parasites. Part 3: Observations on "Fenozan-50f," a difluorinated 3,3'-spirocyclopentane 1,2,4-trioxane. Ann Trop Med Parasitol 1993;87:111–123.

22. Fleck SL, Robinson BL, Peters W, Thévin F, Boulard Y, Glénat C, et al. The chemotherapy of rodent malaria. LIII. "Fenozan B07" (Fenozan 50f), a difluorinated 3,3'-spirocyclopentane 1,2,4-trioxane: comparison with some compounds of the artemisinin series. Am Trop Med Hyg 1997;91:25–32.

23. Posner GH, Oh CH, Gerena L, Milhous WK. Extraordinarily potent antimalarial compounds: new, structurally simple, easily synthesized, tricyclic 1,2,4-trioxanes. J Med Chem 1992;35:2459–2467.

24. Posner GH, Oh CH, Webster K, Ager AL Jr, Rossan RN. New, antimalarial, tricyclic 1,2,4-trioxanes: preclinical evaluation in mice and monkeys. Am J Trop Med Hyg 1994;50:522–526.

25. Posner GH, Cumming JN, Woo SH, Ploypradith P, Xie S, Shapiro TA. Orally active antimalarial 3-substituted trioxanes: new synthetic methodology and biological evaluation. J Med Chem 1998;41:940–951.

26. Zhou W-S, Xu XX. Total synthesis of the antimalarial sesquiterpene peroxide qinghaosu and yingzhaosu A. Acc Chem Res 1994;27:211–216.

27. Jaquet C, Stohler HR, Chollet J, Peters W. Antimalarial activity of the bicyclic peroxide RO 42-1611 (Arteflene) in experimental models. Trop Med Parasitol 1994;45:266–271.

28. Bachi MD, Korshin E, Ploypradith P, Cumming JN, Xie S, Shapiro TA, et al. Synthesis and *in vitro* antimalarial activity of sulfone endoperoxides. Bioorg Med Chem Lett 1998;8:903–906.

29. Bachi MD, Korshin EE. Thiol-oxygen co-oxidation of monoterpenes. Synthesis of endoperoxides structurally related to antimalarial yingzhaosu A. Synlett 1998;122–125.

30. O'Neill PM, Searle NL, Raynes KJ, Maggs JL, Ward SA, Storr RC, et al. A carbonyl oxide route to antimalarial yingzhaosu A analogues: synthesis and antimalarial activity. Tetrahedron Lett 1998;39:6065–6068.

31. Von Seidlin L, Jaffar S, Pinder M, Haywood M, Snounou G, Gemperli B, et al. Treatment of African children with uncomplicated *Falciparum* malaria with a new antimalarial drug, CGP 56697. J Infect Dis 1997;176:1113–1116.

32. Van Vugt M, Wilairatana P, Gemperli B, Gathmann I, Phaipun L, Brockman, A. et al. Looareesuwan S. Efficacy of six doses of artemether–lumefantrine (Benflumetol) in multidrug-resistant *Plasmodium falciparum* malaria. Am J Trop Med Hyg 1999;60:936–942.

33. Looareesuvan S, Wilairatana P, Vaniganonta S, Viravan C, Andrial M. Efficacy and tolerability of a sequential, artesunate suppository plus mefloquine, treatment. Am Trop Med Parasitol 1995;89:469–475.

34. Gomez Landires EA. Efficacy of artesunate suppository followed by oral mefloquine in the treatment of severe *falciparum* malaria in endemic areas where resistance to chloroquine exists in ecuador. Jpn J Trop Med Hyg 1996;24:17–24.

35. Price RN, Nosten F, Luxemburger C, Van Vogt M, Phaipun L, Chongsuphajaisiddhi T, et al. Artesunate/mefloquine treatment of multidrug resistant *falciparum* malaria. Trans R Soc Trop Med Hyg 1997;91:574–577.

36. Sabchrareon A, Attanath P, Charthavanich P, Phanuaksook P, Praringyanupharb V, Poonpanich Y, et al. Comparative clinical trial of artesunate suppositories and oral artesunate in combination with mefloquine in the treatment of children with acute *falciparum* malaria. Am J Trop Med Hyg 1998; 58:11–16.

37. Akompong T, VanWye J, Ghori N, Haldar K. Artemisinin and its derivatives are transported by a vacuolar-network of *Plasmodium falciparum* and their anti-malarial activities are additive with toxic sphingolipid analogues that block the network. Mol Biochem Parasitol 1999;101:71–79.

38. White, N. Antimalarial drug resistance and combination therapy. Phil Trans R Soc London B 1999;354:739–749.

15

Antibiotics and the Plasmodial Plastid Organelle

Barbara Clough and R. J. M. (Iain) Wilson

INTRODUCTION

We are not in a position to say yet what the main function(s) of the apicomplexan plastid is, nor whether it is a realistic target for therapeutics; after all, one could argue it has lain undetected throughout the long quest for antimalarials this century without signaling its presence by the dramatic effect of some specific inhibitor. Thus, to review the effect of antibiotics on the malarial plastid organelle might justifiably be considered premature at present, although this is not the first of its kind *(1–5)*. On the other hand, progress promises to be swift because the ongoing malaria genome sequencing project has the potential to completely describe the organelle's functions within the next year or two. Moreover, the signs are promising that this "new found" organelle will provide novel targets because unforeseen metabolic pathways centered on the plastid have come to light already from scrutiny of the growing chromosomal sequence database *(6)*. It is reasonable, then, to hope that specialized pathways found to operate within the plastid compartment might lend themselves to disruption, with lethal consequences for the organism and minimal effects on the host.

This review will discuss a range of antibiotics with antimalarial activity, whose effects *might* include specific inhibition of the plastid. Frankly, in some cases, the usefulness of these particular compounds to clinicians is questionable in their present state of development. However, the potential of antibiotics as "secondary" antimalarials, used either to forestall the selection of parasites resistant to primary drugs or to treat drug-resistant malaria parasites, is an aspect that perhaps has not been fully exploited. Admittedly, there have been disappointments with drug combinations *(7,8)*, but despite this caveat, we hope the hard lesson learned over recent years of resistance developing following the sole use of individual antimalarials is sufficient to justify the essential future requirement of combination chemotherapy and, here, antibiotics might have a larger role to play. Naturally, treatment with a combination of drugs is more expensive, but at least the pharmacokinetics and safety of most antibacterial agents used in this way have been established previously. As our understanding of the plastid increases, antibiotics might also act as lead compounds for the development of synthetic inhibitors with higher specific activities than the antibiotics presently available.

Mention also should be made at the outset that it has not been possible yet to ascertain directly whether the antimalarial effect of many antibiotics is the result of their

From: *Antimalarial Chemotherapy: Mechanisms of Action, Resistance, and New Directions in Drug Discovery*
Edited by: P. J. Rosenthal © Humana Press Inc., Totowa, NJ

action on the plastid or on the mitochondrion, the other symbiogenic compartment within the cell. Earlier studies posited that the mitochondrion was the target *(9)*, but some reappraisal is now necessary. Inevitably, because both organelles are of prokaryotic origin, some inhibitors (e.g., those blocking protein synthesis) could act at more than one site [but see another cautionary note *(10)*]. The malarial genome sequencing project should come to the rescue, allowing us to identify the characteristic signal sequences used to traffic proteins from the cytosol into the respective symbiogenic organelles and, hence, which functional pathways are specific for each organelle.

ORIGIN OF THE PLASTID ORGANELLE

The plastids carried by plants and algae, even nonphotosynthetic ones, originate from endosymbiosed cyanobacteria *(11)*. These have evolved into semiautonomous, double-membraned organelles, carrying their own genome as well as transcription and translation systems. However, plastid maintenance also depends on the host cell's genome, where hundreds of genes that once were cyanobacterial have been translocated and evolved independently, targeting their cytosolic products back to the organellar compartment. This ergonomically expensive process is favored because the plastid compartment enables host cells to carry out various special, sometimes essential, metabolic pathways (e.g., fatty acid or essential amino acid biosynthesis). These prokaryotic pathways present potential targets for antimalarials.

An apparent complication in the case of apicomplexan parasites is that the plastid is of secondary endosymbiotic origin following phagotrophy, a scenario that has been played out several times in the evolution of so-called "algae" *(11)*. In such cases, the primary endocytobiont—a eukaryote bearing a plastid organelle (probably an algal cell)—was engulfed by another protist, which then usurped the algal cell, utilizing the plastid for its own purposes. For plastid maintenance to continue, this process necessitated a second transfer of cyanobacterial genes, this time from one eukaryotic nucleus to another. There are several well-documented examples *(12)* and the details need not concern us further here. However, one consequence of secondary symbiogenesis, indeed a signature of it, is that the plastid now lies within additional membranes, the number increasing from the original two, to four in *Toxoplasma gondii (13)* and three (arguably by reduction) in *Plasmodium* spp. *(14)*. A reassuring feature that has emerged from studies of these complicated genetic and cellular amalgamations is that many of the basic systems for transport of proteins across the potential membrane barriers remain fundamentally intact in secondary plastids, including those of apicomplexans *(6)*. From the point of view of this review, the membranes around the plastid also remind us that antibiotics with intracellular targets have to be amphipathic in order to gain access.

PLASTID FUNCTIONS

It is reasonable to assume the residual apicomplexan plastid carries out some biosynthetic function(s) typical of other plastids and now essential for the malaria parasite's survival. Hunting in the dark for this function will not be necessary, as it should be revealed by the genome sequencing project. It would be prudent, however, to be appraised of the possibilities by considering what is already known about other plastids—still not necessarily an exhaustive list of functions! The primary candidates are well known to be amino acid, fatty acid, and heme biosynthesis *(15)*. In plastid-

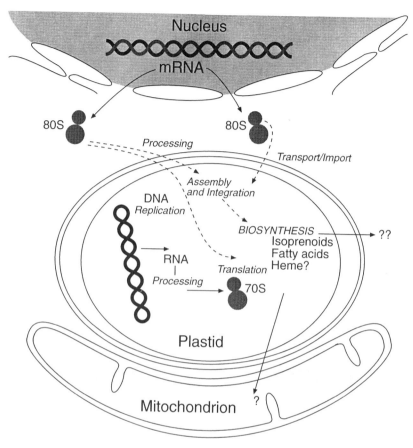

Fig. 1. Diagrammatic representation of the flow of information required for maintenance and biosynthesis in the malarial plastid organelle.

bearing cells, most of the gene products required for these pathways are encoded by the nucleus rather than the plastid genome (Fig. 1). Indeed, relatively few RNAs and proteins are still specified by plastids themselves. In the case of malaria, the sequence of the plastid genome *(16)* shows that its contribution is severely limited—largely specifying selected components required for organellar protein synthesis (rRNAs, tRNAs, RNA polymerase subunits, etc.). The many additional components required for function must be imported from the cytosol and the first examples have now been recorded *(6)*.

That protein synthesis occurs in the malarial plastid is no longer in doubt, active ribosomes having been demonstrated in the organelle by various means *(6,13,17)*. The capacity for plastid protein synthesis seems to be dedicated to the translation of a small number of open reading frames carried on the plastid genome whose products must be regarded as essential. These include a probable molecular chaperone (ClpC) and a gene of unknown function (*ycf*24-ORF 470 in *Plasmodium falciparum*) that is highly conserved in red algal plastids and eubacteria. Thus, it is likely that plastid protein synthesis, although minor in terms of the whole cell, is essential, making it a primary target for antibiotics. Unfortunately, there is no direct evidence yet that the antibiotic inhibitors of protein synthesis mentioned in what follows actually bind to their predicted targets within the organelle. The most convincing evidence that the organelle is susceptible to antibiotics comes from studies of the DNA gyrase inhibitor ciprofloxacin shown specifically to block replication of the 35-kb plastid DNA *(18,19)*.

ANTIBIOTICS: MODE OF ACTION

A striking property of antibiotics that has emerged in the present era of structural research is that they often act as allosteric inhibitors *(20,21)*, blocking conformational switches in proteins and affecting either intermolecular or intramolecular movement. Several examples will be discussed in the first part of this section, which surveys the mode of action of antibiotics, many of whose structures are indicated in Fig. 2. We begin with a brief discussion of antibiotics believed to affect the maintenance of plastid DNA (*see* the subsection Replication) before moving on to those inhibiting the complex processes of organellar transcription (*see* the subsection Transcription) and translation (*see* the subsection Translation); most antibiotics with demonstrable antimalarial activity block protein synthesis (classically) and, in several instances, nucleotide sequence data point to the plastid ribosome as the likely target. We then mention some of the newest findings correlating antibiotics with inhibition of plastid functions (*see* the subsection Proteins Imported into the Plastid) and end (*see* the subsection Clinical Experience with Antibiotics) by surveying the current clinical use of antibiotics.

Replication

DNA gyrase is an essential enzyme in prokaryotes. It controls the level of negative supercoiling of DNA by passing a double-stranded segment through a transient double-stranded break. Its properties are distinct from the type II topoisomerases of eukaryotes *(22)*, including those found in malaria parasites *(23)*. Selective degradation of chloroplast DNA following incubation with bacterial topoisomerase II inhibitors is well known *(24)*, implying that the plastid DNA could be a novel target for antimalarial drugs. Synthetic quinolones, such as ciprofloxacin, inhibit one subunit of DNA gyrase (GyrA), preventing religation of the cut DNA. A similar effect is produced by the peptide antibiotic microcin, which acts on GyrB. The ATP-inhibiting coumarin antibiotics, such as novobiocin as well as the cyclothialidines, also bind to the B-subunit. It has been demonstrated that ciprofloxacin causes selective linearization of the 35-kb plastid DNA of *P. falciparum (18)* within the dose range of several fluoroquinolone drugs shown to be cytotoxic in parasite cultures *(25)*. Of a range of fluoroquinolones including amifloxacin, enoxacin, norfloxacin, ofloxacin, and perfloxacin, ciprofloxacin (Fig. 2A) was the most inhibitory in cultures of *P. falciparum* with median inhibitory concentration (IC_{50}) values of 26 μM and 38 μM for chloroquine-sensitive and chloroquine-resistant strains, respectively *(25)*. Synergy was not observed between different classes of DNA gyrase inhibitors, but ciprofloxacin antagonized some primary antimalarials such as chloroquine and mefloquine in in vitro cultures *(26)*. Ciprofloxacin (25 μM) reduced the copy number of the plastid genome of *T. gondii* by more than 10-fold in vitro *(19)*, resulting in a delayed-death phenotype like that produced by clindamycin (*see* the subsection Spectinomycin).

Transcription

From the sequence of the β-subunit of the plastid-encoded RNA polymerase *P. falciparum* (PEP type; *see* ref. *27*), the enzyme was predicted to be sensitive to rifampicin

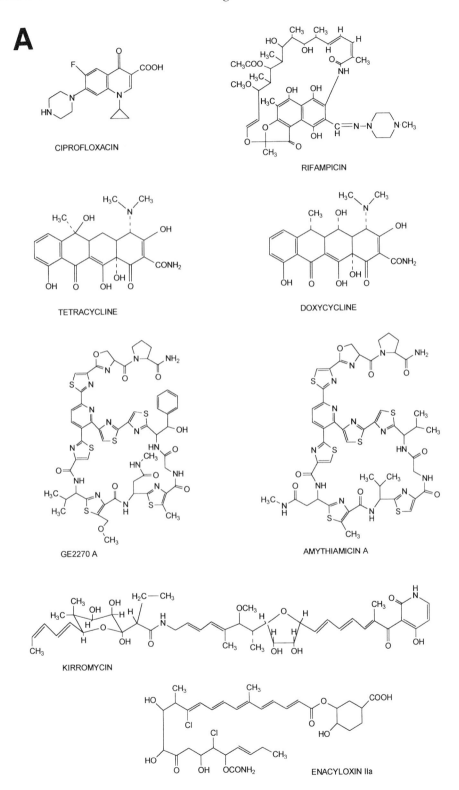

Fig. 2. Published chemical structures of representative antibiotics with antimalarial activity; prepared using the program CHEMDRAW.

B

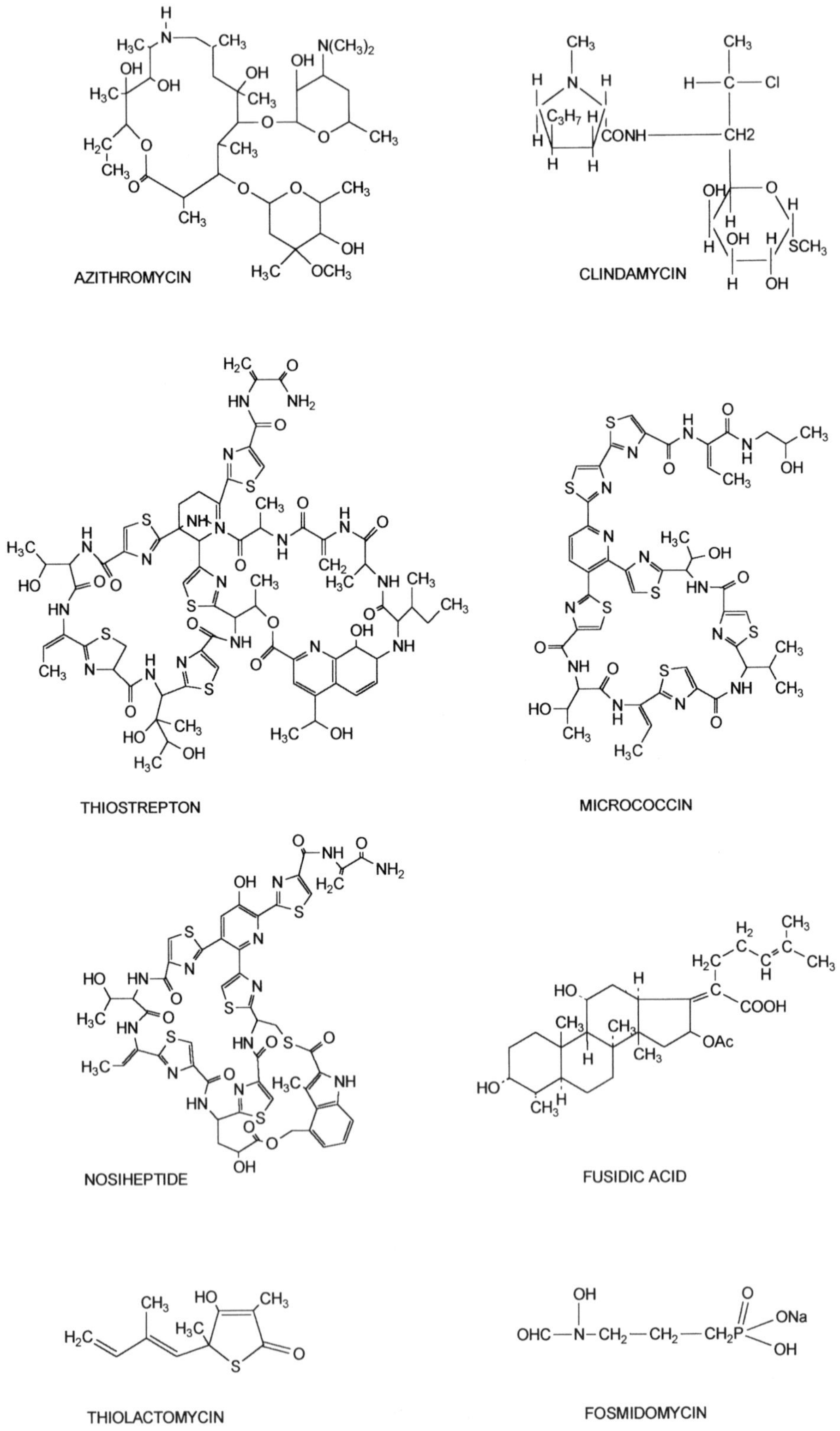

AZITHROMYCIN

CLINDAMYCIN

THIOSTREPTON

MICROCOCCIN

NOSIHEPTIDE

FUSIDIC ACID

THIOLACTOMYCIN

FOSMIDOMYCIN

(28), an antibiotic (Fig. 2A) with antimalarial activity in cultures of *P. falciparum* *(29–31)*. Loss of mRNA specifying the PEP-type RNA polymerase was reported within 6 h of rifampicin being added to parasite cultures *(32)*. By contrast, we found no inhibitory effect with streptolydigin, another antibiotic inhibitor of bacterial RNA polymerase *(31)*. Attempts to produce stable mutants resistant to rifampicin in cultures of *P. falciparum* were unsuccessful in our hands, the resistant parasites that developed always being unstable and lacking mutations in particular "hot spots" previously recorded in the RpoB subunit of rifampicin-resistant bacteria. However, since this work was done, rifampicin resistance in *Escherichia coli* has been correlated with mutations in other regions of the protein *(33)* and so our attempts to equate rifampicin resistance with a modified malarial plastid RpoB subunit must be considered incomplete. Nevertheless, rifampicin has been used clinically as an antimalarial (*see* the section Clinical Experience with Antibiotics).

A second RNA polymerase of the nucleus-encoded single subunit T7-type (NEP type; *see* ref. *27*) found in mitochondria, is expected to emerge from the growing list of *P. falciparum* nuclear genes with recognized organellar leader sequences. It should be noted that in land plants, there is also a plastid version of this second polymerase that preferentially transcribes a subset of plastid maintenance or "housekeeping genes" rather than "photogenes" *(34)*. Whether the plastids of algae (or apicomplexans) also utilize such a polymerase is unknown.

Translation

In prokaryotes, protein synthesis is catalyzed by three elongation factors; EF-Tu (the tRNA binding protein), EF-Ts (the specific nucleotide exchange factor), and EF-G (the translocation factor) (Fig. 3). Both EF-Tu and EF-G are members of the G-protein family of proteins with a conserved structural design. EF-Tu exists in two states: EF-Tu.GDP, the inactive form where the tRNA binding site does not exist because of rotation of domains II and III relative to domain I, and EF-Tu.GTP the active form that binds to aminoacyl (aa)-tRNA *(36)*. In other words, aminoacylation of the 3' end of tRNA regulates a lock and key match with EF-Tu.GTP. Upon binding of the quaternary complex to the A site of the ribosome, GTP is hydrolyzed, releasing EF-Tu.GDP, which is recycled by EF-Ts (catalyzing the exchange of GDP for GTP). Meanwhile, translocation on the ribosome is catalyzed by EF-G; its G domain interacts specifically with the "GTPase-associated site" involving ribosomal protein L11 and the A1067 loop of 23S rRNA *(37)* and possibly also the α-sarcin/ricin loop of 23S rRNA *(38)*. The tip of domain IV of EF-G also interacts with the anticodon arm of the bound tRNA *(39)*. GTP hydrolysis facilitates the exchange of elongation factors in a reciprocating fashion, triggering movement of the ribosome-bound tRNA–mRNA complex to the next mRNA codon and translocation of the peptidyl tRNA to the P site *(39)*.

As is evident from the foregoing, structural information has given considerable insight into the likely mode of action of antibiotics on the prokaryotic 70S ribosome and we have recently examined the potential antimalarial activity of a range of inhibitors of the elongation factors for four reasons. First, a *tuf* gene encoding EF-Tu is still carried on and transcribed from the malarial plastid genome *(16,40)*. Second, elongation is arguably the central step in protein synthesis (apart from the ribosome, EF-Tu is the most important target for inhibitors). Third, a range of structurally distinct antibi-

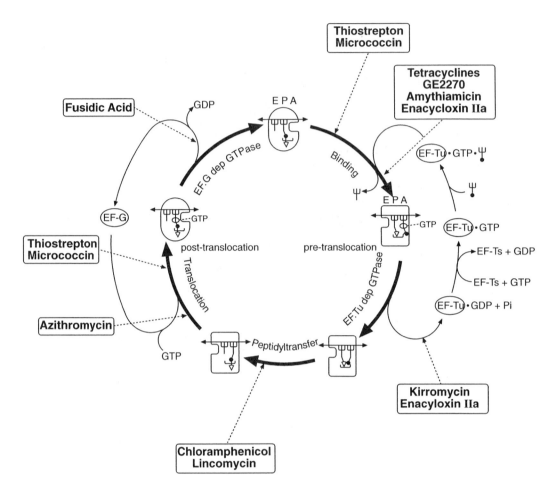

Fig. 3. A representation of the elongation cycle in protein synthesis (modified from ref. *35*) to indicate the points of action of antibiotics with antimalarial activity. Different conformations of the ribosome are indicated, before and after translocation, as well as movement of an amino acid through the aminoacyl (A), peptidyl (P), and exit (E) sites during peptide-bond formation.

otic inhibitors is available with different sites of action. The fourth, and most important reason, was that preliminary experiments with *P. falciparum* cultures found antimalarial effects with classical inhibitors of EF-G, such as fusidic acid *(41)* and thiostrepton *(42,43)*, as well as with kirromycin, the classical inhibitor of EF-Tu *(40)*. The results of our exploratory experiments with these and related antibiotics are mentioned below, along with a wider ranging summary of investigations with other antibiotics.

Aminoacyl–tRNA Binding/EF-Tu

TETRACYCLINES

The tetracyclines (Fig. 2A) act slowly on malaria parasites. Classically, they bind to the 70S prokaryotic ribosome, predominantly on the 30S subunit where there is a unique high-affinity site. This site depends on 16S rRNA (nucleotide A892, *E. coli* numbering), as well as ribosomal proteins S3, S7, S8, S14, and S19, S7 being the most important. Tetracyclines inhibit the binding of aa-tRNA to the A site of the bacterial ribosome and also interact with A2505 and U2504 in the central loop of 23S rRNA in domain V. The antibiotic has good activity against chloroquine-resistant strains of *P. falciparum* and, in this context, it is noteworthy that tetracycline-resistant prokaryotic ribosomes apparently do not exist *(44)*, any change at the unique binding site presumably being lethal. Doxycycline, a modified form of tetracycline (Fig. 2A) with a longer half-life, has been used both in treatment and as a prophylactic (*see* the section Clinical Experience with Antibiotics).

CYCLIC THIOPEPTIDES (GE2270A / AMYTHIAMICIN)

We found inhibition of protein synthesis in cultures of *P. falciparum* incubated with two thiopeptide antibiotics that interfere with the binding of aa-tRNA to EF-Tu, namely GE2770A and amythiamicin A (Figs. 2A and 3). The IC_{50} for amythiamicin A, the more effective, was 10 n*M* *(40)*. Inhibition of hypoxanthine incorporation paralleled that of isoleucine, indicating the likely presence of a second undefined effect on nucleic acid synthesis. The 10-fold difference in activity of amythiamicin and GE2270A may provide information useful for future modifications; the synthetic structures are known *(45,46)*.

KIRROMYCIN / ENACYLOXIN IIA

Despite the absence of crystal structures of EF-Tu complexed with antibiotics, much experimental information is available concerning its interaction with three different types of antibiotic inhibitors; a catalog of mutations in bacterial systems has pinpointed the binding sites for several of them *(47)*. Structurally distinct antibiotics such as kirromycin and enacyloxin IIa (Fig. 2A), although differing in their secondary effects, compete with EF-Ts by binding to a site bridging domains I and III of EF-Tu.GTP.

Kirromycin and its derivatives (e.g., aurodox, efrotomycin) are nontoxic, narrow-spectrum antibiotics once used in veterinary medicine for animal growth enhancement; a median lethal dose (LD_{50}) of over 4g/kg by mouth has been recorded *(48)*, but their activity is strongly affected by membrane selectivity. Kirromycin does not inhibit archaebacterial EF-1α (the cytosolic equivalent of EF-Tu) or eukaryotic protein synthesis directly, but it does affect yeast mitochondrial and chloroplast EF-Tu [50% inhibition at 6 µ*M* in a cell free system *(49)*]. We confirmed the lack of effect on eukaryotic protein synthesis using a myeloma cell line (up to 100 µ*M* kirromycin) but obtained an IC_{50} of 50 µ*M* for kirromycin and several of its derivatives in cultures of *P. falciparum* *(40)*. Inhibition of isoleucine incorporation was evident 5 h after exposure, maximum inhibition being reached within 10 h. This applied to both synchronized rings and schizonts, although transcription of the plastid *tuf* gene is greatest in the late trophozoite and schizont stages. It is not easy to compare kirromycin's inhibitory effect on *P. falciparum* with that on various bacterial systems, as the latter are extremely variable in their sensitivity because of differential permeability: for example, cultures of *P. falciparum* are much more susceptible than *Corynebacterium* spp.

Kirromycin has other effects on cells; in bacteria, EF-Tu acts as a positive regulator of RNA synthesis *(51)* and we noted in both the myeloma cell line and in cultures of *P. falciparum* that RNA synthesis was inhibited upon incubation with kirromycin. In the eukaryotic cell line, inhibition was measurable within 30 min, as observed previously *(51)*. A preliminary finding arguing against a nonspecific effect of kirromycin in cultures of *P. falciparum* is that inhibition was synergistic when kirromycin was combined with tetracycline or myxothiazole (a mitochondrial electron transport inhibitor), but was not with GE2770A (M. Strath et al. National Institute for Medical Research [NIMR], unpublished data).

Superimposition of the predicted amino acid sequence of the *P. falciparum* plastid EF-Tu on the three-dimensional structure of EF-Tu from *Thermus aquaticus*, confirmed that despite extreme sequence divergence compared with other known versions *(13)*, the malarial protein can be folded conventionally *(52)*. The objective of this modeling exercise was to confirm that known binding sites for the various antibiotics mentioned here are all conserved; as indeed they are, except for A237S (*E. coli* numbering) on domain I in the EF-Ts binding region of EF-Tu. In support of this, direct evidence of antibiotic interaction with the malarial protein was obtained with a recombinant version in vitro *(40)*.

A clear candidate for *tuf*M (encoding mitochondrial EF-Tu) has yet to be established in *P. falciparum (52)*, but the 530 loop of the small subunit rRNA that interacts with EF-Tu *(53)* carries the conserved G residue at position 530 (*E. coli* numbering) in both plastid *(54)* and mitochondrial rRNA sequences *(55)*.

Peptidyl Transferase

Another target for antibiotics is close to the "GTPase-associated site" on the 50S ribosomal subunit, the peptidyl transferase loop of domain V of 23S rRNA, the site of peptide bond formation *(56)*. Chloramphenicol and antibiotics such as lincomycin and its more lipid-soluble, chlorinated derivative clindamycin (Fig. 2B) compete with macrolides (e.g., erythromycin, azithromycin [*see* below]) but not tetracycline for binding at this site. Again, one of the nucleotides known from mutations to be critical for binding (A2058 *E. coli* numbering) is conserved on the plastid's 23S rRNA unlike the corresponding mitochondrial rRNA encoded on the 6-kb element *(57)*.

CHLORAMPHENICOL

Chloramphenicol inhibits *P. falciparum* cultures in vitro *(29)* but has no advantage over other antimalarials. However, it has been noted in parasite cultures that a less toxic derivative, thiamphenicol, was more potent as an antimalarial *(9)*. Lincomycin and macrolide antibiotics such as erythromycin compete with chloramphenicol, mainly for binding to the prokaryotic 50S ribosomal subunit, but probably each antibiotic inhibits peptidyltransferase activity in a different way. Unlike the plastid rRNA of *P. falciparum,* reconstructed fragments of mitochondrial rRNA corresponding to the peptidyltransferase region have an altered residue (A2058U, *E. coli* numbering) at the site associated with erythromycin sensitivity *(58)*. By contrast, the residues associated with chloramphenicol sensitivity, 2503-4 and in the 2451 region in *E. coli*, are conserved in both plastid and mitochondrial rRNAs.

CLINDAMYCIN

Clindamycin is effective against *P. falciparum* cultures in the micromolar range *(29)*. The earlier inference that clindamycin and its derivatives inhibit mitochondrial activity in apicomplexans has been reassessed, particular care being taken in studies of its mode of action in *T. gondii (59,60)*. These investigations, which included examination of protein synthesis in resistant mutants, investigation of mitochondrial function (oxygen uptake), and two-dimensional gel analysis of a small subset of proteins believed to be synthesized on mitochondrial ribosomes, led to the conclusion that neither cytoplasmic nor mitochondrial protein synthesis is affected by the antibiotic. By default, the ribosomes enclosed within the plastid compartment were suggested as a possible target of this class of antibiotics. However, appropriate mutations in the rRNA genes carried on the 35-kb plastid DNA of drug-resistant mutants have not been found *(61)*. Nor does the antibiotic inhibit extracellular tachyzoites, although nanomolar concentrations of clindamycin block replication of *T. gondii* in cell cultures. This last effect aroused much curiosity, as the inhibition only becomes apparent several days after treatment. It turns out that this lag correlates with reduced replication and atrophy of parasites that have left the host cell where they were exposed to the antibiotic, and have formed a second parasitophorous vacuole (PV) upon infection of a new cell *(61)*. Whether clindamycin treatment causes a defective PV membrane following invasion is unclear. An odd feature of the PV membrane surrounding *T. gondii* tachyzoites is that it becomes firmly connected with the outer membrane of mitochondria in the host cell by means of the parasite's integral membrane protein ROP2 *(113)*. We have been unable to ascertain if this association is affected by prior treatment with clindamycin.

Translocation/EF-G

AZITHROMYCIN

This antibiotic (Fig. 2B) is a structural analog of erythromycin, with a similar mechanism of action but better pharmacological properties (*see* the section Clinical Experience with Antibiotics).

SPECTINOMYCIN

Evaluation in cultures of *P. falciparum* showed spectinomycin had an IC_{50} of 168 µg/mL *(61)*. In *E. coli*, resistance to spectinomycin (an aminocyclitol antibiotic) has been associated with mutations in the ribosomal protein S5, as well as at nucleotide C1192G,U,A (in descending order of inhibition) in helix 34 of 16S rRNA. This helix is multifunctional, so there is room for speculation concerning the mode of action of spectinomycin, but effects on translocation have been reported. The helix is also involved in termination of translation on UGA codons—a feature of interest in some apicomplexan plastids *(63)*. In chloroplasts of *Chlamydomonas* spp. and plants, mutations on either side of the stem give resistance (nucleotides 1191-3 pair with 1065-7, *E. coli* numbering) *(64)*.

CYCLIC THIOPEPTIDES (THIOSTREPTON/MICROCOCCIN)

Thiopeptide antibiotics inhibit protein synthesis by several routes *(37,44)*, as well as having other complex biological effects *(65)*. The bicyclic thiopeptide antibiotic thiostrepton (Fig. 2B) inhibits various intermediate reactions of protein synthesis dependent on elongation factors. In bacteria, it also affects the synthesis of ppGpp, a regulatory nucleotide produced by ribosomes in association with stringency factor. Although thiostrepton is known classically for its effect on translocation, the primary effect of the antibiotic on cells appears to be inhibition of the binding of aa-tRNA to the ribosomal A site; it also blocks translocation of dipeptidyl-tRNA from the A to the P site (Fig. 3). In cooperative binding with the so-called GTPase domain of 23S rRNA and the proximal part of ribosomal protein L11, thiostrepton binds to a single site on the 50S ribosomal subunit with high affinity ($K_d > 10^{-9}$) *(44)*. Mutations in nucleotides A1067 and/or A1095 (*E. coli* numbering) of the 23S rRNA (Fig. 4), or on one face of the proline-rich helix of L11 (absent from eukaryotic versions)

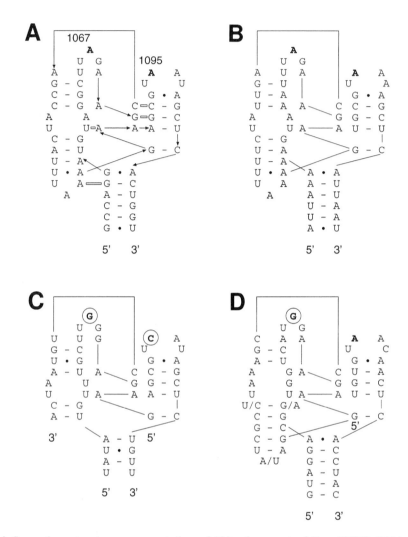

Fig. 4. Secondary structure representation of (**A**) a fragment of *E. coli* 23S rRNA from the GTPase associated domain (nucleotides 1051–1108) based on the new crystal structure of the protein/RNA complex. Lines with arrows indicate 5' to 3' direction of the backbone, horizontal bars are Watson–Crick base pairs, dots are non-Watson–Crick base pairs, open horizontal bars are tertiary bonds between bases, and bases in bold type are those interacting with thiostrepton and micrococcin. Changes to these bases are circled in (**C**) and (**D**). (From ref. *68*).

Comparative sequences from *P. falciparum* are shown for the plastid rRNA (**B**), the corresponding fragment of mitochondrial rRNA (**C**) about which there is now some doubt (*55*), and the alternative forms of cytosolic rRNA (**D**) (*43*).

(*37,66*), confer resistance to thiostrepton as well as to the distantly related cyclic thiopeptide micrococcin (*67*) (Fig. 2B). The crystal/nuclear magnetic resonance (NMR) structures now available for the RNA–protein interaction site (*38,66,68*), do not include thiostrepton, despite the fact that its NMR structure (a "hamburger minus a bite"), is available (*69*). Nevertheless, structural delineation of the "thiostrepton binding pocket" confirms much previous work and has raised the question of whether the thiazole groups of thiostrepton and micrococcin might mimic the multiple proline residues of L11 and compete for a ribosomal or factor binding site *(66)*. Alternatively, thiostrepton might interfere with a conformational transition in the N-terminal region of L11 *(66)*: In mechanistic terms, thiostrepton appears to block reciprocal oscillating conformations of the ribosome, triggered by GTP hydrolysis as the ribosome binds alternatively EF-Tu.GTP or EF-G.GTP. Finally, we note there are functional interactions between the thiostrepton-binding region and the α-sarcin/ricin loop of rRNA, so that antibiotic inhibitors of both domains II and V of 23S rRNA can be linked to the reciprocal binding of the elongation factors *(70)*.

Interest in thiostrepton as a potential antimalarial first emerged from examination of the sequence of the 23S rRNA encoded by the plastid genome of *P. falciparum (71)*. This showed that the two critical nucleotides A1067 and A1095 (*E. coli* numbering) required for high-affinity binding in prokaryotes are conserved (Fig. 4B), whereas modifications may be present in the incompletely known and fragmented mitochondrial sequence as well as in both the C and S cytosolic forms of the large subunit rRNA of *P. falciparum (32)*. Various mutational studies with short transcripts corresponding to the malarial rRNA sequence, combined with physical measurements of thiostrepton binding in vitro *(42,43)*, have clearly correlated thiostrepton binding with the plastid-encoded rRNA. However, the main modification found in the other forms of malarial rRNA (A1067G) produces much less resistance than mutations to C or U *(44)*.

In *P. falciparum* cultures, thiostrepton has an IC_{50} of 3–5 µM *(32,42)*. In one study, more than 10-fold higher concentrations of thiostrepton were required to inhibit total protein synthesis than to inhibit parasite growth *(32)*. Micrococcin (Fig. 2B) produced a similar effect but at approx 100-fold lower concentrations (IC_{50} of 35 n*M*) *(72)*. These studies implicated the plastid organelle as the target by showing within a 6-h incubation that both thiostrepton and rifampicin preferentially blocked synthesis of mRNA period specifying the plastid-encoded organellar RNA polymerase. By contrast, mRNA for merozoite surface antigen 1 (encoded by a nuclear gene) was not affected *(32)*.

We found the thiostrepton-related thiopeptide antibiotic nosiheptide (Fig. 2B) only marginally more effective in vitro (IC_{50} of 2 µ*M*). By contrast, the basic peptide antibiotic viomycin that also somehow blocks translocation was ineffective in cultures of *P. falciparum* (M. Strath et al. NIMR, unpublished data).

FUSIDIC ACID

Fusidic acid (Fig. 2B) is a steroidal antibiotic whose specificity as a classical antibiotic inhibitor of EF-G results from its poor permeability to mammalian cells. We confirmed earlier findings that it is active in cultures of *P. falciparum* at concentrations well within the range achieved by oral dosing (500 mg three times a day [i.e., 80–100 µg/mL]) *(41)*.

Proteins Imported into the Plastid

Aminoacyl-tRNA Synthetases

The plastid genome encodes a minimal set of tRNA genes but aminoacyl-tRNA synthetases encoded in the nucleus must be imported into the organelle. Cytosolic and organellar synthetases are likely to be separate entities and a gene encoding a putative organellar valyl-tRNA synthetase has been identified on chromosome 3 of *P. falciparum (73)*. A number of antibiotic inhibitors, including mupirocin *(74)*, purpuromycin *(75)*, and oxazolidinones *(76)* have been suggested as possible lead compounds to test *(77)*.

Fatty Acid Biosynthesis

THIOLACTOMYCIN

Evidence for the first biosynthetic pathway confined to the plastid (i.e., type II fatty acid biosynthesis), previously found only in bacteria and plastids, has emerged from the *P. falciparum* total genome sequencing project following the identification of several nuclear genes with appropriate N-terminal leader sequences encoding enzymes for this pathway *(6)*. The condensing step in fatty acid biosynthesis is targeted by the antibiotics cerulenin (a nonspecific inhibitor) and thiolactomycin (Fig. 2B), which blocks the prokaryotic type of fatty acid synthetases. Thiolactomycin retarded the growth of *P. falciparum* cultures with an IC_{50} of 50 µM *(6)*; in a standardized plastid test system, the IC_{50} was 2–10 µM *(78)*.

Isoprenoid Biosynthesis

FOSMIDOMYCIN

In *P. falciparum,* two nuclear genes with N-terminal plastid import leader sequences encode the enzymes 1-deoxy-D-xylulose 5-phosphate synthase (DOXP synthase) and DOXP reductoisomerase (see ref. 5). These enzymes catalyze a nonmevalonate, alternative pathway of isoprenoid biosynthesis, previously found only in eubacteria and plants *(79)*. Isoprenoids are used as substrates in diverse pathways and functions (e.g., formation of carotenoids, plastoquinone, terpenoids, and for prenylation of membrane-bound proteins) and could provide a novel target for malarial therapeutics.

Jomaa et al. found that a recombinant version of the newly discovered *P. falciparum* plastid enzyme, DOXP reductoisomerase, is inhibited by fosmidomycin *(80)*. This antibiotic and its derivative FR-900098 suppressed the growth of chloroquine-resistant *P. falciparum* cultures in vitro. Both inhibitors also cured mice infected with *P. vinkei.* Fosmidomycin, a new phosphonic acid antibiotic (Fig. 2B), has been reported to act synergistically with other antimicrobial agents, including tetracycline and nalidixic acid *(81)*. On the other hand, minimal synergy was reported with ciprofloxacin *(82)*.

CLINICAL EXPERIENCE WITH ANTIBIOTICS

A review of malarial chemotherapy a decade ago *(83)* relegated antibiotics to the end of a long list, where they figured as "other compounds of interest." Little has changed *(84)*. It was also pointed out that study of the structure–activity relationships of antibiotics might lead to the synthesis of novel candidate substances, but there has been only a small increase in the range of compounds of potential interest. Discovery of the plastid organelle and its cyanobacterial biosynthetic pathways might focus attention again on the use of antibiotics as investigative tools and as alternative therapeutic agents.

Here, we consider briefly how well-known antibiotics have fared in field trials, with notes on their use and problems as antimalarials, as well as mentioning new entries coming onto the list. Early tests of antibiotics as antimalarials *(85)* found only the tetracyclines and chloramphenicol sufficiently well tolerated and effective to be of potential value. Nowadays, combination treatment of acute infections can be made with antibiotics such as clindamycin, lincomycin, minocycline, doxycycline and azithromycin that act as schizonticides. Doxycycline has been recommended as a prophylactic. Quinine and tetracycline have an additive effect when combined and are used clinically. Minocycline and doxycycline act also on liver stages.

Current Status

Tetracyclines

Tetracycline has good activity against tissue schizonts of drug-resistant strains of *P. falciparum*. Despite this, treatment of acute infections using combination therapy with quinine plus tetracycline has had problems with poor compliance under endemic conditions, resulting, in part, from quinine's side effects (vomiting, tinnitis) *(86,87)*. It has been noted that concommitant *P. vivax* infections were not cured and recommended that primaquine should still be used in such patients. A number of trials have concluded that doxycycline is a useful prophylactic *(88)* and there have been advocates for its wider use *(89)*. However, tetracycline and doxy-cycline are contraindicated in pregnancy and in children less than 8 yr old, and further studies on the safety and toxicity of doxycycline have been recommended because of increasing numbers of reports of photosensitization in travelers *(90,91)*. Doxycycline potentiated the activity of atovaquone in vitro *(92)*, but proguanil was the preferred choice for combination treatment *(93)*. Doxycycline is not regarded as adequate prophylaxis for *P. vivax* *(8)*, but it is currently recommended as the chemoprophylactic agent of choice for those traveling to areas with high levels of multidrug-resistant *P. falciparum* (especially border areas of Thailand).

Clindamycin

Lincomycin and its more lipid-soluble, chlorinated derivative, clindamycin [7(*S*)-chloro-7 deoxy lincomycin] have a history of antimalarial testing *(94)*, as well as clini-cal use in Southeast Asia and Africa *(95)*. In experimental studies in mice, drug-resistant parasites did not emerge rapidly and no cross-resistance with tetracycline antibiotics was found *(96)*. Like other antibiotics, lincosamides on their own are not recommended for treating acute infections of *P. falciparum* and are best accompanied by another fast-acting antimalarial. Caution needs to be exercised with the diarrhea and colitis that can result from the use of clindamycin *(97)*. With these provisos, clindamycin in combina-tion with other drugs has been recommended as safe and effective for uncomplicated infections *(98)* and is routinely used with quinine to treat patients with falciparum malaria who are unable to take tetracycline or doxycycline (children, pregnant women).

Azithromycin

Azithromycin, a semisynthetic analog of erythromycin, has better pharmacokinetics and tolerance. Some have found it an effective prophlyactic antimalarial in field trials and preferable to doxycycline *(99,100)*. For prophylactic use, a daily regimen of 250 mg is required. Recent trials on adults with low levels of immunity in Indonesia, where there is a high incidence of drug-resistant *P. falciparum* parasites, gave an efficacy of only 72% compared with 96% for doxycycline *(101)*.

Azithromycin was not recommended as a prophylactic for nonimmunes, despite good protection (98%) afforded against *P. vivax*, nor has it proved useful in preventing recrudescences when given as a short course in combination with either artemether *(102)* or artesunate *(103)*.

Quinolones

Despite the discovery that DNA gyrase inhibitors act specifically on the plastid DNA, we note that the coumarin antibiotic novobiocin is no longer used to treat infections in humans because of side effects. Unfortunately, the more potent cyclothialidines have reduced antibacterial potency because of problems of permeability and/or cellular pumps. Nevertheless, future developments in such antibiotics may be of interest in the quest for new antimalarials. Exposure of parasites to the fluoroquinolone ciprofloxacin in parasite cultures for 72 h was required to bring the IC_{50} to 1.7 µg/mL, a level within the therapeutic range achieved by oral administration in man *(104,105)*. A combination of ciprofloxacin and tetracycline gave a modest additive effect in *P. falciparum* cultures *(25)*. Clinical trials of norfloxacin were successful in India *(106)* but showed no benefit to patients with multidrug-resistant malaria in Thailand *(107)*. This discrepancy may be associated with the decreased sensitivity found with chloroquine-resistant strains *(25)*. A high oral dose of ciprofloxacin (750 mg every 12 h) was insufficient to control rising parasitemias in Thai patients *(107)*, but we note that of a range of fluoroquinolones tested against *T. gondii* in vivo, trovafloxacin was much more effective than ciprofloxacin *(108)*.

Rifampicin

The antimalarial effect of rifampicin in mice infected with *P. chabaudi (31)* was confirmed in patients with naturally acquired infections of *P. vivax (109)*. It acted slowly and did not produce radical cures, but was well tolerated as a short course and may be of value in combination therapy. Rifampicin is relatively more toxic and more expensive than tetracycline, but can be given to pregnant women and young children. More recent trials in Southeast Asia and Africa with Cotrifazid (a combination of rifampicin, cotrimoxazole and isoniazid) found it effective, even in the treatment of drug-resistant *P. falciparum* in children *(110)*.

CONCLUSION

Following the administration of antibiotics, resolution of malarial infections is slow, both clinically and in cultures of *P. falciparum*. This has been attributed to the combined effect of poor permeability of the antibiotics and inhibition of mitochondrial function *(9)*. Now, however, besides ciprofloxacin *(19)*, we can point to several types of antibiotic (usually not in clinical use) where demonstration of the target *in situ* implicates the plastid organelle rather than the mitochondrion as the potential site of antibiotic activity. Particularly exciting is the discovery of bacteria-like plastid biosynthetic pathways (for fatty acids and isoprenoids) for which antibiotics already exist. On the other hand, the highly divergent nature of the plastid's ribosomal protein and rRNA sequences, as well as the bizarre fragmented rRNAs of the mitochondrion, make the veracity of some other antibiotic targets uncertain. Resolution of this quandary might not be achieved until ribosomes of both organelles have been purified and scrutinized. As a generalization, the present state of knowledge suggests that the plastid rRNA is largely conventional at sites known in other prokaryotes to be essential for sensitivity to antibiotics, the mitochondrial rRNA being less so.

Earlier studies on the effects of oxygen and time dependence on antibiotic inhibitors of *P. falciparum* argued that their effects were on 70S and not 80S ribosomes *(9)*. However, alternative explanations for the effects of some antibiotics cannot be dismissed yet. For example, a slowly developing abnormality of cytosolic ribosomes of *Plasmodium* was noted following treatment with clindamycin *(111)* and it has been suggested from studies with in vitro cultures of *P. falciparum* that the susceptibility of malarial cytosolic ribosomes to some antibiotics may not be like those of other eukaryotes *(10)*. Also, depletion of NTP and dNTP pools in *P. falciparum* has been reported in in vitro cultures 6 h after the addition of antibiotics with ostensibly different types of targets (e.g., doxycycline and ciprofloxacin) *(112)*. Thus we are still in the unenviable position where sometimes distinction between primary and secondary effects remains blurred and where often we are unable to decide whether effects can be attributed specifically to inhibition of the plastid organelle. Resolution of this uncertainty should be possible either by direct tests on fractionated ribosomes (a subject long neglected by malariologists) or by combining the increased knowledge of antibiotic interactions on bacterial ribosomes with the results of the malarial genome sequencing project and analysis of antibiotic-resistant lines of *P. falciparum*.

The discovery of the plastid has highlighted and broadened the therapeutic role of antibiotics that are already useful in malarial chemotherapy and prophylaxis. Further work on the sites of action of antibiotics with antimalarial activity is clearly indicated. Success in this direction would justify more detailed studies of antibiotic structure–function relationships so as to improve their efficacy as antimalarials.

ACKNOWLEDGMENTS

We thank David Roos (Philadelphia) for access to articles prior to publication. Also we should like to thank the British Medical Research Council for long-term support of our work on the malarial plastid. Our close colleagues at NIMR, who have always been a pleasure to work with, also deserve recognition. Finally, we thank Professor Geoffrey Pasvol (Northwick Park Hospital, Harrow, UK) for helpful discussion and comments.

REFERENCES

1. Jeffries AC, Johnson AM. The growing importance of the plastid-like DNAs of the Apicomplexa. Int J Parasitol 1996;26:1139–1150.
2. McFadden GI, Roos DS. Apicomplexan plastids as drug targets. Trends Microbiol 1999;7:328–333.
3. Ridley RG. Planting new targets for antiparasitic drugs. Nature Med 1998;4:894–895.
4. Roos DS, Crawford MJ, Donald RGK, Kissinger JC, Klimcak, LJ, Striepen, B. Origin, targeting, and function of the apicomplexan plastid. Curr Opin Microbiol 1999;2:426–432.
5. Soldati, D. The apicoplast as a potential therapeutic target in *Toxoplasma* and other apicomplexan parasites. Parasitol Today 1999;15:5–7.
6. Waller RF, Keeling, PJ, Donald, RGK, Striepen, B, Handman E, Lang-Unnasch N, et al. Nuclear-encoded proteins target to the plastid in *Toxoplasma gondii* and *Plasmodium falciparum*. Proc Natl Acad Sci USA 1998;95:12,352–12,357.
7. White NJ, Olliaro PL. Strategies for the prevention of antimalarial drug resistance: rationale for combination chemotherapy for malaria. Parasitol Today 1996;12:399–401.
8. Bia FJ. Trends and controversies in the prophylaxis and treatment of malaria. Infect Agents Dis 1992;1:108–113.
9. Divo AA, Geary TG, Jensen JB. Oxygen- and time-dependent effects of antibiotics and selected mitochondrial inhibitors on *Plasmodium falciparum* cultures. Antimicrob Agents Chemother 1985;27:21–27.

10. Budimulja AS, Syafruddin, Tapchaisri P, Wilairat P, Marzuki S. The sensitivity of *Plasmodium* protein synthesis to prokaryotic ribosomal inhibitors. Mol Biochem Parasitol 1997;84:137–141.

11. Delwiche CF, Palmer JD. The origin of plastids and their spread via secondary endosymbiosis. Pl Syst Evol 1997;11(Suppl 11):53–86.

12. McFadden G, Gilson, P. Something borrowed, something green: lateral transfer of chloroplasts by secondary endosymbiosis. Trends Ecol Evol 1995;10:12–17.

13. Kohler S, Delwiche CF, Denny P, Tilney LG, Webster P, Wilson RJM, et al. A plastid of probable green algal origin in apicomplexan parasites. Science 1997;275:1485–1489.

14. Hopkins J, Fowler R, Krishna S, Wilson I, Mitchell G, Bannister L. The plastid in *Plasmodium falciparum* asexual blood stages: a three-dimensional ultrastructural analysis. Protist 1999;150:283–295.

15. McFadden GI, Waller RF. Plastids in parasites of humans. Bioessays 1997;19:1033–1040.

16. Wilson RJM, Denny PW, Preiser PR, Rangachari K, Roberts K, Roy A, et al. Complete gene map of the plastid-like DNA of the malaria parasite *Plasmodium falciparum*. J Mol Biol 1996;261:155–172.

17. Roy A, Cox RA, Williamson DH, Wilson RJM. Protein synthesis in the plastid of *Plasmodium falciparum*. Protist 1999;150:183–188.

18. Weissig V, Vetro-Widenhouse,T.S. and Rowe TC. Topoisomerase II inhibitors induce cleavage of nuclear and 35-kb plastid DNAs in the malarial parasite *Plasmodium falciparum*. DNA Cell Biol 1997;16:1483–1492.

19. Fichera ME, Roos DS. A plastid organelle as a drug target in apicomplexan parasites. Nature 1997;390:407–409.

20. Spahn CMT, Prescott CD. Throwing a spanner in the works: antibiotics and the translation apparatus. J Mol Med 1996;74:423–439.

21. Wilson KS, Noller HF. Molecular movement inside the translational engine. Cell 1998;92:337–349.

22. Lewis RJ, Tsai FTF, Wigley DB. Molecular mechanisms of drug inhibition of DNA gyrase. Bioessays 1996;18:661–671.

23. Rioux, J-F, Gabillot M, Schrevel J, Riou G. Purification and characterization of *Plasmodium bergei* DNA topoisomerases I and II: Drug action, inhibition of decatenation and relaxation, and stimulation of DNA cleavage. Biochemistry 1986;25:1471–1479.

24. Woelfle MA, Thompson RJ, Mosig, G. Roles of novobiocin-sensitive topoisomerase in chloroplast DNA replication in *Chlamydomonas reinhardtii*. Nucl Acids Res 1993;21:4231–4238.

25. Divo AA, Sartorelli AC, Patton CL, Bia FJ. Activity of fluoroquinolone antibiotics against *Plasmodium falciparum* in vitro. Antimicrob Agents Chemother 1988;32:1182–1186.

26. Coyne PE, Gerena L, Milhous WK. Intrinsic antimalarial activity of ciprofloxacin alone or in combination with chloroquine or mefloquine. Am J Trop Med Hyg 1991;45,188.

27. Hajdukiewicz PTJ, Allison LA, Maliga P. The two polymerases encoded by the nuclear and plastid compartments transcribe distinct groups of genes. EMBO J 1997;16:4041–4048.

28. Gardner MJ, Williamson DH, Wilson RJM. A circular DNA in malaria parasites encodes an RNA polymerase like that of prokaryotes and chloroplasts. Mol Biochem Parasitol 1991;44,115–123.

29. Geary TG, Jensen JB. Effects of antibiotics on *Plasmodium falciparum* in vitro. Am J Trop Med Hyg 1983;32:221–225.

30. Geary TG, Divo AA, Jensen JB. Stage specific actions of antimalarial drugs on *Plasmodium falciparum* in culture. Am J Trop Med Hyg 1989;40:240–244.

31. Strath M, Scott-Finnigan T, Gardner M, Williamson D, Wilson I. Antimalarial activity of rifampicin in vitro and in rodent models. Trans R Soc Trop Med Hyg 1993;87:211–216.

32. McConkey GA, Rogers MJ, McCutchan TF. Inhibition of *Plasmodium falciparum* protein synthesis. Targeting the plastid-like organelle with thiostrepton. J Biol Chem 1997;272:2046–2049.

33. Severinov K, Sousko M, Goldfarb A, Nikiforov V. Rif^r mutations in the beginning of the *Escherichia coli rpoB* gene. Mol Gen Genet 1994;244:120–126.

34. Hedtke B, Borner T, Weihe A. Mitochondrial and chloroplast phage-type RNA polymerases in *Arabidopsis*. Science 1997;277:809–811.

35. Hausner T-P, Geigenmuller U, Nierhaus KH. The allosteric three-site model for the ribosome elongation cycle. New insights into the inhibition mechanisms of aminoglycosides, thiostrepton and viomycin. J Biol Chem 1988;263:13,103–13,111.

36. Berchtold H, Reshetnikova L, Reiser COA, Schirmer NK, Sprinzl M, Hilgenfeld R. Crystal structure of active elongation factor Tu reveals major domain rearrangements. Nature 1993;365:126–132.

37. Porse B, Garrett RA. Ribosomal mechanics, antibiotics, and GTP hydrolysis. Cell 1999;97:423–426.

38. Ban N, Nissen P, Hansen J, Capel M, Moore PB, Steitz TA. Placement of protein and RNA structures into a 5Å-resolution map of the 50S ribosomal subunit. Nature 1999;400:841–847.

39. Agrawal RK, Penczek P, Grassucci RA, Frank J. Visualization of elongation factor G on the *Escherichia coli* ribosome: the mechanism of translocation. Proc Natl Acad Sci USA 1998;95:6134–6138.

40. Clough B, Rangachari K, Strath M, Preiser PR, Wilson RJM. Antibiotic inhibitors of organellar protein synthesis in *Plasmodium falciparum*. Protist 1999;150:189–195.

41. Black FT, Wildfang IL, Borgbjerg, K. Activity of fusidic acid against *Plasmodium falciparum* in vitro. Lancet 1985;1:578–579.

42. Clough B, Strath M, Preiser P, Denny P, Wilson RJM. Thiostrepton binds to malarial plastid rRNA. FEBS Lett 1997;406:123–125.

43. Rogers MJ, Bukhman YV, McCutchan TF, Draper DE. Interaction of thiostrepton with an RNA fragment derived from the plastid-encoded ribosomal RNA of the malaria parasite. RNA 1997;3:815–820.

44. Cundliffe, E. Recognition sites for antibiotics within rRNA. In: Hill, WE, et al. (eds). The Ribosome, Structure, Function and Evolution. Washington DC: ASM, 1990, pp. 479–490.

45. Kurz M, Sottani C, Bonfichi R, Lociuro S, Selva E. Revised structure of the antibiotic GE2270A. J Antibiot 1994;47:1564–1567.

46. Shimanaka K, Iinuma H, Hamada M, Ikeno S, S-Tsuchiya S, Arita M, et al. Novel antibiotics, amythiamicins IV. A mutation in the elongation factor Tu gene in a resistant mutant of *B. subtilis*. J Antibiot 1995;48:182–184.

47. Abdulkarim F, Liljas L, Hughes D. Mutations to kirromycin resistance occur in the interface of domains I and III of EF-Tu.GTP. FEBS Lett 1994;352:118–122.

48. Wax R, Maiese W, Weston R, Birnbaum J. Efrotomycin, a new antibiotic from *Streptomyces lactamdurans*. J Antibiot 1976;29:670–673.

49. Parmeggiani A, Swart GWM. Mechanism of action of kirromycin-like antibiotics. Annu Rev Microbiol 1985;39:557–577.

50. Travers A. Control of ribosomal RNA synthesis in vitro. Nature 1973;244:15–17.

51. Schmid B, Anke T, Wolf H. Action of pulvomycin and kirromycin on eukaryotic cells. FEBS Lett 1978;96:189–191.

52. Sato S, Tews I, Wilson RJM. Impact of an endocytobiont on the genome of apicomplexans. Int J Parasitol 2000;30:427–439.

53. Powers T, Noller HF. Evidence for functional interaction between elongation factor Tu and 16S ribosomal RNA. Proc Natl Acad Sci USA 1997;90:1364–1368.

54. Gardner MJ, Feagin JE, Moore DJ, Spencer DF, Gray MW, et al. Organisation and expression of small subunit ribosomal RNA genes encoded by a 35-kilobase circular DNA in *Plasmodium falciparum*. Mol Biochem Parasitol 1991;48:77–88.

55. Feagin JE, Mericle BL, Werner E, Morris M. Identification of additional rRNA fragments encoded by the *Plasmodium falciparum* 6 kb element. Nucl Acids Res 1997; 25:438–446.

56. Douthwaite, S. Functional interactions with 23S rRNA involving the peptidyltransferase center. J Bacteriol 1992;174:1333–1338.

57. Feagin JE. The extrachromosomal DNAs of Apicomplexan parasites. Annu Rev Microbiol 1994;48:81–104.

58. Gillespie DE, Salazar NA, Rehkopf DH, Feagin FE. The fragmented mitochondrial ribosomal RNAs of *Plasmodium falciparum* have short A tails. Nucl Acids Res 1999;27:2416–2422.

59. Pfefferkorn ER, Borotz SE. Comparison of mutants of *Toxoplasma gondii* selected for resistance to azithromycin, spiramycin or clindamycin. Antimicrob Agents Chemother 1994;38:31–37.

60. Beckers CJM, Roos DS, Donald RGK, Luft BJ, Schwab JC, Yang C, et al. Inhibition of cytoplasmic and organellar protein synthesis in *Toxoplasma gondii*: implications for the target of macrolide antibiotics. J Clin Invest 1995;95:367–376.

61. Fichera ME, Bhopale MK, Roos DS. In vitro assays elucidate peculiar kinetics of clindamycin action against *Toxoplasma gondii*. Antimicrob Agents Chemother 1995;39: 1530–1537.

62. McColm AA, McHardy N. Evaluation of a range of antimicrobial agents against the parasitic protozoa, *Plasmodium falciparum*, *Babesia rodhaini* and *Theileria parva* in vitro. Ann Trop Med Parasitol 1984;78:345–354.

63. Lang-Unnasch N, Aiello DP. Sequence evidence for an altered genetic code in the *Neospora caninum* plastid. Int J Parasitol 1999;29:1557–1562.

64. Fromm H, Edelman M, Aviv D, Galun E. The molecular basis for rRNA-dependent spectinomycin resistance in *Nicotiana* chloroplasts. EMBO J 1987;6:3233–3237.

65. Chiou ML, Folcher M, Katoh T, Puglia AM, Vohradsky J, Yun B-S, et al. Broad spectrum thiopeptide recognition specificity of the *Streptomyces lividans* TipAL protein and its role in regulating gene expression. J Biol Chem 1999;274:20578–20586.

66. Wimberley BT, Guyman R, McCutcheon JP, Ramakrishnan V. A detailed view of a ribosomal active site: the structure of the L11-RNA complex. Cell 1999;97:491–502.

67. Rosendahl G, Douthwaite S. The antibiotics micrococcin and thiostrepton interact directly with 23S rRNA nucleotides 1067A and 1095A. Nucl Acids Res 1994;22:357–363.

68. Conn GL, Draper DE, Lattman EE, Gittis AG. Crystal structure of a conserved ribosomal protein–RNA complex. Science 1999;284:1171–1174.

69. Hensens OD, Albers-Schonberg G, Anderson BF. The solution conformation of the peptide antibiotic thiostrepton: a ^{1}H NMR study. J Antibiot 1983;36:799–813.

70. Egebjerg J, Douthwaite S, Garrett RA. Antibiotic interactions at the GTP-ase associated centre within *Escherichia coli* 23S rRNA. EMBO J 1989;8:607–611.

71. Feagin JE, Werner JE, Gardner MJ, Williamson DH, Wilson RJM. Homologies between the contiguous and fragmented rRNAs of the two *Plasmodium falciparum* extrachromosomal DNAs are limited to core sequences. Nucl Acids Res 1992;20:879–887.

72. Rogers MJ, Cundliffe E, McCutchan TF. The antibiotic micrococcin is a potent inhibitor of growth and protein synthesis in the malaria parasite. Antimicrob Agents Chemother 1998;42:715–716.

73. Bowman S, Lawson D, Basham D, Brown D, Chillingworth T, Churcher CM, et al. The complete nucleotide sequence of chromosome 3 of *Plasmodium falciparum*. Nature 1999;400:532–538.

74. Ward A, Campoli-Richards DM. Mupirocin. A review of its antibacterial activity, pharmacokinetic properties and therapeutic use. Drugs 1986;32:425–444.

75. Kirillov S, Vitali LA, Goldstein BP, Monti F, Semenkov Y, Makhno V, et al. Purpuromycin: an antibiotic inhibiting tRNA aminoacylation. RNA 1997;3:905–913.

76. Ford CW, Hamel JC, Stapert D, Moerman JK, Hutchinson DK, Barbachyn MR, et al. Oxazolidinones: new antibacterial agents. Trends Microbiol 1997;5:196–200.

77. Rogers MJ, Li J, McCutchan TF. The *Plasmodium* rRNA genes: developmental regulation and drug target. In: Sherman IW (ed.). Malaria: Parasite Biology, Pathogenesis, and Protection. Washington DC: ASM, 1998, pp. 203–217.

78. Lichtenthaler HK, Feld A, Focke M. Inhibition of early steps of de novo fatty acid biosynthesis by allicin and other xenobiotics. In: Quinn PJ, Harwood JL (eds). Plant Lipid Biochemistry, Structure and Utilization. London: Portland, 1990, pp. 410–413.

79. Rohmer M. Isoprenoid biosynthesis via the mevalonate-independent route, a novel target for antibacterial drugs. Prog Drug Res 1998;50:135–154.

80. Jomaa H, Wiesner J, Sanderbrand S, Altincicek B, Weidemeyer C, Hintz M, et al. Inhibitors of the nonmevalonate pathway of isoprenoid biosynthesis as antimalarial drugs. Science 1999;285:1573–1576.

81. Yokota Y, Murakawa T, Nishida M. In vitro synergism of FR-31564: a new phosphonic acid antibiotic. J Antibiot 1981;34:876–883.

82. Figueredo VM, Neu HC. Synergy of ciprofloxacin with fosfomycin in vitro against *Pseudomonas* isolates from patients with cystic fibrosis. J Antimicrob Chemother 1988;22:41–50.

83. Wernsdorfer WH, Trigg PI. Recent progress of malaria research: chemotherapy. In: Wernsdorfer WH, McGregor IA (eds). Malaria: Principles and Practice of Malariology. Edinburgh: Churchill Livingstone, 1998, pp. 1569–1674.

84. Olliaro PL, Yuthavong, Y. An overview of chemotherapeutic targets for antimalarial drug discovery. Pharmacol Ther 1999;81:91–110.

85. Coatney GR, Greenberg J. The use of antibiotics in the treatment of malaria. Ann NY Acad Sci 1952;55:1075–1081.

86. Fungladda W, Honrado ER, Thimasorn K, Kitayaporn D, Karbwang J, Kamolratanakul P, et al. Compliance with artesunate and quinine + tetracycline treatment of uncomplicated *falciparum* malaria in Thailand. Bull WHO 79 1998;(Suppl 1):15–18.

87. Bunnag D, Karbwang J, Na-Bangchang K, Thanvibul A, Chittamas S, Harinasuta T. Quinine–tetracycline for multidrug resistant *falciparum* malaria. SEA J Trop Med Public Health 1996;27:15–18.

88. Ohrt C, Richie TL, Widjaja H, Shanks GD, Fitriadi J, Fryauff DJ, et al. Mefloquine compared with doxycycline for the prophylaxis of malaria in Indonesian soldiers. Ann Intern Med 1997;126:963–971.

89. Jamieson A. Preferred prophylaxis varies by region. Br Med J 1999;318:1139.

90. Baudon D, Martet G, Pascal B, Bernard J, Keundjian A, Laroche R. Efficacy of daily antimalarial chemoprophylaxis in tropical Africa using either doxycycline or chloroquine-proguanil; a study conducted in 1996 in the French army. Trans R Soc Trop Med Hyg 1999;93:302–303.

91. Schuwerk M, Behrens RH. Doxycycline as first line malarial prophylaxis: How safe is it? J Travel Med 1998;5:102.

92. Yeo AET, Edstein MD, Shanks GD, Rieckmann KH. Potentiation of the antimalarial activity of atovaquone by doxycycline against *Plasmodium falciparum* in vitro. Parasitol Res 1997;83:489–491.

93. Looareesuwan S, Viravan C, Webster HK, Kyle DE, Hutchinson DB, Canfield CJ. Clinical studies of atovaquone, alone or in combination with other antimalarial drugs, for treatment of acute uncomplicated malaria in Thailand. Am J Trop Med Hyg 1996;54:62–66.

94. Seaberg LS, Parquette AR, Gluzman IY, Phillips GW Jr, Brodasky TF, Krogstad DJ. Clindamycin activity against chloroquine-resistant *Plasmodium falciparum*. J Infect Dis 1984;150:904–911.

95. Kremsner PG. Clindamycin in malaria treatment. J Antimicrob Chemother 1990;25:9–14.

96. Jacobs RL, Koontz LC. *Plasmodium berghei*: development of resistance to clindamycin and minocycline in mice. Exp Parasitol 1976;40:116–123.

97. Dhawan VK, Thadepalli H. Clindamycin: a review of fifteen years of experience. Rev Infect Dis 1982;4:1133–1153.

98. Kremsner PG, Winkler S, Brandts C, Neifer S, Bienzle U, Graninger W. Clindamycin in combination with chloroquine or quinine is an effective therapy for uncomplicated *Plasmodium falciparum* malaria in children from Gabon. J Infect Dis 1994;169:467–470.

99. Anderson SL, Oloo AJ, Gordon DM, Ragama OB, Aleman GM, Betman JD, et al. Successful double-blinded, randomized, placebo-controlled field trial of azithromycin and doxycycline as prophylaxis for malaria in Western Kenya. Clin Infect Dis 1998;26:146–150.

100. Sadiq ST, Glasgow KW, Drakeley CJ, Muller O, Greenwood BM, Mabey DC, et al. Effects of azithromycin on malariometric indices in The Gambia. Lancet 1995;346:881–882.

101. Taylor WRJ, Richie TL, Fryauff DJ, Picarima H, Ohrt C, Tang D, et al. Malaria prophylaxis using azithromycin: a double-blind, placebo-controlled trial in Irian Jaya, Indonesia. Clin Infect Dis 1999;28:74–81.

102. Na-Bangchang K, Kanda T, Tipawangso P, Thanavibul A, Suprakob K, Ibrahim, et al. Activity of artemether–azithromycin versus artemether–doxycycline in the treatment of multiple-drug resistant *falciparum* malaria. SEA J Trop Med Public Health 1996;27:522–525.

103. de Vries PJ, Hung LN, Thuy LTD, Long HP, Nam NV, Anh TK, et al. Short course of azithromycin/artesunate against *falciparum* malaria: no full protection against recrudescence. Trop Med Int Health 1999;4:407–408.

104. Krishna S, Davis TME, Chan PCY, Wells RA, Robson KJH. Ciprofloxacin and malaria. Lancet 1988;1:1231–1232.

105. Yeo AET, Rieckmann KH. Prolonged exposure of *Plasmodium falciparum* to ciprofloxacin increases anti-malarial activity. J Parasitol 1994;80:158–159.

106. Sarma PS. Norfloxacin: a new drug in the treatment of *falciparum* malaria. Ann Int Med 1989;111:336–337.

107. Watt G, Shanks GD, Edstein MD, Pavanand K, Webster HK, Wechgritaya S. Ciprofloxacin treatment of drug-resistant *falciparum* malaria. J Infect Dis 1991;164:602–604.

108. Khan AA, Slifer T, Ayaujo FG, Remington JC. Trovafloxacin is active against *Toxoplasma gondii*. Antimicrob Agents Chemother 1996;40:1855–1859.

109. Pukrittayakamee S, Viravan C, Charoenlarp P, Yeaumput C, Wilson RJM, White NJ. Antimalarial effects of rifampicin in *vivax* malaria. Antimicrob Agents Chemother 1994;38:511–514.

110. Goerg H, Ochola SA, Goerg, R. Treatment of malaria tropica with a fixed combination of rifampicin, co-trimoxazole and isoniazid: a clinical study. Chemotherapy 1999;45:68–76.

111. Powers KG, Aikawa M, Nugent KM. *Plasmodium knowlesi*: morphology and course of infection in rhesus monkeys treated with clindamycin and its N-demethyl-4'-pentyl analog. Exp Parasitol 1976;40:13–24.

112. Yeo AET, Rieckmann KH, Christopherson RI. Indirect inhibition by antibiotics of nucleotide and deoxynucleotide biosynthesis in *Plasmodium falciparum*. SEA J Trop Med Public Health 1998;29:24–26.

113. Sinai AP, Webster P, Joiner KA. Association of host cell endoplasmic reticulum and mitochondria with the *Toxoplasma gondii* parasitophorous vacuole membrane: a high affinity interaction. J Cell Sci 1997;110:2117–2128.

16

Fresh Paradigms for Curative Antimetabolites

Pradipsinh K. Rathod

INTRODUCTION

Malaria, Society, and Science

Malaria remains one of the most important infectious diseases of the world. For those who live in tropical countries, obviously, malaria causes an unrelenting health threat. Over 300 million people are infected every year and about 2 million young children die as a result of malaria in Africa every year (1). However, malaria scientists and policy-makers may look at this disease with concern for another reason. As global communities successfully mobilize increasing resources for malaria research, society will expect a proportional decrease in morbidity and mortality from malaria. Otherwise, direct questions will arise about the scientific community's ability to transfer basic knowledge on malaria biology into practical solutions in the field. In the past, public sanitation measures combined with antimalarial drugs offered significant protection against this devastating disease. In the last few decades, though, our ability to control the disease in tropical countries has been unimpressive. The widespread emergence of drug-resistant malarial parasite strains, combined with repeated failure to develop inexpensive, reliable, lasting immunization strategies, has resulted in a global health situation that continues to kill millions of individuals. This, in turn, directly threatens to erode confidence in our technical ability to deal with this disease.

Genomes, Genomics, and Drugs: Upcoming Challenges

Obviously, additional financial resources can be instrumental in generating more data on the biology of the causative agents of malaria. In the last few years, we have witnessed an unprecedented explosion in available DNA sequence information for *Plasmodium falciparum*, which is responsible for the most devastating type of human malaria (2,3). Genomes of other malarial parasites are soon to follow. Such genome sequences, combined with tools designed to look at gene functions and gene expression on a global scale (4,5), provide an opportunity for initiating malaria chemotherapy strategies in an unprecedented number of ways. Targets of future new antimalarial drugs and vaccines must lie in these databases.

However, more data on the biology of the parasite will not automatically result in new, less expensive drugs (or vaccines) if our models for successful treatment strategies are

From: *Antimalarial Chemotherapy: Mechanisms of Action, Resistance, and New Directions in Drug Discovery*
Edited by: P. J. Rosenthal © Humana Press Inc., Totowa, NJ

faulty or incomplete. In the absence of worthy guiding principles, more genome information may actually slow down drug development by diverting limited resources toward unproven, unproductive approaches to cure malaria.

Value of Defined Models

It is more important than ever to understand the molecular basis of efficacy of drugs that have been successful in the past. To deal with the onslaught of functional genomics data that will be upon us, our models for successful drug development need to be current, sophisticated, and testable. Once we have defined the parameters for what constitutes a useful drug target, identification of new targets using functional genomic tools and identifying good drugs will be a welcome challenge.

In this chapter, using *de novo* pyrimidine biosynthesis and folate-based malaria chemotherapy as a model, traditional views of malaria drug development that are on solid footing are considered along with newly recognized elements of successful chemotherapy. Concepts that may be outmoded, or even misleading, are also discussed.

UNDERSTANDING ANTIMETABOLITES
Few Drugs, Fewer Antimetabolites

Chloroquine appeared as an antimalarial agent in the 1940s and established itself as a first-line drug in many countries because of its potency against all forms of human malaria, its low cost, and its authorized use in children as well as pregnant women *(6)*. In many countries, Fansidar® (a combination of pyrimethamine and sulfadoxine) and the old standby quinine have served as second-line drugs. Some other important agents include artemesinin, atovaquone, doxycycline, halofantrine, mefloquine, primaquine, proguanil, and quinidine. Some of these drugs offer significant toxicity and others are only useful as a part of combination chemotherapy *(7)*.

Of all these drugs, only two are simple antimetabolites with a single, defined, genetically proven, drug target: pyrimethamine and sulfadoxine. These compounds were selected in the 1940s for their antimalarial properties *(8)*. Decades later, based on visual comparison of structural formulas, it was correctly predicted that the enzyme dihydrofolate reductase (DHFR) could be inhibited by compounds such as pyrimethamine *(9)*. DHFR from mammals was shown to be about 1000 times less sensitive to pyrimethamine than DHFR from the mouse parasite *P. berghei (9)*. At the time, this was a truly exciting finding because biochemists and pharmacologists were getting their first glimpses into the molecular basis for drug selectivity. Many more years passed before it was shown that parasites that were resistant to pyrimethamine had a DHFR that was less sensitive to pyrimethamine *(10)*, that pyrimethamine-resistant DHFR had point mutations that were shared between resistant strains *(11,12)*, and that transformation of the drug-resistant DHFR gene into drug-sensitive parasites conferred pyrimethamine resistance *(13–16)*. These later studies provided the much needed closure experiments to prove that DHFR alone was the principal target of antifolates such as pyrimethamine.

Antifolate Models: Friend or Foe?

Antifolates such as pyrimethamine were chosen out of thousands of molecules that were either vitamin analogs or analogs of molecules known to be efficacious against other diseases *(8)*. During their development, it was not known what their target was and it was not clear where their selectivity originated. As pointed out earlier, their mechanism of action was determined many years after it was learned that they had potent selective antimalarial activity.

On one hand, there are no antimalarial drugs whose modes of action are understood as clearly as those of the antifolates. At the same time, early successful insights into the mode of action of pyrimethamine may have prematurely lulled us into thinking that we fully understand the molecular basis of why pyrimethamine can be a potent and selective antimalarial agent. If our understanding of the mode of pyrimethamine action is incomplete, we run the serious risk of using incomplete or inaccurate models for future attempts at developing antimalarial agents.

From Correlations to Doctrine

Many of our notions of what it takes to get successful antimalarial drugs come from the action of antifolates. It is very likely that some of these traditional concepts are critical to the success of compounds such as pyrimethamine and sulfadoxine. However, as we will see in subsequent sections of this chapter, there may be more to the success of antifolates than what meets the eye.

Here, each interesting thought about the action of antifolates on malarial parasites is reviewed and compared to what is really known about action of antifolates on malarial parasites. Common generalizations that are supported by these facts are also listed. Subsequently, the relative importance of these generalizations will be critically assessed.

Thought: Dihydrofolate reductase is a proven target of pyrimethamine.
Facts: Transformation of *P. falciparum* and *P. berghei* with mutant forms of DHFR or human DHFR confers pyrimethamine resistance (13–16).
Common generalization: Inhibitors directed at individual enzymes can be good antimalarial drugs.

Thought: Dihydrofolate reductase, the target of pyrimethamine, is an essential enzyme.
Facts: Genetic proof for DHFR being essential is hard to come by, given the limitations of performing molecular genetics in malaria. However, there are pedagogical arguments for thinking that DHFR is essential. Malaria parasites are dependent on thymidylate synthase (TS) for *de novo* pyrimidine biosynthesis (17,18). The TS reaction uses methylenetetrahydrofolate and generates dihydrofolate. Dihydrofolate reductase must be necessary for recycling of dihydrofolate, at least for the TS reaction and possibly other reactions.
Common generalization: Inhibitors of essential enzymes will be good antimalarial drugs.

Thought: The potent antimalarial activity of pyrimethamine is the result of tight-binding of the drug to the proven target.
Facts: Parasites, as well as the purified DHFR enzyme, are inhibited at nanomolar concentrations by pyrimethamine (19,20). Parasites resistant to pyrimethamine show DHFR mutations (13–16, 21). Expression of mutant DHFR domains leads to reduced binding to pyrimethamine (20).
Common generalization: Nanomolar level inhibitors of essential enzymes will be good antimalarial drugs.

Thought: Specificity and lack of toxicity from pyrimethamine comes from poor binding of human DHFR to the antimalarial agent.
Facts: Mouse DHFR binds pyrimethamine 1000-fold more poorly than malarial DHFR (9).
Common generalization: The primary determinant of nontoxicity from antimalarials such as pyrimethamine is poor binding to the host enzyme. Drug development should focus on identification of host–parasite differences in active sites in essential enzymes and drug development efforts should focus on identification of ligands that bind a parasite essential enzyme about 1000 times more tightly than the corresponding host enzyme.

Thought: Drug resistance can arise through point mutations in the target enzyme.

Facts: Resistance to pyrimethamine is associated with specific changes in the DHFR sequence *(11,12)*. Mild resistance can be achieved with a single nucleotide and a single amino acid change; high-level resistance involves alterations in as many as four amino acids in the DHFR sequence. These point mutations are causal because transformation of pyrimethamine sensitive parasites with drug resistant DHFR sequences confers drug-resistance on the parasite.

Common generalization: Point mutations can compromise drug targets. Loss of drugs such as pyrimethamine to drug resistance underscores the need to constantly search for new drug targets.

Thought: Drugs lose efficacy because of resistance. Drug resistance begins primarily because of misuse by the practicing physician or the noncomplying patient.

Facts: Every antimetabolite that has been introduced in the field as a single agent has rapidly succumbed to drug resistance, including pyrimethamine *(10)*. Premature stoppage of treatment can result in subefficacious levels of antimalarial drugs in circulation. Subefficacious levels of drugs in the serum can select incrementally for resistant parasites.

Common generalization: Usage of antimalarial drugs should be tightly controlled to prevent misuse.

Thought: Whenever possible, useful antimalarials should be used as a part of a drug combination to limit the development of drug resistance.

Facts: Drug combinations such as pyrimethamine–sulfadoxine allow the drugs to last longer than when each is used individually. Pyrimethamine and sulfadoxine are synergistic *(21)*.

Common generalization: Synergistic combination of drugs are ideally suited to minimize the development of drug resistance.

Strategies Spawning from Traditional Generalizations

The foregoing generalizations may be considered the bedrock of our views on drug development against malaria and many other infectious diseases. It is not unusual to see research papers or grant proposals begin or end by invoking the importance of one or more of the above principles.

Searches for metabolic pathways and processes that are unique to the parasite *(17,18)*, searches for metabolic steps that are essential to the parasite *(17,18)*, and the search for enzymes that differ between the parasite and the host are all fueled in part by the hope that if one satisfies one or more of the above "criterion" for an important drug target, drug development will be greatly facilitated.

Even after a drug target has been identified, searches for tight-binding ligands using X-ray crystallography *(22–25)*, molecular modeling *(26–28)*, or combinatorial chemistry *(29)* are fueled by the hope that there may be subtle, important differences within the active sites of host and parasite enzymes that may be exploited for selective chemotherapy. Although there is no doubt that all these efforts do help develop good leads for antimalarial drug development, they do not seem to lead to clinically useful drugs fast enough and in a cost-effective manner.

CONFRONTING SHORTCOMINGS

Current Paradigms May Be Ineffective

Above all, current generalizations for drug development have not been useful. No clinically useful antimalarial drugs directed at specific enzymes have been developed through a systematic study of the properties of a particular enzyme or a particular metabolic step. One can argue that this is because the shortage of financial resources or a shortage of scientific groups working on malaria chemotherapy has simply not allowed for a concentrated effort to identify appropriate drug targets and tight-binding enzyme inhibitors. However, even using nucleotide metabolism and folate metabolism as models, one can show that there is not a shortage of suitable drug targets or inhibitors if we define these by prevailing general models for drug development. Where, then, is the problem?

Current Paradigms May Be Outdated

Many of the generalizations listed are not new: They were conceived in the 1940s and 1950s. These ideas were revolutionary for their time. Fifty years ago, we did not know much about the active site of enzymes or the nature of biological catalysis. We did not know much about membrane structures or the control of transport across membrane barriers. We did not know much about replication of the genome and certainly not much about the molecular forces that contribute to variation in genomes and populations. We did not understand mechanisms involved in the transfer of information from DNA to protein or the regulation of these processes. Finally, and very importantly, we knew very little about what makes cells die.

Although our understanding of biology has improved in leaps and bounds, our concepts for what it takes to get a good antimalarial drug has been pretty much static for half a century.

Potential Damage from Outmoded Generalizations

The most obvious result of using incomplete generalizations about drug development may be that resources are dedicated to simple-minded projects that have no realistic chances of delivering successful drugs in a cost-effective manner. Beyond that, if those who make judgments on what is new and worthy of credit (e.g., grant reviewers, editors of journals, patent examiners, venture capitalists, etc.) continue to rely on grossly oversimplified models for drug development, they regularly shortchange good science. When fresh ideas, which directly challenge prevailing views on what it takes to succeed in the pharmaceutical sciences, are kept out of the limelight through institutional misjudgments, there is an indefinite perpetuation of outmoded generalizations.

FRESH, USEFUL CONCEPTS

There are a series of important lessons that arise from studying nucleotide metabolism and folate metabolism that are not part of the standard folklore on drug development. The value of these concepts arise from their utility. In the past, they successfully predicted new lead compounds for potent and selective antimalarial action in a cost-effective manner. They have also helped us predict conditions that lead to emergence of drug resistance. They have helped us identify serious inadequacies of some traditional models for drug development. In the long run, these principles may help plan functional genomics studies that are most likely to identify truly good targets and good drugs for malaria chemotherapy.

Important neglected concepts that should be at the core of our beliefs on successful design of antimetabolites are as follows:

1. Some enzymes make better drug targets than other enzymes because of their role in toxicity and cell death.

2. Host–parasite selectivity of antimetabolites can arise from many mechanisms, above and beyond interactions between a drug and its target.
3. Parasite population dynamics, in addition to mechanism of drug action, determine the initiation of drug resistance.

In the rest of this review, examples from nucleotide metabolism and folate metabolism are used to illustrate the utility of these neglected concepts.

Some Enzymes Make Better Drug Targets Than Other Enzymes

There is no shortage of targets in *de novo* pyrimidine metabolism.

Pyrimidine Biosynthesis in Malaria-Infected Erythrocytes Is Odd

Most of what we know about the metabolic pathways of malaria has been learned from studying the blood-stage form of the parasite. In recent years, this is also the form of the parasite that is most accessible because it can be manipulated in vitro. Mature erythrocytes are devoid of nucleic acids and of free pyrimidine nucleotides. However, human red blood cells are rich in purines such as ATP. The metabolic machinery of malarial parasites reflects this environment. Malarial parasites efficiently salvage purines and are devoid of enzymes for *de novo* purine biosynthesis *(17,30)*. On the other hand, they possess a robust *de novo* pyrimidine biosynthesis apparatus and lack enzymes for the salvage of pyrimidines *(17,30)*.

An Opportunity and a Challenge

A combination of a potent inhibitor of *de novo* pyrimidine biosynthesis and nucleosides ought to have antimalarial activity because proliferating human cells utilize preformed pyrimidines efficiently and malaria parasites do not. Many potent inhibitors of pyrimidine biosynthesis have been tested as antimalarials with limited success *(31–33)*. However, some inhibitors of pyrimidine metabolism are unusually potent *(see* below).

Which De Novo Pyrimidine Enzymes to Target?

Of all the enzymes related to the *de novo* pyrimidine biosynthesis pathway, the two that draw special attention are DHFR and TS. These enzymes historically have proven to be good targets for chemotherapy. Dihydrofolate reductase is the target of anticancer drugs such as methotrexate, antibacterial agents such as trimethoprim, and antiprotozoan agents such as pyrimethamine and cycloguanil. Thymidylate synthase is the target of anticancer agents such as 5-fluorouracil, Z 1694, and 1843U89.

In malarial parasites *(34)*, as in all other protozoans *(35)*, DHFR and TS are part of a single polypeptide that is synthesized from a single RNA molecule. The amino end of each protein folds into a DHFR domain and the carboxyl end of two polypeptides assemble to form a TS homodimer. Clearly, the bifunctional status of malarial DHFR–TS represents a very significant difference in host–parasite biochemistry, but, until recently, it has not been clear how one would exploit this difference for selective chemotherapy.

Good Inhibitors Trigger Nucleotide Ombalances and Cell Death

Why Are DHFR and TS Inhibitors Such Potent Cell Killers?

Normally, DNA contains deoxycytidine (dC) and thymidine (dT) as the pyrimidine nucleosides. However, at a very low frequency, deoxyuridine (dU) can form in DNA molecules as a result of spontaneous hydrolysis of dC residues *(36)*. The resulting dU in DNA has to be promptly excised and the DNA repaired to avoid mutagenesis during replication. In addition, dU can appear in DNA as a result of DNA polymerase accidentally using dUTP as a substrate instead of dTTP. To avoid this problem, cells go to extraordinary efforts to prevent accumulation of dUTP. Cells contain a dUTPase to quickly degrade any dUTP that is formed *(36)*.

In mammalian cells, inhibition of TS activity immediately leads to decreases in TMP and TTP levels and increases in dUMP and dUTP levels. This increase in dUTP overwhelms the standard proofreading and repair mechanisms of the cell and causes excessive incorporation of dU residues into DNA. This, in turn, triggers massive DNA-strand fragmentation and cell death *(37)*. Inhibition of DHFR in mammalian cells, indirectly, leads to the same type of nucleotide imbalances, strand fragmentations, and cell death *(38)*. Therefore, part of the reason that DHFR and TS are such good targets for chemotherapy is that accumulation of the substrate (dUMP) and depletion of product (dTMP), in themselves, are sufficient to trigger cell death. It is not even necessary to fully inhibit TS in order to kill a cell *(39)*.

Selectivity Can Arise from Many Molecular Sources

Exploiting host-parasite differences in enzyme active sites:

Inhibiting Malarial DHFR with Selectivity

A comparison of amino acid sequences between malarial and human DHFR reveals a mere 27% identity *(34)*. This sequence diversity affects the active site. It is known that pyrimethamine binds malarial DHFR as much as 1000 times more tightly than human DHFR *(9)*. The importance of this differential host–parasite binding is underscored by kinetic characterization of mutant DHFR isolated from malarial strains that are pyrimethamine resistant and by transfection studies that show that integration of mutant DHFR–TS sequences into pyrimethamine-sensitive parasites results in resistance to pyrimethamine *(40,41)*.

Recent data on translational control of DHFR–TS suggest that additional factors related to species-specific cellular responses to DHFR and TS inhibitors may play an important role in the selective antimalarial activity of agents directed at this target (Zhang and Rathod, unpublished data; *see* following subsection).

Inhibiting TS with Selectivity

Unlike DHFR, TS is a very conserved enzyme. A comparison of the amino acid coding sequence reveals about 56% identity between human and malarial TS. Furthermore, unlike DHFR enzymes that show very different sensitivities to DHFR inhibitors, to date, all TS enzymes have essentially identical kinetic properties and bind TS inhibitors with equal avidity *(42,43)*. So how can one inhibit malarial TS with selectivity?

Exploiting Host–Parasite Differences Away from Enzyme Active Sites

Selectivity Through Differential Uptake and Metabolism of Pro-Drugs

Thymidylate synthase catalyzes a reaction involving two substrates: dUMP and methylene-tetrahydrofolate (MTHF). There exist substrate analogs of both dUMP and MTHF that inhibit TS enzymes at nanomolar concentrations.

5-Fluoro-2'-deoxyuridylate (5-FdUMP) binds malarial as well as human TS with a K_i of about 1 nM *(42)*. 5-FdUMP cannot be used as a drug itself because it does not permeate cells. Mammalian cells are extremely vulnerable to 5-fluorouracil and to 5-fluoro-2'-deoxyuridine because these preformed pyrimidines can be converted to the toxic 5-FdUMP by salvage pathways. Malarial parasites are inherently resistant to these compounds because they lack the enzymes to activate these molecules to nucleotides *(17,44)*.

5-Fluoroorotate, though, is a potent and selective inhibitor of malarial parasite proliferation. It shows a median inhibitory concentration (IC_{50}) of about 5 n*M* against all malarial strains tested *(44)*. It does not show toxicity to mammalian cells until one uses about 1000 times higher concentrations. 5-Fluoroorotate can cure malaria in mice, whether delivered intraperitoneally or orally *(45)*. 5-Fluoroorotate, after entering malarial parasites, is metabolized to 5-FdUMP and inactivates TS *(46)*.

The potent antimalarial activity of 5-fluoroorotate is likely the result of its selective and efficient transport through the tubovesicular membrane (TVM) network of infected erythrocytes *(47)* and the easy activation of this molecule to nucleotides *(48)*. Mutants resistant to 5-fluoroorotate have decreased ability to take up exogenous 5-fluoroorotate and orotate *(49)*.

Selectivity Through Differential Rescue of Mammalian Cells

Folate-based TS inhibitors like D1694 and 1843U89 arrest mammalian cells with an IC_{50} of about 1–10 n*M (50,51)*. This toxicity can be completely reversed with 10 μ*M* thymidine. The complete lack of toxicity of these folate-based inhibitors in the presence of thymidine underscores the specific and selective activity of the compounds against TS. The compounds do not interfere with any other important function in the cell.

Because malarial parasites cannot utilize exogenous thymidine, a combination of a folate-based TS inhibitor and thymidine was expected to inhibit malarial parasites with absolutely no toxicity to host cells *(52)*.

Recently, 1843U89 was shown to be a potent folate-based inhibitor of purified malarial TS *(43)*. The binding was noncompetitive with respect to methylene–tetrahydrofolate and had a K_i of 1 n*M*. The compound also had potent antimalarial activity in vitro. *Plasmodium falciparum* cells in culture were inhibited by 1843U89 with an IC_{50} of about 70 n*M* and the compound was effective against drug-sensitive and drug-resistant clones. As predicted by the biochemistry of the parasite, the potent inhibition of parasite proliferation by 1843U89 could not be reversed with 10 μ*M* thymidine *(43)*. In contrast, in the presence of 10 μ*M* thymidine, mammalian cells were unaffected by 1843U89 even at concentrations as high as 0.1 m*M*. This greater than 10,000-fold in vitro therapeutic window between malarial and mammalian cells illustrates the powers of understanding differences in host–parasite biochemistry away from the active site of the target enzyme. On this basis, folate-based TS inhibitors may offer a powerful additional tool to combat drug-resistant malaria.

An Opportunity to Interfere with Protein–Protein Interactions

In *P. falciparum*, the DHFR and TS activities that are conferred by a single 70-kDa bifunctional polypeptide (DHFR–TS) assemble into a functional 140-kDa homodimer. In mammals, the two enzymes are smaller distinct molecules encoded on different genes. A 27-kDa amino-terminal domain of malarial DHFR–TS is sufficient to provide DHFR activity, but, until recently, the structural requirements for TS function had not been established.

Although the 3' end of the DHFR–TS gene had high homology to TS sequences from other species, expression of the TS protein fragment failed to yield an active TS enzyme and it failed to complement TS⁻ *E. coli. (53)*. Unexpectedly, even partial 5'-deletion of the full-length DHFR–TS gene abolished TS function on the 3' end. Thus, it was hypothesized that the amino end of the bifunctional parasite protein played an important role in TS function. When the 27-kDa amino-terminal domain (DHFR) was provided in trans, a previously inactive 40-kDa carboxyl domain from malarial DHFR–TS regained its TS function. Physical characterization of the "split enzymes" revealed that the 27-kDa and the 40-kDa fragments of DHFR–TS had reassembled into a 140-kDa hybrid complex *(53)*.

Therefore, in malarial DHFR–TS, there are species-specific physical interactions between the DHFR domain and the TS domain and these interactions are necessary to obtain a catalytically active TS. Interference with these essential protein–protein interactions could lead to new selective strategies to treat parasites resistant to traditional DHFR–TS inhibitors.

It has been argued that electrostatic channeling plays an important role in the kinetics of parasite DHFR–TS. In *Leishmania* and *Toxoplasma*, as much as 80% of dihydrofolate may move directly from TS to DHFR without equilibrating with bulk solvent *(54,55)*. However, the importance of this channeling to malaria pharmacology is probably negligible. The active sites of purified DHFR–TS can accept substrates from bulk solvent, they are fully active when the other site is inhibited, and, in intact parasites, human DHFR can replace the functions of an inhibited malaria DHFR even when the external DHFR is not set up for channeling *(56)*.

Malarial Serine Hydroxymethyltransferase

Three enzymes are involved in methylene–tetrahydrofolate recycling in malaria: TS, DHFR, and serine hydroxymethyltransferase (SHMT). Unlike DHFR–TS, properties of malarial SHMT have remained a mystery for a long time. Recently, the gene for this enzyme was cloned and sequenced, and the SHMT protein from *P. falciparum* was expressed in functional form *(57)*. The genomic sequence had 1485 bp including a 159-bp intron near the 5' end of the gene. The open reading frames coded for a 442 amino acid protein with 38–47% identity to SHMT sequences from other species. The function of this sequence was established through transformation of the malarial SHMT coding sequence in *glyA* mutants of *E. coli*. Expression of malarial SHMT relieved glycine auxotrophy in these mutants and permitted assay of SHMT catalytic activity in bacterial cell lysates.

Thus, it may be possible to attack malarial TS indirectly not just by inhibiting malarial DHFR and attacking *de novo* folate biosynthesis but also by attacking SHMT. The malarial enzyme and the heterologous expression system described earlier will be useful for screening of SHMT inhibitors and for developing new chemotherapeutic strategies directed at malarial TS.

Exploiting Host–Parasite Differences in Cellular Responses to Inhibitors
How do Mammalian Cells Respond to Inhibitors of DHFR and TS?

During cancer chemotherapy, treatment of mammalian cells with inhibitors of DHFR or TS is associated with large accumulation of dead target protein *(58)*. Careful analysis of this phenomenon has revealed that inhibition of TS (or DHFR) triggers production of more TS (or more DHFR, respectively). This induction of protein synthesis appears to be the result of derepression of translation. Mammalian DHFR and TS bind their respective RNAs *(59)*. This controls the amount of DHFR or TS that is made at a given time. The pharmacological interest in such regulation stems from the fact that when the enzyme is inhibited by a drug, the RNA is no longer associated with the protein and is free to synthesize more of the target protein. As a result of such a mechanism operating in mammalian cells, larger quantities of DHFR and TS inhibitors are needed to kill the cells. As protein binds incoming drug, the cells respond by making more target protein. Recently, it was argued that the posttranscriptional increase in TS levels in response to TS inhibitors is primarily the result of stabilization of the target protein and not an increase in protein synthesis *(60)*. However, this study had its own ambiguities, and it may have relied on invalid assumptions (e.g., the rate-limiting step in TS synthesis was expected to be the loading of the ribosomes, it was assumed that a single binding site on the TS RNA was solely responsible for all the translational control of TS, etc.).

Is There Translational Regulation of DHFR–TS in Malaria Parasites?

Because posttranscriptional regulation of TS is seen in *E. coli*, mice, and humans, it is likely that malaria parasites may also use such a mechanism. Whether malaria parasites use translational control mechanisms to regulate DHFR–TS has profound implications on what type of drugs are likely to be effective antimalarials. Given the bifunctional nature of malarial DHFR–TS, there are opportunities for differential host–parasite responses to antimetabolites. If malarial bifunctional DHFR–TS engages in protein–RNA contact, which inhibitors of DHFR or TS would release RNA from protein and, thereby, promote translation of more DHFR–TS? This question is important because compounds that can inhibit DHFR or TS action without inducing synthesis of more target protein are likely to be effective at very low concentrations. This type of analysis also has bearing on whether drug combinations will be synergistic or antagonistic. For instance, if both the DHFR and TS active sites are involved in binding RNA tightly, inhibition of one or the other active site will result in potent antimalarial activity. This is because the free active site in the bifunctional protein will continue to repress translation. However, in this hypothetical example, a combination of DHFR and TS inhibitors would promote protein synthesis and be antagonistic. Preliminary data show that malarial DHFR–TS binds its own RNA tightly and selectively (Zhang and Rathod, unpublished data).

Translational Control of DHFR–TS May Explain Some Mysteries in Malaria.

Malaria parasites have as few as 500 molecules of DHFR–TS per cell, which is about 1000 times less than what is seen in mammalian cells (Zhang and Rathod, unpublished data). This low-level expression of DHFR–TS in the parasite may be the result of very tight autoregulation of DHFR–TS through translational repression.

It may also explain difficulties in overexpressing malarial DHFR–TS in heterologous systems such as *E. coli*. It has generally been assumed that the latter probably has to do with the odd codon usage of malarial genes *(40)*. Although this may be partially true, tight binding of malarial DHFR–TS to RNA would also limit its expression in parasites as well as in heterologous expression systems.

It is not fully understood why compounds such as WR99210 inhibit malarial but not host cell proliferation. Fidock and Wellems *(56)* have clearly demonstrated that transfection of human DHFR into malarial parasites confers 4000-fold resistance to WR99210, leaving little doubt that DHFR is the target of WR99210. However, kinetic studies show that WR99210 is a potent inhibitor of both malarial and host DHFR (Zhang and Rathod, unpublished results). The selective activity of WR99210 may have much to do with differences in cellular responses of mammalian cells versus malaria para-sites to the antifolate. Additionally, the potent and selective activity of pyrimethamine may have to do with more than just tighter binding of this compound to malarial DHFR.

Although it is clear that some mutations in the DHFR–TS region confer higher K_i values for DHFR inhibitors, as one analyzes parasites with many DHFR mutations, there is not a perfect correlation between K_i values and the degree of resistance conferred in the parasite *(40)*. This is true even after one removes the "folate effect" by measuring inhibition of parasite proliferation in folate-free media. It is possible that some point mutations result in weakened translational inhibition and increased target production, which can contribute to resistance.

Population Dynamics Determine Initiation of Drug Resistance

Resistance to traditional established drugs continues to make malaria a serious global threat *(1)*. Resistance against chloroquine first appeared in Southeast Asia and in South America in the late 1950s. Today, chloroquine resistance is prevalent in all tropical and many subtropical countries. In recent years, second-line drugs, such as Fansidar have also failed in many parts of the world. New drugs such as mefloquine and halofantrine have had a very short useful life, especially in Southeast Asia. There is growing evidence that para-sites in some regions of the world, such as Southeast Asia, are developing resistance at a very high rate *(61,62)*. With increased travel between countries and mass migrations across borders, drug resistance in malaria parasites is no longer a localized threat.

Nature of Drug Resistance

Resistance to antimetabolites that have specific protein drug targets appears primarily through point mutations that alter the binding of the drug to the target enzyme. Such changes have been demonstrated for pyrimethamine, sulfadoxine *(63)*, and atovaquone *(64)*. Additional mechanisms may include alterations in folate utilization *(65,66)*.

Chloroquine, mefloquine, and halofantrine have complex and incompletely under-stood mechanisms of action *(67, Ch. 6)* and resistance *(6, Ch. 8)*.

Initiation of Drug Resistance in Malaria

MALARIA VERSUS CANCER

Treating population-based infectious diseases like malaria with chemotherapeutic agents is fundamentally different than treating patient-centered diseases such as cancer or a heart ailment. When a drug fails in cancer treatment, the resistant cells do not pass on to a new patient. In cancer chemotherapy, drug resistance in each patient has to initiate as a *de novo* event. In sharp contrast, when a malaria patient acquires resistance to a drug, that drug-resistance trait can be propagated through a vector to the parasite population at large.

For these reasons, every drug developed for malaria chemotherapy has to be effec-tive not just against one individual or a village but also against parasites infecting all the people in the world for a sustained amount of time.

GENETIC VARIATION

The ability of DNA polymerases to discriminate between nucleoside triphosphate substrates, their ability to correct mistakes through proofreading mechanisms, and the ability of DNA repair enzymes to correct errors in newly synthesized strands together determine the fidelity of DNA replication *(36)*. For most normal cells the error rate is about 10^{-10} per base pair per replication (Table 1). It is such error rates that contribute

Table 1
Comparing Standard Frequencies of Mutations to Parasite Population Sizes

Rates per generation		Parasite population sizes	
		Mosquito Bite	10^2 parasites
Loss of function	10^{-7}		
One nucleotide change	10^{-10}		
		One patient	10^{11} parasites
		A million patients	10^{17} parasites
		The world	10^{19} parasites
Two simultaneous changes	10^{-20}		
		10-yr use of a drug	10^{22} parasites

to genetic diversity and initiation of drug resistance. If a drug can be compromised by a specific type of point mutation, to find one cell that has the appropriate nucleotide substitution at a given base in the parasite genome, one would have to start with a population of at least 10^{10} cells.

PARASITE POPULATION SIZES

A typical patient with serious malaria can have 10^{11} parasites in the body. If the mutation rate in malaria parasites is similar to that in other "standard" organisms, no matter how selective and how safe a drug appears in preclinical trials, if the effectiveness of an antimalarial agent can be compromised by one point mutation, the drug will not be able to reliably cure a single patient and certainly not be able to eradicate a global population of parasites.

If a drug can be compromised by a loss of function mutation (whose frequencies can be as high as 10^{-6} and 10^{-7}), the drug may not even be able to eliminate all parasites in a simple, small-animal model *(45,64)*.

Even for drugs or some drug combinations that require three to four point mutations to be relegated as ineffective *(63)*, if there are incremental benefits to the parasite from single point mutations *(40,63,68)*, it is likely that the drug will be compromised in a relatively short time.

New antimalarial agents that have staying power will be those that require many point mutations simultaneously before they are compromised.

DRUG COMBINATIONS

In many discussions on drug combinations, attention is focused on the importance of synergistic combinations *(69)*. In an individual patient, synergy can be very useful because it decreases potential toxic effects. However, on a population scale, the true power of drug combinations comes from the fact that the frequency of resistance to two compounds that work through independent mechanisms is a multiple of the frequencies of resistance to each compound.

In an experimental system, two nonsynergistic compounds, 5-fluoroorotate and atovaquone, could eliminate exponentially larger populations of parasites compared to each compound alone *(70)*. Drug combinations should not be dismissed or discounted because they lack synergistic effects against small parasite populations.

MULTITARGETING ANTIMETABOLITES

There is a dream for now. Chloroquine proved to be a successful drug on a global scale for decades. This success was not because the actions of chloroquine are unusually specific and not because the drug is unusually nontoxic. Quite to the contrary, the margin of safety for chloroquine is so small that a 10-fold overdose can result in serious toxicity *(71)*. A 10-fold increase in resistance by a parasite is sufficient to make this drug too toxic for therapeutic use *(72)*.

Most likely, the long-term success of chloroquine as a drug came from its ability to act without succumbing to drug resistance against massive numbers of parasites that had huge potential for genetic variation. This staying power probably arises from three factors: (1) the pharmacological properties of chloroquine that allowed for sustained efficacious serum concentrations of the drug from single weekly doses, (2) its ability to kill most if not all parasites within this time frame, and, (3) its mode of action. Although we do not know with certainty the exact means by which choloroquine kills malaria parasites, it is unlikely to be the result of inhibition of a single enzyme, otherwise resistance would have occurred with ease. Chloroquine probably kills through disruptions of many broad processes (Chapter 6). Chloroquine resistance is associated with alterations in not just one or two nucleotides but perhaps dozens of nucleotides, possibly in more than one gene *(72,73*; Fidock and Wellems, private communication; Chapter 8).

How can one dream of having an antimetabolite with the staying power of chloroquine? The answer is multitargeting. If one could design a *single antimetabolite* that simultaneously inhibited more than one malarial enzyme with specificity, the odds of finding a parasite that is able to evade the drug through genetic alterations now reach a maximum of about 10^{-20}. If more than one nucleotide change is necessary for saving a target or if the multitargeting drug can attack three targets, instead of just two, a global parasite population would have a truly difficult time developing drug resistance by altering all targets simultaneously. The beauty of multitargeting with a single agent over drug combinations is that issues of differential pharmakokinetics become irrelevant *(74)*. It is still possible that parasites may develop other mechanisms of resistance to this strategy such as modification of the target or interference with entry of the drug into the parasites, but there are intellectual solutions to these types of problems.

When we have difficulties finding single agents that work with potency and selectivity, what hope is there to develop reagents that successfully multitarget? The development of combinatorial chemistry approaches for finding ligands with appropriate properties and functional genomics tools to find drug targets with the necessary susceptibility patterns should facilitate drug development.

VARIATIONS IN FREQUENCY OF DRUG RESISTANCE IN MALARIA

Recent history teaches us that drug resistance to previously successful antimalarial agents arose from specific parts of the world *(1)*. A traditional explanation for such observations is that parasites in certain places (e.g., Southeast Asia) simply have had greater opportunity for developing resistance because parasites in that part of the world have been exposed to more new drugs than anywhere else. One could also argue that physicians or patients in that part of the world have not used drugs as recommended.

However, another plausible possibility is that parasites in these regions have developed generic mechanisms for *initiating* drug resistance at a more rapid rate than parasites in other parts of the world. To test this hypothesis, different *P. falciparum* clones were treated with two new antimalarial agents: 5-fluoroorotate and atovaquone *(62)*. All parasite populations were equally susceptible in small numbers. However, when large populations of these clones were challenged with either of the two compounds, significant variations in frequencies of resistance became apparent. On one extreme, clone D6 from West Africa, which was sensitive to all traditional antimalarial agents, failed to develop resistance under simple nonmutagenic conditions in vitro. In sharp contrast, the Indochina clone W2, which was known to be resistant to all traditional antimalarial drugs, independently acquired resistance to both new compounds as much as a 1000 times more frequently than D6. Additional clones that were resistant to some (but not all) traditional antimalarial agents, acquired resistance to atovaquone, but not 5-fluoroorotate, at high frequency. These findings were unexpected and surprising based on current views of the evolution of drug resistance in *P. falciparum* populations. Such new phenotypes, named accelerated resistance to multiple drugs (ARMD), raise important questions about the genetic and biochemical mechanisms related to the initiation of drug resistance in malaria parasites. Some potential mechanisms underlying ARMD phenotypes have public health implications that are ominous.

READJUSTING FUTURE RESEARCH PRIORITIES

In recent years, our dominant paradigm for rational drug development involves identification of essential enzymes in the parasite, expression and purification of such enzymes, crystallization and structure determination of these proteins, and searches for tight-binding ligands for such proteins.

Rational drug development cannot be based merely on understanding binding interactions between a drug and a protein. A research program narrowly focused on identification of tight-binding inhibitors to an enzyme easily leads to micromolar inhibitors, and sometimes to nanomolar inhibitors, but rarely to compounds that cure diseases in the field. The more one understands the biology of the parasite and the host, the better the odds of developing truly useful therapeutic strategies that are sound and that are likely to lead to clinical utility.

As we return to more comprehensive views of parasite biology and of drug development, the following deserve at least as much attention as enzyme structure determination.

Host–Parasite Metabolic Pathways

Historically, this is an area of research that is not exactly neglected. It has always been recognized that if one can find a biochemical step or pathway that is unique and essential to the parasite (not found in the host), one can target such a step for selective chemotherapy. However, in addition to knowing which metabolic steps or processes are unique or essential to the parasite, it is equally important to know how dependent the host is on that pathway. There are now numerous examples of pathways that are found both in the host and in the parasite where the pathway is nonessential in the host but is essential in the parasite (e.g., *de novo* pyrimidine metabolism, purine salvage pathway). These considerations can also lead to successful chemotherapeutic strategies.

Transport of Nutrients and Drugs In and Out of Parasites

Information on movement of compounds in and out of cells can be useful in (1) delivery of appropriate drug precursors into parasite cells with selectivity, (2) understanding mechanisms of resistance where the parasite begins to, for instance, utilize exogenous folate that it previously did not import, and (3) anticipating additional mechanisms of drug resistance.

Historically, our understanding of movements of molecules in and out of cells, and within cells, has been extremely limited. Not only do we not know how many different types of metabolic transporters the parasite has, we know very little about where they are located and how essential they are to the parasite for survival. If a drug depends on a nonessential transporter for selectivity or potency, loss of function mutations will readily lead to resistance. Hopefully, these issues will become easier to address as the whole genome of malaria parasites is characterized.

Metabolism of Drugs and Drug Analogs in Parasites

Many antimetabolites that work at nanomolar levels concentrate inside the target cell. This concentration can arise from conversion of a neutral compound into a charged compound that cannot diffuse out of the parasite. Such strategies have been used with great effectiveness in nucleotide metabolism where pyrimidine bases are converted to nucleotides *(46)*. However, we need to know a great deal more about opportunities in malarial parasites to modify pro-drugs, whether they arrive in the form of nucleotide, sugar, lipid, or amino acid precursors. We also need to know how essential these enzymes are to the parasite. As with transporters, a drug that relies on activation by a parasite enzyme would be readily compromised if that enzyme is nonessential to the parasite.

Cellular Responses of Parasites to Antimetabolites

As pointed out in detail earlier, how a cell responds to an antimetabolite (transcriptionally or translationally) can make a big difference in the effectiveness and selectivity of the drug. Whether a cell can or cannot overproduce a specific drug target in response to a drug may be a major determinant in successful chemotherapy. This area of pharmacology is least well understood, but new tools in functional genomics ought to generate a good deal of useful data rapidly.

Resistance to Individual Drugs in Individual Cells

Traditionally, the pharmacology community has placed an unusual importance on identifying host–parasite differences in active sites. Such differences, even when exploitable, may facilitate discovery of ligands that bind with selectivity but they also may make it easy for the parasite to alter the active site without losing catalytic function.

Is it possible that the better drug targets are enzymes that perform difficult chemical tasks, where the active sites are strongly conserved between species and where point mutations that give rise to weaker binding of drug also cause loss of function for the enzyme? Such may be the case with the targets of 5-fluoroorotate (TS; *see* ref. *42*) and difluoromethylornithine (ornithine decarboxylase; *see* ref. *75*). Of course, selectivity for these types of antimetabolites has to come from factors away from the active site of the target enzyme.

Population Responses of Parasites to Antimetabolites

It is now clear that parasite populations do not acquire resistance to drugs at a uniform rate. Even in the absence of pre-existing differences in susceptibility of parasites to a drug, some parasites acquire resistance to some antimetabolites as much as 1000 times faster than to others. Do these parasites which display the ARMD phenotype constitutively mutate at a higher rate or are high rates of mutations induced under drug pressure? If stress plays a role in higher rates of genome alterations, do all classes of drugs induce such changes or just a subset of classes such as antimetabolites directed at nucleotide metabolism? Does the location of the gene for the target make a difference in whether a gene is more likely to mutate? Answers to such questions will play a profound role in selection of strategies for attacking malarial populations.

CONCLUSIONS

Experience to date with inhibitors of *de novo* pyrimidine biosynthesis and folate metabolism is teaching us that:

1. The molecular basis of successful chemotherapy against malaria can be understood at the molecular level.
2. Efficacy against malaria infections can be correctly predicted, if a system is well understood.

As our understanding of cell function has matured in the last 50 yr, our models for successful chemotherapy need to keep pace. Some of the successes in identifying new inhibitors of pyrimidine and folate metabolism have come from deliberately avoiding old, simple generic models and paradigms for drug development. The broader lessons learned from understanding mechanisms of action of effective antimetabolites directed at pyrimidine metabolism ought to be of use in developing other classes of antimetabolites against malaria.

In the future, emerging tools for malaria functional genomics *(4,5)* will undoubtedly offer unexpected views of cellular processes that underlie selective chemotherapy. Our models and paradigms for malaria chemotherapy will continue to improve. Studies on inhibitors of pyrimidine and folate metabolism in malaria, hopefully, will continue to help in this process.

ACKNOWLEDGMENTS

PKR has been supported by grants from the National Institute of Allergy and Infectious Diseases (AI26912 and AI40956) and by a New Initiatives in Malaria Research Award from the Burroughs Wellcome Fund.

REFERENCES

1. Trigg PI, Kondrachine AV. The current global malaria situation. In: Sherman IW (ed). Malaria: Parasite Biology, Pathogenesis, and Protection, Washington DC: ASM, 1998, pp. 11–22.
2. Gardner MJ, Tettelin H, Carucci DJ, Cummings LM, Aravind L, Koonin EV, et al. Chromosome 2 sequence of the human malaria parasite *Plasmodium falciparum* Science 1998;282:1126–1132.
3. Bowman S, Lawson D, Basham D, Brown D, Chillingworth T, Churcher CM, et al. The complete nucleotide sequence of chromosome 3 of *Plasmodium falciparum*. Nature 1999;400:532–538.
4. Wellems TE, Su X-Z, Ferdig M, Fidock DA. Genome projects, genetic analysis and the changing landscape of malaria research. Curr Opin Microbiol 1999;2:415–419.
5. Hayword R, DeRisi J, Alfadhli S, Kaslow D, Brown P, Rathod PK. Shotgun DNA microarrays and stage-specific gene expression in *Plasmodium falciparum* malaria. Mol Microbiol 2000;35:6–14.

6. Krogstad DJ, De D. Chloroquine: Modes of action and resistance and the activity of chloroquine analogs. In: Sherman IW (ed.). Malaria: Parasite Biology, Pathogenesis, and Protection, Washington DC: ASM, 1998, pp. 331–339.

7. Milhous WK, Kyle DE. Introduction to the modes of action of and mechanisms of resistance to antimalarials. In: Sherman IW (ed.). Malaria: Parasite Biology, Pathogenesis, and Protection, Washington DC: ASM, 1998, pp. 303–316.

8. Russell PB., Hitchings GH. 2:4-Diaminopyrimidines as antimalarials. III. 5-Aryl derivatives. J Am Chem Soc 1951;73:3763–3770.

9. Ferone R, Burchall JJ, Hitchings GH. *Plasmodium berghei* dihydrofolate reductase. Isolation, properties, and inhibition by antifolates. Mol Pharmacol 1969;5:49–59.

10. Diggens SM, Gutteridge WE, Trigg PI. Altered dihydrofolate reductase associated with a pyrimethamine-resistant *Plasmodium berghei berghei* produced in a single step. Nature 1970;228:579–580.

11. Peterson DS, Milhous WK, Wellems TE. Molecular basis of differential resistance to cycloguanil and pyrimethamine in *Plasmodium falciparum* malaria. Proc Natl Acad Sci USA 1990;87:3018–3022.

12. Foote SJ, Galatis D, Cowman AF. Amino acids in the dihydrofolate reductase-thymidylate synthase gene of *Plasmodium falciparum* involved in cycloguanil resistance differ from those involved in pyrimethamine resistance. Proc Natl Acad Sci USA 1990;87:3014–3017.

13. van Dijk MR, Waters AP, Janse CJ. Stable transfection of malaria parasite blood stages. Science 1995;268:1358–1362.

14. Donald RG, Roos DS. Stable molecular transformation of *Toxoplasma gondii*: a selectable dihydrofolate reductase-thymidylate synthase marker based on drug-resistance mutations in malaria. Proc Natl Acad Sci USA 1993;90:11,703–11,707.

15. Wu Y, Sifri CD, Lei HH, Su X-Z, Wellems TE. Transfection of *Plasmodium falciparum* within human red blood cells. Proc Natl Acad Sci USA 92:1995:973–977.

16. Waterkeyn JG, Crabb BS, Cowman AF. Transfection of the human malaria parasite *Plasmodium falciparum*. Int J Parasitol 1999;29:945–955.

17. Reyes P, Rathod PK, Sanchez DJ, Mrema JE, Rieckmann KH, Heidrich HG. Enzymes of purine and pyrimidine metabolism from the human malaria parasite, *Plasmodium falciparum*. Mol Biochem Parasitol 1982;5:275–290.

18. Gutteridge WE, Trigg PI. Incorporation of radioactive precursors into DNA and RNA of *Plasmodium knowlesi in vitro*. J Protozool 1970;17:89–96.

19. Chen GX, Mueller C, Wendlinger M, Zolg JW. Kinetic and molecular properties of the dihydrofolate reductase from pyrimethamine-sensitive and pyrimethamine-resistant clones of the human malaria parasite *Plasmodium falciparum*. Mol Pharmacol 1987;31:430–437.

20. Sirawaraporn W, Sirawaraporn R, Cowman AF, Yuthavong Y, Santi DV. Heterologous expression of active thymidylate synthase–dihydrofolate reductase from *Plasmodium falciparum*. Biochemistry 1990;29:10,779–10,785.

21. Chulay JD, Watkins WM, Sixsmith DG. Synergistic antimalarial activity of pyrimethamine and sulfadoxine against *Plasmodium falciparum* in vitro. Am J Trop Med Hyg 1984; 33:325–330.

22. Silva AM, Lee AY, Gulnik SV, Maier P, Collins J, Bhat TN, et al. Structure and inhibition of plasmepsin II, a hemoglobin-degrading enzyme from *Plasmodium falciparum*. Proc Natl Acad Sci USA 1996;93:10,034–10,039.

23. Velanker SS, Ray SS, Gokhale RS, Suma S, Balaram H, Balaram P, et al. Triosephosphate isomerase from *Plasmodium falciparum*: the crystal structure provides insights into antimalarial drug design. Structure 1997;5:751–761.

24. Kim H, Certa U, Dobeli H, Jakob P, Hol WG. Crystal structure of fructose-1,6-bisphosphate aldolase from the human malaria parasite *Plasmodium falciparum*. Biochemistry 1998; 37:4388–4396.

25. Peterson MR, Hall DR, Berriman M, Nunes JA, Leonard GA, Fairlamb AH, et al. The three-dimensional structure of a *Plasmodium falciparum* cyclophilin in complex with the potent anti-malarial cyclosporin A. J Mol Biol 2000;298:123–133.

26. Scheidt KA, Roush WR, McKerrow JH, Selzer PM, Hansell E, Rosenthal PJ. Structure-based design, synthesis and evaluation of conformationally constrained cysteine protease inhibitors. Bioorg Med Chem 1998;6:2477–2494.

27. Shi W, Li CM, Tyler PC, Furneaux RH, Cahill SM, Girvin ME, et al. The 2.0 A structure of malarial purine phosphoribosyltransferase in complex with a transition-state analogue inhibitor. Biochemistry 1999;38:9872–9880.

28. Srivastava IK, Morrisey JM, Darrouzet E, Daldal F, Vaidya AB. Resistance mutations reveal the atovaquone-binding domain of cytochrome b in malaria parasites. Mol Microbiol 1999;33:704–711.

29. Haque TS, Skillman AG, Lee CE, Habashita H, Gluzman IY, Ewing TJ, et al. Potent, low-molecular-weight non-peptide inhibitors of malarial aspartyl protease plasmepsin II. J Med Chem 1999;42:1428–1440.

30. Sherman IW. Purine and pyrimidine metabolism of asexual stages. In: Sherman IW (ed). Malaria: Parasite Biology, Pathogenesis, and Protection, Washington DC: ASM, 1998, pp. 177–184.

31. Seymour KK, Lyons SD, Phillips L, Rieckmann KH, Christopherson RI. Cytotoxic effects of inhibitors of de novo pyrimidine biosynthesis upon *Plasmodium falciparum*. Biochemistry 1994;33:5268–5274.

32. Krungkrai J, Krungkrai SR, Phakanont, K. Antimalarial activity of orotate analogs that inhibit dihydroorotase and dihydroorotate dehydrogenase. Biochem Pharmacol 1992;43:1295–1301.

33. Queen SA, Van der Jagt DL, Reyes P. In vitro susceptibilities of *Plasmodium falciparum* to compounds which inhibit nucleotide metabolism. Antimicrob Agents Chemother 1990;34:1393–1398.

34. Bzik DJ, Li WB, Horii T, Inselburg J. Molecular cloning and sequence analysis of the *Plasmodium falciparum* dihydrofolate reductase–thymidylate synthase gene. Proc Natl Acad Sci USA 1987;84:8360–8364.

35. Coderre JA, Beverley SM, Schimke RT, and Santi DV. Overproduction of a bifunctional thymidylate synthetase–dihydrofolate reductase and DNA amplification in methotrexate-resistant Leishmania tropica. Proc Natl Acad Sci USA 1983;80:2132–2136.

36. Friedberg EC, Walker GC, and Siede, W. DNA Repair and Mutagenesis, 2nd ed., Washington, DC: ASM, 1995.

37. Yoshioka A, Tanaka S, Hiraoka O, Koyama Y, Hirota Y, Ayusawa D, Seno T, et al. Deoxyribonucleoside triphosphate imbalance. 5-Fluorodeoxyuridine-induced DNA double strand breaks in mouse FM3A cells and the mechanism of cell death. J Biol Chem 1987;262:8235–8241.

38. Ingraham HA, Dickey L, Goulian M. DNA fragmentation and cytotoxicity from increased cellular deoxyuridylate. Biochemistry 1986;25:3225–3230.

39. Houghton PJ, Germain GS, Hazelton BJ, Pennington JW, Houghton JA. Mutants of human colon adenocarcinoma, selected for thymidylate synthase deficiency. Proc Natl Acad Sci USA 1989;86:1377–1381.

40. Sirawaraporn W, Sathitkul T, Sirawaraporn R, Yuthavong Y, Santi DV. Antifolate-resistant mutants of *Plasmodium falciparum* dihydrofolate reductase. Proc Natl Acad Sci USA 1997;94:1124–1129.

41. Wu, Y, Kirkman LA, Wellems TE. Transformation of *Plasmodium falciparum* malaria parasites by homologous integration of plasmids that confer resistance to pyrimethamine. Proc Natl Acad Sci USA 1996;93:1130–1134.

42. Hekmat-Nejad M, Rathod PK. Kinetics of *Plasmodium falciparum* thymidylate synthase: interactions with high-affinity metabolites of 5-fluoroorotate and D1694. Antimicrob Agents Chemother 1996;40:1628–1632.

43. Jiang L, Lee, P-C, White J, Rathod PK. "Potent and selective activity of a combination of thymidine and 1843U89, a folate-based thymidylate synthase inhibitor, against *Plasmodium falciparum*". Antimicrob Agents Chemother 2000;44:1047–1050.

44. Rathod PK, Khatri A, Hubbert T, Milhous WK. Selective activity of 5-fluoroorotic acid against *Plasmodium falciparum in vitro*. Antimicrob Agents Chemother 1989;33:1090–1094.

45. Gomez ZM, and Rathod PK. Antimalarial activity of a combination of 5-fluoroorotate and uridine in mice. Antimicrob Agents Chemother 1990;34:1371–1375.

46. Rathod, P. K. Leffers NP, Young RD. Molecular targets of 5-fluoroorotate in the human malaria parasite, *Plasmodium falciparum*. Antimicrob Agents Chemother 1992;36:704–711.

47. Laur SA, Rathod PK, Ghori N, Haldar K. A membrane network for nutrient transport in red cells infected with the malaria parasite. Science. 1997;276:1122–1125.

48. Rathod PK, Reyes P. Orotidylate metabolizing enzymes of the human malarial parasite, *Plasmodium falciparum*, differ from host cell enzymes. J Biol Chem. 1983;258:2852–2855.

49. Rathod PK, Khosla M, Gassis S, Young RD, Lutz C. Selection and characterization of 5-fluoroorotate-resistant *Plasmodium falciparum*. Antimicrob Agents Chemother 1994; 38:2871–2876.

50. Jackman AL, Taylor GA, Gibson W, Kimbell R, Brown M, Calvert AH, et al. ICI D1694, a quinazoline antifolate thymidylate synthase inhibitor that is a potent inhibitor of L1210 tumor cell growth in vitro and in vivo: a new agent for clinical study. Cancer Res. 1991;51:5579–5586.

51. Duch DS, Banks S, Dev IK, Dickerson SH, Ferone R, Heath LS, et al. Biochemical and cellular pharmacology of 1843U89, a novel benzoquinazoline inhibitor of thymidylate synthase. Cancer Res 1993;53:810–818.

52. Rathod PK, and Reshmi, S. Susceptibility of *Plasmodium falciparum* to a combination of thymidine and ICI D1694, a quinazoline antifolate directed at thymidylate synthase. Antimicrob Agents Chemother 38: 1994;476–480.

53. Shallom S, Zhang K, Jiang L, Rathod PK. Essential protein–protein interactions between *Plasmodium falciparum* thymidylate synthase and dihydrofolate reductase domains. J Biol Chem 1999;274:37,781–37,786.

54. Meek TD, Garvey EP, Santi DV. Purification and characterization of the bifunctional thymidylate synthetase–dihydrofolate reductase from methotrexate-resistant Leishmania tropica. Biochemistry 1985;24:678–686.

55. Trujillo M, Donald RG, Roos DS, Greene PJ, Santi DV. Heterologous expression and characterization of the bifunctional dihydrofolate reductase–thymidylate synthase enzyme of *Toxoplasma gondii*. Biochemistry 1996;35:6366–6374.

56. Fidock DA, Wellems TE. Transformation with human dihydrofolate reductase renders malaria parasites insensitive to WR99210 but does not affect the intrinsic activity of proguanil. Proc Natl Acad Sci USA 1997;94:10,931–10,936.

57. Alfadhli S, Rathod PK. *Plasmodium falciparum*: Cloning sequencing and functional expression of serine hydroxymethyltransferase. Mol Biochem Parasitol, 2000; (in press).

58. Chu E, Koeller DM, Casey JL, Drake JC, Chabner BA, Elwood PC, et al. Autoregulation of human thymidylate synthase messenger RNA translation by thymidylate synthase. Proc Natl Acad Sci USA 1995;88:8977–8981.

59. Chu E, Takimoto CH, Voeller D, Grem JL, Allegra CJ. Specific binding of human dihydrofolate reductase protein to dihydrofolate reductase messenger RNA *in vitro*. Biochemistry 1993;32:4756–4760.

60. Kitchens ME, Forsthoefel AM, Rafique Z, Spencer HT, Berger FG. Ligand-mediated induction of thymidylate synthase occurs by enzyme stabilization. Implications for auto-regulation of translation. J Biol Chem 1999;274:12,544–12,547.

61. White NJ. Antimalarial drug resistance: the pace quickens. J Antimicrob Chemother 1992;30:571–585.

62. Rathod PK, McErlean T, Lee PC. Variations in frequencies of drug resistance in *Plasmodium falciparum*. Proc Natl Acad Sci USA 1997;94:9389–9393.

63. Cowman AF. The molecular basis of resistance to the sulfones, sulfonamides, and dihydrofolate reductase inhibitors In Sherman IW (ed.). Malaria: Parasite Biology, Pathogenesis, and Protection, Washington, DC: ASM, 1998, pp. 317–330

64. Vaidya AB. Mitochondrial physiology as a target for atovaquone and other antimalarials. In: Sherman IW (ed.). Malaria: Parasite Biology, Pathogenesis, and Protection, Washington DC: ASM, 1998, pp. 355–368.

65. Milhous WK, Weatherly NF, Bowdre JH, Desjardins RE. In vitro activities of and mechanisms of resistance to antifol antimalarial drugs. Antimicrob Agents Chemother 1985;27:525–530.

66. Wang P, Brobey RK, Horii T, Sims PF, Hyde JE. Utilization of exogenous folate in the human malaria parasite *Plasmodium falciparum* and its critical role in antifolate drug synergy. Mol Microbiol 1999;32:1254–1262.

67. Sullivan DJ Jr, Matile H, Ridley RG, Goldberg DE. A common mechanism for blockade of heme polymerization by antimalarial quinolines. J Biol Chem 1998;273:31,103–31,107.

68. Reynolds MG., Roos DS. A biochemical and genetic model for parasite resistance to antifolates. *Toxoplasma gondii* provides insights into pyrimethamine and cycloguanil resistance in *Plasmodium falciparum*. J. Biol. Chem 1998;273:3461–3469.

69. Canfield CJ, Pudney M, Gutteridge WE. Interactions of atovaquone with other antimalarial drugs against *Plasmodium falciparum in vitro*. Exp Parasitol 1995;80:373–381.

70. Gassis S, Rathod PK. Frequency of drug resistance in *Plasmodium falciparum*: a nonsynergistic combination of 5-fluoroorotate and atovaquone suppresses in vitro resistance. Antimicrob Agents Chemother 1996;40:914–919.

71. Puavilai S, Kunavisarut S, Vatanasuk M, Timpatanapong P, Sriwong ST, et al. Ocular toxicity of chloroquine among Thai patients. Int J Dermatol 1999;38:934–937.

72. Krogstad DJ, Gluzman IY, Kyle DE, Oduola AM, Martin SK, Milhous WK, et al. Efflux of chloroquine from *Plasmodium falciparum*: mechanism of chloroquine resistance. Science 1987;238:1283–1285.

73. Reed MB, Saliba KJ, Caruana SR, Kirk K, Cowman AF. Pgh1 modulates sensitivity and resistance to multiple antimalarials in *Plasmodium falciparum*. Nature 2000;403:906–909.

74. White NJ. Why is it that antimalarial drug treatments do not always work? Ann Trop Med Parasitol 1998;92:449–458.

75. Phillips MA, Coffino P, Wang CC. Cloning and sequencing of the ornithine decarboxylase gene from *Trypanosoma brucei*. Implications for enzyme turnover and selective difluoromethylornithine inhibition. J Biol Chem 1987;262:8721–8727.

17

Iron Chelators

Mark Loyevsky and Victor R. Gordeuk

INTRODUCTION

Over the past two decades, global resistance to both insecticides and antimalarials has emerged, the incidence of malaria has increased, and the disease has become more widespread *(1)*. Although early tests of malaria vaccines in human volunteers may have some promise *(2,3)*, clinically applicable vaccines will not be available for a number of years *(4)* and their importance in controlling malaria is uncertain. In this setting, antimalarial chemotherapy remains the principal means available for reducing the morbidity and mortality of malaria and the task of developing new antimalarial drugs with new mechanisms of action is important *(5)*. Two observations prompted the idea of using iron chelators against malaria infections: the central role of iron for the rapid proliferation of malaria parasites, and the arrest of parasite growth by iron chelators both in vitro and in vivo *(6,7)*. More recently, the iron chelator desferrioxamine (DFO) was found to have antimalarial activity in humans *(8,9)*. Iron chelation may not achieve a defined role in the treatment of malaria until new agents are designed specifically with antimalarial properties.

IRON METABOLISM OF *PLASMODIUM FALCIPARUM*

Acquisition of Iron by the Erythrocytic Parasite

The intraerythrocytic parasite lies within a parasitophorous vacuole. Within the red blood cell, the parasite first appears as a ring form and then matures into a trophozoite. The trophozoite obtains nutrients by ingesting host cell cytoplasm, including hemoglobin, by means of a cytostome *(10)* and may possibly take up molecules from the outer medium directly through a parasitophorous duct *(11,12)*. The heme liberated by the proteolysis of hemoglobin is polymerized in the food vacuole to form hemozoin *(13)*. How the intraerythrocytic phase parasite acquires iron has not yet been determined. Several possible sources have been postulated, including plasma transferrin-bound iron, iron derived from red blood cell host ferritin, iron liberated from the catabolism of host hemoglobin in the food vacuole of the parasite, and a labile intraerythrocytic iron pool.

Plasma Transferrin

In contrast to early clinical studies that suggested a protective effect of iron deficiency against human malaria *(14,15)*, later clinical *(16)* and experimental *(17)* results suggested

From: *Antimalarial Chemotherapy: Mechanisms of Action, Resistance, and New Directions in Drug Discovery*
Edited by: P. J. Rosenthal © Humana Press Inc., Totowa, NJ

that the progression of the disease is independent of the iron status of humans or animals. Similarly, transferrin receptors do not appear to be expressed on mature parasitized erythrocytes (18,19). The possibility that nonspecifically bound transferrin is taken up from plasma into parasitized erythrocytes has been proposed (18,20,21), but the bulk of the evidence indicates that transferrin iron is not taken up by parasitized red cells (17,22).

Erythrocyte Ferritin

Although the mature erythrocyte cannot synthesize ferritin, it does contain residual ferritin that was produced during the earlier erythroblast phase (23). This residual ferritin, if fully saturated with iron, may account for about 4.8 μM iron (24). The acquisition of iron from ferritin that has been transported from the erythrocyte cytoplasm to the parasite's food vacuole is an uninvestigated possibility.

Host Hemoglobin

The intraerythrocytic parasite derives a major portion of amino acids necessary for protein synthesis from the catabolism of host hemoglobin (25–27). The heme released during this process contains a substantial amount of iron, which, if liberated from heme, might be available for the parasite's metabolic needs (17,24). Although firm evidence that the parasite utilizes iron derived from host heme is lacking at present, it is plausible that a small amount of heme in the food vacuole is degraded in a controlled manner to release iron for the metabolic processes of the parasite.

Labile Intraerythrocytic Iron

With evidence against plasma transferrin as the source of iron for the intraerythrocytic trophozoite, it was proposed that the parasite may use a labile pool of iron in the cytoplasm of the erythrocyte for its metabolism (17). In support of this hypothesis, gel filtration and ultrafiltration studies on hemolysates of rat red blood cells parasitized with *P. berghei* revealed a labile pool of iron that is chelatable by preincubation of the intact cells with DFO (17). Further evidence in support of this hypothesis was obtained recently by monitoring the concentration of labile iron in parasitized and nonparasitized erythrocytes with the fluorescent iron-sensing probe, calcein. Labile iron pools were lower in parasitized than nonparasitized erythrocytes, suggesting that labile iron of the host red cell may be either utilized or stored during plasmodial growth (51). Also, lipophilicity, or ability to cross cellular membranes, correlates with the effectiveness of iron chelators to inhibit *P. falciparum* (7,29). On the other hand, two studies found that when iron-chelating agents are introduced into the cytoplasm of erythrocytes but not into the parasite compartment, no plasmodial growth inhibition occurs (12,30). It is possible that both host labile iron and another source of iron, such as host hemoglobin iron, are used by the parasite, and that the abrogation of only one source will not prevent parasite growth.

Metabolic Processes That Are Dependent on Iron

Many enzymes of the erythrocytic malaria parasite are dependent on iron. Table 1 presents a partial listing. From the information provided in Table 1, it can be inferred that the withholding of iron from the parasite by iron chelators may disrupt the metabolism of the parasite by preventing DNA synthesis, inhibiting de novo synthesis of heme, and interfering with normal mitochondrial function and electron transport. In addition, some of the parasite's glycolytic enzymes (37,38) and pentose phosphate shunt enzymes (39) are dependent on iron.

Table 1
Iron-Dependent Enzymes of the Erythrocytic Trophozoite

Enzyme	Function	Ref.
Ribonucleotide reductase	DNA synthesis	*6,31*
Dihydroorotate dehydrogenase	Pyrimidine synthesis	*32,33*
Phosphoenol pyruvate carboxykinase	CO_2 fixation	*32*
Delta-aminolevulinate synthase	Heme synthesis	*34*
Cytochrome oxidase, cytochrome b	Mitochondrial electron transport	*35,36*

ANTIMALARIAL ACTIVITY OF IRON CHELATORS *IN VITRO*

Several classes of iron-chelating compounds have been shown to suppress the growth of *P. falciparum* in erythrocytes in vitro, as shown in Table 2. A number of these compounds are naturally occurring siderophores, molecules produced by microorganisms to acquire iron from the environment. Numerous studies indicate that the degree of antimalarial activity of iron chelators correlates with the degree of lipophilicity, or the ability to cross cell membranes, of the compound *(7,29,42,46)*.

Two Major Mechanisms of Action

The antimalarial iron chelators can be placed into two major categories depending on the predominant mechanism of inhibition of parasite growth: withholding iron from plasmodial metabolic pathways or forming complexes with iron that are toxic to the parasite. For both of these categories, an interaction with iron is the focus of the antimalarial activity.

Withholding Iron from Plasmodial Metabolic Pathways

The mechanism of antimalarial action of iron(III) chelators appears to be the sequestration of iron necessary for plasmodial replication. This effect has been documented for DFO *(6,12,30,53)*, methyl-anthranilic DFO *(12)*, desferrithiocin, desferricrocin *(41)*, α-ketohydroxypyridinones *(45)*, pyridoxal isonicotinoyl hydrazone *(48)*, salicylaldehyde isonicotinoyl hydrazone *(49)*, daphnetin *(47)*, and two aminothiol compounds recently reported to have antimalarial activity *(50)*. The inhibitory action of these compounds on malaria parasite cultures is fully abrogated upon precomplexation with iron.

Forming Toxic Complexes with Iron

Iron(II) chelators seems to have an antiparasitic effect other than the withholding of iron, as the inhibitory effect cannot be abrogated by precomplexation with iron before addition to cultures. In the case of the aromatic metal chelator, 8-hydroxyquinoline, it appears that a complex with iron is formed extracellularly that subsequently enters the parasitized red cell to produce a rapidly lethal free-radical-mediated intracellular reaction *(38,43)*. For the alkylthiocarbamates *(38)*, 2',2'-bipyridyl and certain aminophenols *(51)*, the antimalarial mechanisms are unknown but probably involve free radical reactions.

Potential Major Effects of Withholding Iron

It is plausible that withholding iron may cause malfunction of certain enzymes, for which iron is indispensable. We discuss two possible enzyme targets, but others are also possible (*see* the subsection Metabolic Processes That Are Dependent on Iron, and Table 1).

Table 2
Iron-Chelating Compounds that Inhibit Growth of *P. falciparum* Cultured in Erythrocytes

Class of compound and specific inhibitors	IC$_{50}$[a]	Ref.
A) Agents that inhibit parasite growth by withholding iron		
Hydroxamate siderophores and derivatives		
Desferrioxamine (DFO)	4–35 µM	6
Methyl-anthranilic DFO (MA-DFO)	3–5 µM	12
Circular DFO	5–9 µM	40
Nitrilo-DFO	14–20 µM	40
Desferrithiocin[b]	25 µM	41
Desferricrocin	30–40 µM	41
Reversed siderophores	0.3–70 µM	42
Rhodotorulic acid		43
Mycobactin		43
Catecholamide and catecholate siderophores		
Vibriobactin	2–5 µM	44
Parabactin	2–3 µM	44
Gamma amino butyric acid (GABA)	4–5 µM	44
N4-nonyl, N1, N8-*bis* (2.3-dihydroxybenzoyl) spermidine hydrobromide (compound 7)	0.17–1.0 µM	36
α-ketohydroxypyridinones		
Deferiprone	15–45 µM	45
CP96	5–45 µM	46
Dihydroxycoumarins		
Daphnetin (ash tree bark extract)	25–40 µM	47
Polyanionic amines		
HBED	5 µM	29
Acylhydrazones		
Pyridoxal isonicotinoyl hydrazone (PIH)	30 µM	48
Salicylaldehyde isonicotinoyl hydrazone (SIH)	18–30 µM	49
2-Hydroxy-1-naphthylaldehyde m-fluorobenzoyl hydrazone (HNFBH)	0.17–0.26 µM	49
Aminothiols		
Ethane-1,2-*bis*(N-1-amino-3-ethylbutyl-3-thiol) (BAT)	6–9 µM	50
N',N',N'-tris(2-methyl-2-mercaptopropyl)-1,4,7 -triazacyclononane (TAT)	3–4 µM	50
Aminophenols		
Aminophenol II	0.5–0.7 µM	51
Bis-cyclic imides		
Dexrazoxane[c]	32–36 µM	28
B) Agents that inhibit parasite growth by forming toxic complexes with iron		
2,2'-Bipyridyl	12–14 µM	52
8-Hydroxyquinoline	8.3 nM	38

[a]Concentrations of iron chelator that produce 50% growth inhibition after 48–72 h of culture.
[b]Effective against both erythrocytic and hepatic stages of the parasite.
[c]Effective against hepatic stage but not erythrocytic stage of the parasite.

Ribonucleotide Reductase

One of the trophozoite enzymes essential for DNA synthesis is ribonuc'. reductase, an iron-containing enzyme that catalyzes the reduction of ribonucleo. diphosphates to deoxyribonucleoside diphosphates, the precursors of DNA *(54)*. In fa. the function of ribonucleotide reductase is rate limiting for DNA synthesis *(55–57)*. 1 vitro, iron chelation reversibly inhibits ribonucleotide reductase *(54–56)* and produces a potent inhibition of DNA synthesis in various cellular systems *(55)*. Thus, iron chelators such as DFO may exert their antiplasmodial action through the inhibition of parasite ribonucleotide reductase activity by binding the essential component, iron *(6,58)*. In addition, exposure to DFO leads to decreased levels of mRNA for the small B2-subunit of ribonucleotide reductase in *P. falciparum* parasites cultured in erythrocytes *(35)*.

Delta-Aminolevulinate Synthase

Plasmodium falciparum and other plasmodial species synthesize heme *de novo*, despite the fact that the parasite is located within the red blood cell, a virtual "red sea" of hemoglobin. The *de novo* synthesis of heme might represent a novel target for antimalarial therapy *(34,59)*. To synthesize heme, it appears that the parasite synthesizes the first enzyme in the pathway, delta-aminolevulinate synthase. It also appears that other enzymes in the heme synthetic pathway, such as delta-aminolevulinate dehydrase, coproporphyrinogen oxidase and ferrochelatase, are of host origin and are transported into the parasite from the host red blood cell compartment *(34)*. In human erythroid cells, iron chelators cause a downregulation in delta-aminolevulinate synthase synthesis *(60)*, resulting in a reduced ability to synthesize heme. Iron chelators might exert a similar effect in the erythrocytic trophozoite, which could prevent cytochrome synthesis.

Physical Properties That Affect the Antimalarial Activity of Iron Chelators

The iron withheld by iron chelators in the process of inhibiting the growth of intraerythrocytic malaria parasites most likely resides within the parasitic compartment of the infected red blood cell *(12,17,30)*. One would thus predict that an effective antimalarial iron chelator would have the ability to cross lipid membranes well, would have a high affinity for iron(II) or iron(III), and would selectively bind iron as compared to other trace metals *(44,46)*.

Lipophilicity

The direct positive correlation between the degree of lipophilicity of a compound and its inhibitory action against malaria has been demonstrated experimentally for the reversed siderophores *(42)* the N-alkyl derivatives of 3-hydroxypyridine-4-one *(46)* and several aminothiol compounds *(50)*.

Affinity for Iron

A high affinity for iron is an important prerequisite of antimalarial activity of an iron-chelating drug *(7,44,46)*. The affinity constants of antimalarial iron chelators for iron(III) range from 10^{24} for acetomethoxy-calcein to 10^{28} for the acylhydrazones *(61)*, 10^{31} for DFO *(62)*, 10^{36} for hydroxypyridine-4-ones *(46)*, and 10^{38} for the 8-hydrohyquinolines *(63)*.

Selectivity for Iron Versus Other Cations

The selectivity of a chelator for iron versus other cations has importance for two reasons. First, malaria parasites have a limited capability to recover after iron eprivation compared to mammalian cells *(7)*, making it reasonable to target iron as ompared to other essential metals for which the ability to recover from deprivation las not been studied. Second, removal by iron chelators of the other biometals, such as zinc, calcium, and magnesium, may be detrimental for the mammalian host as well. In this regard, the hydroxamate siderophores have a favorable profile, for their affinity for iron is at least one order of magnitude greater than their affinity for zinc and several orders of magnitude higher than for calcium *(66)*.

Number of Coordination Sites

The iron atom has six coordination sites, and hexadentate chelators would be expected to form the most stable complexes with the metal. Pentadentate and quadridentate chelators may leave one or two coordination sites of the iron atom unbound and potentially available to participate in toxic reactions that could damage host tissues. Tridentate and bidentate chelators could fully occupy the coordination sites of iron by forming 2:1 or 3:1 complexes with the metal, but, especially at low chelator concentrations, partial dissociation from iron might occur and expose coordination sites to participate in toxic reactions.

Information on Specific Antimalarial Iron Chelators

Desferrioxamine

Desferrioxamine is the only agent now available for clinical use as an iron chelator in most countries. DFO is a naturally occurring trihydroxamic acid derived from cultures of *Streptomyces pilosus*; it is remarkably safe and nontoxic. As shown in Table 2, when given as a single agent, DFO suppresses the growth of *P. falciparum* in parasitized erythrocytes in vitro in concentrations achieved and tolerated in the blood of patients.

The antimalarial activity of DFO appears to be related to its ability to enter the erythrocytic trophozoite and to chelate a pool of parasite-associated iron. It has been suggested that DFO may enter the parasite directly through a parasitophorous duct that invaginates from the red cell membrane and communicates with the parasitophorous vacuole *(11)*, thus bypassing the host red cell cytoplasm *(12)*.

Experiments with synchronized in vitro cultures of *P. falciparum* showed that DFO has a cytocidal effect on late trophozoites and early schizonts and that the critical duration of exposure may be as short as 6 h at this stage of parasite development *(53)*. Ultrastructural lesions included the breakdown of the nuclear envelope into small membranous fragments and progressive vacuolization of the nucleoplasm. Other organelles, including food vacuoles and mitochondria, were not visually affected, although the most recent biochemical data indicate that the levels of mRNAs encoding cytochrome c oxidase and cytochrome b are affected *(35)*.

Desferrioxamine has an additive inhibitory effect on the in vitro growth of *P. falciparum* when it is combined with classical antimalarials *(21)*, although, in a single report, it failed to enhance the activity of chloroquine *(64)*. It has been reported that zinc–DFO complexes have greater antiparasitic activity than DFO alone on *P. falciparum* cultured in erythrocytes. A potential explanation for this observation is that Zn–DFO may penetrate the cell membranes and exchange bound zinc for ferric ions because the affinity of DFO for iron is greater than its affinity for zinc *(65)*.

In summary, the available studies indicate that the action of DFO on the intraerythrocytic parasite is both stage-specific and cytocidal. In contrast, in mammalian cells this compound displays only a cytostatic inhibitory effect, which is reversed upon the removal of the drug from the suspension *(40,66)*. The differential effect of DFO on malaria-infected erythrocytes and mammalian cells provides the basis for the selective action of DFO as an antimalarial.

N-Terminal Derivatives of Desferrioxamine

One of the major disadvantages of DFO as an antimalarial agent is its poor permeability into parasitized red cells. To improve its permeability, two classes of modified hydroxamate-based chelators were synthesized, the N-terminal derivatives of DFO and the reversed siderophores *(12,40,42)*. Methylanthranilic DFO, the most lipophilic (and most membrane-permeant) member of the N-terminal derivatives of DFO, reduces parasite proliferation with a median inhibitory concentration (IC_{50}) of 4 ± 1 μM. The parental DFO, the most hydrophilic of these compounds, displays an IC_{50} of 21 ± 7 μM. Cyclic DFO and nitrilo-DFO, N-terminal derivatives with intermediate hydrophilicity, have intermediate IC_{50}'s of 7 ± 2 and 17 ± 3 μM, respectively. Methylanthranilic DFO has strikingly selective activity against malaria parasites as compared to mammalian cells. This agent inhibits the proliferation of mammalian cells (human K562 erythroleukemia cells and human HEPG2 hepatocarcinoma cells) with an IC_{50} of >100 μM, but as noted earlier, inhibits the growth of malaria parasites with an IC_{50} of only 4 ± 1 μM.

Reversed Siderophores

The "reversed siderophores" were produced by modifying ferrichrome molecules in a way that preserved their iron-binding properties but replaced their hydrophilic envelopes with lipophilic ones to facilitate penetration into infected erythrocytes *(42,67)*. Because the function of the modified compounds was iron withholding from cells versus the original function of iron delivery *(68)*, they were named reversed siderophores *(42)*. The permeation properties of these compounds across biological membranes were increased while fully retaining iron(III)-binding capacity *(7)*. In vitro, reversed siderophores have a cytotoxic effect on rings and cytostatic effects on trophozoites and schizonts. In contrast, DFO has major cytotoxic effects only on trophozoites and early schizonts *(12,66)*. This differential pattern of inhibition might be related to different abilities of two classes of chelators to interfere with iron metabolism in the parasites and to different speeds of permeation to the parasitic compartments of the infected red blood cells *(66,69)*.

Hydroxypyridin-4-ones

Hydroxypyridin-4-ones are neutral bidentate ligands with a high specificity for ferric iron. The stability constant for the iron complex ($\log \varepsilon K_a = 37$) is six orders of magnitude higher than that of DFO. Unlike DFO, hydroxypyridinones are effective to treat iron overload when administered orally *(70,71)*. In vitro, they exhibit a dose-related suppression of *P. falciparum* growth *(45,72)*. The dimethyl compound of this group, 1,2-dimethyl-3-hydroxypyrid-4-one, also known as deferiprone (L1 or CP20), inhibits the growth of *P. falciparum* by more than 50% at concentrations ranging from 5 to 100 μM, when exposure to the chelator is continuous *(45,46)*.

Acylhydrazones

Two members of the acylhydrazone family *(73)*, salicylaldehyde isonicotinoyl hydrazone (SIH) and 2-hydroxy-1-naphthylaldehyde *m*-fluorobenzoyl hydrazone (HNFBH), were tested on malaria cultures in vitro, either as single drugs or in combination with DFO *(49)*. SIH and HNFBH were very efficient in suppressing para-site growth at all developmental stages, with mean (± SD) IC$_{50}$'s of 24 ± 6 µM and 0.21 ± 0.04 µM, respectively. SIH and HNFBH produced a dose-dependent inhibition of growth when parasitized cells were continuously exposed to these agents.

Aminothiols

Two compounds from a family of multidentate aminothiol chelators, BAT [ethane-1,2-bis(N-1-amino-3-ethylbutyl-3-thiol)] and TAT [N',N',N'-tris(2-methyl-2-mercapto-propyl)1,4,7-triazacyclononane], inhibit the growth of *P. falciparum* cultured in erythrocytes *(50)*. The IC$_{50}$'s are 7.6 ± 1.2 µM for BAT and 3.3 ± 0.3 µM for TAT. Both agents appear to affect the trophozoite and schizont stages of parasite develop-ment, and they display selective cytotoxicity to malaria parasites versus mammalian cells. The inhibitory effects of these aminothiols seem to be related mainly to their iron-withholding action, because precomplexation with iron fully reverses the anti-parasitic effect *(50)*. In addition to their iron-binding properties, the aminothiols are capable of preventing free-radical formation (M. Loyevsky, unpublished observations). This feature is most likely the result of the thiol groups present in the molecules and suggests that these compounds may have promise in blocking the oxidative damage to tissues that occurs in patients with severe malaria.

Aminophenols

A pentadentate aminophenol ligand, aminophenol II [N,N'-*bis*(hydroxybenzyl)-N-4-benzyldiethylenetriamine], was recently shown to inhibit the growth of *P. falciparum* cultured in erythrocytes *(51)*. The IC$_{50}$ concentration determined in 48-h assays was 0.6 ± 0.1 µM. Aminophenol II binds both iron(II) and iron(III) at physiologic pH, but the selectivity and specificity of iron binding by aminophenol II or the affinity constants for iron(II) and iron(III) at physiologic pH are not known. Because aminophenol II can coordinate with five of the six coordination sites of iron, it likely forms a 1:1 complex with iron, but some more complex ratio is possible.

Iron Chelator Combinations

Desferrioxamine and Reversed Siderophores

The combination of DFO with the more lipophilic and more permeant reversed siderophore, RSFilem2, produced a strong synergistic inhibitory effect *(66)*. This effect may result from the different speeds of permeation of the two chelators through the host and parasite cell membranes. The rapidly permeating lipophilic agent RSFilem2 irreversibly affects ring-stage parasites whereas the slowly permeating but persistent DFO mainly arrests the development of mature parasite stages *(66,73)*.

Desferrioxamine and Acylhydrazones

Both SIH and HNFBH potentiate the antimalarial effect of DFO in vitro *(49)*. For the combination of SIH and DFO, the synergistic inhibitory effect may be explained by free shuttling of SIH through the membranes, withholding iron from critical intrapara-sitic sources, exiting from the cell as an the iron-chelator complex, and conveying iron to the slowly permeating DFO. DFO has a greater affinity constant for iron and may, therefore, serve as an iron sink *(7,49)*.

When DFO was combined with deferiprone, an additive interaction on plasmodial growth suppression was observed (G. Mabeza, unpublished observations), implying that the two iron(III) chelators do not antagonize the effects of each other but rather complement them.

DESFERRIOXAMINE AND 2',2'-BIPYRIDYL

As single agents, both DFO and 2',2'-bipyridyl independently inhibit the growth of *P. falciparum* in culture, with IC_{50}'s of 5.2 µ*M* and 12.4 µ*M*, respectively *(52)*. The combination of DFO (2 µ*M*) with 2',2'-bipyridyl at various concentrations leads to a relative increase in parasitemia compared to 2',2'-bipyridyl alone, suggesting that these compounds have antagonistic effects. DFO might successfully compete with 2',2'-bipyridyl for iron binding by virtue of its greater affinity for iron (K_a of 10^{31} for DFO versus K_a of 10^{28} for 2',2'-bipyridyl), and thereby prevent the formation of toxic 2',2'-bipyridyl-iron complexes.

Effect of Iron Chelators on the Hepatic Phase of **P. falciparum**

The studies summarized in Table 2 and demonstrating a suppressive effect on the growth of *P. falciparum* by iron chelators were performed on the erythrocytic phase of the life cycle of the parasite. It was also reported that DFO, desferrithiocin, and dexrazoxane are able to inhibit the growth of the exoerythrocytic hepatic phase of *P. falciparum* or *P. yoelii* in a culture system employing human or mouse hepatocytes *(28,74)*. These studies suggest that iron chelation represents a potential antimalarial strategy with effectiveness against both the erythrocytic and hepatic phases of the parasite. Dexrazoxane is an iron-chelating pro-drug that must undergo intracellular hydrolysis to bind iron *(75,76)*. As a single agent, dexrazoxane inhibits synchronized cultures of *P. falciparum* in human erythrocytes only at suprapharmacologic concentrations (>200 µ*M*). In contrast, pharmacologic concentrations of dexrazoxane (50–200 µ*M*) as a single agent inhibit the progression of *P. yoelii* from sporozoites to schizonts in cultured mouse hepatocytes by 45% to 69% *(28)*.

ANTIMALARIAL ACTIVITY OF IRON CHELATORS IN LABORATORY ANIMALS

Studies of Iron Chelators as Single Agents

Desferrioxamine

In the only animal study investigating iron chelation therapy to suppress parasitemia with *P. falciparum (77)*, DFO was active against the erythrocytic phase of the parasite in Aotus monkeys. Similar observations were made with *P. berghei* and *P. vinckei* infections in rodents *(17,29,78,79)*. These animal studies demonstrated an antimalarial effect of DFO at doses that overlap with acceptable doses in humans (up to 100–150 mg/kg/d). Continuous subcutaneous infusions or divided doses of DFO were more effective than single daily doses in reducing parasitemia and mortality. The antimalarial effect of DFO administered in liposomes was studied in *P. vinckei*-infected mice *(79)*. Suppression of parasitemia and long-term survival (>1 mo after infection) of mice were obtained by subcutaneous injections of liposomal DFO prior to infection (d –1 and 0, 400 or 800 mg DFO/kg/d). In a separate experiment, long-term survival was also obtained by treatment with liposomal DFO on d 7 and 8 after infection in doses of 400 mg/kg/d. Thus, liposomes appear to be suitable carrier systems for DFO in experimental murine malaria and this form of therapy may lead to cure in this setting.

Deferiprone

Although in vitro studies suggest that the oral administration of hydroxypyridinone (deferiprone) in safe doses might result in a clinically detectable antimalarial effect, the single reported animal study of deferiprone proved to be negative. Deferiprone in three divided doses of 300 mg/kg/d for 13 d did not suppress *P. berghei* infection in six female Wistar rats. The lack of effectiveness of deferiprone in this animal model, as compared to the studies in vitro, was attributed to intermittent attainment of suppressive plasma concentrations with the subcutaneous or oral mode of administration and to the relatively low lipophilicity of deferiprone, which would limit entry into the red cell under these circumstances *(80)*.

Reversed Siderophores

To achieve sustained blood levels of the highly lipophilic reversed siderophore, RSFileu$_{m2}$, the agent was delivered in fractionated coconut oil (miglyol 840) via subcutaneous injections to mice infected with *P. vinckei petteri*. The chelator was administered at a dosage of 370 mg/kg every 8 h, and no adverse reactions were observed. Repeated injections of the reversed siderophore over a 56-h period were associated with a significant delay in the increase in parasitemia compared to the controls. Parasitemia relapsed in all mice 24 h after ceasing the treatment *(81)*.

Studies of Iron Chelator Combinations

Desferrioxamine and SIH were administered as a combination to Swiss mice infected with *P. vinckei petteri* or *P. berghei*. The drugs were delivered by several routes: single intraperitoneal injection, multiple intraperitoneal injections, or subcutaneous insertion of a drug-containing polymeric device designed for slow, continuous drug release over 7 d. As single agents administered in doses of 125–500 mg/kg/d in these manners, all three agents led to delays and reductions in peak parasitemias and to reduced mortality. The combination of DFO and SIH led to greater speed of drug action and greater inhibition of parasitemia than either agent alone. The antimalarial action of this combination was greatest when the drugs were slowly released into the circulation by means of a biodegradable polymer that was implanted subcutaneously *(82)*.

IRON CHELATION THERAPY FOR HUMAN MALARIA

The first use of an iron chelator for human malaria can be attributed to the Chinese who used the bark of ash trees, which are rich in coumarins, as a folk remedy for malaria. One of these coumarins, a dihydroxycoumarin named daphnetin, is an iron chelator with moderate antimalarial activity in vitro (Table 2) *(47)*. More recently, Traore and colleagues reported the administration of DFO with chloroquine to six patients with uncomplicated falciparum malaria, and there was no evidence of toxicity *(83)*. Larger clinical trials of the use of DFO in adults with uncomplicated malaria have now been conducted in Thailand and Zambia.

Iron Chelators in Adults with Asymptomatic P. falciparum Infection
DFO

DFO (100 mg/kg/d by continuous 72-h subcutaneous infusions) was administered to 65 adult subjects in Zambia with asymptomatic infection with *P. falciparum.* Two randomized, double-blind, placebo-controlled, crossover trials were performed *(8,97)*. Compared to placebo, DFO treatment significantly enhanced the rate of parasite clearance. Serum concentrations of DFO + ferrioxamine (the iron complex of DFO) were measured in 26 subjects. Mean ± SEM steady-state concentrations were 6.9 ± 0.6 μM at 36 h and 7.7 ± 0.7 μM at 72 h. These levels are at the lower end of the range of values reported for the IC_{50} for DFO against *P. falciparum* as determined in vitro (Table 2). Although results obtained with low levels of parasitemia in partially immune adults cannot necessarily be extrapolated to patients with severe infection, these findings suggested that iron chelation may be a potential chemotherapeutic strategy for human infection with *P. falciparum*.

Deferiprone

A prospective, double-blind, placebo-controlled crossover trial of deferiprone was conducted in 25 adult Zambians with asymptomatic *P. falciparum* parasitemia *(106)*. Deferiprone was administered daily for 3 or 4 d in divided doses of 75 or 100 mg/kg body weight per day. No reduction in asexual intraerythrocytic parasites was observed during or after deferiprone treatment. The mean peak plasma concentration of deferiprone (108.2 ± 24.9 mol/L) achieved was within the range demonstrated to inhibit the growth of *P. falciparum* in vitro. However, the times to reach peak plasma levels and to clear the drug from the plasma were short, and plasma levels of deferiprone were only in the range of a modest antimalarial effect for much of the time between the oral doses used in these studies. Because of the risk of neutropenia and other adverse effects with higher doses or prolonged use of the chelator, additional trials of deferiprone as an antimalarial would not seem to be justified.

Desferrioxamine in Symptomatic, Uncomplicated Falciparum and Vivax Malaria

Fourteen adult males with *P. falciparum* infection and 14 adult males with *P. vivax* infection were given DFO, 100 mg/kg/d, as a continuous intravenous infusion for three consecutive days. DFO as a single agent reduced parasitemia to zero within 57 h for the falciparum group and 106 h for the vivax group. DFO was, in general, well tolerated, but about one-third of the subjects experienced transient visual blurring. Recrudescence was observed in all subjects, occurring on the average 10 d after start of therapy in the falciparum group and 15 d in the vivax group. This study demonstrated that iron chelation with DFO is effective as a single agent in both uncomplicated falciparum and vivax malaria and that this therapy can clear moderate degrees of parasitemia. It also showed that the dose and duration of iron chelation therapy employed in this study failed to achieve a radical cure *(86)*.

Desferrioxamine and Artesunate

Although the combination of DFO and artemisinin derivatives might be expected to be antagonistic, no evidence of adverse interaction was found in a small cohort of patients with either uncomplicated or severe malaria who received both DFO and artesunate *(87)*.

Effect of Desferrioxamine on Recovery from Coma and on Mortality in Children with Cerebral Malaria

The obstruction of the cerebral microvasculature by *P. falciparum*-infected erythrocytes leading to ischemia and microhemorrhage may contribute to the development of cerebral malaria *(88–91)*. Free hemoglobin can serve as a biologic Fenton reagent to provide iron for electron transfer and the generation of the hydroxyl radical *(92)*. DFO inhibits peroxidant damage to lung tissue in mice *(93)*, to the myocardium in rabbits *(94)*, and to the central nervous system in cats *(95)*. Iron chelation with DFO may protect against damage to the central nervous system by (1) enhancing parasite clearance through withholding iron from a vital metabolic pathways of the parasite, (2) inhibiting iron-induced peroxidant damage to cells and subcellular structures of the brain, and (3) enhancing Th-1 cell-mediated immunity *(96)*.

A prospective, randomized, double-blind trial of DFO or placebo added to standard quinine therapy was first conducted in 83 Zambian children. The goal was to determine if iron chelation speeds recovery of full consciousness in cerebral malaria *(84)*. Each child received quinine, 10 mg/kg, every 8 h for 5 d and a single dose of sulfadoxine–pyrimethamine, 25/1.2 mg/kg. In addition, either DFO, 100 mg/kg/d, or placebo were given as a 72-h intravenous infusion. The addition of DFO to the conventional therapy shortened the rate of clearance of parasitemia and the rate of recovery of full consciousness in children with deep coma, each by about two-fold.

To examine the effect of iron chelation on mortality in cerebral malaria, 352 children were enrolled into a second clinical trial of DFO in addition to standard quinine therapy at two centers in Zambia, one rural and one urban *(98)*. The study design was the same as the first study except that a loading dose of quinine was given (20 mg/kg). Overall mortality was 18.3% (32/175) in the DFO plus quinine group and 10.7% (19/177) in the placebo plus quinine group ($p = 0.074$). At the rural study site, mortality was 15.4% (18/117) with DFO compared to 12.7% (15/118) with placebo ($p = 0.78$). At the urban site, mortality was 24.1% (14/58) with DFO and 6.8% (4/59) with placebo ($p = 0.061$). Among survivors, there was a trend to faster recovery from coma in the DFO group. This study did not provide evidence for a beneficial effect on mortality in children with cerebral malaria when DFO was added to quinine in a regimen that included a loading dose of quinine. Indeed, at one of two research sites, there was a trend to higher mortality with DFO. The lack of a positive effect of DFO on both parasite clearance and recovery from coma in this study, in contrast to earlier work *(84)*, may be attributable to the impact of a loading dose of quinine used in the present study but not in the previous one (i.e., a relatively delayed beneficial effect of DFO in cerebral malaria was masked by substantial beneficial effect of the quinine loading dose).

Iron Chelators and Immunity in the Setting of Malaria

Two different studies of Zambian children who were enrolled in placebo-controlled trials of DFO in addition to quinine for cerebral malaria suggested a possible effect of iron chelation on Th-1-mediated immune function *(85,96)*. In one study, serum levels of neopterin, an indirect marker of Th-1 cell-mediated immune function *(99,100)*, did not change significantly in children receiving DFO plus quinine but did decline significantly in children receiving placebo plus quinine. In the same study, serum concentrations of NO_2^-/NO_3^-, the stable end products of NO degradation, increased significantly with DFO plus quinine but not placebo plus quinine *(96)*. These observations made in patients are compatible with in vitro results, demonstrating that DFO enhances neopterin formation by positively modulating interferon-gamma (IFN-γ) activity *(101)*. In another study, serum concentrations of interleukin-4 (IL-4), a Th-2-related cytokine, increased with placebo plus quinine but not DFO plus quinine *(85)*.

Taken together, these studies raise the possibility that the possible beneficial effect of iron chelation therapy seen in one study *(84)* may have resulted from a strengthening of Th-1 cell-mediated immune function by enhancing IFN-γ activity, as reflected by neopterin and NO formation, and a reduction in the production of Th-2-mediated cytokines such as IL-4. Therefore, DFO may direct the immune response toward a Th-1 effector mechanism, which may be beneficial in the early phase of parasitic infections.

It remains to be determined whether the inconsistent beneficial effect of iron chelators in cerebral malaria is the result of immune modulation in the central nervous system, to the chelation of iron and prevention of toxic hydroxyl radical formation in this compartment, or to a combination of both mechanisms *(102–104)*.

CONCLUSIONS AND DIRECTIONS FOR THE FUTURE

The discussion in this chapter is based on early and fragmentary knowledge of the iron metabolism of *P. falciparum* and the clinical role of iron chelators as antimalarials. Advances are needed in two broad areas, namely understanding the iron metabolism of the malaria parasite and developing iron chelators designed for the treatment of malaria rather than iron overload *(105)*. Specific areas that require work include (1) the determination of the source of the iron that is essential for the growth of the intraerythrocytic parasite, (2) the identification of the metabolic pathways with which iron chelation interferes, and (3) the design of iron-chelating compounds that are effective orally, safe for a short course of antimalarial therapy, and specifically targeted to bind parasite-associated iron and provide antioxidant protection to host tissues. In addition, it is important to further investigate the potential influence of iron chelators in enhancing host immunity.

REFERENCES

1. Clyde DF. Recent trends in the epidemiology and control of malaria. Epidemiol Rev 1987;9:219–243.
2. Patarroyo ME, Amador R, Clavijo P, Moreno A, Guzman F, Romero P, et al. A synthetic vaccine protects humans against challenge with asexual blood stages of *Plasmodium falciparum* malaria. Nature 1988;332:158–161.
3. Stoute JA, Slaoui M, Heppner DG, Momin P, Kester KE, Desmons P, et al. A preliminary evaluation of a recombinant circumsporozoite protein vaccine against *Plasmodium falciparum* malaria. N Engl J Med 1997;336:86–91.
4. Tanner M, Teuscher T, Alonso PL. SPf66—the first malaria vaccine. Parasitol Today 1995;11:10–13.
5. WHO Scientific Group. Advances in Malaria Chemotherapy. WHO Tech Rep Series No. 711. Geneva: World Health Organization, 1984.
6. Raventos-Suarez C, Pollack S, Nagel RL. *Plasmodium falciparum*: inhibition of in vitro growth by desferrioxamine. Am J Trop Med Hyg 1982;31:919–922.
7. Cabantchik ZI, Glickstein H, Golenser J, Loyevsky M, Tsafack, A. Iron chelators: mode of action as antimalarials. Acta Haematol 1996;95:70–77.
8. Gordeuk VR, Thuma PE, Brittenham GM, Biemba G, Zulu S, Simwanza G, et al. Iron chelation as a chemotherapeutic strategy for falciparum malaria. Am J Trop Med Hyg 1993;48:193–197.
9. Mabeza G, Loyevsky M, Gordeuk VR, Weiss G. Iron chelation therapy for malaria: a review. Pharmacol Ther 1999;81:53–75.
10. Aikawa, M. Fine structure of malaria parasites in the various stages of development. In: Wernsdorfer WH, McGregor I (eds.). Principles and Practice of Malariology. Edinburgh: Churchill Livingstone, 1988, pp. 97–130.

11. Pouvelle B, Spiegel R, Hsiao L, Howard RJ, Morris RL, Thomas AP, et al. Direct access to serum macromolecules by intraerythrocytic malaria parasites. Nature 1991;353:73–75.

12. Loyevsky M, Lytton SD, Mester B, Libman J, Shanzer A, Cabantchik ZI. The antimalarial action of Desferal involves a direct access route to erythrocytic (*Plasmodium falciparum*) parasites. J Clin Invest 1993;91:218–224.

13. Slater AF, Cerami A. Inhibition by chloroquine of a novel heme polymerase enzyme activity in malaria trophozoites. Nature 1992;355:167–169.

14. Murray MJ, Murray AB, Murray MB, Murray CJ. The adverse effect of iron repletion on the course of certain infections, Br Med J 1978;2:1113–1115.

15. Oppenheimer SJ, Gibson FD, MacFarlane SB, Moody JB, Harrison C, Spencer A, et al. Iron supplementation increases prevalence and effects of malaria: report on clinical studies in Papua New Guinea. Trans R Soc Trop Med Hyg 1986;80:603–612.

16. Harvey PW, Heywood PF, Nesheim MC, Galme K, Zegans M, Habicht, J-P, et al. The effect of iron therapy on malarial infection in Papua New Guinean schoolchildren. Am J Trop Med Hyg 1989;40:12–18.

17. Hershko C, Peto TE. Deferoxamine inhibition of malaria is independent of host iron status. J Exp Med 1988;168:375–387.

18. Pollack S, Schnelle, V. Inability to detect transferrin receptors on *P. falciparum* parasitized red cells. Br J Haematol 1988;68:125–129.

19. Sanchez-Lopez R, Halder K. A transferrin-independent iron uptake activity in *Plasmodium falciparum*-infected and uninfected erythrocytes. Mol Biochem Pharmacol 1992;55:9–20.

20. Pollack S, Flemming J. *P. falciparum* takes up iron from transferrin. Br J Haematol 1984;58:289–293.

21. van Zyl RL, Havlik I, Hempelman E, MacPhail AP, McNamara, L. Malaria pigment and extracellular iron: possible target for iron chelating agents. Biochem Pharmacol 1993;45:1431–1436.

22. Peto TE, Thompson JL. A reappraisal of the effects of iron and desferrioxamine on the growth of *Plasmodium falciparum* "*in vitro*": the unimportance of serum iron. Br J Haematol 1986;63:273–280.

23. Cazzola M, Arioso P, Barosi G, Bergamaschi G, Dezza L, Ascari E. Ferritin in the red cells of normal subjects and patients with iron deficiency and iron overload. Br J Haematol 1983;53:659–665.

24. Gabay T, Ginsburg H. Haemoglobin denaturation and iron release in acidified red blood cell lysate—a possible source of iron for intraerythrocytic malaria parasites. Exp Parasitol 1993;77:261–272.

25. Gamboa de Dominguez N, Rosenthal PJ. Cysteine proteinase inhibitors block early steps in hemoglobin degradation by cultured malaria parasites. Blood 1996;87:4448–4454.

26. Kolakovich KA, Gluzman IY, Duffin KL, Goldberg DE. Generation of hemoglobin peptides in the acidic digestive vacuole of *Plasmodium falciparum* implicates peptide transport in amino acid production. Mol Biochem Parasitol 1997;87:123–135.

27. Francis SE, Banerjee R, Goldberg DE. Biosynthesis and maturation of the malaria aspartic hemoglobinases plasmepsins I and II. J Biol Chem 1997;272:14,961–14,968.

28. Loyevsky M, Sacci JB Jr, Boehme P, Weglicki W, John C, Gordeuk VR. *Plasmodium falciparum* and *Plasmodium yoelii*: effect of the iron chelation prodrug dexrazoxane on in vitro cultures. Exp Parasitol 1999;91:105–114.

29. Yinnon AM, Theanacho EN, Grady RW, Spira DT, Hershko C. Antimalarial effect of HBED and other phenolic and catecholic iron chelators. Blood 1989;74:2166–2171.

30. Scott MD, Ranz A, Kuypers FA, Lubin BH, Meshnick SR. Parasite uptake of desferrioxamine: a prerequisite for antimalarial activity. Br J Haematol 1990;75:598–603.

31. Wrigglesworth JM, Baum H. The biochemical functions of iron. In: Jacobs A, Worwood M (eds). Iron in Biochemistry and Medicine II, New York: Academic, pp. 29–86, 1980.

32. Bezkorovainy A. Biochemistry of Nonheme Iron. New York: Plenum, 1980.

33. Scheibel LW, Sherman IW. Metabolism and organellar function during various stages of the life cycle: proteins, lipids, nucleic acids and vitamins. In: Wernsdorfer W, McGregor I (eds.). Malaria: Principles and Practice of Malariology, New York: Churchill Livingstone, p. 219, 1988.

34. Bonday ZQ, Taketani, S. Gupta PD, Padmanaban G. Heme biosynthesis by the malarial parasite. Import of delta-aminolevulinate dehydrase from the host red cell. J Biol Chem 1997;272:21,839–21,846.

35. Moormann AM, Hossler PA, Meshnick SR. Deferoxamine effects on *Plasmodium falciparum* gene expression. Mol Biochem Parasitol 1999;98:279–283.

36. Pradines B, Ramiandrasoa F, Basco LK, Bricard L, Kunesh G, Le-Bras J. In vitro activities of novel catecholate siderophores against *Plasmodium falciparum*. Antimicrob Agents Chemother 1996;40:2094–2098.

37. Scheibel LW, Adler A, Trager W. Tetraethylthiuram disulfide (Antabuse) inhibits the human malaria parasite *Plasmodium falciparum*. Proc Natl Acad Sci USA 1979;76: 5303–5307.

38. Scheibel LW, Adler A. Anti-malarial activity of selected aromatic chelators. Mol Pharmacol, 1980;18:320–325.

39. Bailey-Wood R, Blayney LM, Muir JR, Jacobs A. The effects of iron deficiency on rat liver enzymes. Brit J Exp Pathol 1975;56:193–198.

40. Glickstein H, Breuer B, Loyevsky M, Konijn A, Libman J, Shanzer A, et al. Differential cytotoxicity of iron chelators on malaria-infected cells versus mammalian cells. Blood 1996;87:4871–4878.

41. Fritsch G, Sawatzki G, Treumer J, Jung A, Spira DT. *Plasmodium falciparum*: inhibition in vitro with lactoferrin, desferrithiocin and desferricrocin. Exp Parasitol 1987;63:1–9.

42. Shanzer,A., Libman J, Lytton SD, Glickstein H, Cabantchik ZI. Reversed siderophores act as anti-malarial agents. Proc Natl Acad Sci USA 1991;88:6585–6589.

43. Scheibel LW, Stanton GG. Anti-malarial activity of selected aromatic chelators IV. Cation uptake of *Plasmodium falciparum* in the presence of oxines and siderochromes. Mol Pharmacol 1986;30:364–369.

44. Scheibel LW, Rodriguez S. Anti-malarial activity of selected aromatic chelators. V. Localization of 59Fe in *Plasmodium falciparum* in the presence of oxines. Prog Clin Biol Res 1989;313:119–149.

45. Heppner DG, Hallaway PE, Kontoghiorghes GJ, Eaton JW. Antimalarial properties of orally active iron chelators. Blood 1988;72:358–361.

46. Hershko C, Theanacho EN, Spira DT, Peter HH, Dobbin P, Hider RC. The effect of N-alkyl modification on the antimalarial activity of 3-hydroxyppyridin-4-one oral iron chelators. Blood 1991;77:637–643.

47. Yang Y, Ranz A, Pan HZ, Zhang ZN, Lin XB, Meshnick SR. Daphnetin: a novel antimalarial agent with in vitro and in vivo activity. Am J Trop Med Hyg 1992;46:15–20.

48. Clarke CJ, Eaton JM. Hydrophobic iron chelators as new antimalarial drugs. Clin Res 1990;38:300A.

49. Tsafack A, Loyevsky M, Ponka P, Cabantchik ZI. Mode of action of iron (III) chelators as anti-malarials. IV. Potentiation of desferal action by benzoyl and isonicotinoyl hydrazone derivatives. J Lab Clin Med 1996;127:575–582.

50. Loyevsky M, John C, Zaloujnyi I, Gordeuk V. Aminothiol multidentate chelators as antimalarials. Biochem Pharmacol 1997;54:451–458.

51. Loyevsky M, John C, Dickens B, Hu V, Gordeuk VR. Chelation of iron within the erythrocytic *Plasmodium falciparum* parasite by iron chelators. Mol Biochem Parasitol 101: 1999;.43–59.

52. Jairam KT, Havlik I, and Monteagudo FSE. Possible mechanism of action of desferrioxamine and 2,2'-bipyridyl on inhibiting the *in vitro* growth of *Plasmodium falciparum* (3 strain), Biochem Pharmacol 1991;8:1633–1634.

53. Whitehead S, Peto TE. Stage-dependent effect of deferoxamine on growth of *Plasmodium falciparum* in vitro. Blood 1990;76:1250–1255.
54. Reichard P, Ehrenburg A. Ribonucleotide reductase—a radical enzyme. Science 1983; 221:514–519.
55. Cavanaugh PF, Porter CW, Tukalo D, Frankfurt DS, Pavelic ZP, Bergeron RJ. Characterization of L1210 cell growth inhibition by the bacterial iron chelators parabactin and compound II, Cancer Res 1985;45:4754–4759.
56. Nyholm S, Mann GJ, Johansson AG, Bergeron RJ, Graslund A, Thelander, L. Role of ribonucleotide reductase in inhibition of mammalian cell growth by potent iron chelators. J Biol Chem 1993;268:26,200–26,205.
57. Rubin H, Salem HS, Li LS, Yang FD, Mama S, Wang ZM, et al. Cloning, sequence determination, and regulation of the ribonucleotide reductase subunits from *Plasmodium falciparum*: a target for antimalarial therapy. Proc Natl Acad Sci USA 1993;90:9280–9284.
58. Hoffbrand AV, Ganeshaguru K, Hooton JW, Tattersall MH. Effect of iron deficiency and desferrioxamine on DNA synthesis in human cells. Br J Haematol 1976;33:517–526.
59. Surolia N, Padmanaban G. *De novo* biosynthesis of heme offers a new chemotherapeutic target in the human malarial parasite. Biochem Biophys Res Commun 1992;187:744–750.
60. Fuchs O, Ponka P. The role of iron supply in the regulation of 5-aminolevulinate synthase mRNA levels in murine erythroleukemia cells. Neoplasma 1996;43:31–36.
61. Ponka P, Richardson DR, Edward JT, Chubb FL. Iron chelators of the pyridoxal isonycotinoyl hydrazone class. Relationship of the lipophilicity of the apochelator to its ability to mobilize iron from reticulocytes in vitro. Can J Physiol Pharmacol 1994;72:659–666.
62. Goodwin JF, Whitten CF. Chelation of ferrous sulfate solutions by desferrioxamine B. Nature 1965;205:281–283.
63. Albert, A. Selective Toxicity. New York: Chapman & Hall, 1981.
64. Basco LK, Le Bras J. *In vitro* activity of chloroquine and quinine in combination with desferrioxamine against *Plasmodium falciparum*. Am J Haematol 1993;42:389–391.
65. Chevion M, Chuang L, Golenser J. Effects of zinc–desferrioxamine on *Plasmodium falciparum* in culture. Antimicrob Agents Chemother 1995;39:1902–1905.
66. Lytton SD, Mester B, Libman J, Shanzer A, Cabantchik ZI. Mode of action of iron(III) chelators as antimalarials. II. Evidence for differential effects on parasite iron-dependent nucleic acid synthesis. Blood 1994;84:910–915.
67. Cabantchik ZI. Iron chelators as antimalarials—the biochemical basis of selective cytotoxicity. Parasitol Today 1995;11:73–78.
68. Neilands JB. Siderophores: structure and function of microbial iron transport compounds. J Biol Chem 1995;270:26,723–26,726.
69. Lytton SD, Mester B., Dayan I, Glickstein H, Libman J, Shanzer A, et al. Mode of action of iron (III) chelators as antimalarials: I. Membrane permeation properties and cytotoxic activity. Blood 1993;81:214–221.
70. Porter JB, Gyparaki M, Huehns ER, Hider RC. The relationship between the lipophilicity of hydroxypyrid-4-one iron chelators and cellular iron metabolism using an hepatocyte culture model. Biochem Soc Trans 1986;14:1180 (abstract).
71. Kontoghiorghes GJ, Hoffbrand AV. Orally active alpha ketohydroxyl pyridine iron chelators intended for clinical use: in vivo studies in rabbits. Br J Haematol 1986;62:607–613.
72. Pattanapanyasat K, Thaithong S, Kyle DE, Udomsangpetch R, Yongvanitchit K, Hider RC, et al. Flow cytometric assessment of hydroxypyridone iron chelators on in vitro growth of drug-resistant malaria. Cytometry 1997;27:84–91.
73. Golenser J, Tsafack A, Amichai Y, Libman J, Shanzer A, Cabantchik ZI. Antimalarial action of hydroxamate-based iron chelators and potentiation of desferrioxamine action by reversed siderophores. Antimicrob Agents Chemother 1995;39:61–65.
74. Stahel E, Mazier D, Guillouzo A, Miltgen P, Landau I, Mellouk S, et al. Iron chelators: in vitro inhibitory effect on the liver stage of rodent and human malaria. Am J Trop Med Hyg 1988;39:236–240.

75. Hasinoff BB. The interaction of the cardioprotective agent ICRF-187 ((+)-1,2-bis(3,5-dioxopiperazinyl-1-yl)propane; its hydrolysis product (ICRF-198); and other chelating agents with the Fe (III) and Cu (II) complexes of adriamycin. Agents Action 1989;26:378–385.

76. Hasinoff BB, Reiders FX, Clark V. The enzymatic hydrolysis-activation of the adriamycin cardioprotective agent (+)-1,2-bis(3,5-dioxopiperazinyl-1-yl)propane. Drug Metab Dispos 1991;19:74–80.

77. Pollack S, Rossan RN, Davidson DE, Escajadillo A. Desferrioxamine suppresses *Plasmodium falciparum* in Aotus monkeys. Proc Soc Exp Biol Med 1987;184:162–164.

78. Fritsch G, Treumer J, Spira DT, Jung A. *Plasmodium* vinckei: suppression of mouse infections with deferoxamine B. Exp Parasitol 1985;60:171–174.

79. Postma NS, Hermsen CC, Zuidema J, Eling WM. *Plasmodium* vinckei: optimization of desferrioxamine B delivery in the treatment of murine malaria. Exp Parasitol 1998:89:323–330.

80. Hershko C, Gordeuk VR, Thuma PE, Theanacho EN, Spira DT, Hider RC, et al. The anti-malarial effect of iron chelators in animal models and in humans with mild falciparum malaria. J Inorg Biochem 47:1992;267–277.

81. Lytton SD, Loyevsky M, Mester B, Libman J, Landau I, Shanzer A, et al. In vivo antima-larial action of a lipophilic iron (III) chelator: suppression of *Plasmodium* vinckei infec-tion by reversed siderophore. Am J Hematol 1993;43:217–220.

82. Golenser J, Domb A, Teomim D, Tsafack A, Nisim O, Ponka P, et al. The treatment of animal models of malaria with iron chelators by use of a novel polymeric device for slow drug release. J Pharmacol Exp Therap 1997;281:1127–1135.

83. Traore O, Carnevale P, Kaptue-Noche L, M'Bede J, Desfontaine M, Elion J, et al. Pre-liminary report on the use of desferrioxamine in the treatment of *Plasmodium falciparum* malaria. Am J Hematol 1991;37:206–208.

84. Gordeuk VR, Thuma PE, Brittenham GM, McLaren C, Parry D, Backenstose AR, et al. Effect of iron chelation therapy on recovery from deep coma in children with cerebral malaria. New Engl J Med 1992;327:1473–1477.

85. Thuma PE, Weiss G, Herold M. Gordeuk V. Serum neopterin, interleukin-4 and inter-leukin-6 concentrations in cerebral malaria patients and the effect of iron chelation therapy. Am J Trop Med Hyg 1996;54:164–168.

86. Bunnag D, Poltera AA, Viravan. C., Looaresuwan S, Harinasuta T, Schundlery, C. Plasmodicidal effect of desferrioxamine in human vivax or falciparum malaria from Thai-land. Acta Trop 1992;52:59–67.

87. Looaresuwan S, Wilairatana P, Vannaphan S, Gordeuk VR, Taylor TE, Meshnick SR, et al. Co-administration of desferrioxamine B with artesunate in malaria: an assess-ment of safety and tolerance. Ann Trop Med Parsaitol 1996;90:551–554.

88. MacPherson GG, Warrell MJ, White NJ, Looareesuwan S, Warrell DA. Human cerebral malaria: a quantitative ultrastructural analysis of parasitized erythrocyte sequestration. Am J Pathol 1985;119:385–401.

89. Oo MM, Aikawa M, Than T, Aye TM, Myint PT, Igarashi I, et al. Human cerebral malaria: a pathological study. J Neuropathol Exp Neurol 1987;46:223–231.

90. Aikawa M, Iseki M, Barnwell JW, Taylor D, Oo MM, Howard RJ. The pathology of human cerebral malaria. Am J Trop Med and Hyg 1990;43(Suppl):30–37.

91. Berendt AR, Ferguson DJ, Gardner, J, Turner G, Rowe, A, McCormick C, Ret al. Mole-cular mechanisms of sequestration in malaria. Parasitology 1994;108:519–528.

92. Sadrzadeh SM, Graf E, Panter SS, Hallaway PE, and Eaton JW. Hemoglobin: a biologic Fenton reagent. J Biol Chem 1984;259:14,354–14,356.

93. Ward PA, Till GO, Kunkel R, Beauchamp C. Evidence for role of hydroxyl radical in complement and neutrophil-dependent injury. J Clin Invest 1983;72:369–371.

94. Ambrosio, G, Zweier JL, Jacobus WE, Weisfeldt ML, Flaherty JT. Improvement of post-ischemic myocardial function and metabolism induced by administration of deferoxamine

at time of reflow: role of iron in the pathogenesis of reperfusion injury. Circulation 1987;76:906–915.

95. Sadrzadeh SM, Anderson DK, Panter SS, Hallaway PE, Eaton JW. Hemoglobin potentiates central nervous system damage. J Clin Invest 1987;79:662–664.

96. Weiss G, Thuma P, Mabeza G, Werner ER, Herold M, Gordeuk VR. Modulatory potential of iron chelation therapy on nitric oxide formation in cerebral malaria. J Infect Dis 1997;175:226–230.

97. Gordeuk VR, Thuma PE, Brittenham GM, Zulu S, Simwanza G, Mhangu A, et al. Iron chelation with deferoxamine B in adults with asymptomatic *Plasmodium falciparum* parasitemia. Blood 1992;79:308–312.

98. Thuma PE, Mabeza GF, Biemba G, Bhat GJ, McLaren C, Moyo VM, et al. Effect of iron chelation therapy on mortality in Zambian children with cerebral malaria. Trans R Soc Trop Med Hyg 1998;92:214–218.

99. Huber C, Batchelor JR, Fuchs D, Hausen A, Lang A, Niederwieser D, et al. Immune response associated production of neopterin. J Exp Med 1984;160:310–316.

100. Fuchs D, Hausen A, Reibnegger G, Werner ER, Deitrich MP, Wachter, H. Neopterin as a marker of activated cell-mediated immunity: application on HIV infection. Immunol Today 1988;9:150–155.

101. Weiss G, Fuchs D, Hausen A, Reibnegger G, Werner ER, Werner-Felmayer G, et al. Iron modulates interferon-gamma effects in human myelomonocytic cell line THP-1. Exp Hematol 1992;20:605–610.

102. Halliwell B, Gutteridge JMC, Cross CE. Free radicals, antioxidants and human disease. Where are we now? J Lab Clin Med 1992;119:598–620.

103. Gordeuk VR, Thuma PE, McLaren CE, Biemba G, Zulu S, Poltera AA, et al. Transferrin saturation and recovery from coma in cerebral malaria. Blood 1995;85:3297–3301.

104. Rosen GM, Pou S, Ramos CL, Cohen MS, Britigan BE. Free radicals and phagocytic cells. FASEB J 1995;9:200–209.

105. Cabantchik ZI, Moody-Haupt S, Gordeuk VR. Iron chelators as anti-infectives; malaria as a paradigm. FEMS Immunol Med Microbiol 1999;26:289–298.

106. Thuma PE, Olivieri NF, Mabeza GF, Biemba G, Parry D, Zulu S, et al. Assessment of the effect of the oral iron chelator deferiprone on asymptomatic *Plasmodium falciparum* parasitemia in humans. Am J Trop Med Hyg 1998;58:358–364.

18

Protease Inhibitors

Philip J. Rosenthal

INTRODUCTION

Extensive evidence demonstrates that proteases play important roles during the malaria parasite life cycle. Initial studies of partially purified protease activities and of the biological effects of protease inhibitors have now been complemented by molecular and biochemical analyses of important proteases of all four major catalytic classes. With these detailed characterizations of plasmodial proteases, we are poised to develop specific inhibitors of these enzymes with the potential for potent antimalarial activity.

PROTEASES AS CHEMOTHERAPEUTIC TARGETS

Plasmodial proteases are appealing new targets for antimalarial chemotherapy because of their critical functions and the significant efforts toward the inhibition of other proteases that have already taken place. In erythrocytic parasites, proteases appear to be required for the degradation of hemoglobin by trophozoites, the rupture of the erythrocyte by mature schizonts, and the invasion of erythrocytes by free merozoites (Fig. 1). Studies with protease inhibitors and analyses of the life cycle stage-specific expression of proteases have identified candidate protease activities (Table 1) and, in a number of cases, well-characterized enzymes that appear to be responsible for key proteolytic events (Table 2). Although studies evaluating the antimalarial effects of protease inhibitors are limited to date, experience with other systems suggests that inhibitors of essential plasmodial proteases can be developed as antimalarial drugs.

Hundreds of proteases have been well characterized in other biological systems (1). Potent inhibitors of all four major mechanistic classes of proteases have been developed. In addition, major pharmaceutical efforts have led to the discovery and development of protease inhibitors as potential and, in some cases, available drugs for human diseases. Two cases are noteworthy in this regard. Inhibitors of angiotensin-converting enzyme, which were designed based on natural inhibitors from snake venom, are among the most important cardiovascular drugs currently in use (2). Inhibitors of the human immunodeficiency virus (HIV) aspartic protease, which were developed from existing renin inhibitors, are valuable components of our antiviral armamentarium (3). Many other host and microbial proteases are currently under study as potential targets of chemotherapy. Thus, antimalarial protease inhibitor discovery need not occur in a vacuum. Rather, it should ideally benefit from advances made with other proteases.

From: *Antimalarial Chemotherapy: Mechanisms of Action, Resistance, and New Directions in Drug Discovery*
Edited by: P. J. Rosenthal © Humana Press Inc., Totowa, NJ

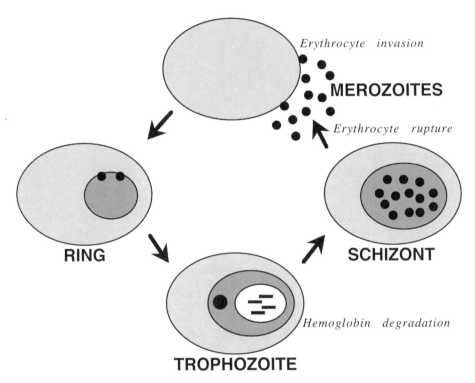

Fig. 1. Erythrocytic life cycle of malaria parasites. Processes that require protease activity, and thus are potential targets for protease inhibitors, are labeled in italics.

This is a key consideration, as funding for antimalarial drug development is limited, and "piggybacking" onto existing industrial drug discovery efforts may be the most effective means of developing new antimalarial drugs.

BIOLOGICAL ROLES OF PROTEASES OF MALARIA PARASITES

Studies with protease inhibitors and erythrocytic malaria parasites have identified three processes that clearly require protease activity: hemoglobin degradation, erythrocyte invasion, and erythrocyte rupture. In addition, it is likely that other biological processes in erythrocytic parasites and in other parasite stages require protease activity. Key proteases probably include degradative enzymes that cleave target proteins (e.g., hemoglobin, erythrocyte cytoskeletal proteins) at multiple sites and processing enzymes that cleave only a single site in a protein (e.g., merozoite surface protein-1 [MSP-1]). For both cases, available evidence suggests that multiple proteolytic activities are required for normal parasite development.

Hemoglobin Degradation

Malaria parasites take up erythrocyte hemoglobin and digest it in acidic food vacuoles (*see* also Chapter 4). Parasites utilize amino acids from hemoglobin for nutritional purposes, as they have limited capacity to take up or synthesize certain essential amino acids. Hemoglobin degradation may also serve to create space within the erythrocyte for the growing malaria parasite. Although the basis for hemoglobin degradation and

Table 1
Effects of Peptide Protease Inhibitors on the Life Cycle of Malaria Parasites

Life-cycle stage	Biological process	Effective inhibitors	Protease class implicated[a]	Ref.
Trophozoite	Hemoglobin hydrolysis	Leupeptin, E-64	Cysteine	*5,7–9,64*
		Pepstatin	Aspartic	*6,8,53*
Schizont	Erythrocyte rupture	Chymostatin	Serine	*18,31*
		Leupeptin	Cysteine	*18,30,31*
Merozoite	Erythrocyte invasion	Chymostatin	Serine	*17–19,21,30,31*

Note: Only results that were seen consistently in multiple studies are shown.
[a]Principal class inhibited, although some of the compounds also inhibit other classes.

Table 2
Well Characterized Proteases of Malaria Parasites

Protease	Class	Putative role	Sequence described?	Species studied[a]
Falcipains	Cysteine	Hemoglobin hydrolysis	Yes	Pf, Pv, Po, Pm, P, M, A
Plasmepsins	Aspartic	Hemoglobin hydrolysis	Yes	Pf, Pv, Po, Pm, M
Falcilysin	Metallo	Hemoglobin hydrolysis	Yes	Pf
Aminopeptidase	Metallo	Hemoglobin hydrolysis	Yes	Pf, M
PVHSP28	Metallo	Unknown	Yes	Pv
Pf68	Cysteine	Erythrocyte rupture	No	Pf, M
Pf76	Serine	Erythrocyte invasion	No	Pf, M
Pfsub-1	Serine	Erythrocyte invasion	Yes	Pf
Pfsub-2	Serine	Erythrocyte invasion	Yes	Pf

[a]Pf, *P. falciparum*; Pv, *P. vivax*; Po, *P. ovale*; Pm, *P. malariae*; P, primate malaria species; M, murine malaria species; A, avian malaria species.

the biochemical mechanism of this process are incompletely understood, the process has profound implications for antimalarial chemotherapy. Hemoglobin degradation releases free heme; effects on the disposition of heme probably explain the action of chloroquine and other quinoline antimalarials (*see* Chapter 6). Interactions with heme and the subsequent release of free radicals may also explain the action of artemisinin and its analogs (*see* Chapter 10). Relevant to this chapter, inhibition of the hydrolysis of globin is toxic to malaria parasites.

Multiple proteases appear to hydrolyze hemoglobin and globin fragments in the food vacuole. As of now, four food vacuole proteases have been well characterized (*see* Chapter 4). It has been suggested that two aspartic proteases, plasmepsin I and plasmepsin II, are responsible for initial cleavages of hemoglobin, that the cysteine protease falcipain-2 cleaves relatively large globin fragments, and that the newly identified metalloprotease falcilysin cleaves smaller peptides. Small globin peptides are then likely transported to the parasite cytosol, where a cytosolic aminopeptidase and probably other proteases complete the hydrolysis of globin to free amino acids.

The pathway of hemoglobin digestion may not be fully ordered, however. The precise roles of different proteases in hydrolyzing hemoglobin are uncertain, and results evaluating the hydrolysis of native hemoglobin by these proteases have varied depending on the reaction conditions studied. Under nonreducing conditions, plasmepsin I most efficiently cleaved native hemoglobin, plasmepsin II cleaved hemoglobin at the same peptide bond but preferred denatured globin as a substrate, and falcipain cleaved denatured globin but not native hemoglobin *(4)*. However, under mild reducing conditions, falcipain-2 cleaved both native and denatured hemoglobin (*see* section "Falcipains and Other Cysteine Proteases").

Both cysteine *(5)* and aspartic *(6)* protease inhibitors have been shown to block hemoglobin degradation by cultured malaria parasites. However, evaluations of the effects of protease inhibitors on hemoglobin degradation have led to results that are somewhat difficult to reconcile. Incubation of cultured *Plasmodium falciparum* parasites with cysteine protease inhibitors led to the accumulation of large quantities of undegraded hemoglobin in the food vacuole *(5,7–9)*, suggesting that falcipain-2 is required for initial steps in hemoglobin digestion. In additional studies with cultured parasites, the cysteine protease inhibitor E-64, but not the aspartic protease inhibitor pepstatin, inhibited the dissociation of the hemoglobin tetramer *(9)*, the release of heme *(9)*, the initial processing of α- and β-globin *(10)*, and the formation of the hemoglobin breakdown product hemozoin *(11)*. In other studies, however, pepstatin *(6)* and specific plasmepsin inhibitors *(12)* blocked the degradation of hemoglobin and formation of hemozoin by cultured parasites much more effectively than the cysteine protease inhibitor leupeptin. Both effects of cysteine protease inhibitors *(5)* and aspartic protease inhibitors *(12)* on hemoglobin processing were reversible after the washout of inhibitors. These studies are difficult to interpret, as inhibitory effects on hemoglobin processing cannot easily be separated from overall toxicity of the studied inhibitors. Thus, specific agents might inhibit hemoglobin processing only as a consequence of the inhibition of another parasite process. In the one study that attempted to separate overall parasite toxicity from that specifically resulting from effects on hemoglobin degradation, E-64, but not pepstatin, inhibited hemozoin formation at concentrations that did not affect parasite uptake of hypoxanthine *(11)*.

The full elucidation of the specific roles of multiple parasite proteases in hemoglobin degradation will require additional study. Conclusions consistently supported by available data are that the plasmepsins act early in the hemoglobin degradation process, that falcipain-2 plays a key role in digesting globin, and that the specific inhibition of either of these classes of proteases is toxic to cultured parasites. In addition, falcilysin appears to hydrolyze small globin peptides, and the final steps of hemoglobin hydrolysis probably involve a cytosolic aminopeptidase. Relevant to the consideration of protease inhibitors as antimalarial drugs, multiple proteases that act at different points in the hemoglobin degradation pathway are potential chemotherapeutic targets.

Erythrocyte Invasion

The invasion of erythrocytes by merozoites includes a series of discrete steps *(13)*. In this process, the merozoite attaches reversibly to erythrocyte receptors, realigns itself such that its apical end apposes the erythrocyte membrane, forms an irreversible tight junction, and then enters the erythrocyte within the parasitophorous vacuole. The contents of three different types of secretory organelles (rhoptries, micronemes, and dense granules) are released from the apical end of merozoites during this process, and these contents are believed to include proteases that facilitate erythrocyte entry *(14–16)*.

Results have been somewhat inconsistent, but the clearest available evidence suggests a role for serine proteases in erythrocyte invasion. In studies with cultured parasites, serine protease inhibitors blocked erythrocyte invasion by merozoites of *P. knowlesi (17,18)*, *P. falciparum (7,19,20)*, and *P. chabaudi (21)*. Erythrocyte invasion was consistently blocked by inhibitors of chymotrypsin-like (chymostatin), but not trypsin-like (aprotinin, antipain, α-1-antitrypsin, soybean trypsin inhibitor) serine proteases. In *P. knowlesi*, chymostatin did not block initial erythrocyte binding or junction formation, but subsequent invasion was strongly inhibited *(18)*. Additionally supporting a role for chymotrypsin-like proteases in erythrocyte invasion, pretreatment of human erythrocytes with chymotrypsin *(7)* or pretreatment of murine erythrocytes with a purified *P. chabaudi* serine protease *(21)* reversed the inhibition of invasion by serine protease inhibitors. Also, treatment of intact erythrocytes with chymotrypsin induced conformational changes in the integral membrane protein band 3, suggesting that a serine protease facilitates invasion by altering the erythrocyte membrane and underlying cytoskeleton *(22)*.

Inhibitors of cysteine and trypsin-like serine proteases also blocked erythrocyte invasion in some studies *(7,17,19,20)*, but the only studies that evaluated invasion of isolated merozoites, thus clearly distinguishing effects on erythrocyte rupture from effects on invasion, showed no inhibition of invasion by the cysteine and trypsin-like protease inhibitor leupeptin *(18)*, the cysteine protease inhibitor E-64 *(21)*, or the aspartic protease inhibitor pepstatin *(18,21)*. Both chymostatin and leupeptin also inhibited the invasion of merozoites after introduction to lysed and then resealed erythrocytes *(7)* and altered the morphology of the rhoptry organelle of mature *P. knowlesi* schizonts *(23)*. These results suggest that parasite proteases required for erythrocyte invasion are active prior to erythrocyte rupture. Inhibitors of the calcium-dependent cysteine protease calpain and the aminopeptidase inhibitor bestatin also inhibited the invasion of erythrocytes by *P. falciparum* in one study *(20)*. In summary, plasmodial chymotrypsin-like protease activity appears to be required for erythrocyte invasion. Other activities may also be involved in this process.

A number of proteins of mature schizonts and merozoites are proteolytically processed immediately before or during erythrocyte invasion. The best characterized such protein is merozoite surface protein-1 (MSP-1). At approximately the time of erythrocyte rupture, initial proteolytic cleavages generate four polypeptide fragments that are joined in a noncovalent complex and bound to the merozoite surface by a glycosylphosphatidylinositol-anchored carboxy-terminal 42-kDa fragment *(13)*. The nature of the proteolytic activity responsible for these cleavages is uncertain. At some point after merozoite release, an additional processing step yields a 19-kDa membrane-bound fragment *(24)*. This last cleavage appears to be necessary for the invasion of erythrocytes by merozoites, as antibodies directed against the 42-kDa fragment that inhibit its processing block erythrocyte invasion *(25,26)*. This final MSP-1 processing event appears to be the result of the action of a membrane-bound calcium-dependent serine protease, as it is inhibited by chelating agents, reversed by added calcium, and also inhibited by the serine protease inhibitor phenylmethyl sulfonylfluoride (PMSF), but not inhibitors of other proteolytic classes *(27)*. Interestingly, although the ultimate MSP-1 processing site has a chymotrypsin-like cleavage sequence, processing was not inhibited by chymostatin, suggesting involvement of another type of serine protease (*see* "Serine Proteases").

Another protein that is proteolytically processed at the time of merozoite release is the serine-repeat antigen (SERA or P126), a candidate vaccine component *(28)* that shares features of cysteine proteases (*see* "Plasmodial Cysteine and Aspartic Protease-Like Proteins"). SERA is processed into multiple fragments that are released into culture media *(29)*. The processing of SERA by cultured *P. falciparum* was altered by leupeptin, which caused the accumulation of a new processing intermediate, and it was unaffected by chymostatin or antipain *(30)*. These results suggest that a cysteine protease activity is required for the processing of SERA, which may be required for erythrocyte invasion or rupture.

Erythrocyte Rupture

The mechanism of rupture of erythrocytes by mature schizonts is poorly understood, but this process also appears to require protease activity. Potential roles for proteases include the hydrolysis of erythrocyte cytoskeletal proteins to facilitate egress from the host cell and the processing of parasite proteins. Available studies suggest that both serine and cysteine proteases are required for erythrocyte rupture. In studies with *P. falciparum*, this process was markedly inhibited by a combination of peptide inhibitors of all four major protease classes *(31)*. The inhibitor combination caused the accumulation of mature, unruptured schizonts (segmenters) in parasite cultures. The most marked inhibitions of erythrocyte rupture with *P. falciparum (30,31)* and *P. knowlesi (18)* were caused by leupeptin and chymostatin. However, in some studies with *P. knowlesi (17)* and *P. falciparum (7)*, neither leupeptin nor chymostatin markedly inhibited this process.

Erythrocyte membrane and cytoskeletal proteins are altered by plasmodial infection *(32,33)*, and parasite proteases that hydrolyze these proteins have been identified. A *P. lophurae* aspartic protease activity cleaved spectrin and band 3 *(34)*. An activity of *P. falciparum* and *P. berghei* that was inhibited by both chymostatin and leupeptin hydrolyzed spectrin and band 4.1 *(35)*. A *P. chabaudi* serine protease cleaved band 3 *(21)*. Recently, the aspartic protease plasmepsin II was shown to be present in parasite fractions enriched for spectrin-hydrolyzing activity and to localize to the periphery of mature schizont-stage parasites *(36)*. In addition, recombinant plasmepsin II cleaved spectrin, actin, and band 4.1 at neutral pH, and the cleavage site in spectrin for the recombinant enzyme was identical to that of the enriched parasite fractions.

In summary, studies with protease inhibitors suggest that cysteine and serine proteases are required for erythrocyte rupture. Studies with isolated proteases have demonstrated the hydrolysis of erythrocyte components by serine and aspartic proteases. Thus, it appears that cysteine, serine, and aspartic proteases may all play roles in erythrocyte rupture by mature schizonts.

Other Processes

Proteases likely play multiple additional functions within the life cycles of malaria parasites. In particular, potential roles for proteases in nonerythrocytic life-cycle stages have not been explored in detail. These stages must invade cells and degrade host tissues in fashions analogous to those of erythrocytic parasites, and it is likely that they utilize the same or related proteases to perform similar tasks. Thus, it is possible that protease inhibitors that prevent the growth of erythrocytic parasites may also act on other life-cycle stages.

Roles for Host Proteases in the Life Cycle of Malaria Parasites

The human bloodstream serine protease and plasminogen activator urokinase was recently shown to bind to the surface of *P. falciparum*-infected erythrocytes *(37)*. The depletion of urokinase from parasite culture medium inhibited erythrocyte rupture by mature schizonts, and this inhibition was reversed by the addition of exogenous urokinase. These data suggested that host urokinase activity is required for erythrocyte rupture. However, specific inhibitors of urokinase did not block the erythrocytic development of *P. falciparum* or the rupture or invasion of erythrocytes by these parasites *(38)*. In addition, murine malaria parasites infecting mice deficient in urokinase, tissue plasminogen activator, or plasminogen replicated as efficiently as those infecting wild-type mice, arguing against a role for host plasminogen activators in the parasite life cycle.

After being taken up in an anopheline mosquito blood meal, malaria parasites come in contact with multiple insect proteases, including trypsin, chymotrypsin, and aminopeptidase activities *(39)*. "Early" trypsins, which are constitutively expressed and so present at the time of blood meal ingestion, appear to induce expression of two "late" trypsins, which are believed to to play a key role in the breakdown of blood components *(40)*. The insect trypsins and other proteases may also be responsible for cleavages that are required for parasite development in the mosquito midgut. For example, in *P. gallinaceum,* which, unlike human malaria parasites, is transmitted by *Aedes* mosquitoes, a chitinase used by the parasite to cross the peritrophic matrix that surrounds the blood meal is activated by mosquito trypsin *(41)*. Inhibition of the trypsin activity by protease inhibitors *(42)* or trypsin-specific antibodies *(43)* blocked the infectivity of *P. gallinaceum* parasites for *Aedes* mosquitoes, and this effect was negated by exogenous chitinase. These data suggest that inhibitors of mosquito proteases might effectively block parasite transmission if they could be introduced into mosquitoes at the time of blood meal ingestion. This raises the possibility of including a transmission-blocking protease inhibitor in a chemoprophylactic regimen.

PROTEASE TARGETS

Important advances over about the last decade have led to the biochemical and molecular characterization of a number of plasmodial proteases. Although the biological role is not fully characterized for any of these enzymes, plausible hypotheses exist to explain their functions. Many of the plasmodial proteases that have been characterized appear to have necessary roles in the erythrocytic life cycle; thus, they are potential chemotherapeutic targets.

Falcipains and Other Cysteine Proteases

A recent affinity purification of the principal *P. falciparum* trophozoite cysteine protease has provided, for the first time, the amino-terminal sequence of this enzyme and yielded the surprising result that it is not encoded by the previously identified *P. falciparum* cysteine protease gene (now termed falcipain-1 *[44,45]*). Thus, although the falcipain-1 gene is transcribed in erythrocytic parasites and the recombinant enzyme has been shown to degrade hemoglobin *(46)*, the function of the protease is uncertain. The principal trophozoite cysteine protease is encoded by the newly identified falcipain-2 gene *(45)*. Falcipain-2 is a fairly typical papain-family cysteine protease *(5,45)*. As is typical for this mechanistic class, it has an acidic pH optimum and its activity is enhanced by reducing agents *(45,47)*.

Falcipain-2 activity is most prominent in trophozoites, the erythrocytic stage during which most hemoglobin degradation occurs *(45,48)* and has been localized to the parasite food vacuole, the site of hemoglobin degradation *(4,45)*. Falcipain-2 has a cathepsin L-like substrate specificity *(47)*, but clear differences between falcipain-2 and host cysteine proteases are seen in the hydrolysis of peptide substrates and inhibition by peptide inhibitors *(45)*.

Falcipain-2 shares similarity in sequence with other papain-family proteases *(45)*. In a GenBank BLAST search, its sequence was most similar to that of falcipain-1, but identity of mature protease domains was less than 50%. Falcipain-2 is much more similar in sequence to a putative third *P. falciparum* cysteine protease, identified by the Sanger Centre genome sequencing project, and provisionally named falcipain-3. However, falcipain-2 alone is responsible for over 90% of trophozoite cysteine protease activity *(45)*, and no clear role for other cysteine proteases in hemoglobin degradation has been documented. Importantly, older studies of "trophozoite cysteine protease" activity or "falcipain" activity should now be appreciated to pertain principally to falcipain-2. Partial or complete sequences of falcipain homologs from nine other plasmodial species, including all species that infect humans, are available, and the sequences of these proteases are well conserved *(49)*. However, preliminary analysis suggests that all of these enzymes are homologs of falcipain-1, not falcipain-2, and so it is a priority to identify homologs of falcipain-2 in other plasmodial species.

Falcipain-2 inhibitors block the hydrolysis of hemoglobin by cultured *P. falciparum* parasites, causing the accumulation in the food vacuole of large quantities of undegraded globin and a subsequent block in parasite development *(5,9)*. Thus, falcipain-2 appears to be required for the degradation of hemoglobin by erythrocytic parasites. Falcipain-2 does not cleave native hemoglobin in a nonreducing environment *(4,45)*, but it does cleave this substrate under mildly reducing conditions (approx 0.5–1 mM glutathione) that are predicted to be present in the food vacuole *(45)*. Falcipain-2 more rapidly cleaves denatured globin, suggesting that once initial cleavages of the hemoglobin tetramer have taken place, the cysteine protease plays a major role in hydrolyzing globin to small peptides.

Additional cysteine protease activities have been identified in mature erythrocytic parasites. An M_r 68,000 cysteine protease was purified from schizonts and merozoites of *P. berghei* and *P. falciparum* *(50,51)*. Antisera directed against the *P. berghei* protease localized to the merozoite apex, suggesting a role in erythrocyte invasion. An M_r 35,000–40,000 cysteine protease that differed from falcipain-2 in size and stage specificity was identified in mature schizonts *(48)*. The precise biochemical features and biological roles of these proteases are not known. A number of cysteine protease sequences and sequence fragments have recently been identified by the *P. falciparum* genome sequencing project. Some of these sequences likely encode proteases that were previously identified biochemically. The sequence information should be a valuable tool for the determination of the biological roles of additional cysteine proteases.

Plasmepsins

Plasmepsins I and II are located in the *P. falciparum* food vacuole, have acidic pH optima, and share significant sequence homology with other aspartic proteases *(4,52–55)* (*see* also Chapter 4). The enzymes are biochemically similar, but not identical; in evaluations of globin cleavage, substrate preferences of the two enzymes were distinct *(4,56)*. The plasmepsins are synthesized as proenzymes, which are integral membrane proteins that are cleaved to soluble forms under acidic conditions *(57)*. The synthesis and processing of both plasmepsins peaks in trophozoites, but plasmepsin I is also synthesized, processed, and presumably active in young ring-stage parasites *(57)*. Homologs of the *P. falciparum* plasmepsins have recently been identified in the three other human malaria parasites *(58)* and in the rodent parasite *P. berghei (59)*. Only one aspartic protease has been identified in each of these species; the biochemical properties of the proteases were quite similar to those of the *P. falciparum* plasmepsins. Additional *P. falciparum* aspartic proteases may also be present, including additional food vacuole activities identified biochemically *(60)* and a recently identified plasmepsin homolog that contains substitutions of universally conserved aspartic protease amino acids *(61)*, but nonetheless appears to have proteolytic activity (*see* Chapter 4). Also, the *P. falciparum* genome sequencing project has identified additional aspartic protease sequences *(59)*, and the characterization of the biological functions of the different proteases is a high priority.

Plasmepsins I and II are hemoglobinases capable of cleaving native hemoglobin at multiple sites *(4)*. In in vitro studies, both aspartic proteases initially cleaved native hemoglobin at a peptide bond that is a hinge region of the molecule *(4)*. This cleavage apparently alters the structure of the substrate to expose other sites for additional cleavages by the plasmepsins, falcipain-2, and possibly other proteases *(62)*. Both plasmepsin I *(63)* and plasmepsin II *(54,55)* have been heterologously expressed, and native and recombinant enzymes have been characterized biochemically. The substrate specificities of plasmepsin I and plasmepsin II differ somewhat, and each appears to cleave different sites in globin after the initial cleavage of hemoglobin *(4)*. Aspartic protease inhibitors, including pepstatin *(8,64)* and more specific plasmepsin inhibitors *(53,63,65,66)*, are toxic to cultured malaria parasites, suggesting that the plasmepsins are appropriate chemotherapeutic targets.

Serine Proteases

As noted earlier, the serine protease inhibitor chymostatin consistently blocks merozoite invasion of erythrocytes, strongly suggesting that a serine protease is required for this process. A candidate chymostatin-sensitive invasion protease is an M_r 76,000 serine protease of schizonts and merozoites of *P. falciparum (67)* and *P. chabaudi (21)*. This protease is bound in an inactive form to the merozoite membrane by a glycosyl-phosphatidylinositol anchor, and activated by phosphatidylinositol-specific phospholipase C *(67)*. The purified *P. chabaudi* and *P. falciparum* proteases cleaved the erythrocyte membrane protein band 3 *(21,68)*. Another merozoite-specific *P. falciparum* serine protease of similar size that does not require activation by phospholipase C has also been identified *(48)*.

Genes encoding two *P. falciparum* serine proteases have recently been identified. Pfsub-1 *(69)* and Pfsub-2 *(70,71)* encode subtilisin-like serine proteases with similarities in sequence to bacterial subtilisins. These genes probably do not encode the membrane-anchored serine protease discussed earlier *(67)*, because they appear to have different sizes, subtilisins are not generally inhibited by chymostatin, their sequences do not predict glycosyl-phosphatidylinositol anchored proteins, and Pfsub-1 could not be identified by the substrate gel electrophoresis technique that identified the other proteases

(48,67,69,70). The predicted sequences of Pfsub-1 and Pfsub-2 have 48% amino acid similarity in the active-site region, but are otherwise quite different *(70)*. Both proteases are expressed in erythrocytic-stage parasites as proforms and concentrated in dense granules. Pfsub-1 is proteolytically processed in two autocatalytic steps, yielding a 47-kDa form that accumulates in dense granules and then is released from merozoites in a soluble form at the time of erythrocyte invasion *(69,72)*. The autocatalytic cleavage sites are at aspartate residues, an unusual specificity for subtilisins *(72)*. Pfsub-2 is a much larger protein that is synthesized in schizonts and processed as a merozoite integral membrane protein *(70,71)*. The biological roles of Pfsub-1 and Pfsub-2 are unknown. Of note, the terminal processing of MSP-1, which is required for erythrocyte invasion, is mediated by a calcium-requiring serine protease that is inhibited by PMSF but not diisopropyl fluorophosphate (DFP) or chymostatin (see "Erythrocyte Invasion"). These biochemical features are suggestive of a subtilisin and also consistent with the observation that Pfsub-1 did not react with DFP. However, the substrate specificity of Pfsub-1 argues against a role for this enzyme in the secondary processing of MSP-1. Nonetheless, available data suggest that Pfsub-1 and Pfsub-2 are processing enzymes that are required for the cleavage of plasmodial proteins, including, perhaps, MSP-1, and thus that they are logical chemotherapeutic targets.

Metalloproteases

Three plasmodial metalloprotease genes have been identified. A *P. falciparum* food vacuole metalloprotease, falcilysin, has recently been characterized *(73)*. The sequence of falcilysin shows that it is a member of the M16 family of metallopeptidases. Falcilysin cannot cleave native hemoglobin or denatured globin, but it cleaves relatively small (up to 20 amino acid) hemoglobin fragments at polar residues. Thus, it appears to act downstream of the plasmepsins and falcipain-2 in the hydrolysis of hemoglobin. A *P. vivax* heat-shock protein has been noted to contain metalloprotease sequence motifs *(74)* and to exhibit metalloprotease activity *(75)*. The predicted *P. vivax* protein is much smaller than falcilysin, and it belongs to a different metalloprotease family.

A third metalloprotease gene was identified in *P. falciparum*. This gene predicts a metalloprotease that is about the size of falcilysin, but belongs to the M1 family, which includes a large number of aminopeptidases *(76)*. Antisera raised against a peptide encoded by this gene identified two schizont proteins, possibly two processed forms of the protease. The antiserum also immunoprecipitated schizont aminopeptidase activity that was purified from extracts of schizont-stage parasites *(76)*. This aminopeptidase is probably the same enzyme previously identified in parasite but not food vacuole lysates of *P. falciparum*, *P. chabaudi*, and *P. berghei (77–79)*. This aminopeptidase had maximal activity against leucine and alanine monopeptides, had a neutral pH optimum, and was inhibited by both the aminopeptidase inhibitor bestatin and metal chelators *(77,78,80)*. Recent studies suggest that the ultimate steps in hemoglobin hydrolysis occur in the parasite cytoplasm, as the incubation of hemoglobin with *P. falciparum* food vacuole lysates generated multiple peptide fragments but not free amino acids *(79)*. The neutral metalloaminopeptidase likely plays a part in the hydrolysis of globin peptides after they are transported from the food vacuole. The aminopeptidase inhibitors nitrobestatin and bestatin blocked the growth of cultured *P. falciparum* parasites, suggesting that the aminopeptidase is another potential chemotherapeutic target *(80)*.

Plasmodial Cysteine and Aspartic Protease-Like Proteins

The serine-repeat antigen (SERA) is under study as a potential component of a malaria vaccine. Portions of SERA *(28)* and its homolog SERPH *(81)* have limited sequence homology with cysteine proteases, particularly near highly conserved active-site residues. The "protease domain" of these proteins is located within a much larger protein without apparent similarity to cysteine proteases. Recent studies have identified eight contiguous SERA genes on *P. falciparum* chromosome 2 *(82)* and multiple SERA homologs from other plasmodial species *(83,84)*. SERAs can be subdivided into proteins that have replaced the canonical active-site cysteine with a serine and others that have conservation of all active-site cysteine protease residues *(84)*. Three of the eight gene sequences on chromosome 2 show conservation of papain-family active-site amino acids. It is likely that a subset of SERAs are unusual cysteine proteases. As cysteine protease inhibitors block erythrocyte rupture *(18,31)* and the SERAs are located in the parasitophorous vacuole that surrounds mature schizonts *(29)*, these proteins may be responsible for proteolytic cleavages required for this process.

A *P. falciparum* gene predicting a plasmepsin homolog that is expressed in erythrocytic parasites has recently been identified *(61)*. Similar to the case of some of the SERA proteins, the plasmepsin homolog has substitutions of universally conserved aspartic protease amino acids. Thus, it either is a protease with a unique catalytic mechanism (as suggested in preliminary studies; *see* Chapter 4) or it has a different biological function.

ANTIMALARIAL EFFECTS OF PROTEASE INHIBITORS

Protease inhibitors have been valuable reagents for studying the biological roles of proteases of malaria parasites. Evaluations of protease inhibitors as potential antimalarial drugs are fairly limited to date. However, increasing evidence suggests that inhibitors of cysteine and aspartic proteases that degrade hemoglobin have potent antimalarial activity and may be appropriate antimalarials (Table 3). In addition, recent advances in the characterization of other hemoglobinases and in proteases that are required for erythrocyte rupture or invasion suggest that inhibitors of many of these enzymes may also demonstrate antiparasitic activity.

Cysteine Protease Inhibitors

Inhibitors of falcipain-2 prevent the degradation of hemoglobin by *P. falciparum*, cause undegraded hemoglobin to accumulate in the parasite food vacuole, and block parasite development *(5,7,8,64)*. Initial studies with generic peptide cysteine protease inhibitors including leupeptin and E-64 were followed by studies with more specific protease inhibitors. Selected peptidyl fluoromethyl ketones *(47,85,86)* and vinyl sulfones *(87,88)* inhibited falcipain-2 and blocked *P. falciparum* development at nanomolar concentrations (Table 3). The degree of inhibition of falcipain-2 correlated with the extent of biological effects, supporting the conclusion that the protease inhibitors exerted their antimalarial effects directly via the inhibition of falcipain-2 and a consequent block in hemoglobin hydrolysis *(86)*. Analysis of the structural requirements for falcipain-2 inhibition by the peptidyl inhibitors identified leucine–homophenylalanine peptides as excellent inhibitors. In addition, the presence of amino-terminal groups that improved aqueous solubility and bulky carboxy-terminal groups improved activity *(88)*. Both fluoromethyl ketones *(89)* and vinyl sulfones *(88)* also cured mice infected with

Table 3
Evaluations of Protease Inhibitors as Antimalarial Drugs

Target protease	Biological role	Inhibitor	Antimalarial effects		Ref.
			In vitro[a] (μM)	In vivo[b] (mg/kg/d)	
Falcipain-2	Hemoglobin degradation	Fluoromethylketones			
		Z-Leu-Tyr-CH$_2$F	0.059		85
		Z-Phe-Arg-CH$_2$F	0.064		86
		Mu-Phe-HPh-CH$_2$F	0.004	200–400 sc	89
		Vinyl sulfones			
		Mu-Leu-HPh-VSPh	0.004		87
		N-Me-pipu-Leu-HPhVSPh	0.002	100–200 po	88
		N-Me-pipu-Leu-HPhVS-2Np	0.0004	100–200 po	88
		Oxalic bis ((2-hydroxy-1-naph-thylmethylene)hydrazide)	7		93
		1-(2,5-dichlorophenyl)-3-(4-quinolinyl)-2-propen-1-one	0.23		94
		7-chloro-1,2-dihydro-2-(2,3-dimethoxy-phenyl)-5,5-dioxide-4-(1H,10H)-phenothiazinone	2		95
Plasmepsin I	Hemoglobin degradation	SC-50083	2–5		53
Plasmepsin II	Hemoglobin degradation	Ro 40-4388	0.25		63
		Compound 7	20		65
Plasmepsins I and II	Hemoglobin degradation	Compounds 9–11	1–2		66
Falcipain-2 and plasmepsins	Hemoglobin degradation	N-Me-pipu-Leu-HPhVSPh plus pepstatin	Synergy[c]	20 ip plus 40 ip	103
Pf68	Erythrocyte invasion	GlcA-Val-Leu-Gly-Lys-NHC$_2$H$_5$	900		100

[a]IC$_{50}$ values for the inhibition of development or uptake of [^{3}H]hypoxanthine by cultured P. falciparum parasites.

[b]Dosages that cured the majority of mice of otherwise lethal infections with P. vinckei; sc, subcutaneous; po, oral; ip, intraperitoneal.

[c]The two compounds were markedly synergistic, with potent inhibition of parasite development by combinations including nanomolar concentrations of each compound.

otherwise lethal malaria infections. Morpholine urea–phenylalanine–homophenyla-lanine fluoromethyl ketone cured 80% of mice treated subcutaneously with 100 mg/kg four times per day for 4 d and N-methyl piperazine urea–leucine–homophenylalanine–naphthyl vinyl sulfone cured about 40% of mice treated orally with 50–100 mg/kg twice a day for 4 d.

Peptidyl falcipain-2 inhibitors do not appear to be ideal candidate drugs for three reasons. First, their peptide nature might allow rapid hydrolysis by host proteases. Second, their irreversible mode of action may increase toxicity resulting from the creation of complexes that stimulate autoimmune or other toxic reactions. Third, the compounds are relatively nonselective, and toxicity might be engendered by the inhibi-tion of host cysteine proteases. Recent studies suggest that, despite these theoretical limitations, small peptidyl vinyl sulfone inhibitors of falcipain-2 and other protozoan cysteine proteases have resonable toxicity and pharmacokinetic profiles *(90)*. Hydroly-sis of the peptidyl inhibitors may have been limited by the inclusion of non-native amino acids, most commonly homophenylalanine, at the P1 position. Toxicity may have been limited by differences in the availability of the inhibitor to host and parasite targets. In the case of malaria parasites, inhibitors are delivered directly to the food vacuole, the site of action of falcipain-2, once they are transported into the erythrocyte or cross the relatively leaky *(91)* erythrocyte membrane. Similar host papain-family proteases are principally compartmentalized in lysosomes, which do not appear to be as accessible to peptidyl inhibitors. This conclusion is supported by the in vitro and in vivo evaluations of inhibitors of falcipain-2 and the related *Trypanosoma cruzi* protease cruzain. Vinyl sulfone inhibitors of these enzymes cured experimental infections at concentrations that caused no apparent toxicity to host mice *(88,92)*.

Attempts to develop nonpeptide inhibitors of falcipains are also underway. A modeled structure of falcipain-1 allowed the computational screening of a database of small com-pounds for their potential to inhibit the activity we now know to be that of falcipain-2 *(93)*. Biochemical evaluation of a small set of compounds selected by the computational screen identified a low micromolar lead compound. This compound also inhibited the development of cultured parasites at low micromolar concentrations. Subsequent itera-tive cycles of synthesis and screening identified chalcones *(94)* and phenothiazines *(95)* that inhibited falcipain-2 and blocked the development of cultured parasites at nanomolar to low micromolar concentrations. Falcipain-2 was also strongly inhibited by a confor-mationally constrained pyrrolidinone aldehyde *(96)*. Recent work, as discussed earlier, has identified falcipain-2 as the gene encoding the principal trophozoite cysteine protease. Modeling studies of falcipain-2 are currently underway. Fortunately, in contrast to experience with falcipain-1 *(46)*, falcipain-2 is amenable to high-yield expression in a bacterial system *(45)*. Expression of active falcipain-2 will simplify biochemical studies and structure determination, and solution of the structure of falcipain-2 should expedite ongoing drug discovery efforts. In the meantime, additional studies of the antimalarial properties of peptide-based and nonpeptide falcipain-2 inhibitors are underway.

Aspartic Protease Inhibitors

The generic aspartic protease inhibitor pepstatin causes marked morphological changes and a block in the development of cultured parasites *(8,64)*. However, pepstatin does not clearly exert its antimalarial effects via the inhibition of the plasmepsin hemoglobinases.

Pepstatin does not cause the accumulation of undegraded hemoglobin in the parasite food vacuole, as seen with cysteine protease inhibitors *(8,64)*. In addition, pepstatin exerts its antimalarial effects principally during the ring and schizont stages, rather than during the trophozoite stage, when most hemoglobin degradation takes place *(8,64)*. These results suggest that pepstatin may not act directly via the inhibition of hemoglobin degradation, perhaps because it cannot access the plasmepsins in the food vacuole. However, the potent effects of pepstatin argue for a key aspartic protease function in ring-stage and schizont-stage parasites, perhaps related to the recently identified role for plasmepsin II in the processing of erythrocyte cytoskeletal proteins in schizonts *(36)*.

Recent studies have focused on the antimalarial effects of more specific inhibitors of the plasmepsins. These have been facilitated by the development of efficient systems for the heterologous expression of plasmepsin I *(63,97)* and plasmepsin II *(54)*. The determination of the structure of plasmepsin II *(65)* has expedited the discovery of inhibitors of this enzyme, and combinatorial approaches have recently identified potent and selective inhibitors *(66,98,99)*. In most cases, inhibitor specificity has differed markedly between the two plasmepsins, although peptidomimetic inhibitors with low nanomolar activity against both proteases have been reported *(66)*. Some inhibitors of plasmepsin I *(53,63)*, plasmepsin II *(65)*, and both proteases *(66)* also blocked the development of cultured malaria parasites at nanomolar–micromolar concentrations (Table 3). As is the case with pepstatin, these compounds do not appear to cause the accumulation of undegraded hemoglobin in treated parasites, and it is as yet unclear whether they exert their antimalarial effects directly via the inhibition of hemoglobin digestion. No studies of the in vivo antimalarial activity of plasmepsin inhibitors have yet been reported.

Serine Protease Inhibitors

Studies of the antimalarial effects of peptide serine protease inhibitors have yielded valuable insights into the roles of serine proteases in the parasite life cycle. The studies discussed earlier suggest that chymostatin-inhibitable protease activity is required for both erythrocyte rupture by mature schizonts and erythrocyte invasion by free merozoites. In addition, a chymostatin-insensitive serine protease activity, possibly that of Pfsub-1 or Pfsub-2, appears to be responsible for the secondary processing of MSP-1 that is required for erythrocyte invasion. One report describes the antimalarial effects of a group of peptidyl ethylamide inhibitors of the M_r 68,000 cysteine protease of schizonts and merozoites *(100)*. The most potent inhibitor tested, GlcA–valine–leucine–glycine–lysine–NHC_2H_5, inhibited the activity of the cysteine protease at high micromolar concentrations and blocked erythrocyte invasion by *P. falciparum* merozoites, although millimolar concentrations of the compound were required for this antiparasitic effect. Ongoing characterizations of plasmodial serine proteases should aid efforts to develop specific inhibitors of these enzymes as antimalarial drugs.

Aminopeptidase Inhibitors

A plasmodial metalloaminopeptidase appears to play a role in the hydrolysis of small globin fragments into free amino acids in the parasite cytosol. The aminopeptidase inhibitors bestatin and nitrobestatin inhibited the activity of the purified aminopeptidase *(77,78,80)*. The inhibitors also blocked the development of cultured *P. falciparum* and *P. chabaudi* parasites at micromolar concentrations *(80)*. As was the case with inhibition of the enzyme, nitrobestatin was more potent that bestatin.

Proteasome Inhibitors.

A full proteosome of malaria parasites has not yet been reported, although a proteasome S4 ATPase was recently identified in *P. falciparum (101)*. The proteosome inhibitor lactacystin inhibited the development of cultured *P. falciparum* parasites *(101,102)*. Lactacystin also inhibited the development of *P. berghei* in mice, although the therapeutic index of this therapy was low *(102)*.

Protease Inhibitor Combinations

As discussed earlier, cysteine and aspartic proteases appear to act cooperatively in hemoglobin degradation. The two classes of proteases acted synergistically to degrade hemoglobin in vitro *(53)*. Inhibitors of the two classes also inhibited the metabolism and development of cultured parasites *(8,103)* and the progression of murine malaria in a synergistic manner *(103)*. Thus, it may be appropriate to use protease inhibitor combinations to treat malaria.

SUMMARY

This is an exciting time for those interested in characterizing the biological roles of plasmodial proteases and in evaluating the potential of these enzymes as targets for new antimalarial drugs. A number of key proteases of all four major mechanistic classes have now been identified, and these enzymes are increasingly well characterized both molecularly and biochemically. The *P. falciparum* genome sequencing project has recently identified sequences that likely encode additional proteases, and more protease sequences can be expected. Parasite proteolytic mechanisms are clearly more complex than initially envisioned. Extensive efforts will be needed to dissect the specific roles of multiple similar enzymes over the life cycle of the parasite. Fortunately, powerful new tools for studying plasmodial proteases are now available, including plasmodial transfection systems, specific protease inhibitors, and, quite soon, a complete *P. falciparum* genome sequence. It is anticipated that these tools will allow the characterization of the specific roles of multiple plasmodial proteases. Concurrently, significant efforts are being made in the evaluation of new classes of protease inhibitors as potential drugs. Enthusiasm in this area is not principally directed toward inhibitors of plasmodial proteases, but progress will nonetheless expedite efforts to develop new modes of antimalarial therapy. It is anticipated that progress in the understanding of the biology of plasmodial proteases and the development of protease inhibitors will feed into rational strategies toward the identification of inhibitors of essential plasmodial proteases as new antimalarial drugs.

REFERENCES

1. Barrett AJ, Rawlings ND, Woessner JF. Handbook of Proteolytic Enzymes. San Diego: Academic, 1998.
2. Jackson EK, Garrison JC. Renin and angiotensin. In: Hardman JG, Limbird LE (eds.). Goodman and Gilman's The Pharmacological Basis of Therapeutics. New York: McGraw-Hill, 1996, pp. 733–758.
3. Deeks SG, Smith M, Holodniy M, Kahn JO. HIV-1 protease inhibitors. A review for clinicians. JAMA 1997;277:145–153.
4. Gluzman IY, Francis SE, Oksman A, Smith CE, Duffin KL, Goldberg DE. Order and specificity of the *Plasmodium falciparum* hemoglobin degradation pathway. J Clin Invest 1994;93:1602–1608.

5. Rosenthal PJ, McKerrow JH, Aikawa M, Nagasawa H, Leech JH. A malarial cysteine proteinase is necessary for hemoglobin degradation by *Plasmodium falciparum*. J Clin Invest 1988;82:1560–1566.

6. Goldberg DE, Slater AF. G., Cerami A, Henderson GB. Hemoglobin degradation in the malaria parasite *Plasmodium falciparum*: an ordered process in a unique organelle. Proc Natl Acad Sci USA 1990;87:2931–2935.

7. Dluzewski AR, Rangachari K, Wilson RJ. M, Gratzer WB. *Plasmodium falciparum*: protease inhibitors and inhibition of erythrocyte invasion. Exp Parasitol 1986;62:416–422.

8. Bailly E, Jambou R, Savel J, Jaureguiberry G. *Plasmodium falciparum*: differential sensitivity in vitro to E-64 (cysteine protease inhibitor) and pepstatin A (aspartyl protease inhibitor). J Protozool 1992;39:593–599.

9. Gamboa de Domínguez ND, Rosenthal PJ. Cysteine proteinase inhibitors block early steps in hemoglobin degradation by cultured malaria parasites. Blood 1996;87:4448–4454.

10. Kamchonwongpaisan S, Samoff E, Meshnick SR. Identification of hemoglobin degradation products in *Plasmodium falciparum*. Mol Biochem Parasitol 1997;86:179–186.

11. Asawamahasakda W, Ittarat I, Chang C-C, McElroy P, Meshnick SR. Effects of antimalarials and protease inhibitors on plasmodial hemozoin production. Mol Biochem Parasitol 1994;67:183–191.

12. Bray PG, Janneh O, Raynes KJ, Mungthin M, Ginsburg H, Ward SA. Cellular uptake of chloroquine is dependent on binding to ferriprotoporphyrin IX and is independent of NHE activity in *Plasmodium falciparum*. J Cell Biol 1999;145:363–376.

13. Barnwell JW, Galinski MR. Invasion of vertebrate cells: erythrocytes. In: Sherman IW (ed). Malaria: Parasite Biology, Pathogenesis, and Protection. Washington DC: ASM, 1998, pp. 93–120.

14. Sam-Yellowe TY, Shio H, Perkins ME. Secretion of *Plasmodium falciparum* rhoptry protein into the plasma membrane of host erythrocytes. J Cell Biol 1988;106:1507–1513.

15. Torii M, Adams JH, Miller LH, Aikawa M. Release of merozoite dense granules during erythrocyte invasion by *Plasmodium knowlesi*. Infect Immun 1989;57:3230–3233.

16. Torii M, Aikawa M. Ultrastructure of asexual stages. In: Sherman IW (ed.). Malaria: Parasite Biology, Pathogenesis, and Protection. Washington DC: ASM, 1998, pp. 123–134.

17. Banyal HS, Misra GC, Gupta CM, Dutta GP. Involvement of malarial proteases in the interaction between the parasite and host erythrocyte in *Plasmodium knowlesi* infections. J Parasitol 1981;67:623–626.

18. Hadley T, Aikawa M, Miller LH. *Plasmodium knowlesi*: studies on invasion of rhesus erythrocytes by merozoites in the presence of protease inhibitors. Exp Parasitol 1983;55:306–311.

19. Dejkriengkraikhul P, Wilairat P. Requirement of malarial protease in the invasion of human red cells by merozoites of *Plasmodium falciparum*. Z Parasitenkd 1983;69:313–317.

20. Olaya P, Wasserman M. Effect of calpain inhibitors on the invasion of human erythrocytes by the parasite *Plasmodium falciparum*. Biochem Biophys Acta 1991;1096:217–221.

21. Braun-Breton C, Blisnick T, Jouin H, Barale JC, Rabilloud T, Langsley G, et al. *Plasmodium chabaudi* p68 serine protease activity required for merozoite entry into mouse erythrocytes. Proc Natl Acad Sci USA 1992;89:9647–9651.

22. McPherson RA, Donald DR, Sawyer WH, Tilley L. Proteolytic digestion of band 3 at an external site alters the erythrocyte membrane organisation and may facilitate malarial invasion. Mol Biochem Parasitol 1993;62:233–242.

23. Bannister LH, Mitchell GH. The fine structure of secretion by *Plasmodium knowlesi* merozoites during red cell invasion. J Protozool 1989;36:362–367.

24. Blackman MJ, Whittle H, Holder AA. Processing of the *Plasmodium falciparum* major merozoite surface protein-1: identification of a 33-kilodalton secondary processing product which is shed prior to erythrocyte invasion. Mol Biochem Parasitol 1991;49:35–44.

25. Blackman MJ, Heidrich H-G, Donachie S, McBride JS, Holder AA. A single fragment of a malaria merozoite surface protein remains on the parasite during red cell invasion and is the target of invasion-inhibiting antibodies. J Exp Med 1990;172:379–382.

26. Blackman MJ, Scott-Finnigan TJ, Shai S, Holder AA. Antibodies inhibit the protease-mediated processing of a malaria merozoite surface protein. J Exp Med 1994;180:389–393.

27. Blackman MJ, Holder AA. Secondary processing of the *Plasmodium falciparum* merozoite surface protein-1 (MSP1) by a calcium-dependent membrane-bound serine protease: shedding of MSP1$_{33}$ as a noncovalently associated complex with other fragments of the MSP1. Mol Biochem Parasitol 1992;50:307–316.

28. Bzik DJ, Li W-B, Horii T, Inselburg J. Amino acid sequence of the serine-repeat antigen (SERA) of *Plasmodium falciparum* determined from cloned cDNA. Mol Biochem Parasitol 1988;30:279–288.

29. Delplace P, Fortier B, Tronchin G, Dubremetz J, Vernes A. Localization, biosynthesis, processing and isolation of a major 126 kDa antigen of the parasitophorous vacuole of *Plasmodium falciparum*. Mol Biochem Parasitol 1987;23:193–201.

30. Debrabant A, Delplace P. Leupeptin alters the proteolytic processing of P126, the major parasitophorous vacuole antigen of *Plasmodium falciparum*. Mol Biochem Parasitol 1989;33:151–158.

31. Lyon JA, Haynes JD. *Plasmodium falciparum* antigens synthesized by schizonts and stabilized at the merozoite surface when schizonts mature in the presence of protease inhibitors. J Immunol 1986;136:2245–2251.

32. Weidekamm E, Wallach DF, Lin PS, Hendricks J. Erythrocyte membrane alterations due to infection with *Plasmodium berghei*. Biochim Biophys Acta 1973;323:539–546.

33. Yuthavong Y, Wilairat P, Panijpan B, Potiwan C, Beale GH. Alterations in membrane proteins of mouse erythrocytes infected with different species and strains of malaria parasites. Comp Biochem Physiol [B] 1979;63:83–85.

34. Sherman IW, Tanigoshi L. Purification of *Plasmodium lophurae* cathepsin D and its effects on erythrocyte membrane proteins. Mol Biochem Parasitol 1983;8:207–226.

35. Deguercy A, Hommel M, Schrevel J. Purification and characterization of 37-kilodalton proteases from *Plasmodium falciparum* and *Plasmodium berghei* which cleave erythrocyte cytoskeletal components. Mol Biochem Parasitol 1990;38:233–244.

36. Le Bonniec S, Deregnaucourt C, Redeker V, Banerjee R, Grellier P, Goldberg DE, et al. Plasmepsin II, an acidic hemoglobinase from the *Plasmodium falciparum* food vacuole, is active at neutral pH on the host erythrocyte membrane skeleton. J Biol Chem 1999;274:14,218–14,223.

37. Roggwiller E, Fricaud A-C, Blisnick T, Braun-Breton C. Host urokinase-type plasminogen activator participates in the release of malaria merozoites from infected erythrocytes. Mol Biochem Parasitol 1997;86:49–59.

38. Rosenthal PJ, Semenov A, Ploplis VA, Plow EF. Plasminogen activators are not required in the erythrocytic life cycle of malaria parasites. Mol Biochem Parasitol 1998;97:253–257.

39. Rosenfeld A, Vanderberg JP. Identification of electrophoretically separated proteases from midgut and hemolymph of adult *Anopheles stephensi* mosquitoes. J Parasitol 1998;84:361–365.

40. Muller HM, Catteruccia F, Vizioli J, della Torre A, Crisanti A. Constitutive and blood meal-induced trypsin genes in *Anopheles gambiae*. Exp Parasitol 1995;81:371–385.

41. Shahabuddin M, Toyoshima T, Aikawa M, Kaslow DC. Transmission-blocking activity of a chitinase inhibitor and activation of malarial parasite chitinase by mosquito protease. Proc Natl Acad Sci USA 1993;90:4266–4270.

42. Shahabuddin M, Criscio M, Kaslow DC. Unique specificity of in vitro inhibition of mosquito midgut trypsin-like activity correlates with in vivo inhibition of malaria parasite infectivity. Exp Parasitol 1995;80:212–219.

43. Shahabuddin M, Lemos FJ, Kaslow DC, Jacobs-Lorena M. Antibody-mediated inhibition of *Aedes aegypti* midgut trypsins blocks sporogonic development of *Plasmodium gallinaceum*. Infect Immun 1996;64:739–743.

44. Rosenthal PJ, Nelson RG. Isolation and characterization of a cysteine proteinase gene of *Plasmodium falciparum*. Mol Biochem Parasitol 1992;51:143–152.

45. Shenai BR, Sijwali PS, Singh A, Rosenthal PJ. Characterization of native and recombinant falcipain-2, a principal trophozoite cysteine protease and essential hemoglobinase of *Plasmodium falciparum*. J Biol Chem 2000;275:29,000–29,010.

46. Salas F, Fichmann J, Lee GK, Scott MD, Rosenthal PJ. Functional expression of falcipain, a *Plasmodium falciparum* cysteine proteinase, supports its role as a malarial hemoglobinase. Infect Immun 1995;63:2120–2125.

47. Rosenthal PJ, McKerrow JH, Rasnick D, Leech JH. *Plasmodium falciparum*: inhibitors of lysosomal cysteine proteinases inhibit a trophozoite proteinase and block parasite development. Mol Biochem Parasitol 1989;35:177–184.

48. Rosenthal PJ, Kim K, McKerrow JH, Leech JH. Identification of three stage-specific proteinases of *Plasmodium falciparum*. J Exp Med 1987;166:816–821.

49. Rosenthal PJ. Conservation of key amino acids among the cysteine proteinases of multiple malarial species. Mol Biochem Parasitol 1996;75:255–260.

50. Bernard F, Schrevel J. Purification of a *Plasmodium berghei* neutral endopeptidase and its localization in merozoite. Mol Biochem Parasitol 1987;26:167–174.

51. Grellier P, Picard I, Bernard F, Mayer R, Heidrich H-G, Monsigny M, Schrevel J. Purification and identification of a neutral endopeptidase in *Plasmodium falciparum* schizonts and merozoites. Parasitol Res 1989;75:455–460.

52. Goldberg DE, Slater AF. G., Beavis R, Chait B, Cerami A, Henderson GB. Hemoglobin degradation in the human malaria pathogen *Plasmodium falciparum*: a catabolic pathway initiated by a specific aspartic protease. J Exp Med 1991;173:961–969.

53. Francis SE, Gluzman IY, Oksman A, Knickerbocker A, Mueller R, Bryant ML, et al. Molecular characterization and inhibition of a *Plasmodium falciparum* aspartic hemoglobinase. EMBO J 1994;13:306–317.

54. Hill J, Tyas L, Phylip LH, Kay J, Dunn BM, Berry C. High level expression and characterisation of plasmepsin II, an aspartic proteinase from *Plasmodium falciparum*. FEBS Lett 1994;352:155–158.

55. Dame JB, Reddy GR, Yowell CA, Dunn BM, Kay J, Berry C. Sequence, expression and modeled structure of an aspartic proteinase from the human malaria parasite *Plasmodium falciparum*. Mol Biochem Parasitol 1994;64:177–190.

56. Luker KE, Francis SE, Gluzman IY, Goldberg DE. Kinetic analysis of plasmepsins I and II, aspartic proteases of the *Plasmodium falciparum* digestive vacuole. Mol Biochem Parasitol 1996;79:71–78.

57. Francis SE, Banerjee R, Goldberg DE. Biosynthesis and maturation of the malaria aspartic hemoglobinases plasmepsins I and II. J Biol Chem 1997;272:14,961–14,968.

58. Westling J, Yowell CA, Majer P, Erickson JW, Dame JB, Dunn BM. *Plasmodium falciparum*, *P. vivax*, and *P. malariae*: a comparison of the active site properties of plasmepsins cloned and expressed from three different species of the malaria parasite. Exp Parasitol 1997;87:185–193.

59. Humphreys MJ, Moon RP, Klinder A, Fowler SD, Rupp K, Bur D, et al. The aspartic proteinase from the rodent parasite *Plasmodium berghei* as a potential model for plasmepsins from the human malaria parasite, *Plasmodium falciparum*. FEBS Lett 1999;463:43–48.

60. Vander Jagt DL, Hunsaker LA, Campos NM, Scaletti JV. Localization and characterization of hemoglobin-degrading aspartic proteinases from the malarial parasite *Plasmodium falciparum*. Biochem Biophys Acta 1992;1122:256–264.

61. Berry C, Humphreys MJ, Matharu P, Granger R, Horrocks P, Moon RP, et al. A distinct member of the aspartic proteinase gene family from the human malaria parasite *Plasmodium falciparum*. FEBS Lett 1999;447:149–154.

62. Francis SE, Sullivan DJ, Goldberg DE. Hemoglobin metabolism in the malaria parasite *Plasmodium falciparum*. Annu Rev Microbiol 1997;51:97–123.

63. Moon RP, Tyas L, Certa U, Rupp K, Bur D, Jacquet C, Matile H, et al. Expression and characterisation of plasmepsin I from *Plasmodium falciparum*. Eur J Biochem 1997;244:552–560.

64. Rosenthal PJ. *Plasmodium falciparum*: effects of proteinase inhibitors on globin hydrolysis by cultured malaria parasites. Exp Parasitol 1995;80:272–281.

65. Silva AM, Lee AY, Gulnik SV, Majer P, Collins J, Bhat TN, et al. Structure and inhibition of plasmepsin II, a hemoglobin-degrading enzyme from *Plasmodium falciparum*. Proc Natl Acad Sci USA 1996;93:10,034–10,039.

66. Haque TS, Skillman AG, Lee CE, Habashita H, Gluzman IY, Ewing TJ, et al. Potent, low-molecular-weight non-peptide inhibitors of malarial aspartyl protease plasmepsin II. J Med Chem 1999;42:1428–1440.

67. Braun-Breton C, Rosenberry TL, Pereira da Silva L. Induction of the proteolytic activity of a membrane protein in *Plasmodium falciparum* by phosphatidyl inisitol-specific phospholipase C. Nature 1988;332:457–459.

68. Roggwiller E, Bétoulle MEM, Blisnick T, Braun Breton C. A role for erythrocyte band 3 degradation by the parasite gp76 serine protease in the formation of the parasitophorous vacuole during invasion of erythrocytes by *Plasmodium falciparum*. Mol Biochem Parasitol 1996;82:13–24.

69. Blackman MJ, Fujioka H, Stafford WH, Sajid M, Clough B, Fleck SL, et al. A subtilisin-like protein in secretory organelles of *Plasmodium falciparum* merozoites. J Biol Chem 1998;273:23,398–23,409.

70. Barale JC, Blisnick T, Fujioka H, Alzari PM, Aikawa M, Braun-Breton C, et al. *Plasmodium falciparum* subtilisin-like protease 2, a merozoite candidate for the merozoite surface protein 1-42 maturase. Proc Natl Acad Sci USA 1999;96:6445–6450.

71. Hackett F, Sajid M, Withers-Martinez C, Grainger M, Blackman MJ. PfSUB-2: a second subtilisin-like protein in *Plasmodium falciparum* merozoites. Mol Biochem Parasitol 1999;103:183–195.

72. Sajid M, Withers-Martinez C, Blackman MJ. Maturation and specificity of *Plasmodium falciparum* subtilisin-like protease-1, a malaria merozoite subtilisin-like serine protease. J Biol Chem 2000;275:631–641.

73. Eggleson KK, Duffin KL, Goldberg DE. Identification and characterization of falcilysin, a metallopeptidase involved in hemoglobin catabolism within the malaria parasite *Plasmodium falciparum*. J Biol Chem 1999;274:32,411–32,417.

74. Fakruddin JM, Biswas S, Sharma YD. Identification of a *Plasmodium vivax* heat-shock protein which contains a metalloprotease sequence motif. Mol Biochem Parasitol 1997;90:387–390.

75. Fakruddin JM, Biswas S, Sharma YD. Metalloprotease activity in a small heat shock protein of the human malaria parasite *Plasmodium vivax*. Infect Immun 2000;68:1202–1206.

76. Florent I, Derhy Z, Allary M, Monsigny M, Mayer R, Schrevel J. A *Plasmodium falciparum* aminopeptidase gene belonging to the M1 family of zinc-metallopeptidases is expressed in erythrocytic stages. Mol Biochem Parasitol 1998;97:149–160.

77. Vander Jagt DL, Baack BR, Hunsaker LA. Purification and characterization of an aminopeptidase from *Plasmodium falciparum*. Mol Biochem Parasitol 1984;10:45–54.

78. Curley GP, O'Donovan SM, McNally J, Mullally M, O'Hara H, Troy A, et al. Aminopeptidases from *Plasmodium falciparum*, *Plasmodium chabaudi*, and *Plasmodium berghei*. J Eukaryot Microbiol 1994;41:119–123.

79. Kolakovich KA, Gluzman IY, Duffin KL, Goldberg DE. Generation of hemoglobin peptides in the acidic digestive vacuole of *Plasmodium falciparum* implicates peptide transport in amino acid production. Mol Biochem Parasitol 1997;87:123–135.

80. Nankya-Kitaka MF, Curley GP, Gavigan CS, Bell A, Dalton JP. *Plasmodium chabaudi chabaudi* and *P. falciparum*: inhibition of aminopeptidase and parasite growth by bestatin and nitrobestatin. Parasitol Res 1998;84:552–558.

81. Knapp B, Nau U, Hundt E, Küpper HA. A new blood stage antigen of *Plasmodium falciparum* highly homologous to the serine-stretch protein SERP. Mol Biochem Parasitol 1991;44:1–14.

82. Gardner MJ, Tettelin H, Carucci DJ, Cummings LM, Aravind L, Koonin EV, et al. Chromosome 2 sequence of the human malaria parasite *Plasmodium falciparum*. Science 1998;282:1126–1132.

83. Kiefer MC, Crawford KA, Boley LJ, Landsberg KE, Gibson HL, Kaslow DC, et al. Identification and cloning of a locus of serine repeat antigen (SERA)-related genes from *Plasmodium vivax*. Mol Biochem Parasitol 1996;78:55–65.

84. Gor DO, Li AC, Wiser MF, Rosenthal PJ. Plasmodial serine repeat antigen homologues with properties of schizont cysteine proteases. Mol Biochem Parasitol 1998;95:153–158.

85. Rockett KA, Playfair JHL, Ashall F, Targett GAT, Angliker H, Shaw E. Inhibition of intraerythrocytic development of *Plasmodium falciparum* by proteinase inhibitors. FEBS Lett 1990;259:257–259.

86. Rosenthal PJ, Wollish WS, Palmer JT, Rasnick D. Antimalarial effects of peptide inhibitors of a *Plasmodium falciparum* cysteine proteinase. J Clin Invest 1991;88:1467–1472.

87. Rosenthal PJ, Olson JE, Lee GK, Palmer JT, Klaus JL, Rasnick D. Antimalarial effects of vinyl sulfone cysteine proteinase inhibitors. Antimicrob Agents Chemother 1996;40:1600–1603.

88. Olson JE, Lee GK, Semenov A, Rosenthal PJ. Antimalarial effects in mice of orally administered peptidyl cysteine protease inhibitors. Bioorg Med Chem 1999;7:633–638.

89. Rosenthal PJ, Lee GK, Smith RE. Inhibition of a *Plasmodium vinckei* cysteine proteinase cures murine malaria. J Clin Invest 1993;91:1052–1056.

90. McKerrow JH. Development of cysteine protease inhibitors as chemotherapy for parasitic diseases: insights on safety, target validation, and mechanism of action. Int J Parasitol 1999;29:833–837.

91. Kutner S, Baruch D, Ginsburg H, Cabantchik ZI. Alterations in membrane permeability of malaria-infected human erythrocytes are related to the growth stage of the parasite. Biochem Biophys Acta 1982;687:113–117.

92. Engel JC, Doyle PS, Hsieh I, McKerrow JH. Cysteine protease inhibitors cure an experimental *Trypanosoma cruzi* infection. J Exp Med 1998;188:725–734.

93. Ring CS, Sun E, McKerrow JH, Lee GK, Rosenthal PJ, Kuntz ID, et al. Structure-based inhibitor design by using protein models for the development of antiparasitic agents. Proc Natl Acad Sci USA 1993;90:3583–3587.

94. Li R, Kenyon GL, Cohen FE, Chen X, Gong B, Dominguez JN, et al. *In vitro* antimalarial activity of chalcones and their derivatives. J Med Chem 1995;38:5031–5037.

95. Domínguez JN, López S, Charris J, Iarruso L, Lobo G, Semenov A, et al. Synthesis and antimalarial effects of phenothiazine inhibitors of a *Plasmodium falciparum* cysteine protease. J Med Chem 1997;40:2726–2732.

96. Scheidt KA, Roush WR, McKerrow JH, Selzer PM, Hansell E, Rosenthal PJ. Structure-based design, synthesis and evaluation of conformationally constrained cysteine protease inhibitors. Bioorg Med Chem 1998;6:2477–2494.

97. Tyas L, Gluzman I, Moon RP, Rupp K, Westling J, Ridley RG, et al. Naturally-occurring and recombinant forms of the aspartic proteinases plasmepsins I and II from the human malaria parasite *Plasmodium falciparum*. FEBS Lett 1999;454:210–214.

98. Carroll CD, Patel H, Johnson TO, Guo T, Orlowski M, He ZM, et al. Identification of potent inhibitors of *Plasmodium falciparum* plasmepsin II from an encoded statine combinatorial library. Bioorg Med Chem Lett 1998;8:2315–2320.

99. Carroll CD, Johnson TO, Tao S, Lauri G, Orlowski M, Gluzman IY, et al. Evaluation of a structure-based statine cyclic diamino amide encoded combinatorial library against plasmepsin II and cathepsin D. Bioorg Med Chem Lett 1998;8:3203–3206.

100. Mayer R, Picard I, Lawton P, Grellier P, Barrault C, Monsigny M, et al. Peptide derivatives specific for a *Plasmodium falciparum* proteinase inhibit the human erythrocyte invasion by merozoites. J Med Chem 1991;34:3029–3035.

101. Certad G, Abrahem A, Georges E. Cloning and partial characterization of the proteasome S4 ATPase from *Plasmodium falciparum*. Exp Parasitol 1999;93:123–131.

102. Gantt SM, Myung JM, Briones MR, Li WD, Corey EJ, Omura S, et al. Proteasome inhibitors block development of *Plasmodium* spp. Antimicrob Agents Chemother 1998;42:2731–2738.

103. Semenov A, Olson JE, Rosenthal PJ. Antimalarial synergy of cysteine and aspartic protease inhibitors. Antimicrob Agents Chemother 1998;42:2254–2258.

19

Inhibitors of Phospholipid Metabolism

Henri Joseph Vial and Michèle Calas

INTRODUCTION

Malaria remains one of the most widespread parasitic tropical diseases. All inhabitants in endemic zones are infected from birth to death and can only survive because of the premunition they acquire during the first 5 yr of life, a period during which mortality from malaria is very high. The selection of drug-resistant parasites and insecticide-resistant mosquitoes can be held responsible for this depressing picture, which has ruined the hope for malaria eradication and led to a very serious situation. Developed countries are not exempt: The number of imported cases has increased because of expanding international transport. *Plasmodium falciparum* accounts for the majority of infections and is the most lethal form *(1,2)*.

The development of a vaccine against malaria has so far not fulfilled expectations in field trials *(3,4)*, and differences in the biology of major malaria vectors preclude the development of simple, universally applicable strategies for malaria control *(5)*. Consequently, curative or preventive malaria chemotherapy is an essential arm in the battle against this major endemic disease. In many areas, the mounting problem of antimalarial drug resistance is now manifested as multidrug resistance. Induction of resistance is rapid for molecules with similar mechanisms of action. This pleads for new pharmacological models, which would allow selection of molecules with a novel mechanism of action that could delay the appearance of resistance.

The past 20 yr have witnessed a very impressive increase in our knowledge regarding *Plasmodium* with attention focused on specific parasite molecules that are essential keys to the parasite life cycle or pathogenesis of the disease. Some reports have summarized these potentially unique parasite characteristics that have provided valid pharmacological targets or may provide targets for the development of future chemotherapeutics *(6–8)*. However, these results have not yet led to the development of new drugs.

The present chapter describes a new approach to malaria chemotherapy that targets the phospholipid metabolism of the intraerythrocytic malarial parasite, which is crucial for its intense membrane biogenesis and, consequently, is a prerequisite for its development and growth. This approach has required extensive fundamental research (metabolic pathways and their limiting steps, characteristics of enzymes and transporters, pharmacological studies, synthesis of new molecules, structure–activity relationships). With these elements now at our disposal, we are optimistic about the possibility of developing a new antimalarial drug.

From: *Antimalarial Chemotherapy: Mechanisms of Action, Resistance, and New Directions in Drug Discovery*
Edited by: P. J. Rosenthal © Humana Press Inc., Totowa, NJ

PHOSPHOLIPID METABOLISM AS A NOVEL PHARMACOLOGICAL TARGET

Lipids are major constituents of biological membranes. The lipid content of malarial-infected erythrocytes is considerably higher than that of normal erythrocytes, because they have three concentric membranes (host cell, parasitophorous vacuole, and parasitic plasma membranes) and many membrane-limited intraparasitic organelles. Membrane biogenesis accompanying parasite growth requires parasite-driven lipid synthesis because the erythrocyte lacks this capacity. Of principal interest is the fact that *Plasmodium* membranes are essentially composed of phospholipids (PLs) whose content in erythrocytes after infection is increased by 500%, whereas *Plasmodium* does not contain or synthesize cholesterol. Consequently, asexual intraerythrocytic proliferation of the parasite (the phase associated with clinical symptoms of the disease) is accompanied by the synthesis of a considerable quantity of PLs needed for the production of *Plasmodium* membranes.

In-depth investigations of PL metabolism were undertaken to identify the specific requirements of the parasite for this metabolism along with potential targets for chemotherapeutic interference. *Plasmodium* has been shown to contain enzymes of PL metabolism that are specific to higher eukaryotes such as mammals (e.g., *de novo* synthesis of phosphatidylcholine [PC] and phosphatidylethanolamine, the "Kennedy pathway") as well as enzymes described in prokaryotes (such as *de novo* synthesis of phosphatidylserine). The lipidic metabolism of serine, involving intensive direct decarboxylation into ethanolamine *(9)*, also seems to be unique to the malarial parasite (Fig. 1). Two PL enzymes from *P. falciparum* have so far been cloned and their products functionally characterized (reviewed in ref. *10*).

This very high PL biosynthetic capacity occurs at the expense of plasma-derived precursors (fatty acid, choline, ethanolamine, serine and inositol) *(10–13)*. Our group was thus intrigued by the idea of blocking the entry of PL precursors inside the erythrocyte to modify plasmodial PL metabolism. This led to new antimalarial pharmacological strategies involving analogous polar head groups acting by substitution, competition *(14–16)*, or utilization of unnatural fatty acids *(17,18)*.

The biosynthesis of PC in *Plasmodium* is of particular interest because it is the most abundant lipid, accounting for half of the total PL in parasite membranes. The most promising drug interference is blockage of the choline transporter that provides the intracellular parasite with choline, a precursor required for synthesis of this major parasite PL. This target is easily accessible from the extracellular milieu and constitutes a limiting step in this metabolic pathway.

Choline Entry Is Increased upon Malarial Infection

Data on levels of choline-containing metabolites and characteristics of enzymatic activities indicate that, under physiological conditions, the PC biosynthesis rate depends on the extracellular choline concentration. Choline was found to be almost exclusively present in the host erythrocyte fraction *(96%)* and absent in the parasite, where phosphorylcholine predominates *(13,19)*.

In normal erythrocytes, choline entry occurs by a facilitated-diffusion system involving a membrane carrier *(20)*. Choline also enters *P. knowlesi*-infected erythrocytes via a saturable carrier that possesses the same high affinity as that of normal simian erythrocytes (K_T around 10 μM). The major difference involves a 10-fold increase in the transport

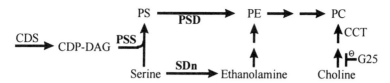

Fig. 1. Pathways of phosphatidylcholine (PC) and phosphatidylethanolamine (PE) biosynthesis in *Plasmodium*. PS: phosphatidylserine, CDP–DAG: cytidinediphosphate diacylglycerol; PSS: PS synthase; PSD: PS decarboxylase; SDn: serine decarboxylase; CDS: CDP–DAG synthase; CCT: cytidylylcholine transferase; G25: antimalarial drug.

rate. A major factor is that after *Plasmodium* infection, choline entry remains totally controlled, with no significant passive diffusion, as revealed by the absence of entry at 4°C and complete inhibition by choline analogs *(21)*. The increased choline pathway is thus distinct from the new permeation pathway, which has been largely documented *(22,23)*. The choline carrier in infected erythrocytes has characteristics that are quite distinct from that of the nervous system (e.g., sodium dependence, absence of stereospecificity, and distinct effect of nitrogen substitution), which indicates a possible discrimination between the antimalarial activity (choline transport in the erythrocyte) and the toxic effect (cholinergic effect on the nervous system) [ref. *24*, and Vial et al., unpublished data])

The increased choline entry could correspond to hyperfunctioning of the native choline carrier after *Plasmodium* infection. This might result from major modifications of the carrier environment in infected membranes owing to general disturbance of the membrane properties or of the carrier protein (e.g., by phosphorylation, glycosylation, etc.). The other alternative to be considered is an augmentation of the active carrier number after infection either by deciphering pre-existing carriers (e.g., present at the reticulocyte stage) or by parasite neosynthesis. The fact that the rate constant of inactivation by N-ethylmaleimide (NEM) was not modified after infection, whereas there was a marked increase in the V_{max}, strongly supports these hypotheses. Insertion of new proteins (synthesized by the parasite itself) in the erythrocyte membrane is one possibility. In this case, it is particularly noteworthy that the main characteristics of the newly synthesized carrier (affinity, effectors, asymmetry, rate-limiting step) are very close to that of the normal cell. No information is currently available concerning the nature and structure of the carrier, which is likely an outstanding pharmacological target (*see* "Chemical Synthesis").

Other questions concern the mechanisms of choline entry in the parasite. The parasite must also have the ability to transport choline beyond the parasite vacuolar membrane, through its own plasma membrane. The presence, at high density in the former, of a high-conductivity channel that is permeable to a range of structurally unrelated cations and anions *(25)* might serve this purpose. It is also possible that the parasite encodes and targets the appropriate protein *(24)*.

CHEMICAL SYNTHESIS OF INHIBITORS OF PHOSPHOLIPID METABOLISM

Rationale Based on Choline Analogy

From a molecular point of view, the pharmacological approach is based on the capacity for a molecule to mimic choline and competitively bind to the choline carrier, thus inhibiting choline transport within infected red cells (Fig. 2). The target recognizes

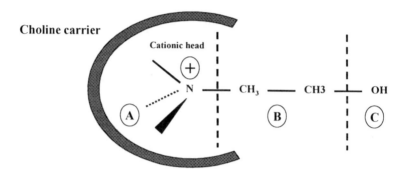

Fig. 2. Design of choline analogs for antimalarial properties.

and interacts with choline or its analog by electrostatic attraction. In terms of molecular recognition, the competitor must possess a positively charged moiety to bind to the same site as choline. For example, it should be a quaternary ammonium salt such as choline (first generation of compounds) or a compound containing a basic function ($pKa > 9$) that must be protonated at a physiological pH (e.g., an amine, amidine, or guanidine function [second-generation of compounds]).

More than 420 choline analogs have been synthesized and their structures optimized using quantitative structural–activity criteria (QSAR). First-generation compounds (G25 as a lead) most notably contain a quaternary ammonium for high antimalarial activity. Newly synthesized bioisosteres of quaternary ammonium (MS1, M53, and M60 are lead compounds) revealed better absorption and lower toxicity. New active molecules with higher intestinal absorption are currently being synthesized and a pro-drug program aimed at increasing oral absorption of quaternary ammonium compounds (first-generation leader products) is currently being developed (TE4c and TE4g, current lead compounds).

First-Generation Compounds: Mono and Bis Quaternary Ammonium Salts

In terms of molecular recognition, the choline molecules are divided into three parts: quaternary ammonium, the hydroxyl group, and the chain between the nitrogen and the hydroxyl group (Fig. 2). In order to optimize the competitor structure, each part was progressively modified, applying pharmacochemistry principles (homology, structure rigidification, additional interaction, etc.). The 280 quaternary ammonium salts (263 specifically synthesized for this purpose) were distributed into 10 families and their structures were optimized to get the best antimalarial activity. The median inhibitory concentration (IC_{50}) values were improved from 10^{-6} M to 10^{-12} M. We now have 37 molecules with an in vitro IC_{50} against *P. falciparum* lower than 20 nM and 17 with an IC_{50} lower than 2 nM (refs. *26–28*; Vial et al., unpublished results). The following subsection describes the essential structural parameters involved in this potent antimalarial activity.

The Lipophily of Nitrogen Substituents is a Crucial Parameter for Antimalarial Activity

The hydrophobic environment of the cation plays an important role in the strengthening of the bond to the target, and the volume of the cation meets very strict requirements to adapt to the active site. The nitrogen atom must be substituted with groups bulkier than methyl to adapt to the active site. Plotting IC_{50} values as a function of the polar head volume (Fig. 3) revealed maximal activity for a polar head volume ranging between 200 and 350 Å^3 (e.g., the volume of a *N*-methylpyrrolidinium or a tripropylammonium group).

Duplication of Molecules Considerably Increased Antimalarial Activity

Another important and decisive observation was that a molecular variation involving duplication of pharmacophoric groups ("twin-drug") considerably increased the antimalarial activity and led to very potent antimalarial activities. Bis-ammonium salts were generally 100-fold more active than mono-ammonium salts. This huge increase in activity is not unusual for bivalent ligands able to bind adjacent target proteins or subsites, regardless of whether they are identical or not *(29–31)*. Binding of a bivalent ligand to vicinal recognition sites may involve distinct steps. Only the simultaneous occupation of vicinal sites (which may or may not be identical) by one bivalent ligand could enhance the activity (case iv of Fig. 4). Indeed, if both charged centers are held by the receptive protein or subunit, simultaneous dissociation of both centers from the targets is highly improbable, and as long as one center is held, reattachment of the second is more probable owing to the proximity of the cationic head and the receptive site, allowing a high local concentration of the free recognition unit in the vicinity of the neighboring site *(26)*.

On the Spacer or Chain-Length Modification

For optimal antimalarial activity, one of the nitrogen substituents must be a long hydrophobic chain. For monoquaternary ammonium salts, optimum activity was noted for 12 methylene groups ($IC_{50} \approx 10^{-7}$ M). In the case of bisquaternary ammonium salts, the longer the hydrophobic alkyl interchain, the better the antimalarial activity (up to 21 methylene groups, $IC_{50} = 3 \times 10^{-12}$ M). All attempts at functionalization of the long lipophilic chain, or its rigification, led to a decrease in antimalarial activities. In both quaternary ammonium series, the presence of a second lipophilic chain ($C_{12}H_{25}$) on nitrogen atoms caused a dramatic decrease in activity. Finally, the presence of an hydroxyl function, present in the choline, is not necessary for antimalarial activity.

Compound G25 (Fig. 5) *(32)* was chosen as a lead compound because of its intrinsically potent antimalarial activity, both in vitro and in vivo, and because of its ease of synthesis and low cost of production (ref. *26* and Calas et al., unpublished data). Potent antimalarial activities are obtained for bis-quaternary ammonium salts (IC_{50} lower than 1 n*M*) with a polar head volume ranging between 200 and 350 A^3. Structure–activity-relationship studies have provided a rough topographic model of the ligand-binding site and suggest the presence of two anionic sites (with a radius of the globular pocket of 4 ± 0.4 Å) in the target (likely the choline carrier). Between these sites, there is a long hydrophobic domain corresponding to a length of at least 14 methylene groups (higher than 20 Å) (*see* Fig. 4).

The compounds exhibit outstanding in vivo antimalarial activity, even against human malaria after parenteral (but not oral) administration (*see* Table 1). However, quaternary ammonium salts do not easily go through the intestinal barrier, and probably less than 5% of compound could be orally absorbed. Indeed, the presence of a permanent cationic charge in the molecule hampers its permeability through the intestinal barrier and hinders further development of such compounds because oral administration appears to be a prerequisite for a widespread use in the treatment of uncomplicated malaria. The quaternary ammonium structure is also probably responsible for the relatively high toxicity of the present compounds, which most likely result from a cholinergic nicotinic effect.

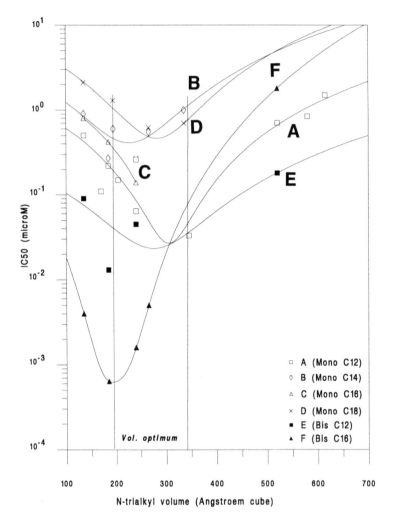

Fig. 3. In vitro antimalarial activity (IC$_{50}$) depends on the polar head volume. IC$_{50}$ values of N-dodecylammonium salts (plot A), N-tetradecylammonium salts (plot B), N-hexadecylammonium salts (plot C), N-octadecylammonium salts (plot D), 1,12-dodecamethylenebisammonium salts (plot E), and 1,16-hexadecamethylenebisammonium salts (plot F) as a function of the polar head volume. The polar head volume was calculated using a molecular modeling software program (TSAR, Oxford Molecular). The best volume fitting the active site was between 200 and 350 Å^3.

Second-Generation Compounds: Difunctional Bioisosteric Analogs of G25 (Series M and MS)

To remedy the low oral absorption of quaternary ammonium salts, the cationic heads of G25 were replaced by groups that could create the same bonds with the target. The generic structure of the antimalarial compounds includes two basic head groups that are the proto-nated form (BH$^+$) of a basic function (B, such as amine, amidine, or guanidine), separated by a lipophilic spacer. These functions, being protonated at physiological pH, mimic the cationic head of choline. Because of the equilibrium between protonated and unprotonated forms, the compounds can diffuse more easily through the tissues owing to the neutral form.

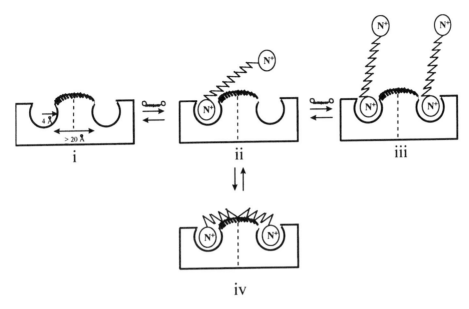

Fig. 4. Schematic description of potential steps involved in the binding of a bivalent ligand to vicinal recognition sites. Case i represents two unoccupied vicinal sites; case ii, univalent binding of a bivalent ligand; case iii, the occupation of vicinal recognition sites by individual bivalent ligands; case iv, bridging of vicinal sites (which may or may not be identical) by one bivalent ligand.

1,16 hexamethylene bis (N-methyl pyrrolidinium) dichloride	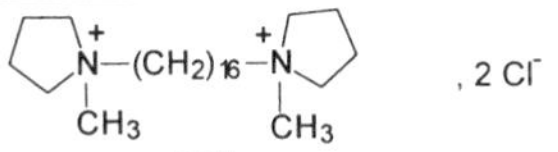 G25
1,1'-(1,12-dodecanediyl) bis-(4-methyl-2-(1H) pyridinimine) dibromhydrate	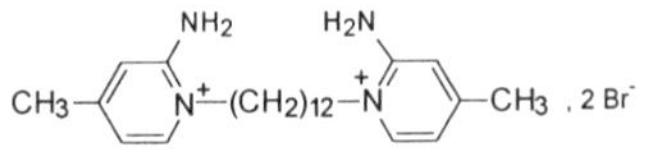 MS1

Fig. 5. Structure of first- (G25) and second- (MS1) generation lead compounds.

The modification of a quaternary ammonium to a tertiary amine, similarly substituted, resulted in a 100-fold decrease of activity ($IC_{50} \approx 10^{-7}$ M). On the other hand, replacing the quaternary ammonium moiety by an amidine or guanidine function led to the recovery of potent antimalarial activities. The 83 molecules (among them 80 synthesized) were allocated to 4 chemical families. The IC_{50} values ranged from 10^{-6} M to 10^{-10} M, with 33 molecules with a IC_{50} lower than 20 nM and 21 lower than 2 nM.

Two series of amidine compounds were synthesized. In series M, the amidine function is not conjugated, and N atoms may be substituted by R alkyl groups. Series MS includes aromatic amidines in which the amidine function is present in the 2-imino-1,2-dihydropyridine group. In its protonated form, this cationic head is composed of the 2-aminopyridinium cation, which is substituted by various R groups.

Radical R belongs to the pharmacophoric polar head, and because of its nature and size, it modulates the overall lipophilicity of the molecule, with optimal availability.

Table 1
Essential Biological Parameters of Lead Compounds

				Compounds				
	CQ	G25	MS1	M53	M60	TE4c	TE4g
IC_{50} in vitro against *P. falciparum*	30 nM	0.6 nM	0.5 nM	2 nM	3.8 nM	4.4 nM	2.3 nM
Active against resistant *P. falciparum* isolates	No	Yes	Yes	Yes	Yes	Yes	
In vitro activity against *P. vivax*		Yes	Yes	Yes	Yes	Yes	
Acute toxicity in mice (LD_{50}), ip	70 mg/kg	1.3 mg/kg	30 mg/kg	50 mg/kg	45 mg/kg	100 mg/kg	45 mg/kg
Semichronic toxicity in mice (scLD_{50}), ip	nt	1.2 mg/kg	7.8 mg/kg	34 mg/kg	30 mg/kg	50 mg/kg	
Acute toxicity (mice) po (LD_{50})	270 mg/kg	130 mg/kg	365 mg/kg	900 mg/kg	450 mg/kg	1000 mg/kg	650 mg/kg
Semi-chronic toxicity in mice (scLD_{50}), po		70 mg/kg	> 90 mg/kg	165 mg/kg	200 mg/kg	≈ 300 mg/kg	
ED_{50} against *P. vinckei* (mice), ip	3 mg/kg	0.22 mg/kg	1.6 mg/kg	3.4 mg/kg	2.8 mg/kg	0.95 mg/kg	< 1.5 mg/kg

Therapeutic index (TI) = scLD$_{50}$/ED$_{50}$ in mouse, ip	23[c]	5	10	11	≈ 50	> 30
ED$_{50}$ against *P. vinckei* (mice), po		≈ 90 mg/kg	62 mg/kg	85 mg/kg	≈ 6 mg/kg	< 20 mg/kg
Therapeutic index (TI) = scLD$_{50}$/ED$_{50}$ in mouse, po	5	< 4	2.7	2.4	≈ 50	> 30
Half-time of elimination $t_{1/2}$ (e)	5 h	10.5 h	16 h	> 35 h	nt	
Relative bioavailability = AUC po/AUC ip	1.7%	3.1%	5.2%	nt		
In vivo activity against *P. falciparum*/Aotus	Yes, im at ≤0.03 mg/kg TI$_{mk}$>50	Yes, im at 1.5 mg/kg	nt	nt	Yes, im at 2 mg/kg	
Mutagenic activity (Ames)	No	No	nt	nt	nt	

Note: ED, efficient dose; LD, lethal dose; ip, intraperitoneal; im, intramuscular; po, per os; nt, not tested: Acute toxicity is determined after one single dose and semichronic (sc) toxicity after a twice daily administration for 4 d, usually in malaria-infected animals. TI is the LD$_{50}$/ED$_{50}$ ratio and AUC is the area under the curve. Co is the seric concentration of the elimination phase extrapolated to time 0.

[a] In this case, the effect was determined against *P. berghei* after ip parasite inoculation, which could overestimate TI.

For series of bis amidines and bis guanidines possessing the same internitrogen spacer, $(CH_2)_{12}$, the basicity of cationic heads (pK_a values) was found to be strongly correlated with in vitro antimalarial activity (not shown). In amidine (M and MS series) and guanidine series, the positive charges are strongly delocalized and the ability of these groups to form hydrogen or ionic bonds is higher than that of tertiary amines and quaternary ammoniums. The pK_a values of these compounds does not only indicate the percentage of the compound protonated at physiologic pH but also its ability to form strong bonds with the target.

For this second generation of active molecules, MS1, M53, and M60 were selected as lead compounds. Only MS1 is shown here (Fig. 5) *(33)*. The new compounds (MS1 lead compound) exhibit potent in vitro and in vivo antimalarial activity and are better tolerated and better absorbed after oral administration (*see* Vial et al., unpublished data). However, one of the main drawbacks of bis-cationic salts used in therapy is still their weak oral absorption due to their positive charge. Despite this improvement obtained with second-generation compounds, third-generation molecules were designed to improve oral bioavailability.

Third-Generation Compounds

An alternative approach to enhance the oral bioavailability of these antimalarial compounds involves the synthesis of nonionic pro-drugs that in vivo can lead to a quaternary ammonium salt. The pro-drug concept concerns any compound that undergoes biotransformation prior to exhibiting its pharmacological effects. It has been widely applied to overcome problems such as a lack of solubility, lack of bioavailability or lack of stability. It is thus of potential pharmacological interest because it may be an aid in overcoming the membrane barrier or providing a drug with a more appropriate pharmacokinetic profile. The pro-drug approach is more discriminating than modifying the global lipophilicity of a molecule, which can lead to all tissues being nonspecifically exposed to higher levels of drug.

Pro-drug strategies were applied both to quaternary ammonium compounds and amidine and guanidine derivatives (not shown here). The neutral pro-drug forms can easily diffuse across biological membranes and, thus, be efficiently absorbed. The active cationic form is later generated in the blood circulation.

We will only briefly discuss the precursors of thiazolium *(34)*, which have given promising results, even against human malaria in monkeys.

Precursors of Thiazolium Salts for Delivery of Vitamin B₁ in Humans

This pro-drug concept has already been successfully developed to administer ammonium salts in the oral mode. As an example, thiamine (B_1 vitamin), which is weakly absorbed orally (because of its permanent charge), can be delivered as a neutral disulfide pro-drug (sulbutiamine, Arcalion®) or thioester (acétiamine, Algo-nevriton® or Vitanevril®). The bioprecursors undergo an in vivo rearrangement under the action of glutathione or thioesterase, leading to active ionized thiamine (Fig. 6) *(35,36)*. Recently, such a strategy has been used to improve delivery of DOPA in the brain *(37)*.

Precursors of Thiazolium Salts to Deliver Bis-quaternary Ammonium Salts as Antimalarials

We have developed a program based on this strategy and have synthesized both types of neutral pro-drugs: disulfides (TS) and thioesters (TE) and their corresponding

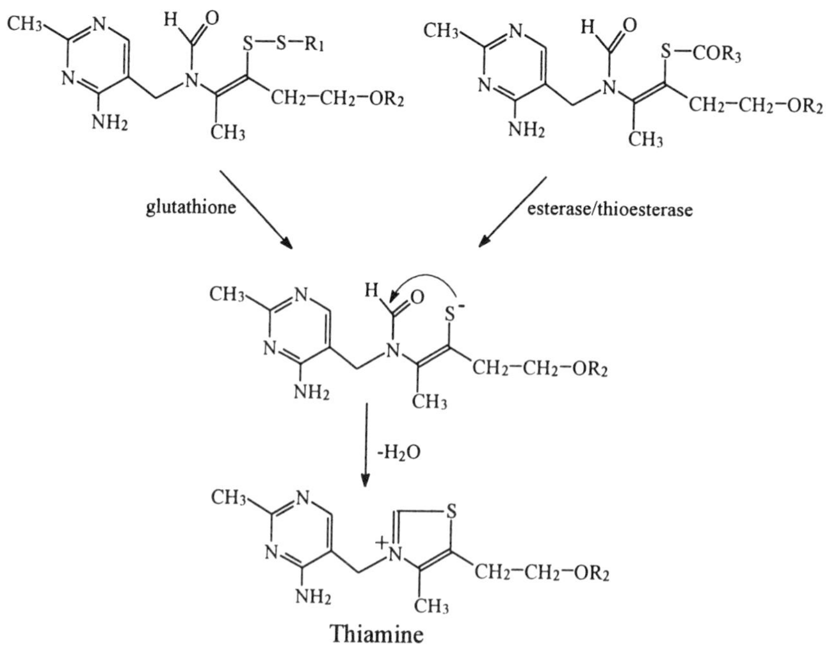

Fig. 6. Neutral disulfide or thioester pro-drugs of thiamine.

quaternarized drugs (T). Thiazolium cycles take the place of polar heads of G25 (first generation) or MS1 (second generation), with the long lipophilic chain on either nitrogen atoms or carbon atoms. Twenty-seven compounds were synthesized in these series (TS and TE) with various substituants to modify the physicochemical properties and improve antimalarial activity along with tolerance.

When tested in vitro against *P. falciparum*, after one cycle of contact with the compounds, TE and TS bioprecursors were as active as their corresponding drugs, which suggests a quantitative pro-drug/drug transformation. As for quaternary ammonium compounds, *bis*-thiazolium forms (T3 and T4, IC_{50} = 2.25 and 0.65 nM) were much more active than corresponding monoquaternary thiazolium salts (T1 and T2, IC_{50} = 70 and 75 nM). Moreover a similar compound, with an alkyl group instead of RS (or RCO), which cannot undergo enzymatic cleavage leading to thiazolium, is totally inactive (TM1, IC_{50}> 10 µM). This result suggests that the antimalarial activity is the result of the quaternary ammonium compounds formed in vivo and not to the open-ringed derivatives, an aspect that is currently being investigated. Biological, pharmacological, and toxicological data on current lead compounds TE4c and TE4g are given in Table 1.

Thiazolium compounds thus have the same antimalarial activity pattern as first- and second-generation compounds. The bis compounds exhibited the same range of activity (i.e., the nanomolar range) as G25. In vivo, pro-drugs revealed better toleration and absorption than the quaternary ammonium. TS3b, TE4c, and TE4g pro-drugs also possessed in vivo antimalarial activity against *P. vinckei*, with a therapeutic index higher than compounds of the two first generations. Recent results indicated that TE4c was also active in vivo in Aotus monkeys infected with the human parasite. This approach has been validated with both series. A judicious choice of the substituent improved the solubility in water and stability of pro-drugs.

OVERVIEW OF THE BIOLOGICAL POTENCY AGAINST MALARIA

In Vitro Efficacy and Cytotoxic Versus Cytostatic Effect

The new molecules show powerful antimalarial activity with 50% inhibitory concentrations (IC_{50}) in the nanomolar range against *P. falciparum* during its intraerythrocytic stage. In vitro and in vivo experiments showed sharp dose-response curves (IC90/IC10 ≈ 10–20), indicating a very specific target that is directly associated with *Plasmodium* development (instead of a nonspecific generalized toxic effect). Irrespective of the compounds, inhibitions were complete and very steep curves were obtained with activity occurring over 1.5 orders of magnitude.

Compounds are much more active against native parasites, with the most sensitive form the trophozoite stage. This specificity corresponds to the most intense phase of PL biosynthesis activity during the parasite cycle, thus corroborating the mechanism of action. At this stage, compounds exert a rapid and irreversible cytotoxic effect, because, for mature stages, complete clearance of parasitemia was observed after only 5 h of contact with the drugs.

Compounds Are Similarly Effective Against Pharmacoresistant and Multiresistant P. falciparum *(Clones and Isolates)*

In vitro antimalarial activity of PL metabolism inhibitors against resistant or multiresistant *P. falciparum* isolates were studied by several independent laboratories. The most complete studies were carried out by Pascal Ringwald (OCEAC, Yaoundé, Cameroon), who has evaluated the in vitro antimalarial activity of compounds G25, MS1, M53, and T3 against multiresistant *P. falciparum* isolates from Cameroon (more than 170). Rather than assessing the pro-drug, we tested the quaternarized derivative (T3) because, according to the mechanism of action, it should be the active component present in the plasma compartment.

G25, M53, and T3 were found to be highly effective against *P. falciparum* isolates, even against chloroquine-resistant isolates. The IC_{50} varied only to a minor extent between the various isolates (not shown). No in vitro cross-resistance was observed between these compounds and six established antimalarials (chloroquine, mefloquine, halofantrine, quinine, cycloguanil, artemether). Finally, there was the same pattern of behavior in the in vitro antimalarial activity of the three series of compounds, strongly supporting the hypothesis that they share a similar mechanism of action. Compounds are thus equally effective against strains or isolates resistant to current antimalarials, highlighting their importance in the setting of multidrug resistance.

Effect on Development of Sexual Stages in Culture and on Transmission (P. berghei *and* P. falciparum)

Malaria-control policies must take into account the gametocytocidal or gametocyte transmission-enhancing properties of drugs. For example, chloroquine can enhance gametocyte infectivity, thereby enhancing transmission. Conversely, combining an effective chemotherapeutic with gametocytocidal properties (e.g., artemisinin) with vector-control intervention is likely, at least in some situations, to be a highly effective malaria-control strategy *(38,39)*.

Effects on development of sexual stages in culture and on transmission were studied by the Dutch groups of C. Janse (University of Leiden, *P. berghei*) and W. Eling (University of Nijmegen, *P. falciparum*). G25 did not stimulate gametocyte production or enhance infectivity, like some others antimalarial drugs. Conversely, G25 likely represses gametocyte activation, and after standard blood treatment, infective *P. falciparum* gametocytes would be less able to infect the mosquito host. In addition, G25 prevents growth of the parasite oocyst in the mosquito, which could diminish transmission. The gametocytocidal IC_{50} of G25 was equal to the minimum inhibitory concentration for asexual stages of *P. falciparum* isolates. G25 treatment thus impaired the infectiousness of developing gametocytes and reduced sporogony, particularly when given during a late phase of maturation.

In Vivo Antimalarial Curative Activity (Rodent Malaria)

Most molecules tested revealed in vivo antimalarial activity in mice infected with *P. berghei*, *P. vinckei*, or *P. chabaudi*. Parasites invading mature erythrocytes (*P. vinckei* and *P. chabaudi*) were found to be much more sensitive than reticulocyte-invading parasites (*P. berghei* and *P. yoelii*). Rapid total disappearance of parasitemia was observed, indicating rapid antimalarial efficacy in vivo (therapeutic index in the 5–50 range). After a 4-d treatment, compounds exerted their antimalarial in vivo activity over a narrow concentration range. G25 was able to cure *P. chabaudi* infection at very high parasitemia (at least up to 11%), with an ED_{50} (efficient dose) of 0.3 mg/kg.

In Vivo Antimalarial Activity Against P. falciparum in Aotus Monkeys

In collaboration with Dr. S. Herrera (Cali, Colombia), 17 monkeys have already been treated with G25 at different initial parasitemia levels (up to 23%) and with various doses (between 0.2 and 0.01 mg/kg). Under these conditions, only two monkeys died after treatment, one due to a too low dose (0.01 mg/kg, which probably corresponds to the threshold of sensitivity of a *falciparum*-infected monkey to G25), and the second one whose parasitemia leveled off quickly (from 5% to 19% in 2 d). When the therapeutic window was reduced from 8 to 4 d, anti-PL effector treatment also fully succeeded in curing *P. falciparum*-infected Aotus monkeys. In this case there was also no recrudescence. Doses as low as 0.03 mg/kg of G25 succeeded in curing *P. falciparum*-infected Aotus monkeys without recrudescence (six monkeys). The maximal tolerable dose for these monkeys is around 1.5 mg/kg, corresponding to a therapeutic index higher than 50, revealing the very high efficiency of G25 against *P. falciparum* in vivo.

MS1, one lead compound of second-generation active compounds, was also capable of curing highly infected *P. falciparum* Aotus monkeys. Seven monkeys (at high initial parasitemia, 4–22%) were treated at 2 or 1.5 mg/kg, twice a day, intramuscularly for 4 or 8 d. For all of them, MS1 led to a parasitemia decrease. Clearance was not complete in only one monkey, whose initial parasitemia was very high (*17%*); the monkey died very rapidly with a parasitemia of 14%, 3 d after the beginning of treatment. The six other monkeys were definitively cured without recrudescence. This notably included heavily parasitized monkeys (e.g., 17% and 22% initial parasitemia) that were treated for only 4 d or with a lower dose, 1.5 mg/kg. At very high initial parasitemia, 5 d therapy was required to obtain complete parasite clearance and absence of recrudescence.

TE4c, a third-generation compound at 2 mg/kg (not tested at lower doses), also succeeded in curing *P. falciparum*-infected Aotus monkeys without recrudescence. The maximal tolerable dose of TE4c for the monkey is around 100 mg/kg, corresponding to a therapeutic index of higher than 50, revealing the very high in vivo efficiency of anti-PL effectors against *P. falciparum*.

In Vitro and In Vivo Efficacy of Phospholipid Inhibitors Against P. vivax-*type Parasites*

Experiments carried out by A. Thomas and C. Kocken (BPRC, Rijwik, NL) clearly showed that *P. vivax* and *P. cynomolgi* are very susceptible to the three distinct PL inhibitor classes of drugs: quaternary ammonium (G25), amidines (M53, M60), and thiazolium pro-drugs or metabolites (TE4c, T3), with IC_{50}'s very close to those against *P. falciparum* (nanomolar range).

The lead compound G25 was further evaluated in vivo against *P. cynomolgi*, which is phylogenetically very closely linked to *P. vivax*. Five *P. cynomolgi*-infected rhesus monkeys were treated with G25 twice daily at 0.145 mg/kg intraperitoneally, when parasitemia ranged from 0.2%–0.5%. All treated monkeys were rapidly and successfully cleared of parasitemia without recrudescence, whereas the five control monkeys had peak parasitemias ranging from 5%–10% 3.5 d after the onset of treatment. The control monkeys had the first recrudescence at d 10 or 11, but most notably, no parasites were detected in G25-treated monkeys, indicating that no recrudescence appeared in any of the G25 treated monkeys.

Hence, quaternary ammonium (G25), amidines (M53, M60), and thiazolium pro-drugs or metabolites (TE4c, T3) could also be very useful against human vivax malaria.

MECHANISM OF ACTION

The mode of action is probably through inhibition of *de novo* PC biosynthesis, as shown by the early effect on PC biosynthesis and the very close correlation between their PL antimetabolic and antimalarial activities. The compounds are specific to mature parasites (trophozoites) (i.e., the most intense phase of PL biosynthesis during the erythrocytic cycle).

Specificity of Action with Respect to Plasmodium *PL Metabolism*

The compounds tested show a specificity of action in two respects: specificity for the biosynthesis of PC from choline (among other PLs) and specificity relative to the synthesis of other macromolecules (nucleic acids and proteins).

There is a very close correlation between the antimalarial activity of the compounds expressed as IC_{50} and the PC_{50} (phosphatiolyl choline) (i.e., the concentration that inhibit by 50% the biosynthesis of phosphatidylcholine (PC) [not shown]). The PC_{50} are in the same order of magnitude as the K_i obtained for the choline transporter. An excess of choline causes a significant shift in the PC metabolism inhibition curves (not shown).

Selective Uptake of Compounds by Infected Erythrocytes

Synthesis of radiolabeled bis-quaternary ammonium derivatives related to G25 allowed us to characterize the interaction of the compounds with malarial-infected erythrocytes.

Compound VB5, a benzophenone photoreactive derivative of G25, was concentrated inside infected erythrocytes to a very large extent with a cellular accumulation ratio higher than 55. This accumulation is specific to infected erythrocytes and temperature dependent. After fractionation of *P. falciparum*-infected erythrocytes, VB5 was recovered in erythrocytic cytosol and its membrane *(65%)*, whereas 35% of the compound was in parasite membranes. No saturable component was observed until a concentration of 0.25 mM VB5. [^{125}I]PL53, a *p*-azidophenyl photoligand derivative of G25, showed interaction with a 56 kDA protein present only in the membranous fraction of infected erythrocytes (Cathiard et al., unpublished results).

Thus, as chloroquine *(40)* and artemisinine *(41)*, anti-PL effectors selectively accumulate in infected erythrocytes. This selective accumulation of compounds could be part of the mechanism of action of our compounds and could be the source of specificity of the compounds that affect only infected erythrocytes.

HIGHER SENSITIVITY OF HUMAN MALARIA THAN MURINE MALARIA TO ANTI-PL EFFECTORS

We noted a high discrepancy for the in vivo antimalarial activity of anti-PL effectors when the compounds were tested in the murine model (*P. chabaudi* or *P. vinckei*) and in the monkey model (*P. falciparum*), with a therapeutic index ranging from 5–50 to higher than 50, respectively. This difference likely results from a lower susceptibility of murine parasites. By contrast, the remarkable in vivo antimalarial activity against *P. falciparum* has to be related to the very high activity obtained in vitro (nanomolar range).

The low in vivo antimalarial activity of anti-PL effectors against *P. vinckei* or *P. berghei* likely results from the low susceptibility of murine parasites (as observed in vitro with *P. berghei*) rather than from unfavorable pharmacokinetics of these compounds, as noted in ex vivo tests (G25 or MS1) (not shown).

This difference in parasite susceptibility to our compounds when comparing murine and human models greatly questions the relevance of the murine model for in vivo screening of compounds and casts doubt on the possibility for anticipating the antimalarial activity of our compounds in vivo against *P. falciparum*. This indicates that the in vivo antimalarial activity against human malaria in monkeys could be much better than in the infected rodent model.

TOXICOLOGY AND PHARMACOKINETIC PROPERTIES

In Vitro Specificity of Action Relative to Other Cell Systems

There is a total absence of correlation between concentrations producing 50% inhibition of parasite growth in vitro (IC_{50}) and concentrations affecting the viability of mammalian cell lines (e.g., human megakaryocytes, lymphoblastoid and macrophage cell lines, all of them showing rapid division) with an in vitro selectivity index of 300–38,000. These results provide evidence that structural prerequisites for the inhibition of PL metabolism are highly specific to infected cells and certain compounds can now be divested of toxic effects.

Toxicity, Genotoxicity, and Pharmacokinetic Properties

The essential parameters of the main lead compounds are shown in Table 1. The acute toxicity levels of the compounds (expressed as LD_{50}) were determined after one single-drug administration. Subacute toxicity was evaluated after twice daily administration for 4 consecutive days to detect any possible cumulative toxicity compared to acute toxicity. The tested compounds (G25 and MS1) did not show mutagenic activity in the Ames test, using *Salmonella typhimurium*, even in the presence of metabolic activation.

Ex vivo bioassay tests were developed to quantitate the plasma concentration of candidate antimalarial agents after administration in various animals (Ancelin et al., unpublished results). These bioassay tests are very helpful to obtain useful information regarding plasma levels and pharmacokinetic characteristics of compounds after administration in animals (especially on the elimination half-time, $t_{1/2}$, or extrapolated concentration to zero time, C_0, or maximal serum concentration, C_{max}) and to predict their in vivo antimalarial activity. This bioassay can be used to estimate the drug concentration of active ingredients without using sophisticated methods or equipment and can be applied to various animal species.

Pharmacokinetics determined using the bioassay method in mouse, dog, and monkey indicated that compounds exhibited a very fast distribution (<1 h), half-time of elimination of 5–35 h, and plasma levels that appear to be quite advantageous related to the in vitro IC_{50} against *P. falciparum*.

EXPLORING RESISTANCE REVERSION AND RESISTANCE INDUCTION

Anti-PL effectors cannot reverse chloroquine or mefloquine resistance of *P. falciparum*. Interaction between anti-PL effectors and chloroquine/mefloquine are additive and no synergy is observed (experiments carried out by Dr. J. Lebras and Dr. L. Basco, Paris).

In vitro experiments using *P. falciparum* under drug pressure did not lead to the appearance of a clone resistant to G25 (Dr. P. Ringwald, IRD, Yaoundé, Cameroon, 3 mo of drug pressure, and Dr. P. Rathod, Catholic University, Washington, D.C., USA, 50 d trial).

CONCLUSION AND PROSPECTS

This original pharmacological approach targeting a specific metabolic pathway of *P. falciparum* has now been fully validated with malaria-infected mice and Aotus monkeys infected with virulent *P. falciparum* isolates. This unique mechanism of action should make the molecules active against polypharmacoresistant isolates of *P. falciparum* and limits the risk of emergence of cross-resistance. Overall, the three compound generations meet the essential characteristics of potent and realistic antimalarials as shown in Table 2. Both series of pro-drugs showed improved acute tolerance and absorption. The most interesting results with these new agents concern their in vivo activity against *P. vinckei,* which is better than G25. At the present time, these compounds possesses the highest activity ever obtained in both modes. The current strategy is to choose one compound to be assessed in preclinical studies. We consider that oral administration is highly practical for dispensaries in endemic countries that often do not have adequate facilities to safely give drug injections, and it is indispensable for prophylactic or curative treatments for travelers. The goal of our program is to obtain an oral formulation of our compounds. Three patents have been taken out covering the new chemical structures and the therapeutic application.

The program still also includes basic studies on the regulation of PL metabolism and mechanisms involved in possible acquisition of resistance against PL effectors (until now no evidence of such a process has been found). The pharmacological target is sufficiently promising that it is now time to invest in studies on its identification, isolation, and molecular characterization.

Table 2
Essential Characteristics of the Pharmacological Approach

Efficacy of product candidates

- Potent in vitro activity against *P. falciparum* (IC_{50} < 5 nM).
- Compounds are equally effective against multiresistant *P. falciparum* malaria (strains and isolates).
- Active in vitro against sexual stages of *P. falciparum* (or *P. berghei*) with IC_{50} close to that against asexual stages and ability to impair zygote/ookinete development.
- Strong evidence of an original mode of action (phospholipid metabolism inhibition).
- Efficacy has been observed ex vivo and in vivo on *P. vinckei* and *P. chabaudi* in mice (but murine parasites are much less sensitive [by 20-fold] to anti-PL effectors than *P. falciparum*).
- Curative in vivo against human *P. falciparum* malaria in Aotus monkeys without recrudescence.
- Compounds are likely also effective against *P. vivax* and similar parasites.
- The bioavailability of the compounds was found to be advantageous (slow blood clearance and no significant concentration in tissues).
- Attempts to induce drug resistance have failed after 3 months under drug pressure.
- In vitro and in vivo antibabesia activity (*B. divergens*, *B. canis*).

Safety

- High in vitro selectivity against hematozoan parasites as compared to mammalian cell lines.
- All leading molecules show a very good therapeutic index (LD_{50}/ED_{50}) of 6–50 in mice, but higher than 50 in monkeys. Human malaria parasites are much more sensitive (by 20-fold) to the compounds than rodent malaria parasites.
- Genotoxicity has been tested for the first two generations of compounds.

Chemistry

- Most of them are stable and water soluble.
- Industrial-scale synthesis should be easy and inexpensive.
- Third-generation compounds (bioprecursors) have recently been synthesized in order to improve oral absorbtion.

ACKNOWLEDGMENTS

These studies were supported by the European Communities (INCO–DC), CNRS (GDR 1077), MENESR, AUPELF–UREF, and the WHO/TDR Special Programme. The pharmacological model is currently being developed with the following partners: A. Thomas and C. Kocken (BPRC–Rijswik, Netherlands), S. Herrera (Universitad del Valle, Cali, Colombia), P. Ringwald (OCEAC, Yaoundé, Cameroon), J. Bourguignon (CNRS, Strasbourg, France), and W. Eling (Nijmegen, Netherlands), who are gratefully acknowledged for their appreciated expertise and skillful work.

REFERENCES

1. Butler D, Maurice J, O'Brien C. Time to put out malaria control on the global agenda. Nature 1997;386:535–540.
2. WHO. WHO Report on Infectious Diseases: Removing Obstacles to Healthy Development. Geneva: World Health Organization, 1999.
3. Engers H, Godal T. Malaria vaccine development: current status. Parasitol Today 1998;14:56–64.

4. Tanner M, Teuscher T, Alonso PL. SPf66 - The first malaria vaccine. Parasitol Today 1995;11:10–13.

5. Collins F, Paskewitz M. Malaria: current and future prospects for control. Ann Rev Entomol 1995;40:195–219.

6. Vial H. Recent developments and rationale towards new strategies for malarial chemotherapy (A large review). Parasite 1996;3:3–23.

7. Sherman I. Malaria, Parasite Biology, Pathogenesis and Protection. Washington DC: ASM, 1998.

8. Olliaro PL, Yuthavong Y. An overview of chemotherapeutic targets for antimalarial drug discovery. Pharmacol Ther 1999;81:91–110.

9. Elabbadi N, Ancelin ML, Vial HJ. Phospholipid metabolism of serine in *Plasmodium*-infected erythrocytes involves phosphatidylserine and direct serine decarboxylation. Biochem J 1997;324:435–445.

10. Vial H, Ancelin M. Malarial lipids. In: Sherman I (ed). Malaria: Parasite Biology, Biogenesis, Protection. American Association of Microbiology, Washington DC, 1998, pp. 159–175.

11. Holz GG. Lipids and the malaria parasite. Bull WHO 1977;55:237–248.

12. Sherman IW. Metabolism. In: Peters W, Richards WHG (ed), Antimalarial drugs. New York: Springer-Verlag, 1984, pp. 31–81.

13. Vial HJ, Ancelin ML. Malarial lipids, an overview. In: Avila JL, Harris JR (eds). Subcellular Biochemistry. New York: Plenum, 1992, pp. 259–306.

14. Vial HJ, Thuet MJ, Ancelin ML, Philippot JR, Chavis C. Phospholipid metabolism as a new target for malaria chemotherapy. Mechanism of action of D-2-amino-1-butanol. Biochem Pharmacol 1984;33:2761–2770.

15. Ancelin ML, Vial HJ, Philippot JR. Inhibitors of choline transport into *Plasmodium*-infected erythrocytes are effective antiplasmodial compounds *in vitro*. Biochem Pharmacol 1985;34:4068–4071.

16. Ancelin ML, Vial HJ. Quaternary ammonium compounds efficiently inhibit *Plasmodium falciparum* growth *in vitro* by impairment of choline transport. Antimicrob Agents Chemother 1986;29:814–820.

17. Beaumelle BD, Vial HJ. Correlation of the efficiency of fatty derivatives in suppressing *Plasmodium falciparum* growth in culture with their inhibitory effect on acyl-CoA synthetase activity. Mol Biochem Parasitol 1988;28:39–42.

18. Krugliak M, Deharo E, Shalmiev G, Sauvain M, Moretti C, Ginsburg H. Antimalarial effects of C18 fatty acids on *Plasmodium falciparum* in culture and on *Plasmodium vinckei petteri* and *Plasmodium yoelii nigeriensis* in vivo. Exp Parasitol 1995;81:97–105.

19. Ancelin ML, Vial HJ. Regulation of phosphatidylcholine biosynthesis in *Plasmodium*-infected erythrocytes. Biochim Biophys Acta 1989;1001:82–89.

20. Ellory JC, Young JD. Red cell membrane, a methological approach. London, Academic Press, 1982.

21. Ancelin ML, Parant M, Thuet MJ, Philippot JR, Vial HJ. Increased permeability to choline in simian erythrocytes after *Plasmodium knowlesi* infection. Biochem J 1991;273:701–709.

22. Elford B, Cowan G, Ferguson D. Parasite-regulated membrane transport processes and metabolic control in malaria-infected-erythrocytes. Biochem J 1995;308:361–374.

23. Ginsburg H, Kirk K. Membrane transport in Malaria-infected erythrocytes. In: Sherman I (ed). Malaria: Parasite Biology, Biogenesis, Protection. American Association of Microbiology, 1998, pp. 219–232.

24. Vial H., et al Transport of phospholipid synthesis precursors and lipid trafficking into malarial-infected erythrocytes. In: Transport and Trafficking in the Malaria-Infected Erythrocytes. Novartis Foundation Symposium No. 226. 1999, pp. 74–88.

25. Desai SA, Rosenberg RL. Pore size of the malaria parasite's nutrient channel. Proc Natl Acad Sci (USA) 1997;94:2045–2049.

26. Calas M, Ancelin ML, Cordina G, Portefaix P, Piquet G, Vidal-Sailhan V, Vial H. Antimalarial activity of compounds interfering with *Plasmodium falciparum* phospholipidic metabolism: comparison between mono and bisquaternary ammonium salts. J Med Chem 2000;43:505–516.
27. Calas M, Cordina G, Bompart J, Ben Bau M, Jei T, Ancelin ML, Vial H. Antimalarial activity of molecules interfering with *Plasmodium falciparum* phospholipid metabolism. Structure–activity relationship analysis. J Med Chem 1997;40:3557–3566.
28. Ancelin M, Calas M, Bompart J, Cordina G, Martin G, Ben Bari M, et al. Antimalarial activity of 77 phospholipid polar head analogs: close correlation between inhibition of phospholipid metabolism and *in vitro Plasmodium falciparum* growth. Blood 1998;91:1426–1437.
29. Costa T, Wuster M, Harz A, Shigomohigashi Y, Chen HC, Rodbard D. Receptor binding and biological activity of bivalent enkephalins. Biochem Pharmacol 1985;34:25–30.
30. Portoghese P. Bivalent ligands in the development of selective opioid receptor antagonists. Trends Med Chem 1987;10: 327–336.
31. Portoghese PS. Bivalent ligands and the message-address concept in the design of selective opioid receptor antagonists. Trends Pharmacol Sci 1989;10:230–235.
32. Vial HJ, Calas M, Ancelin M, Giral L. Agents antipaludéens et antibabésioses et compositions pharmaceutiques les contenant, USA, Japan, Europe, Fr. Patent 2,751,967.
33. Vial HJ, Calas M, Bourguignon JJ, Ancelin M, Giral L. Bis-2-aminopyridine: leur procédé de préparation et leur application, France, USA, Japan, Europe, Fr. Patent 2,725,718.
34. Vial HJ, Calas M, Bourguignon J, Ancelin ML, Vidal V, Rubi E. Précurseurs de sels de bis-ammonium quaternaire et leurs applications comme prodrogues ayant une activité antiparasitaire. Fr. Patent 9909471, 1999.
35. Bitsch R, Wolf M, Möller J, Heuzeroth L, Gruneklee D. Bioavailability assessment of the lipophilic benfothiamine as compared to a water-soluble thiamine derivative. Ann Nutr Metab 1991;5:292–296.
36. Baker H, Franck O. Absorption, utilisation and clinical effectiveness of allithiamines compared to water-soluble thiamine. J Nutr Sci Vitaminol 1976;22(suppl):63–68.
37. Ishikura T, Senou T, Ishihara H, Kato T, Ito T. Drug delivery to the brain. DOPA prodrugs based on a ring-closure reaction to quaternary thiazolium compounds. Int J Pharm 1995;116:5–63.
38. Molyneux D, Floyd K, Barnish G, Fèvre E. Transmission control and drug resistance in malaria: a crucial interaction. Parasitol Today 1999;15:238–240.
39. Buckling A, Ranford-Cartwright LC, Miles A, Read AF. Chloroquine increases *Plasmodium falciparum* gametocytogenesis in vitro. Parasitology 1999;118(Pt 4):339–346.
40. Bray PG, Janneh O, Raynes KJ, Mungthin M, Ginsburg H, Ward SA. Cellular uptake of chloroquine is dependent on binding to ferriprotoporphyrin IX and is independent of NHE activity in *Plasmodium* falciparum. Cell Biol 1999;145:363–376.
41. Meshnick SR, Taylor TE, Kamchonwongpaisan S. Artemisinin and the antimalarial endoperoxides: from herbal remedy to targeted chemotherapy. Microbiol Rev 1996;60:301–315.

20

Development of New Malaria Chemotherapy by Utilization of Parasite-Induced Transport

Annette M. Gero and Alexander L. Weis

INTRODUCTION

This chapter focuses on the changes in the transport of solutes across the malaria-infected erythrocyte membrane and the possibility of exploiting this process for selective chemotherapy.

During its development in the host erythrocyte, the malarial parasite causes profound alterations in the permeability of the host cell membrane. New transport pathways are induced by the parasite into the host erythrocyte membrane and these transporters have properties significantly different than those of the host cell. In this chapter, we look at our current knowledge of how these parasite induced transporters can be used in the development of new chemotherapeutic agents. Two mechanisms will be discussed: first, the means by which cytotoxic compounds can be directed into the parasite-infected erythrocyte through parasite-induced transporters, thereby enhancing their selective chemotherapeutic potential, and second, the potential for developing antiparasitic agents that block parasite induced transporters and thereby deprive the parasite of essential nutrients or biochemical functions.

One of the intriguing aspects of parasitism is the complexity of the interactions between parasite and host, and the methods by which parasites exploit their hosts and their environment to satisfy their own needs for growth and reproduction. The induction of transporters is one such example. When the malarial parasite, *Plasmodium falciparum*, invades the human erythrocyte, it develops over a period of 48 h and, subsequently, reproduces itself manyfold. The intraerythrocytic development of the parasite imposes on the host cell a major new demand for the supply of nutrients and disposal of waste products. To satisfy these demands, the intraerythrocytic parasite causes profound alterations in the permeability of the host erythrocyte membrane and it is now clear that parasite-mediated transport systems are quite different from those of the uninfected erythrocyte.

There have been many investigations of the transport of solutes and nutrients into *Plasmodium*-infected erythrocytes, as well as into the isolated malaria parasite itself. Solute trafficking in nonhuman malarias has been previously reviewed *(1)* and the more recent work on transport in *P. falciparum* malaria is discussed in Chapter 3 and in recent comprehensive reviews *(2–5)*.

From: *Antimalarial Chemotherapy: Mechanisms of Action, Resistance, and New Directions in Drug Discovery*
Edited by: P. J. Rosenthal © Humana Press Inc., Totowa, NJ

The traditional view of how compounds gain access to the intraerythrocytic parasite is that solutes enter or leave the parasite-infected cells via the erythrocyte cytoplasm. In passing between internal parasite and the external plasma, compounds have to cross a series of three membranes: the host erythrocyte membrane (EM), the parasitophorous vacuole membrane (PVM) and the parasite plasma membrane (PPM) (Fig. 1).

Alternative models have been suggested by which solutes may enter or leave the parasite within the red cell (Fig. 1). These models suggest that the parasite may have direct access to the extracellular milieu. This could be via a "metabolic window" formed at a point of close apposition of the host erythrocyte membrane, the parasitophorous vacuole membrane and the parasite plasma membrane (6) or via a membranous "duct" (a tubular structure formed as a continuation of the host erythrocyte membrane and parasitophorous vacuole membrane (refs. 7 and 8; see Chapter 3). Irrespective of the routes by which solutes enter and leave the intracellular parasite, the induction of transport pathways in *Plasmodium*-infected erythrocytes that are different from those in other mammalian cells offer potential opportunities for antimalarial chemotherapy. Potential antimalarials might include toxic compounds that are selectively transported into the parasite-infected erythrocytes by the induced transport systems as well as compounds that inhibit the parasite-induced transporters.

What Are the Altered /Induced Transporters in Plasmodium-Infected Erythrocytes?

The membranes of normal mammalian cells, including erythrocytes, are endowed with many solute transporters that mediate the movement of ions and molecules between the plasma and the cell cytosol. Following malarial infection of the erythrocyte, there appear to be at least two types of change in transport. For some solutes, there is simply an increased flux via transport pathways with properties similar to those of the endogenous host cell transporters. For example, some nutrients show a marked elevation in transport rates, but this is via a pathway with kinetic and pharmacological properties similar to those of the corresponding transporter of uninfected erythrocytes (9). However, for many nutrients, hours after invasion of the erythrocyte (usually at the trophozoite stage), new "induced" permeation pathways with functional characteristics quite different from those of the normal host transporters appear. Studies in a number of laboratories have established that these transporters have a greatly enhanced permeability to a wide variety of compounds that include many essential for the survival of the parasite (1). Compounds with increased transport include small carbohydrates (e.g., pentitols, pentoses, hexitols, hexoses) (10,11), polyamines (12), purine and pyrimidine nucleosides (13–15), most amino acids, sodium, potassium, calcium, zinc, iron, small peptides (16–18) and several antimalarial drugs. Lactate also is effluxed through these transporters as a waste product (19–21).

The kinetic and pharmacological properties of these transporters in *Plasmodium*-infected cells are quite different from those of the normal red cells. Several of the pharmacological properties that have important chemotherapeutic implications are as follows. (1) The parasite-induced pathways are not saturable for substrate concentration ranges up to millimolar concentrations and show an apparent preference for hydrophobic solutes over similarly sized hydrophilic solutes (11,21). (2) The pathways are not inhibited by the classical inhibitors that inhibit the corresponding transport pathways in mammalian cells (such as cytochalasin B and nitrobenzyl-thioinosine, which inhibit mammalian glucose and nucleoside transport, respectively) (13,15). (3) The pathways

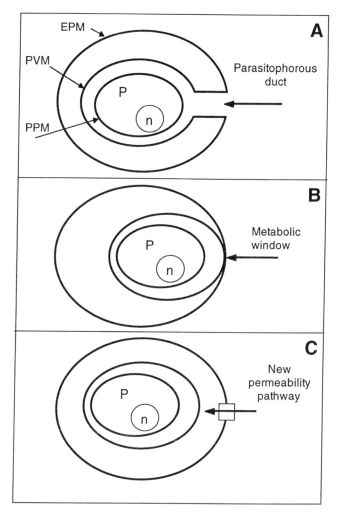

Fig. 1. Models of "parasite-induced" solute transport in *P. falciparum*-infected erythrocytes. Schematic diagrams showing several proposed models for solute transport pathways in *P. falciparum*-infected erythrocytes. **(A)** parasitophorous duct; **(B)** metabolic window; **(C)** new permeability pathway (NPP). EPM, erythrocyte plasma membrane; PVM, parasite vacuolar membrane; PPM, parasite plasma membrane; P, parasite; n, nucleus.

are not stereospecific (as in mammalian cells) and hence do not discriminate between the sterioisomers of physiological compounds such as arabitol *(11)*, alanine *(21,22)*, nucleosides *(23,24)*, or lactate *(20)*. These characteristics indicate that the transporter may be a pore or, more likely, a channel, rather than a conventional carrier.

Recently it has been suggested that much of the malaria-induced transport is actually via one common pathway or transport system *(21)*. The induced transport of monovalent anions and cations, amino acids, sugars, and nucleosides were all shown to be blocked by a series of anion transport inhibitors, with the same order of inhibitor potency for each solute. Furthermore, dose-response curves for the effect of these inhibitors on the malaria-induced transport of choline (a monovalent cation) were superimposable on those for the pyrimidine nucleoside, thymidine (a relatively hydrophobic nonelectrolyte).

If there is a single major pathway that mediates the *Plasmodium*-induced influx of these disparate solutes, its characteristics are quite unlike those of any transport system known to be present in normal human erythrocytes, but are similar to those of anion-selective channels in other cell types *(21,25)*.

Clearly, the transport system has a very broad substrate specificity. It is strongly anion selective: its permeability to monovalent anions is some 1000 times higher than its permeability to monovalent cations, with electroneutral zwitterions and uncharged molecules (such as nucleosides) falling in between. The pathway is non-saturable within physiological substrate concentration ranges and it shows an apparent preference for hydrophobic solutes over similarly sized hydrophilic solutes *(11,21)*.

Considering the importance of the parasite-induced transporter and the need to develop new antimalarials, it is noteworthy that the inhibition of the induced transporter is fatal to the parasite. However, additional transport mechanisms have also been characterized (Chapter 3), and any transport pathways might be targets for chemotherapy.

INHIBITION OF THE INDUCED TRANSPORTER

The concept that the blocking of the induced transporter by an added compound could inhibit parasite growth has been studied by various groups using a diverse armory of compounds ranging from phlorizin to anion transport blockers to inhibitors of carboxylic acid translocating systems (Fig. 2).

Inhibition by Phlorizin

Some of the earliest observations suggesting that the induced transporter may have a role as a potential chemotherapeutic target were reported by Kutner et al. *(26)*. They found that phlorizin (phloretin-2-β-glucoside) inhibited the in vitro growth of *P. falciparum* with a median inhibitory concentration (IC_{50}) of 16 µ*M*. The susceptibility to phlorizin was apparent at the trophozoite stage and onward and required 2–8 h of drug exposure for an irreversible effect. However, most significantly, they also observed that phlorizin inhibited the parasite-induced transporter with an IC_{50} of 17 µ*M*, a value that is virtually identical to that for inhibition of parasite growth. Subsequent studies with a range of phlorizin derivatives indicated that substitution in the 3-position of the dihydrochalcone ring yielded a wide spectrum of inhibitory activity, with the nitro and isothiocyano derivatives the most potent compounds *(27)*.

On the basis of these observations, Kutner et al. *(26)* suggested that the antimalarial action of phlorizin was associated, at least in part, with inhibition of the solute transporter of the host cell membrane induced by the invasion of the parasite. Although the drug inhibited parasite growth, the phlorizin could be washed out of the cells, albeit with difficulty, thereby reversing the effect of the drug. This implied that even temporary blocking of the transporter had detrimental effects on parasite growth and survival.

Inhibition by Anion Transport Blockers

Kirk et al. *(21)* subsequently showed that a number of anion transport blockers potently inhibited the transport of a wide range of solutes into erythrocytes infected in vitro with *P. falciparum*. The most effective blockers were 5-nitro-2-(3-phenyl-propylamino) benzoic acid (NPPB), furosemide, and niflumate; all three blocked the parasite-induced transport of a range of solutes including monovalent anions and

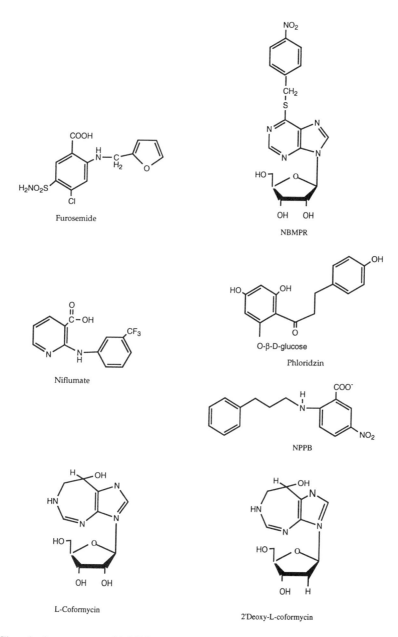

Fig. 2. Chemical structures of inhibitors of the parasite-induced transporter or of the parasite adenosine deaminase.

cations, neutral amino acids, sugars, and nucleosides. The IC_{50} values for the inhibition of induced choline influx were 20 μM for niflumate, 5 μM for furosemide, and 0.8 μM for NPPB. For each class of solutes tested for inhibition of induced transport, the order of potency of the inhibitors was always NPPB> furosemide> niflumate. Kirk et al. *(21)* concluded that the simplest explanation consistent with their observations was that the induced transport of a wide range of ions and solutes occurred via a single pathway. This pathway also showed marked functional similarities to chloride channels in other cell types. Furosemide also had a toxic effect on parasites grown in vitro. The totality of these findings raised the possibility that these channels, with their anion selectivity, were important for the growth of the parasite, and, hence, inhibition of the channels could open the way for new pharmacological approaches.

At the same time, Gero's group found that infection of erythrocytes by *P. falciparum* induced a permeation pathway for nucleoside uptake *(13)*. This permeation was characterized by the fact that it mediated the transport of L-adenosine, the nonphysiological isomer of D-adenosine *(28)*. This pathway induced by the parasite was very specific, as L-adenosine was not transported into normal human erythrocytes or many other mammalian cell types. Furthermore, the uptake of L-adenosine into *P. falciparum*-infected erythrocytes was potently inhibited by both phlorizin (IC_{50}, 3 μM) and furosemide (IC_{50}, 1 μM), consistent with prior studies *(21,26)*. Piperine also had a substantial inhibitory effect on L-adenosine transport (IC_{50}, 13 μM). A similar effect was reported in mouse erythrocytes infected with *P. yoelii*; the parasite-induced flux of L-adenosine was inhibited by furosemide (IC_{50}, 15 μM) *(23)*. However, the most significant aspect of the observations of Upston and Gero *(28)* was that parasite infection results in the induction of a system that allows the uptake of a nonphysiological stereoisomer, L-adenosine. This observation provides a new, pharmacological approach based on the potential of using toxic L-nucleoside analogs to specifically target the parasite without interfering with host cell metabolism.

Inhibition by Aromatic Acid Derivatives

A number of aromatic acid derivatives have also been shown to be effective in blocking permeation pathways and/or inhibiting parasite growth. These groups of compounds include cinnamic acid derivatives *(29)* and arylaminobenzoates *(30)*.

Cinnamic acid derivatives (CADs) are known inhibitors of monocarboxylate transport across mammalian membranes. These derivatives inhibited the growth of intraerythrocytic *P. falciparum* in culture (IC_{50}, 50 μM–1.1 mM) *(29)*. The CADs also inhibited the translocation of a number of different types of solutes, and this inhibition correlated with effects on parasite growth. The impairment of parasite growth by the CADs may have been the result of inhibition of processes such as lactate transport; lactate production in parasite-infected erythrocytes is up to 100-fold greater than that in uninfected erythrocytes. CADs thus provide another experimental tool for defining the properties of induced permeation pathways, and the feasibility of then using these pathways as pharmacological loci, although they are too toxic to be considered potential drugs.

Kirk and Horner *(30)* have also studied a series of arylaminobenzoates that are analogs of the chloride channel blocker NPPB. These derivatives effectively blocked induced solute transport; with choline as the marker solute, transport was substantially inhibited (IC_{50} values all in the very low micromolar range). The four most potent transport inhibitors also potently inhibited parasite growth as measured by [^{3}H] hypoxanthine incorporation. However, the feasibility of using such compounds as potential antimalarials is questionable because their in vitro effectiveness is reduced by serum components. At 2% serum, IC_{50} values were 17–30 μM and at 8.5% serum, the compounds had little effect at concentrations up to 50 μM. Kirk and Horner *(30)* concluded that "if induced transport inhibitors of this type are to be of value as antimalarials, it will be necessary to dissociate the interaction of the inhibitors with the induced-transport pathway from their binding to serum components."

Inhibition by Sulfonyl Ureas

Another quite different group of compounds that may have some antimalarial potential by virtue of their blocking-induced permeation pathways are the sulfonyl ureas. Sulfonyl ureas such as glibenclamide and the structurally related compounds meglitinide and tolbutamide are used in the treatment of diabetes because they stimulate insulin release from the pancreas. Their action has been attributed to effects on various ion channels; glibenclamide has recently been shown to potently inhibit a chloride channel.

All three sulfonyl ureas inhibited the influx of choline into parasite-infected erythrocytes, the most effective being glibenclamide with an IC_{50} of 11 μM *(25)*. Glibenclamide and meglitinide also inhibited parasite growth, as measured by [^{3}H] hypoxanthine incorporation, but as with the arylaminobenzoates, their effectiveness was reduced by serum components. To be useful as antimalarials such compounds need to be modified to ensure preferential binding to the induced transporters in the presence of serum.

Protease Inhibitor Pepstatin A

The parasite degrades host cell proteins, predominantly hemoglobin, for its amino acid requirements; this is carried out by a range of proteases within the parasite acidic food vacuole (Chapter 4). Not surprisingly, protease inhibitors are lethal to the parasite and could provide a different form of chemotherapeutic attack on the parasite *(31; see* Chapter 18, this volume). However, such inhibitors must first gain entry into the infected erythrocyte. Saliba and Kirk *(32)* have noticed an interesting effect involving the protease inhibitor pepstatin A. They observed that furosemide protected the parasite against pepstatin A. Furosemide, an inhibitor of the induced transporter as noted previously, has a cytotoxic effect itself, but at sublethal concentrations, it exerted a protective effect against the cytotoxic effect of pepstatin A. The IC_{50} value for inhibition of parasite growth by pepstatin increased from 9 μM in the absence of furosemide to 70 μM in the presence of 500 μM furosemide. A possible explanation is that the protease inhibitor enters the parasitized erythrocyte via a furosemide-sensitive transport pathway. Important implications of this finding is that quite large solutes may enter via this permeation pathway and that, as a consequence, this permeation pathway may be used as a means of targeting the parasite-infected cell by a very wide range of cytotoxic agents.

CHEMOTHERAPY BY TARGETING DRUGS THROUGH TRANSPORTERS

Although many compounds have been shown to be transported through the parasite-induced transporter, only purine nucleosides have been investigated as chemotherapeutic agents employing this pathway. Unlike mammalian cells, the parasite lacks the ability to synthesize purines *de novo* and must salvage its purines for growth and reproduction. Hence, it must acquire its purines by means of salvage mechanisms, and this involves the induced transporter. Much of the parasite's purine requirements are salvaged as nucleosides, presenting the opportunity to target toxic analogs of purines to infected cells.

Nucleoside Analogs as Chemotherapeutic Agents

Many cytotoxic nucleoside derivatives that are valuable anticancer and antiviral drugs have been shown to have potent activity against *P. falciparum* by interfering with the synthesis of nucleic acids *(33–35, see* Chapter 16). Unfortunately, nucleosides are also toxic to normal cells and they rely on the rapid proliferation of pathogens or tumors for selective activity.

Nucleosides such as 5-fluoro-2'-deoxy-uridine (FdUrd), 6-thio-guanosine, and 6-mercapto-purine-riboside are used clinically but must be first phosphorylated within the cell to their respective nucleotides (e.g., 5FdUMP) for pharmacological activity. Nucleotides are anionic or polyanionic compounds that cannot cross through cellular membranes. On the other hand, nucleosides and their analogs are neutral molecules that can enter cells and assume their therapeutic role after intracellular phosphorylation.

Nucleoside Transport in Normal Cells

The nucleoside transporter in mammalian cells has been well characterized *(36,37)* and its gene recently cloned *(38)*. In erythrocytes, nucleosides are transported by a plasma membrane protein. Transport is reversible, energy independent, and nonconcentrative, and the substrate specificity is broad in that ribosides and deoxyribosides of both purines and pyrimidines and structurally diverse cytotoxic nucleosides are transported. This transporter is potently inhibited by the adenosine analogs nitrobenzyl thioinosine (NBMPR) and nitrobenzyl thioguanosine (NBTGR) and by a variety of vasodilators such as dipyridamole and dilazep, which are structurally unrelated *(36)*. In human erythrocytes, the inhibition of nucleoside transport by NBMPR is the result of the extremely tight but reversible binding of NBMPR (K_D, 0.3–1 nM) to specific membrane binding sites that are either at the transport site or are part of the transport protein *(36)*.

Characteristics of the Mechanisms of Transport for Nucleosides or Bases into Parasite-Infected Erythrocytes

In the 1970s, studies on rodent and duck *Plasmodium*-infected cells suggested that fundamental changes occurred in the uptake and incorporation of labeled purine nucleosides and bases into *P. lophurae-* and *P. berghei*-infected erythrocytes when compared to uninfected erythrocytes *(39–41)*. In particular, in infected erythrocytes adenosine, hypoxanthine, and inosine appeared to enter the cells through a common permeation site *(39,41)*. In addition NBMPR failed to block the incorporation of adenosine into nucleic acids of *P. berghei* parasites isolated from erythrocytes by saponin lysis *(40,42)*.

More recently, the transport of adenosine has been followed over short periods in *P. falciparum-* and *P. yoelii*-infected erythrocytes *(13,14,43,44)*. When erythrocytes were infected there was a marked change in the transport characteristics for nucleosides (such as adenosine and the cytotoxic adenosine analog, tubercidin). Furthermore, the nucleoside transport inhibitors, NBMPR, NBTGR, dipyridamole, and dilazep were ineffective at blocking a large component of the transport of nucleosides into infected cells at concentrations 10,000-fold higher than that required to block transport in normal erythrocytes. In *P. falciparum*-infected erythrocytes, the lack of inhibition by these compounds was related to the stage of development of the intraerythrocytic parasite and was most pronounced in the mature trophozoite stage, when the metabolic activity of the parasite is at its maximum. The changes following infection suggested that an altered or new nucleoside transport mechanism, which had low sensitivity to NMBPR, had been introduced into the host cell membrane *(24)*. Thus, the altered nucleoside transporters in *Plasmodium*-infected cell membranes offered an excellent target for a new chemotherapeutic approach potentially without the problem of toxic side effects to the host.

Two approaches utilizing these concepts have been subsequently investigated as antimalarial regimes; these are presented in the following subsections.

Antimalarial Regime with a Toxic Nucleoside Plus a Transport Inhibitor

The first approach consists of a regime of simultaneous administration of two compounds: a toxic nucleoside that destroys the viability of the intraerythrocytic malarial parasite and a nucleoside transport inhibitor that protects normal host cells from the toxicity of the first compound (Fig. 3). The feasibility of this regime has been successfully demonstrated in mice infected with *P. yoelii* or *P. berghei* by the coadministration of a lethal concentration of a cytotoxic nucleoside, such as tubercidin or sangivamycin, in combination with NBMPR. This drug combination administered over 4 consecutive days was not toxic to noninfected control mice, but in the infected mice, the treatment significantly decreased parasitemias and doubled survival times *(43–45)*.

Antimalarial Regime with Toxic Compounds That Enter Only Infected Cells via the Parasite-Induced Transporter

The second approach involves cytotoxic nucleosides that are unable to enter normal cells through the endogenous nucleoside transporter, but that can specifically enter infected cells via the parasite-induced transporter. An initial comparison of biochemical characteristics of the transport of nucleosides in normal and infected cells has revealed that there are some important structural components of a nucleoside that are necessary for both their toxicity and their ability to be transported through the altered membrane transporter. Alteration of the purine ring of a nucleoside (particularly at the 6-, 7-, or 8-position [e.g., tubercidin and sangivamycin]) can change its role from physiological to cytotoxic. In particular, the change from the normal D-isomer, to the enantiomer L-form produces radical alterations of transport ability. Initial studies *(23,28)* showed that infected cells had the unique ability to transport L-nucleosides compared to normal mammalian cells. The transport of L-nucleosides into parasites was not blocked by NBMPR but was inhibited by furosemide *(23,28)*, substantiating that these isomers were transported through the parasite-induced transporter *(46)*. It was also established that the L-isomers of physiological nucleosides, both purines and pyrimidines (i.e., L-adenosine, L-guanosine, L-thymidine, L-cytidine, and L-uridine and their 2'-deoxyribo- analogs) were readily transported through the parasite-induced transporter. On the basis of these observations, L-nucleoside pro-drugs were designed to be transported specifically into parasite-infected cells.

Metabolism of L-Nucleosides

A major advantage in the development of a L-nucleoside antimalarial is that L-nucleosides can be metabolized by the enzymes of the parasite but not by those of the erythrocyte or any other mammalian cells *(28)*. Many enzymes of the parasite are significantly different to the corresponding enzymes in the host, both quantitatively and qualitatively, such as the enzymes of purine salvage *(47)*, pyrimidine *de novo* biosynthesis *(48)*, and exonucleases, nucleosidases, and phosphodiesterases. It appears that the substrate specificity of many of these enzymes is significantly different from the host. Relevant to this discussion, the parasite enzymes can metabolize L-nucleoside pro-drugs, whereas the host enzymes cannot.

One example that has been investigated in detail is adenosine deaminase (ADA). ADA has much higher enzyme activity in *P. falciparum*-infected cells [specific activity 28,500 nmol/mg/h, compared to 37 nmol/mg/h in human erythrocytes *(49)*] and

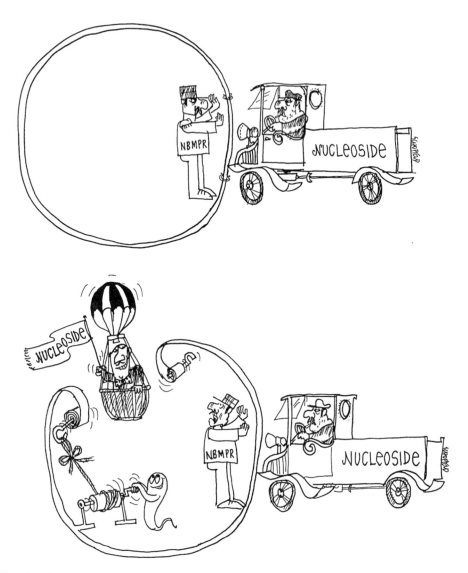

Fig. 3. Diagrammatic representation of the two-drug regime utilizing the nucleoside transporter induced in the membrane of the malaria infected erythrocyte. (Reprinted from *Parasitology Today*, vol. 8, Gero and Upston, Altered membrane permeability: a new approach to malaria chemotherapy, pp. 283–286 [1992], with permission from Elsevier Science.)

significant differences in its substrate specificities compared with the human enzyme *(50–52)*. It was shown that L-adenosine (6-amino-purine-L-riboside) was deaminated by parasite ADA and that all synthetic L-nucleoside analogs which have substituents in the 6-position can also be metabolized. This introduces the concept that a L-nucleoside altered on the 6-position could be designed as an antimalarial drug.

L-Nucleosides cannot be metabolized by mammalian cell lysates indicating that even if such compounds could enter normal host cells, they would not be metabolized to the toxic compound. These concepts have led to the design of several groups of L-nucleoside antimalarials.

There are three different groups of L-nucleoside pro-drugs that have been investigated for potential antimalarial activity. These groups are L-analogs of known toxic D-nucleosides, L-analogs as adenosine deaminase inhibitors and L-nucleosides as a carrier to selectively deliver a toxic moiety or molecule.

L-Analogs of Known Toxic D-Nucleosides

Transport and toxicity studies of a large number of L-nucleosides showed that L-enantiomers of physiological D-nucleosides entered infected erythrocytes and parasites, but they exhibited no antimalarial effects. However, L-enantiomers of toxic D-nucleosides, such as 6-thio-L-guanosine, 6-thio-L-inosine, and L-sangivamycin inhibited both wild-type and resistant strains of *P. falciparum* in vitro, with ID_{50} values of 160 µ*M*, 200 µ*M*, and 25 µ*M*, respectively *(53)*. None of these compounds entered normal cells, thus increasing the therapeutic index over the D-analogs. 6-Thio-L-inosine and 6-thio-L-guanosine were not metabolized by the parasite suggesting that their action was by direct inhibition of the parasite ADA. The D-nucleoside analogs of these compounds successfully eliminated *P. knowlesi* infections in monkeys *(54)* but have the disadvantage of being toxic to normal cells. However, as L-enantiomers would enter only parasite-infected erythrocytes, toxicity against the host should be avoided.

Although the mechanism of action of toxic D-nucleosides depends on their phosphorylation to the corresponding nucleotide, it is apparent that, unlike the case with some virally infected cells, L-nucleosides cannot be phosphorylated in parasite-infected erythrocytes *(28,55,56)*. Hence in the case of the toxic L-nucleosides mentioned earlier (e.g., 6-thio-L-adenosine, 6-thio-L-guanosine, and L-sangivamycin), they may exert their effects through a different mechanism other than phosphorylation. L-Toyocamycin and L-nebularine , although toxic to malaria parasites in their D configuration, had no effect against infected cells *(53)*.

L-Analogs as Adenosine Deaminase Inhibitors

Parasite adenosine deaminase is present at high activity and has a different substrate specificity to that of the mammalian enzyme *(47,49)*. It can deaminate L-adenosine to L-inosine, whereas the mammalian enzyme cannot. Potent known inhibitors of the mammalian ADA such as 2'-D'-deoxycoformycin and D-coformycin also inhibit the parasite ADA *(50,51)*. *P. falciparum* ADA exhibited a K_i for 2'-deoxy-D-coformycin of 11.5 p*M*, comparable to that for erythrocyte ADA (15 p*M*) *(57)*. Previous observations showed that ADA inhibitors eliminated *P. knowlesi* infections in monkeys *(54)*. However, preliminary data suggested that 2'-deoxy-D-coformycin does not confer similar toxicity to cultures of *P. falciparum* *(58)*. 2'-Deoxy-D-coformycin is an ubiquitous inhibitor of ADAs *(59)*, which are present in most human tissues and cell lines including erythrocytes and lymphocytes. The design of an antimalarial targeting ADA as an activator or inhibitor, would need to be strictly specific for *P. falciparum* ADA.

Recently it has been shown that two L-nucleoside structural analogs of 2'-deoxy-D-coformycin, namely L-isocoformycin and L-coformycin, were specific inhibitors of *P. falciparum* ADA and have no effect on host ADA *(53,60)*. *P. falciparum* ADA exhibited a K_i for L-coformycin of 250 p*M*, and 7 p*M* for L-isocoformycin. Thus, a minor modification to a single hydroxyl group on the purine ring of L-coformycin enhanced the efficacy of the inhibitor some 35-fold. Like 2'-deoxy-D-coformycin, L-coformycin and L-isocoformycin were competitive inhibitors of *P. falciparum* ADA.

Furthermore, the results show that L-isocoformycin and L-coformycin were able to discriminate between host and parasite ADAs. In addition, a second advantage of these inhibitors is that, being L-nucleosides, they are unable to enter normal mammalian cells *(60)*.

L-Nucleosides That Act as a "Carrier" to Selectively Deliver a Second Compound, Such as a Cytotoxic Nucleotide into the Infected Cell*

These compounds are dinucleoside monophosphate dimers in which L-nucleosides are used to selectively deliver a toxic D-nucleoside (tide) into the parasite-infected erythrocyte. They are dimers of two nucleosides conjugated through the 3'- and 5'-OH to a phosphate group. For the structure–activity relationship study, a number of 3'–3' and 5'–5' dimers were also prepared. The L-nucleosides were used in pure α or β anomeric forms. The antimalarial evaluation demonstrated that the β - L-nucleoside containing dimers were usually more active than the α - L-nucleoside containing dimers. The dinucleoside monophosphate dimer is metabolized by the parasite enzymes *in situ,* releasing the nucleotide as the suicidal form of the active drug (Fig. 4). These compounds exhibit significant toxicity to *P. falciparum* in vitro in the ID_{50} range 1–10 μM.

The carrier moiety of the dimer can consist of L-isomers of any of the physiological purines or pyrimidines. The toxic D-nucleotides that have been attached to the L-nucleoside carrier consist of 5-fluoro-2-D-deoxyuridine or purine nucleosides such as D-tubercidin.

This presents the concept of using either a toxic purine or a toxic pyrimidine as a potential chemotherapeutic agent by virtue of their attachment to an L-nucleoside, as a "carrier" for selective transport into only parasite-infected erythrocytes.

As discussed earlier, for purine requirements, the parasite relies primarily on salvage pathways. However, to meet its requirements for pyrimidines, the parasite uses *de novo* biosynthesis. This suggests that inhibitors of pyrimidine biosynthesis may serve as attractive molecular targets in antimalarial drug design *(48)*. This is certainly not a new concept, but, until now, there has been no way to selectively deliver a cytotoxic pyrimidine biosynthesis inhibitor to the malarial parasite without producing significant host toxicity. Thus, although drugs such as the cancer chemotherapeutics 5-fluorouracil and 5-fluoro-2'deoxyuridine, which block thymidine biosynthesis by inhibition of the enzyme thymidylate synthase, also inhibit the growth of *Plasmodium (61)*, they do so at the expense of excessive toxicity to the host. Hence, a "magic bullet" such as the L-nucleoside dimers would deliver a cytotoxic pyrimidine to the parasite via the parasite-infected host cell without affecting the function of healthy cells.

The dimers that consist of combinations of L-purine nucleosides such as L-adenosine, L-deoxy adenosine, and L-guanosine linked via a phosphate group to 5-fluoro-2'-deoxy-uridine (FdUrd; D-isomer) (Fig. 4), are more toxic to the parasite than FdUrd alone (ID_{50} = 35 μM), indicating the potential of releasing the toxic drug in its nucleotide form (5FdUMP) *in situ* in the malarial cell. Normally, 5FdUrd is metabolized to 5FdUMP, which is the cytotoxic form, as a result of potent inhibition of thymidylate synthetase *(62)*, but it is also toxic to the host. However, L-nucleoside dinucleoside monophosphate dimers can deliver the cytotoxic pyrimidine nucleotide selectively to the parasite. Analysis by high-performance liquid chromatography (HPLC) confirmed that

---

*Note: A number of patents covering these compounds have been filed by Lipitek International and The University of New South Wales.

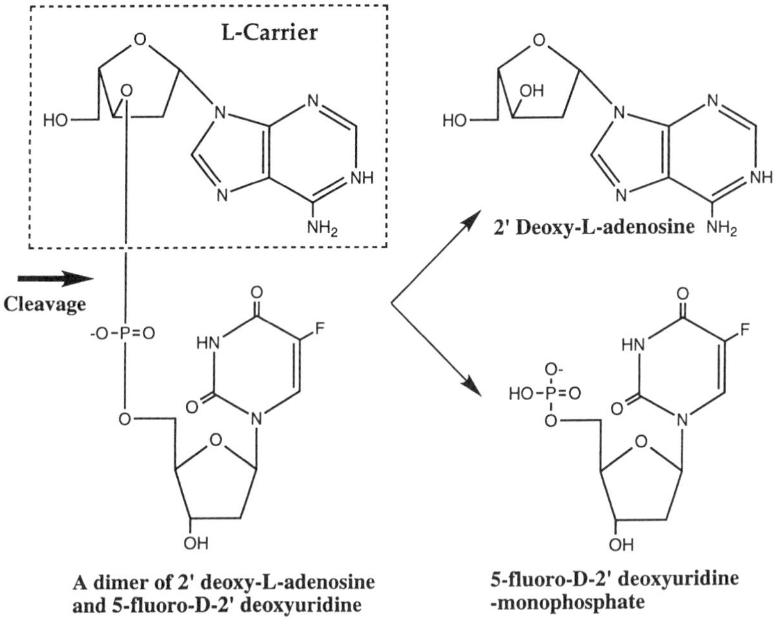

Fig. 4. Structure and cleavage products of one example of an L-dinucleoside monophospate dimer.

the dinucleoside monophosphate dimers were metabolized, releasing the toxic D-nucleotide and the L-nucleoside in these cells (Fig. 5). A major advantage is that the dimer carrying the toxic nucleotide could not enter normal cells. Additionally, even if the dimer could enter normal cells, HPLC analysis indicated that no metabolism or cleavage of the dimers occurred in lysates of uninfected red cells or lymphocytes (Gero and Weis, unpublished data).

A further major advantage of the dinucleoside monophosphate dimers is that after cleavage by the parasite, neither of the products of these pro-drugs (the L-nucleoside carrier or the toxic mononucleotides) can re-enter uninfected host cells if they were to be released into the serum. L-adenosine is excreted unchanged in the urine of mice approx 21 h after administration *(63)*. When evaluated for toxicity in mice, the dinucleoside monophosphate dimers were found to be nontoxic to healthy animals, even at the highest dose tested (400 mg/kg).

Recent work by Dunn, Weis, and Gero has shown that furosemide inhibits the transport of these dimers, confirming their transport through the parasite-induced transporter. Additionally, furosemide (10 µ*M*) reduced parasite death when incubated in vitro in combination with the dimers.

Future Potential for the Design of Antimalarials Based on the Parasite-Induced Transporter

As dinucleoside monophosphate dimers readily enter the parasite-infected erythrocyte through the induced transporter, the question arises as to how large a molecule can be transported via this system to target the parasite. It has been shown that infected erythrocytes are permeable to dipeptides and tripeptides *(16–18)*. Parasite growth is also inhibited by various antibodies and peptides containing 28 to 32 amino acid residues *(64)* and antisense oligonucleotides *(65)*. Clearly, all these various compounds

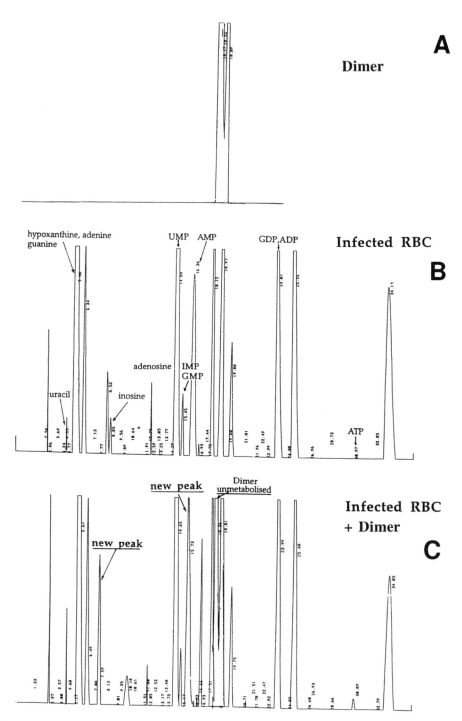

Fig. 5. Analysis by (HPLC) of a dinucleoside monophosphate dimer after incubation with a preparation of *P. falciparum*-infected erythrocytes. (**A**) The ultraviolet detection of the compound alone at 254 nm eluted from a nucleotide column. (**B**) The spectrum of malaria infected erythrocytes. (**C**) The spectrum of infected erythrocytes incubated with the dimer, showing transport of the dimer into the infected cell and two additional peaks of the two metabolic products, the structures of which are shown in Fig. 4.

must enter the parasite-infected cell to exert their effects. These various observations suggest that a range of compounds of quite different sizes are accommodated by changes in the permeability of the host cell.

Furthermore, the characteristics of the parasite-induced transporter, particularly the ability to transport L-nucleosides, suggest the possibility of a completely new range of antimalarials. For example, conjugation of known antimalarials to an L-nucleoside carrier would provide even greater antimalarial efficacy and specificity. Conjugation of an L-nucleoside to other pro-drugs (other than a nucleotide) could result in an entirely new battery of antimalarials that act as suicide inhibitors by virtue of their metabolism specifically within the parasite. The list of possible permutations and combinations of carrier plus toxic moiety is long. The development of the L-nucleosides dimers illustrates that alterations caused by the parasite can be exploited in the design of compounds that will, in turn, selectively destroy it.

In summary, the altered permeability of the parasite-infected erythrocyte offers the potential of developing a very wide range of antimalarials to target this alteration in the parasitized cell as a new and innovative form of chemotherapy. The observations to date suggest that a wide range of solutes, of quite different structures and quite different sizes, can permeate the parasitized cell, and it may be that future antimalarials of this type can be even more diverse in structure and form than those developed to date.

ACKNOWLEDGMENTS

We are grateful to Elena Gorovits for her extensive contribution to this work and her comments on the manuscript.

Research in this area carried out in the author's laboratories was supported by the US Army Medical Research and Material Command Grant DAMD 17-97-C-7014, the UNDP/World Bank/WHO Special Programme for Research and Training in Tropical Diseases, and the National Health and Medical Research Council of Australia. The views, opinions, and/or findings contained herein are those of the authors and should not be construed as an official Department of the Army position, policy, or decision unless designated by other documentation.

REFERENCES

1. Sherman IW. Mechanisms of molecular trafficking in malaria. Parasitol 1988;96:857–881.
2. Ginsburg H. Alterations caused by the intraerythrocytic malaria parasite in the permeability of its host cell membrane. Comp Biochem Physiol 1990;95:31–39.
3. Cabantchik ZI. Properties of permeation pathways induced in the human red cell membrane by malaria parasites. Blood Cells 1990;16:421–432.
4. Gero AM, Kirk K. Nutrient transport pathways in *Plasmodium*-infected erythrocytes: what and where are they? Parasitol Today 1994;10:395–399.
5. Ginsburg H, Kirk K. Membrane transport in the malaria infected erythrocyte. In: Sherman IW (ed). Malaria Parasite Biology, Pathogenesis, and Protection. Washington DC: ASM, 1998, pp. 219–232.
6. Bodammer JE, Bahr GF. The initiation of a "metabolic window" in the surface of host erythrocytes by *Plasmodium berghei* NYU-2. Lab Invest 1973;28:708–718.
7. Pouvelle B, Spiegel R, Hsiao I, Howard RJ, Morris RL, Thomas A, et al. Direct access to serum macromolecules by intraerythrocytic malaria parasites. Nature 1991;353:73–75.
8. Lauer SA, Rathod PK, Ghori N, Haldar K. A membrane network for nutrient import in red cells infected with the malaria parasite. Science 1997;276:1122–1125.

9. Ancelin ML, Parant M, Thuet MJ, Philippot JR, Vial HJ. Increased permeability to choline in simian erythrocytes after *Plasmodium knowlesi* infection. Biochem J 1991;273:701–709.

10. Ginsburg H, Krugliak M, Eidelman O, Cabantchik ZI. New permeability pathways induced in membranes of *Plasmodium falciparum* infected erythrocytes. Mol Biochem Parasitol 1983;8:177–190.

11. Ginsburg H, Kutner S, Krugliak M, Cabantchik ZI. Characterization of permeation pathways appearing in the host membrane of *Plasmodium falciparum* infected red blood cells. Mol Biochem Parasitol 1985;14:313–322.

12. Singh S, Puri SK, Sing SK, Srivastava R, Gupta RC, Pandey VC. Characterisation of simian malarial parasite (*Plasmodium knowlesi*)-induced putrescine transport in rhesus monkey erythrocytes. A novel putrescine conjugate arrests in vitro growth of simian malarial parasite (*Plasmodium knowlesi*) and cures multidrug resistant murine malaria (*Plasmodium yoelii*) infection in vivo. J Biol Chem 1997;272:13,506–13,511.

13. Gero AM, Bugledich EM. A., Paterson ARP, Jamieson GP. Stage-specific alteration of nucleoside membrane permeability and nitrobenzylthioinosine insensitivity in *Plasmodium falciparum* infected erythrocytes. Mol Biochem Parasitol 1988;27:159–170.

14. Gero AM, Scott HV, O'Sullivan WJ, Christopherson RI. Antimalarial action of nitro-benzylthioinosine in combination with purine nucleoside antimetabolites. Mol Biochem Parasitol 1989;34:87–98.

15. Gero AM, Wood AM, Hogue DL, Upston JM. Effect of diamide on nucleoside and glucose transport in *Plasmodium falciparum* and Babesia bovis infected erythrocytes. Mol Biochem Parasitol 1991;44:195–206.

16. Elford BC, Ferguson DJP. Secretory processes in *Plasmodium*. Parasitol Today 1993;9:80–81.

17. Elford BC, Cowan GM, Ferguson DJP. Parasite-regulated membrane transport processes and metabolic control in malaria-infected erythrocytes. Biochem J 1995;308:361–374.

18. Atamna H, Ginsburg H. The malaria parasite supplies glutathione to its host cell—investigation of glutathione metabolism in human erythrocytes infected with *Plasmodium falciparum*. Eur J Biochem 1997;250:670–679.

19. Kanaani J, Ginsburg H. Transport of lactate in *Plasmodium falciparum*-infected human erythrocytes. J Cell Physiol 1991;149:469–476.

20. Cranmer SL, Conant AR, Gutteridge WE, Halestrap AP. Characterization of the enhanced transport of L- and D-lactate into human red blood cells infected with *Plasmodium falciparum* suggests the presence of a novel saturable lactate proton cotransporter. J Biol Chem 1995;270:15,045–15,052.

21. Kirk K, Horner HA, Elford BC, Ellory JC, Newbold CI. Transport of diverse substrates into malaria-infected erythrocytes via a pathway showing functional characteristics of a chloride channel. J Biol Chem 1994;269:3330–3347.

22. Elford BC, Pinches RA, Newbold CI, Ellory JC. Heterogeneous and substrate-specific membrane transport pathways induced in malaria-infected erythrocytes. Blood Cells 1990;16:433–435.

23. Gati WP, Lin AN, Wang TI, Young JD, Paterson ARP. Parasite-induced processes for adenosine permeation in mouse erythrocytes infected with the malarial parasite *Plasmodium yoelii*. Biochem J 1990;272:277–280.

24. Gero AM, Upston JM. Altered membrane permeability: a new approach to malaria chemotherapy. Parasitol Today 1992;8:283–286.

25. Kirk K, Horner HA, Spillett DJ, Elford BC. Glibenclamide and meglitinide block the transport of low molecular weight solutes into malaria-infected erythrocytes. FEBS Lett 1993;323:123–128.

26. Kutner S, Breuer WV, Ginsburg, H, Cabantchik ZI. On the mode of action of phlorizin as an antimalarial agent in in vitro cultures of *Plasmodium falciparum*. Biochem Pharmacol 1987;36:123–129.

27. Silfen J, Yanai P, Cabantchik ZI. Bioflavonoid effects on *in vitro* cultures of *Plasmodium falciparum*. Biochem Pharmacol 1998;27:4269–4276.

28. Upston JM, Gero AM. Parasite-induced permeation of nucleosides in *Plasmodium falciparum* malaria. Biochim Biophys Acta 1995;1236:249–258.
29. Kanaani J, Ginsburg H. Effects of cinnamic acid derivatives on *in vitro* growth of *Plasmodium falciparum* and on the permeability of the membrane of malaria-infected erythrocytes. Antimicrob Agents Chemother 1992;36:1102–1108.
30. Kirk K, Horner HA. In search of a selective inhibitor of the induced transport of small solutes in *Plasmodium falciparum*-infected erythrocytes: effects of arylaminobenzoates. Biochem J 1995;311:761–768.
31. Rosenthal PJ. Proteases of malaria parasites: new targets for Chemotherapy. Emerg Infect Dis 1998;4:49–57.
32. Saliba KJ, Kirk K. Uptake of an antiplasmodial protease inhibitor into *Plasmodium falciparum*-infected human erythrocytes via a parasite-induced pathway. Mol Biochem Parasitol 1998;94:297–301.
33. Coomber D, O'Sullivan WJ, Gero AM. Adenosine analogues as antimetabolites against *Plasmodum falciparum* malaria. Int J Parasitol 1994;24:357–365.
34. Rathod PK, Khosla M, Gassis S, Young RD, Lutz C. Selection and characterisation of 5-fluoroorotate-resistant *Plasmodium falciparum*. Antimicrob Agents Chemother 1994;38: 2871–2876.
35. Queen SA, Vander Jagt DL, Reyes P. *In vitro* susceptibilities of *Plasmodium falciparum* to compounds which inhibit nucleotide metabolism. Antimicrob Agents Chemother 1990;34: 1393–1398.
36. Paterson ARP, Cass CE. Transport of nucleoside drugs in animal cells. In: Goldman ID (ed.). Membrane Transport in Antineoplastic Agents. International Encyclopaedia of Pharmacology Therapy, Section 118, Pergamon Press, Oxford, UK, 1986, pp. 309–329.
37. Plagemann PGW, Wohlhueter RM. Permeation of nucleosides, nucleic acid bases, and nucleotides in animal cells. Curr Topics Membrane Trans 1980;14:225–330.
38. Griffiths M, Beaumont N, Yao SYM, Sunduram M, Boumah CE, Davies A, et al. Cloning of a human nucleoside transporter implicated in the cellular uptake of adenosine and chemotherapeutic drugs. Nature Med 1997;3:89–93.
39. Tracey SM, Sherman IW. Purine uptake and utilisation by the avian malarial parasite *Plasmodium lophurae*. J Protozool 1972;19:541–549.
40. Van Dyke K. Purines and Pyrimidines in malarial cells. [Commentary.] Blood Cells 1990;16:485–495.
41. Hansen SD, Sleeman HK, Pappas PW. Purine base and nucleoside uptake in *Plasmodium berghei* and host erythrocytes. Parasitology 1980;66:205–212.
42. Van Dyke K, Trush MA, Wilson ME, Stealey PK. Isolation and analysis of nucleotides from erythrocyte-free malarial parasites (*Plasmodium berghei*) and potential relevance to malaria chemotherapy. Bull WHO 1977;55:253–264.
43. Gati WP, Stoyke AF, Gero AM, Paterson ARP. NBMPR—insensitive nucleoside permeation in mouse erythrocytes infected with *Plasmodium yoelii*. Biochim Biophys Res Commun 1987;145:1134–1141.
44. Gero AM, Wood AM. In: (Harkness, RA, Ellion GB, Zollner N (eds.). Purine and Pyrimidine Metabolism in Man. (Vol.VII) New York: Plenum, 1991, Part A, pp. 169–173.
45. Gero AM. Nucleosides and parasites: a novel approach to chemotherapy. Paths Pyrimidines 1995;3:61–67.
46. Gero AM, Hall ST. *Plasmodium falciparum*: transport of entantiomers of nucleosides into Sendai-treated trophozoites. Exp Parasitol 1997;86:228–231.
47. Gero AM, O'Sullivan WJ. Purines and pyrimidines in malarial parasites. Blood Cells 1990;16:467–484.
48. Seymour KK, Lyon SD, Phillips L, Rieckmann KH, Christopherson RJ. Cytotoxic effects of inhibitors of the *de novo* pyrimidine biosynthesis upon *Plasmodium falciparum*. Biochemistry 1994;33:5268–5274.

49. Reyes P, Rathod PK, Sanchez DJ, Mrema JE. K., Rieckman KH, Heidrich HG. Enzymes of purine and pyrimidine metabolism from the human malaria parasite, *Plasmodium falciparum*. Mol Biochem Parasitol 1982;5:275–290.

50. Daddona PE, Wiesmann WP, Lambros C, Kelley WN, Webster HK. Human malaria parasite adenosine deaminase. Characterisation in host enzyme-deficient erythrocyte culture. J Biol Chem 1984;259:1472–1475.

51. Schmandle CM, Sherman IW. Characterization of adenosine deaminase from the malarial parasite, *Plasmodium lophurae*, and its host cell, the duckling erythrocyte. Biochem Pharmacol 1983;32:115–122.

52. Wiesmann WP, Webster HK, Lambros C, Kelley WN, Daddona PE. Adenosine deaminase in malaria infected erythrocytes: unique parasite enzyme presents a new therapeutic target. Prog Clin Bio Res 1984;165:325–342.

53. Gero AM, Perrone G, Brown D, Hall ST, Chu CK. L-Purine nucleosides as selective antimalarials. Nucleosides Nucleotides 1999;18(4/5):885–890.

54. Webster HK, Wiesmann WP, Pavia CS. Adenosine deaminase in malaria infection: Effect of 2'deoxycoformycin *in vivo*. In: De Bruyn CHMM, et al. (eds). Advances in Experimental Medicine and Biology, Vol 165A. Purine Metabolism in Man IV. New York: Plenum, 1984, pp. 225–229.

55. Spadari S, Maga G, Focher F, Ciarocchi G, Manservigi R, Arcamone F, Iafrate E, Manzini S, Garbesi A, Tondelli L. L-Thymidine is phosphorylated by herpes simplex type 1 thymidine kinase and inhibits viral growth. J Med Chem 1992;35:4214–4220.

56. Verri A, Montecucco A, Gosselin G, Boudou V, Spadari, S, Focher F. L-ATP is recognised by some human and viral enzymes:does chance drive enzymatic enantioselectivity? Biochem J 1999;337:585–591.

57. Agarwal RP, Spector T, Parks RE. Jr. Tightbinding inhibitors—IV. Inhibition of adenosine deaminases by various inhibitors. Biochem Pharmacol 1977;26:359–367.

58. Roth E Jr, Ogasawara N, Schulman S. The deamination of adenosine and adenosine monophosphate in *Plasmodium falciparum*-infected human erythrocytes: in vitro use of 2'deoxycoformycin and AMP deaminase-deficient red cells. Blood 1989;74:1121–1125.

59. Gallagher KP, McClanahan TB, Martin BJ, Saganek LJ, Ignasiak DP, Mertz TE, et al. Does adenosine deaminase inhibition protect ischemic myocardium? Adv Exp Med Biol 1994;370:291–294.

60. Brown DM, Netting AG, Chun BK, Yongseok C, Chu CK, Gero AM. L-Nucleoside analogues as potential antimalarials that selectively target *Plasmodium falciparum* adenosine deaminase. Nucleotides Nucleosides 1999;18(11/12):2521–2532.

61. Rathod P, Leffers, N, Young R. Molecular targets of 5 fluoroorotate in the human malarial parasite *Plasmodium falciparum*. Antimicrob Agents Chemother 1992;36:704–711.

62. Périgaud C, Gosselin G, Imbach J-L. Nucleoside analogues as chemotherapeutic agents: a review. Nucleosides Nucleotides 1992;11:903–945.

63. Jurovcik M, Holy A, Shorm F. The utilization of L-adenosine by mammalian tissues. FEBS Lett 1971;18:274.

64. Ghosh JK, Shaool D, Guillaud P, Cicéron L, Mazier D, Kustanovich I, et al. Selective toxicity of dermaseptin S3 toward intraerythrocytic *Plasmodium falciparum* and the underlying molecular basis. J Biol Chem 1997;272:31609–31616.

65. Barker RH Jr, Metelev V, Rapaport E, Zamecnik P. Inhibition of *Plasmodium falciparum* malaria using antisense oligodeoxynucleotides. Proc Natl Acad Sci USA 1996;93:514–518.

Index